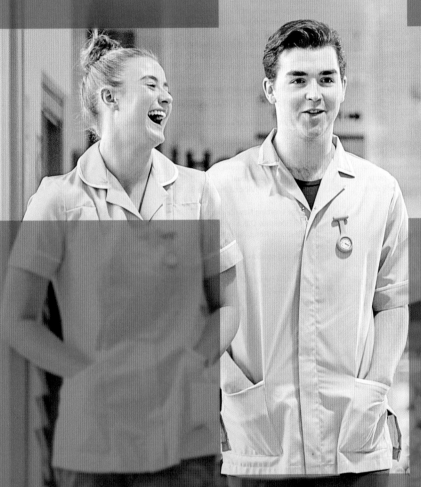

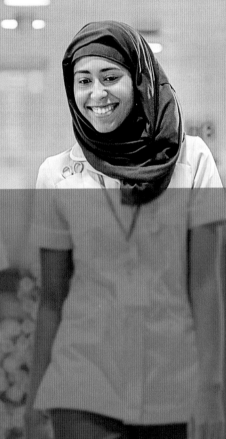

Essential Clinical Skills

ENROLLED NURSES

JOANNE **TOLLEFSON** | GAYLE **WATSON**

EUGENIE **JELLY** | KAREN **TAMBREE**

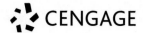

Essential Clinical Skills: Enrolled Nurses
5th Edition
Joanne Tollefson
Gayle Watson
Eugenie Jelly
Karen Tambree

Head of content management: Dorothy Chiu
Senior content manager: Sophie Kaliniecki
Content developer: Stephanie Davis
Project editor: Raymond Williams
Text designer: Nikita Bansal
Cover design: Danielle Maccarone
Editor: Leanne Peters
Proofreader: James Anderson
Indexer: Max McMaster
Permissions/Photo researcher: Wendy Duncan
Cover: iStock.com/sturti
Typeset by KnowledgeWorks Global Ltd

Any URLs contained in this publication were checked for currency during the production process. Note, however, that the publisher cannot vouch for the ongoing currency of URLs.

Fourth edition published by Cengage in 2019.

Every effort has been made to review and confirm the accuracy of content in this publication. By following the instructions contained herein the reader willingly assumes all risks in connection with such instructions. The reader should review procedures, treatments, drug dosages or legal content. Neither the authors nor the publisher assume any liability for injury or damage to persons or property arising from any error or omission. Inclusion of proprietary names for any drugs or devices should not be interpreted as a recommendation

Acknowledgements
Appendix:© Nursing and Midwifery Board of Australia. Please see www. nursingmidwiferyboard.gov.au for up to date information, standards and guidelines for Australian nurses and midwives.

For product information and technology assistance,
in Australia call 1300 790 853;
in New Zealand call 0800 449 725

For permission to use material from this text or product, please email aust.permissions@cengage.com

National Library of Australia Cataloguing-in-Publication Data
ISBN: 9780170454087
A catalogue record for this book is available from the National Library of Australia.

Cengage Learning Australia
Level 7, 80 Dorcas Street
South Melbourne, Victoria Australia 3205

Cengage Learning New Zealand
Unit 4B Rosedale Office Park
331 Rosedale Road, Albany, North Shore 0632, NZ

For learning solutions, visit cengage.com.au

Printed in China by 1010 Printing International Limited.
3 4 5 6 7 25 24

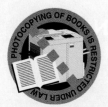

CONTENTS

Guide to the text

As you read this text you will find a number of features in every chapter to enhance your study of essential clinical skills and help you understand how the theory is applied in the real world.

PART OPENING FEATURES

Chapter list outlines the chapters contained in each part for easy reference.

> PART **2**
>
> ## ASSESSMENT
>
> **2.1** HEAD-TO-TOE ASSESSMENT
> **2.2** RISK ASSESSMENT AND RISK MANAGEMENT
> **2.3** TEMPERATURE, PULSE AND RESPIRATION (TPR) MEASUREMENT
> **2.4** BLOOD PRESSURE MEASUREMENT
> **2.5** PULSE OXIMETRY
> **2.6** BLOOD GLUCOSE MEASUREMENT
> **2.7** NEUROLOGICAL OBSERVATION
> **2.8** NEUROVASCULAR OBSERVATION
> **2.9** PAIN ASSESSMENT
> **2.10** 12-LEAD ECG RECORDING
>
> **Note:** These notes are summaries of the most important points in the assessments/procedures and are not exhaustive on the subject. References of the materials used to compile the information have been supplied. The student is expected to have learnt the material surrounding each skill as presented in the references. No single reference is complete on each subject.

CHAPTER OPENING FEATURES

Identify Indications sections identify the clinical reasons to perform the skill outlined in the chapter.

> CHAPTER **2.1**
>
> ## HEAD-TO-TOE ASSESSMENT
>
> ### IDENTIFY INDICATIONS
>
> The indication to perform a head-to-toe assessment is usually contact with a healthcare facility or with healthcare workers in the community. If the patient presents to a healthcare facility, there is concern about their health and they should be assessed accordingly. The patient may be presenting to the healthcare facility for admission, and the admission procedure of most facilities includes a thorough assessment. The purpose of a health history is to formulate a database incorporating historical and current data, and to provide an opportunity for the nurse to develop a trusting relationship with the patient. The interview provides information on the patient's perception of their health concerns and learning needs. The head-to-toe assessment should also be conducted any time the patient's condition changes. This allows the nursing staff to report accurately and adequately to the doctor. Such an assessment provides data on which nursing interventions are based and is a key nursing action. The collection and organisation of information about the patient assists the nurse to identify existing or potential healthcare problems and to make decisions based on accurate information to help the patient return to a better state of health.
>
> A briefer head-to-toe assessment should also be conducted when completing other routine assessments, such as vital signs, to gain an overall assessment of the patient's status or to gain further information when these might vary from previous readings (North, 2017). The nurse should also complete a brief head-to-toe assessment as part of the shift handover, or soon after the commencement of their shift (Haugh, 2015).

FEATURES WITHIN CHAPTERS

Gather equipment sections list and explain each item of equipment you will need to perform the clinical skill.

GATHER EQUIPMENT

Gather equipment prior to starting the procedure to maximise efficiency, reduce apprehension on the patient's part and increase confidence in the nurse. The following equipment is required for head-to-toe assessment:

- sphygmomanometer, stethoscope and blood pressure (BP) cuff of appropriate size
- pulse oximeter
- thermometer, penlight torch and watch

- weighing scales
- height stick
- relevant facility forms.

To prepare the environment, ensure that the ambient temperature is comfortable and without draughts, there is sufficient light for the nurse to be able to examine the patient, the area is made private and there is provision for privacy and warmth.

Challenge the theory you have learnt by considering the **NEW Critical thinking boxes**, perhaps in a group discussion.

CRITICAL THINKING

NEW

Growth and Development

1. Access the intranet at your work placement and review the relevant documents relating to Skills 7.2 to 7.4.
   How do you think these forms/paperwork may vary within the following types of facilities:
   - public hospital
   - private hospital
   - aged care facility
   - community nursing?
2. Consider how you would adapt a patient teaching session for a child aged 5 compared to an adult aged 30.
3. Explain why nursing care plans should be individualised to each patient's personal needs and their stage of growth and development.

Chapter linkages refer you back to important foundational skills and highlight the connection between similar tasks, procedures and skills.

Analyse in-depth **Case studies** that present issues in context, encouraging you to integrate and apply the concepts discussed in the chapter to the workplace.

Nurses must assess their patients for risk and choose to use a critical aseptic field as opposed to a general aseptic field if there is an increased chance of infection. If a critical aseptic field is required, don surgical gloves using open gloving as per **Skill 4.9**.

Refer to **Skill 4.2** for further description of basic wound dressing technique. This basic dressing technique (standard aseptic technique) and general aseptic field can be adapted for more complex wounds and procedures (e.g. **Skills 4.3, 4.5 and 4.6**) that require critical aseptic fields and a surgical aseptic

CASE STUDY

1. Using a nursing history and assessment form from your facility, complete a basic assessment on a family member. Practise the required assessment skills, and collect information about their health history. Follow the processes of professional and effective patient communication when completing this procedure.
2. Evelyn Deer is a 31-year-old woman admitted to your day surgery ward this morning for a right knee arthroscopy

procedure. She is athletic and plays team netball, is generally fit and well, and does not have any significant medical history She has been fasting. Her observations are within the normal adult range. Besides completing her vital signs, what other head-to-toe assessments will you perform?

Note: These notes are summaries of the most important points in the assessments/procedures, and are not exhaustive on the subject. The naming of documents or charts may differ from state to state, and facility to facility. In all possible situations the guidelines of the ACSQHC are used when describing national charts or documents (e.g. the ACSQHC Observation and Response Chart is named the Adult Observation and Response Chart in WA, and the Rapid Detection and Response Observation Chart in SA). References of the materials used to compile the information have been supplied. The student is expected to have learned the material surrounding each skill as presented in the references. No single reference is complete on the subject.

END-OF-CHAPTER FEATURES

At the end of each chapter you will find several tools to help you to review, practise and extend your knowledge of the key learning outcomes.

Extend your understanding through the suggested **recommended readings** relevant to each chapter.

At the end of each chapter you'll find an **essential skills competency table** for you to review, practise and record your growing competency for each clinical skill.

- The key **performance criteria** for an entire skill are listed, not just a task or procedure, and the relevant **NMBA National Competency Standards** are included.

- There is space for students and clinical facilitators to record your performance and progress.

- **Signature section** for students and clinical facilitators to record assessment.

ESSENTIAL SKILLS COMPETENCY

Neurological Observation
Demonstrates the ability to effectively assess the neurological status of the patient

Criteria for skill performance (Numbers indicate *Enrolled Nurse Standards for Practice*, 2016)	Y (Satisfactory)	D (Requires development)
1. Identifies indication (8.3, 8.4)		
2. Gathers equipment (1.2, 1.6, 4.4, 6.4, 8.4, 9.4): ▪ sphygmomanometer, BP cuff and stethoscope ▪ thermometer, watch with a second hand ▪ pulse oximeter ▪ penlight torch ▪ pen ▪ neurological observation sheet (e.g. Glasgow Coma Scale)		
3. Performs hand hygiene (1.2, 1.4, 1.8, 3.9, 6.4, 9.4)		
4. Evidence of therapeutic communication with the patient; gives explanation of procedure, gains patient consent (2.1, 2.3, 2.4, 2.5, 6.3)		
5. Demonstrates problem-solving abilities; e.g. modifies questions with regard to age, culture and existing physical conditions, can describe warning postures (4.1, 4.2, 8.3, 8.4, 9.4)		
6. Assesses level of consciousness (1.2, 1.4, 3.2, 4.1, 4.2, 6.6, 7.1, 8.4, 9.4)		
7. Assesses orientation of the patient (1.2, 1.4, 3.2, 4.1, 4.2, 6.6, 7.1, 8.4, 9.4)		
8. Assesses motor response (1.2, 1.4, 3.2, 4.1, 4.2, 6.6, 7.1, 8.4, 9.4)		
9. Assesses pupillary activity (1.2, 1.4, 3.2, 4.1, 4.2, 4.4, 6.4, 6.6, 7.1, 8.4, 9.4)		
10. Assesses muscle strength and tone (1.2, 1.4, 3.2, 4.1, 4.2, 6.3, 6.6, 7.1, 8.4, 9.4)		
11. Assesses vital signs (1.2, 1.4, 3.2, 4.1, 4.2, 4.4, 6.4, 6.6, 7.1, 8.4, 9.4)		
12. Performs hand hygiene (1.2, 1.4, 1.8, 3.9, 6.4, 9.4)		
13. Cleans, replaces and disposes of equipment appropriately (1.2, 1.4, 3.9, 6.5, 9.4)		
14. Documents relevant information (1.2, 1.3, 1.8, 3.2, 5.3, 6.6, 7.1, 7.2, 7.3, 7.4, 7.5)		
15. Demonstrates ability to link theory to practice (8.3, 8.4, 8.5, 9.4)		

Student:

Clinical facilitator: Date:

Guide to the online resources

FOR THE INSTRUCTOR

Cengage is pleased to provide you with a selection of resources
that will help you to prepare your lectures and assessments,
when you choose this textbook for your course.
Log in or request an account to access instructor resources at
au.cengage.com/instructor/account for Australia or
nz.cengage.com/instructor/account for New Zealand.

COMPETENCY MAPPING GRID

The **Mapping grid** is a simple grid that shows how the content of this book relates to the units of competency
needed to complete the HLT54121 Diploma of Nursing.

INSTRUCTOR RESOURCES PACK

Premium resources that provide additional instructor support
are available for this text, including
Sample lesson plans
Sample care plans
Case studies plus case archive database
Downloadable logbook
Artwork from text

These resources save you time and are a convenient way to add
more depth to your classes, covering additional content and with an
exclusive selection of engaging features aligned with the text.
The Instructor Resource Pack is included for institutional adoptions
of this text when certain conditions are met.
The pack is available to purchase for course-level adoptions
of the text or as a standalone resource.
Contact your Cengage learning consultant for more information.

SAMPLE LESSON PLANS

Sample lesson plans provide a practical tool for your students to review and create sample lesson plans for a
classroom.

CASE STUDIES PLUS CASE ARCHIVE DATABASE

Case studies plus case archive database contains case studies that link the theory to real-world situations and
can be utilised in both the classroom and online student activities. Comprehensive solutions to each case study
question have been supplied for your use.

SAMPLE CARE PLANS

Sample care plans provide a practical tool for your students to review and create care plans as they would in the workplace.

DOWNLOADABLE LOGBOOK

The **downloadable logbook** is designed to record a students evidence of experience. The word format enables instructors to edit and customise to your institutions requirements.

ARTWORK FROM THE TEXT

Add the **digital files** of graphs, tables, pictures and flow charts into your learning management system, use them in student handouts, or copy them into your lecture presentations.

INTRODUCTION

The Nursing and Midwifery Board of Australia (NMBA) (2016) Standards for Practice – Enrolled Nurses (see the Appendix) were developed to guide workplace performance and are the minimum requirements for registration as a nurse. Nursing 'Industry Reference Committees' have also liaised with the Australian Nursing and Midwifery Accreditation Council and used these standards to develop the Diploma of Nursing qualification for use by the vocational education and training sector in enrolled nursing course content and for assessment of student performance. The Diploma of Nursing qualification has embedded these industry benchmarks. Students and qualified enrolled nurses can achieve competence in these required standards through the consistent application of knowledge, skills and attitudes required to operate effectively within the workplace (NCVER, n.d.). The nurse should also be able to transfer skills and knowledge gained to new situations and environments.

Essential Clinical Skills for Enrolled Nurses outlines and explains the practical actions for completing skills that contribute to the development of satisfactory performance, underlying knowledge and required clinical competence as an enrolled nurse (EN). Each chapter contains descriptions of nursing skills and underlying knowledge required within core units of the Diploma of Nursing course, and some of the elective units. Many of the skills are also required within some units of the Advanced Diploma of Nursing course.

NEW TO THIS EDITION

All the skills in this edition have been extensively reviewed and edited, not only to reflect current industry standards of practice, but also national standards and recommendations from government bodies such as the Australian Commission on Safety and Quality in Health Care and the National Health and Medical Research Council.

All skills within this text, along with the attached skills grids, have been revised and updated according to current industry standards. More images have also been included. We have recognised the impact of COVID-19 on the nursing workplace, and the consequent impact on infection control. A greater focus has been placed on donning and doffing throughout this text to support student development of these key skills when performing other procedures and improve their infection control practices.

Critical Thinking and Lifespan boxes have been included throughout the text to expand student skills and understanding of different care situations. The lifespan development helps students recognise the different situations between paediatric and adult patients.

Over 50% of the case studies are new or updated. The case studies are designed to reinforce the students' underlying knowledge of the relevant skill and the ability to apply this to a clinical situation. Further online resources are also available on the book's companion website.

Clinical skills assessment

Clinical skills performance is only one aspect of the overall competency of an individual nurse. Assessment in the VET sector (Department of Training and Workforce Development, 2016) describes competence as being able to consistently apply knowledge and skills to required workplace standards. When implementing relevant skills and knowledge, students should also be able to plan and integrate several tasks when delivering nursing care; recognise their own scope of practice; meet workplace responsibilities and expectations; and respond appropriately to unexpected outcomes or occurrences. Performance evidence that contributes towards a student's competence can be collected using many different methods, including observation of performed skills during nursing skills laboratories, in simulation-based assessments and the workplace (i.e. during clinical placement experience).

Students are novice practitioners (Benner, 1984) who benefit from guidelines and direction, and who need to have complex interactions simplified into recognisable and achievable steps to enhance learning and reduce distress. With the skills broken down into steps, the student is more able to concentrate on the complexities of the situation than if the task were an overwhelming whole. Initially, these skills are taught in the safety of the laboratory using demonstrations and discussions from a skilled and current nursing practitioner. They should then be used together as part of simulation scenarios to reinforce skill development, build critical thinking skills and the student's ability to individualise patient care. The skills and the linked theory can be read, digested, conceptualised and discussed before the student completes required simulation-based assessments or attempts the use of a new skill in the workplace and on a vulnerable person. This increases student confidence and fosters critical thinking around the skill.

Using this clinical skills manual

This text has been developed as a guide to be used by enrolled nursing students when they are learning new skills. Students can use the skills grids to assess their own performance, gain feedback on their performance and maintain a personal record of skills they have practised. Theory about each skill can help build and consolidate knowledge about how or why a skill is implemented.

The skill descriptions are generic and can be adapted to meet organisation policies, different workplace situations and patient needs. Organisational policies and procedures must always be checked before undertaking any procedure as they may create variations on how a skill is completed. It is designed to support the learning of skills required in the different units of competence in the Diploma of Nursing in the Health Training Package.

This text can be used in skills laboratories, simulation scenarios, classroom lectures and clinical placement in conjunction with demonstrations and discussions of the various aspects of a skill. The individual skills grids can give structure to a skill that is being learnt by the student. The theory provided before each skills grid is general and needs to be adapted to, and integrated with, the specific context (i.e. what type of facility, its geographical location, the staff available, shift, time of day, day of the week, season) and the individual differences between patients (taking into consideration the age and developmental stage of the patients, their culture, gender, wellness, needs and desires, diagnosis, stress levels and ability to communicate).

The theory underlying the skills has been gleaned from a number of sources. This includes fundamental nursing texts, searches of various databases and government, medical and health related websites (including publicly available nursing clinical practice guidelines). Recent evidence-based material was used. The databases searched included ProQuest Health, CINAHL and Cochrane Library. Some nursing care skills have limited evidence, or research-based references, and the information is based on clinical practice experience validated by peer input and review. The information presented in each skill set is not exhaustive in relation to the subject but does give the student and assessor a mutual, basic understanding of the procedure.

Guidelines for lecturers, clinical facilitators and preceptors

Lecturers, clinical facilitators and preceptors need to be skilled nurses, who are also emotionally intelligent, confident of their own abilities, understanding of how students learn and aware of their own need for professional development. They need to draw on these attributes to create safe and positive student learning opportunities that will support enrolled nursing students in gaining not only their required skills, but also a positive vision of their own career path. Experienced nurses, lecturers, preceptors and clinical facilitators are able to integrate theoretical principles and knowledge with realistic practical application to a patient situation, and thus become positive role models for students developing these same clinical skills.

This text is not designed to be used as an actual assessment tool, as each education facility will have its own moderated and validated assessment tool for use in clinical, laboratory and simulation settings. It is designed to support these tools by providing a guideline for how different skills should be completed when collecting evidence of student performance. The skills grids can be used by students to assess their own performance, and gain formative learning or peer assessment input during the practice of their skills. The grids also provide a quick reference point to refresh what is required to complete a nursing skill when used on clinical placement. Columns are provided for individual clinical skills to provide feedback to the student being assessed as 'Satisfactory' or 'Requires Development'. This skill achievement would then be recorded within the educational institution's documentation for skills required. Competence would be achieved when all required skills and knowledge for the unit of competence have been consistently and satisfactorily demonstrated over a period of time.

Each exemplar in the skills grid is linked to one or more of the interpretative cues in the Enrolled Nurse Standards for Practice (NMBA, 2016). The number of the appropriate professional standard indicator has been recorded beside each exemplar. This facilitates linking the student's performance with the relevant standard. The lecturer, facilitator or preceptor can gather many cues in relation to one competency standard before giving the student feedback on their performance. The student may then be given a verbal or written observation of their progress for each professional standard indicator.

Theoretical knowledge of a procedure should be reviewed both before and after the procedure to ascertain the student's level of understanding of the implemented nursing care, which will vary according to the context and the individual patient. When a student has implemented patient care and the relevant skills, the facilitator/preceptor needs to promote student self-assessment and reflection on their performance, provide immediate constructive feedback about the student's performance and ascertain their reasons for the actions they performed. Feedback should be fair, relevant to their scope and experience plus enable the student to determine when they have met industry standards or areas that require improvement and how they can improve. Always create a plan with a student to engender their trust in the learning environment and support them to improve their clinical skills.

Students should be given feedback on their ability to interact with the patient, to solve problems, manage their time and resources, as well as performing the procedure competently , cleaning up afterwards and completing documentation. The two or three pages that make up the theoretical section of each skill give an overview of the procedure and the items within each guideline that are mandatory for the enrolled nursing student to know. As noted at the end of these sections, the notes are summaries of the most important points in the procedure and are not exhaustive on the subject. The student is expected to have read widely, attended laboratory and classroom sessions and absorbed the material from them, and discussed concerns with the lecturer, clinical facilitator or preceptor, to broaden their knowledge prior to implementing a skill in the clinical setting.

Criteria for skill performance

The criteria for skill performance have been broken into arbitrary sections. However, the entire skill should be seamless. Students should not be assessed on their first attempt to complete a procedure. Practice improves performance and fosters confidence in the student. The levels for completion – `Satisfactory' and `Requires Development' – are meant as a guide for the student in their progress towards becoming a confident and competent enrolled nurse practitioner. Bondy (1983) describes degrees of performance in clinical skill development and avoiding subjectivity. These concepts have been recognised, but simplified to reflect VET sector outcomes, within the two outcomes used in the grids. A brief description of the levels for completion follows:

- *Satisfactory* indicates that the student is able to complete the procedure/skill efficiently and without any prompts or assistance from the clinical facilitator on more than one occasion. This student can discuss the theory as it relates to the practical situation for the individual patient. The clinical facilitator would feel confident that the student is able to perform this procedure, or one similar, without supervision.
- *Requires development* indicates that the student is unable to complete the procedure without assistance (e.g. moderate amounts of verbal prompting, supervision to enable student competence and confidence, or physical assistance to complete the skill) from the clinical facilitator. This student has difficulty linking theoretical knowledge to practical situations. The clinical facilitator would not allow this student to complete this or a similar procedure without supervision.

As stated above, each number in the skills grid relates to one or more of the EN standards for practice. This helps to link the skill to the relevant standards indicator element. This text contains the major skills taught in core units and some elective units of the undergraduate enrolled nurse programs throughout Australia. It also includes some of the skills that are part of the Advanced Diploma of Nursing. It is designed to be used throughout the entire program, both on clinical placement and in theory-building encounters during each semester. At the end of their course, students will have a personal record of the skills they have practised throughout their nursing education.

Enrolled Nurse Standards for Practice

At the time of publication the current version of the Australian Nursing and Midwifery Accreditation Council Enrolled Nurse Standards for Practice is available on the Nursing and Midwifery Board of Australia website at http://www.nursingmidwiferyboard.gov.au/Codes-Guidelines-Statements/Codes- Guidelines.aspx. Check the website to ensure you are referring to the most current standards.

For further information, visit the Australian Nursing and Midwifery Accreditation Council website at http://www.anmac.org.au.

References

Benner, P. (1984). *From Novice to Expert: Excellence and Power in Clinical Nursing Practice*. Menlo Park, CA: Addison-Wesley.

Bondy, K.N. (1983). Criterion-referenced definitions for rating scales in clinical evaluation. *Journal of Nursing Education*, 22(9), pp. 376–82.

Department of Training and Workforce Development. (2016). *Assessment in the VET Sector* (2nd ed.). Government of Western Australia https://www.dtwd.wa.gov.au/sites/default/files/uploads/Assessment%20in%20the%20VET%20Sector%20-%202016%20-%20Final.pdf

National Centre for Vocational Education and Research (NCVER). (n.d.). *Glossary of terms*. Retrieved from http://www.voced. edu.au/content/glossary-term-competency

Nursing and Midwifery Board of Australia (NMBA). (2016). *Enrolled Nurse Standards for Practice*. Dickson, ACT: NMBA.

ABOUT THE AUTHORS

Joanne Tollefson (RN, BGS, MSc, PhD) was Senior Lecturer in the School of Nursing Sciences at James Cook University. She is a registered nurse with many years of clinical experience in several countries and extensive experience in nursing education at both the hospital and tertiary levels. Her research interests include competency-based education and clinical assessment, development of reflective practitioners for a changing work environment, chronic pain and arbovirus disease in the tropics. She is a two-time recipient of the National Awards for Outstanding Contributions to Student Learning (Carrick Award, 2007 and Australian Teaching and Learning Council Award, 2008). Since retirement, she has maintained an interest in nursing through researching, writing and editing nursing textbooks.

Gayle Watson (RN, BNurs (Hons), MEd Studies, Cert IV T&D) has more than 30 years' experience in nursing and nursing education, with a focus on the VET sector. She has actively worked in the delivery of the Diploma of Nursing, along with development of program delivery and giving feedback as part of statewide meetings to the planned 2021 update of the Diploma of Nursing qualification. Her background teaching experience includes classroom, nursing laboratory, simulation laboratory and clinical placement areas. She is currently employed in a senior academic and leadership role in the nursing portfolio at North Metropolitan TAFE (WA). During recent years Gayle has focused on applying her research and study interests of education into establishing enrolled nursing education that promotes active and engaged learners who become not just competent beginner practitioners, but lifelong learners.

Eugenie Jelly (RN, BAppSc[NsgEd], MEdMgt) is a hospital-trained registered nurse whose career progressed into the educational sphere, supported by tertiary academic studies in that area. Her teaching experience of over 40 years includes both registered and enrolled nursing programs within hospital-based schools of nursing, university and the TAFE sector. Her work within TAFE has included curriculum development, resource and assessment development, course coordination and teaching in the classroom, nursing laboratory and clinical area. She works currently with an active focus on the supervision/facilitation of nursing students on clinical placement, along with other nursing laboratory and classroom teaching.

Karen Tambree (RN, BNurs, GradCertTEd) has worked as a nurse for more than 40 years. Her area of expertise is palliative care and oncology, both paediatric and adult. Karen has worked in both the university and TAFE sector. Within the university sector Karen has lectured within both the undergraduate and master's levels, and has been involved in nurse education within the TAFE sector for over 15 years. She is experienced in nursing course development, resource development and leadership. She has taught within the classroom, nursing laboratory and clinical supervision. Karen originally trained as an enrolled nurse and later completed a Bachelor of Nursing and Graduate Certificate in Tertiary Education. Karen is currently employed within one of Perth's university nursing programs.

ACKNOWLEDGEMENTS

The publisher would like to acknowledge Toni Bishop for her contribution to the development of Essential Clinical Skills.

The authors and publishing team would like to thank the following reviewers for their incisive and helpful comments:

- Amanda Beetson, TAFE QLD South West
- Kylie Brennan, TAFE NSW Ultimo
- Ingrid Devlin, Health Skills Australia
- Leanne Ferris, Manager for Curriculum and Compliance with Mater Education Limited
- Annelize Grech, RDNS and Silverchain Training
- Michelle Hay-Chapman, Charlton Brown
- Hellene Heron, TAFE SA
- Shalet Mamachan, Job Training Institute, Dandenong
- Susan Nursey, Skills Training Australia
- Kathy Pearce, Charles Sturt University and TAFE Western
- Vicki Smith, TAFE Gold Coast
- Carmel Storer, GoTAFE Benalla Campus
- Diane Taylor, TAFE East Coast
- Herma Waters, ANMF (HERC)

ACKNOWLEDGEMENTS

The publisher would like to acknowledge Toni Bishop for her contribution to the development of essential skills.

The authors and publishing team would like to thank the following reviewers for their incisive and helpful comments:

- Amanda Reeson, TAFE QLD South West
- Kylie Brennan, TAFE NSW Ill000
- Ingrid Devlin, Health Skills Australia
- Leanne Petrie, Manager for Curriculum and Compliance with Mater Education Limited
- Anneke Groot, BHSS and Silverchain Training
- Michelle ... Chapman, Charlton ...
- Helen ...
- Niall ...
- Susan ..., Sally Training Australia
- Kathy Penny, Charles Sturt University and TAFE Western
- Vicki Smith, TAFE Gold Coast
- Carmel ..., ... TAFE ... campus
- Diane ..., TAFE East Coast
- Fiona ..., ACNP HED...

HAND HYGIENE

1.1 HAND HYGIENE

Note: These notes are summaries of the most important points in the assessments/procedures and are not exhaustive on the subject. References of the materials used to compile the information have been supplied. The student is expected to have learnt the material surrounding each skill as presented in the references. No single reference is complete on each subject.

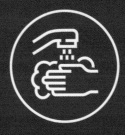

CHAPTER 1.1

HAND HYGIENE

IDENTIFY INDICATIONS

Hand hygiene is a basic infection-control measure that reduces the number of microorganisms on the hands, therefore reducing the risk of transferring microorganisms to a patient. Hand hygiene encompasses both handwashing and use of an alcohol-based hand rub (ABHR). Hand hygiene reduces the risk of cross-contamination; that is, spreading microorganisms from one patient to another. This reduces the risk of infection among health care workers and transmission of infectious organisms to oneself and others. A current national priority in place by the Australian Commission on Safety and Quality in Health Care (ACSQHC, 2019) is to reduce the number of healthcare-associated infections (HCAIs). The COVID-19 coronavirus pandemic reinforces the importance of hand hygiene.

Hand Hygiene Australia recommends '5 Moments for Hand Hygiene':
1. before touching a patient
2. before a procedure
3. after a procedure or body fluid exposure risk
4. after touching a patient
5. after touching a patient's surroundings.

Hand hygiene must also be performed before putting on gloves and after the removal of gloves.

Contact with contaminated hands is a primary source of hospital-acquired infection. Not only does the nurse need to be diligent in handwashing, but also in educating both patients and family members of the importance of effective hand hygiene.

GATHER EQUIPMENT

- *Running water* that can be regulated to warm is most important. Warm water damages the skin less than hot water, which opens pores, removes protective oils and causes irritation. Cold water is less effective at removing microorganisms and can be uncomfortable.
- *The sink* should be of a convenient height and large enough that splashing is minimised since damp uniforms/clothing allow microbes to travel and grow.
- *Soap or an antimicrobial solution* is used to cleanse the hands. The choice is dictated by the condition of the patient – antimicrobial soap is recommended if the nurse will attend immuno-suppressed patients or the pathogens present are virulent.
- *A convenient dispenser* (preferably non-hand-operated) increases hand hygiene compliance.
- *Paper towels* are preferred for drying hands because they are disposable and prevent the transfer of microorganisms. Ensure the paper towels are removed without contaminating the remaining paper towels, which could lead to cross-infection.

PERFORM HAND HYGIENE

Prepare and assess hands

Preparation of hands includes inspection for any lesions, open cuts and abrasions. Removal of jewellery ensures the principles of 'bare below elbow' are followed. These precautions protect both the nurse and the patient and will determine whether further precautions are needed; for example, gloving or non-contact (some agencies prevent nurses with open lesions from caring for high-risk patients). Jewellery harbours microorganisms. Removing jewellery will reduce the potential risk of infection. A simple wedding band may be left on, but must be moved about on the finger during hand hygiene so that soap/gel and friction are applied to the metal and to the underlying skin to dislodge dirt and microorganisms. Following the policy of the organisation so that the touching of hair or clothing does not later contaminate clean hands. Long or artificial nails, or nails with chipped or old nail polish, have been linked to outbreaks of infection and should all be removed (National Health and Medical Research Council, 2019).

Turn on the water flow

Using whatever mechanism is available (hand, elbow, knee or foot control), establish a flow of warm water. Flowing water rinses dirt and microorganisms from the skin and flushes them into the sink.

Thoroughly wet hands and apply soap

Do not touch the inside or outside of the sink. The sink is contaminated and touching it will transfer microorganisms onto the nurse's hands. Wet hands to above the wrists, keeping hands lower than elbows to prevent water from flowing onto the arms and, when contaminated, back onto the clean hands. Add liquid soap or an antimicrobial cleanser. Five millilitres is sufficient to be effective; less does not effectively remove microbes. More soap would be wasteful of resources. Lather hands to above the wrists.

Clean under the fingernails

Under the nails is a highly soiled area and high concentrations of microbes on hands come from beneath fingernails. The area under the nails should be cleansed thoroughly.

Wash hands

Lather and wash your hands for a period of not less than 30 seconds before care or after care if touching 'clean' objects (clean materials, limited patient contact such as pulse-taking), and 1 to 2 minutes if engaged in 'dirty' activities (Hand Hygiene Australia, 2017), such as direct contact with excreta or secretions. A surgical handwash will take 3 to 6 minutes, depending on policies.

Rub one hand with the other, using vigorous movements since friction is effective in dislodging dirt and microorganisms. Pay particular attention to palms, backs of hands, knuckles and webs of fingers. Dirt and microorganisms lodge in creases of the hands and fingers. Lather and scrub up over the wrist, and onto the lower forearm if doing a longer wash to remove dirt and microorganisms from this area. The wrists and forearms are considered less contaminated than the hands, so they are scrubbed after the hands to prevent the movement of microorganisms from a more contaminated to a less contaminated area. Repeat the wetting, lathering with additional soap and rubbing if hands have been heavily contaminated.

Rinse hands

Rinse the hands and fingers under running water to wash microorganisms and dirt from skin, and prevent residual soap from irritating the skin.

Dry hands

Using paper towels, dry hands commencing at the fingers, hands and then the forearm. Dry well to prevent chafing. Damp hands are a source of microbial growth and transfer, as well as contributing to chafing and then lesions of the hands.

Turn off taps

Using dry paper towels, turn hand-manipulated taps off, taking care not to contaminate hands on the sink or taps. Carefully discard paper towels so that hands are not contaminated. Turn off other types of taps with foot, knee or elbow as appropriate. After several washes, hand lotion should be applied to prevent chafing. Frequent hand hygiene can be very drying and chafed skin becomes a reservoir for microorganisms.

ALTERNATIVE HAND HYGIENE

Apply alcohol-based hand rub as required

ABHR is now considered the gold standard of care for hand hygiene. Hand hygiene using a waterless, ABHR has been demonstrated to reduce the microbial load on hands when 5 mL of the 70% ethanol-based solution is vigorously rubbed over all hand and finger surfaces (pay the same attention to the palms, back of the hands, finger webs, knuckles and wrists as during the traditional handwash) for 30 seconds. The use of such a rub is effective for minimally contaminated hands. It increases compliance and reduces skin irritation. Thorough handwashing is still required for contaminated hands or following 'dirty' activities (Hand Hygiene Australia, 2017).

Hands must be visibly clean and dry prior to using the ABHR.

Further information

The National Hand Hygiene Initiative has an online learning package accessible from the site for correct handwashing, with the ability to create a certificate once you have studied the package. This certificate can be used as an assessment tool and some hospitals require students to present it before commencing clinical practice in that area.

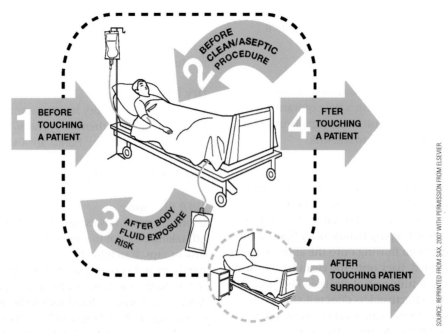

SOURCE: REPRINTED FROM SAX, 2007 WITH PERMISSION FROM ELSEVIER.

FIGURE 1.1.1 5 Moments for Hand Hygiene

CASE STUDY

During the COVID-19 global pandemic, hand hygiene was the key message sent from the World Health Organization (WHO) and health authorities worldwide.

Answer the following questions as an enrolled nurse working in a tertiary hospital in Australia.

1. Where would you find the relevant information on the precautions you need to take when nursing a patient with COVID-19?

2. Why is hand hygiene so important in reducing the spread of COVID-19?
3. For how long should you wash your hands?
4. When would you use an alcohol-based hand gel as opposed to performing a soap and water wash?

Note: These notes are summaries of the most important points in the assessments/procedures, and are not exhaustive on the subject. The naming of documents or charts may differ from state to state, and facility to facility. In all possible situations the guidelines of the ACSQHC are used when describing national charts or documents (e.g. the ACSQHC Observation and Response Chart is named the Adult Observation and Response Chart in WA, and the Rapid Detection and Response Observation Chart in SA). References of the materials used to compile the information have been supplied. The student is expected to have learned the material surrounding each skill as presented in the references. No single reference is complete on the subject.

CRITICAL THINKING

What would be the implications of not performing appropriate hand hygiene in both the hospital and community settings?

REFERENCES

Australian Commission on Safety and Quality in Health Care (ACSQHC). (2019). *Preventing and Controlling Healthcare-Associated Infection Standard*. https://www.safetyandquality. gov.au/standards/nsqhs-standards/preventing-and-controlling-healthcare-associated-infection-standard

Hand Hygiene Australia. (2017). http://www.hha.org.au
National Health and Medical Research Council. (2019). *Australian Guidelines for the Prevention and Control of Infection in Healthcare*. https://www.nhmrc.gov.au/health-advice/public-health/preventing-infection

RECOMMENDED READINGS

Australian Commission on Safety and Quality in Health Care (ACSQHC). (2017). *National Hand Hygiene Initiative*. https://www.safetyandquality.gov.au/our-work/healthcare-associated-infection/hand-hygiene
Australian Commission on Safety and Quality in Health Care (ACSQHC). (2019). *Hand Hygiene*. https://www.safetyandquality. gov.au/our-work/infection-prevention-and-control/national-hand-hygiene-initiative-nhhi/what-hand-hygiene

Gray, S., Ferris, L., White, L.E., Duncan, G. & Baumle, W. (2018). *Foundations of Nursing: Enrolled Nurses* (2nd ANZ ed.). Melbourne: Cengage.
World Health Organization (WHO). (2009). WHO guidelines on hand hygiene in health care. In *World Alliance for Patient Safety. First Global Patient Safety Challenge Clean Care is Safer Care* (1st ed.). Geneva: World Health Organization Press.

CHAPTER 1.1

ESSENTIAL SKILLS COMPETENCY

Hand Hygiene

Demonstrates the ability to effectively reduce the risk of infection by appropriate hand hygiene

Criteria for skill performance	Y	D
(Numbers indicate *Enrolled Nurse Standards for Practice*, 2016)	(Satisfactory)	(Requires development)
1. Identifies indication (8.3, 8.4)		
2. Gathers equipment (1.2, 6.4, 8.4, 9.4): ■ warm running water ■ soap ■ paper towels		
3. Prepares and assesses hands (1.2, 1.4, 8.2, 8.3, 8.4, 9.4)		
4. Turns on and adjusts water flow and water temperature (1.2, 1.3, 1.4, 1.8, 3.2, 3.9, 4.4, 6.4, 8.4, 9.4)		
5. Wets hands, applies soap (1.2, 1.3, 1.4, 1.8, 3.2, 3.9, 8.4, 9.4)		
6. Cleans under the fingernails when required (1.2, 1.3, 1.4, 1.8, 3.2, 3.9, 8.4, 9.4)		
7. Thoroughly washes hands (1.2, 1.3, 1.4, 3.2, 3.9, 8.4, 9.4)		
8. Rinses hands (1.2, 1.3, 1.4, 1.8, 3.2, 3.9, 8.4, 9.4)		
9. Turns off the water if elbow taps used; if ordinary taps, turns off after drying hands (1.2, 1.3, 1.4, 1.8, 3.2, 3.9, 4.4, 6.4, 8.4, 9.4)		
10. Dries hands (1.2, 1.3, 1.4, 1.8, 3.2, 3.9, 8.4, 9.4)		
11. Uses alcohol-based hand rub as an alternative to hand hygiene, when appropriate (1.2, 1.3, 1.4, 1.8, 3.2, 3.9, 8.4, 9.4)		
12. Demonstrates ability to link theory to practice (8.3, 8.4, 8.5, 9.4)		

Student:

Clinical facilitator: Date:

PART 2

ASSESSMENT

Note: These notes are summaries of the most important points in the assessments/procedures and are not exhaustive on the subject. References of the materials used to compile the information have been supplied. The student is expected to have learnt the material surrounding each skill as presented in the references. No single reference is complete on each subject.

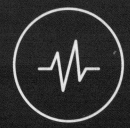

CHAPTER 2.1

HEAD-TO-TOE ASSESSMENT

IDENTIFY INDICATIONS

The indication to perform a head-to-toe assessment is usually contact with a healthcare facility or with healthcare workers in the community. If the patient presents to a healthcare facility, there is concern about their health and they should be assessed accordingly. The patient may be presenting to the healthcare facility for admission, and the admission procedure of most facilities includes a thorough assessment. The purpose of a health history is to formulate a database incorporating historical and current data, and to provide an opportunity for the nurse to develop a trusting relationship with the patient. The interview provides information on the patient's perception of their health concerns and learning needs. The head-to-toe assessment should also be conducted any time the patient's condition changes. This allows the nursing staff to report accurately

and adequately to the doctor. Such an assessment provides data on which nursing interventions are based and is a key nursing action. The collection and organisation of information about the patient assists the nurse to identify existing or potential healthcare problems and to make decisions based on accurate information to help the patient return to a better state of health.

A briefer head-to-toe assessment should also be conducted when completing other routine assessments, such as vital signs, to gain an overall assessment of the patient's status or to gain further information when these might vary from previous readings (North, 2017). The nurse should also complete a brief head-to-toe assessment as part of the shift handover, or soon after the commencement of their shift (Haugh, 2015).

GATHER EQUIPMENT

Gather equipment prior to starting the procedure to maximise efficiency, reduce apprehension on the patient's part and increase confidence in the nurse. The following equipment is required for head-to-toe assessment:

- sphygmomanometer, stethoscope and blood pressure (BP) cuff of appropriate size
- pulse oximeter
- thermometer, penlight torch and watch

- weighing scales
- height stick
- relevant facility forms.

To prepare the environment, ensure that the ambient temperature is comfortable and without draughts, there is sufficient light for the nurse to be able to examine the patient, the area is made private and there is provision for privacy and warmth.

PERFORMING HEAD-TO-TOE ASSESSMENT

Hand hygiene

Perform hand hygiene before touching the patient or the patient's surrounds and prior to any procedure involving patient contact to reduce the possibility of cross-contamination. Hand hygiene is the most effective method of infection control as it removes transient organisms from the hands of the nurse.

Give a clear explanation of the procedure and establish therapeutic communication

Discuss the procedure and gain the patient's consent. Giving a clear explanation is required to gain legal consent and to address policy requirements. It will also assist the patient to cooperate with the procedure, allay anxiety and assist in establishing a therapeutic relationship.

The initial action of introducing yourself to the patient and gaining their consent will help the patient to feel relaxed during the assessment. The more relaxed the patient is, the more information will be obtained, and the easier and more accurate the assessment will be. Most patients on admission to hospital or other healthcare facilities are anxious, and establishing therapeutic relationships with newly admitted patients should be a priority of the nurse. Thorough explanations of procedures to be undertaken and of hospital routines and regulations that affect the patient, honest answers to questions and a sincere attitude to the patient will foster an effective relationship. The patient's privacy is maintained during the health history by using a soft voice for questioning and discussion plus pulling the curtains, closing the door and ensuring the patient is covered with a sheet when not assessing that body area (Gray et al., 2018).

Obtain the patient's health history

The health history is obtained early in the assessment procedure unless the patient is in acute distress – for example, has severe pain or respiratory distress – when an abbreviated nursing history will be obtained. The patient is the person who can most accurately describe symptoms, give their history and share their problems and perceptions. They are, thus, the primary informant. If someone else – for example, a parent or spouse – gives the information for the health history, they are considered a secondary source and this should be noted during documentation. The information given by the patient is subjective data; that is, information that only the patient can supply, such as reports of pain, depression and other symptoms that are not verifiable by another person. This history consists of the demographics of the patient – that is, their age, date of birth, gender identity, occupation, marital or family status, current medical problems, medications being taken and reasons for taking them, allergies, patterns of daily living and other current data that may affect the care given during hospitalisation. Historical data includes information about past events such as their experiences with previous hospitalisation and illness, mental health issues, exposure to infections, previous experience of surgery or anaesthesia, family history, history of medication or alcohol use, social history, cultural background and, again, any pertinent information that might impact on their nursing care.

Much data can be gathered from the patient during the interview. The level of anxiety, mood, level of discomfort, communication and intellectual ability, interpersonal relationships and some idea of body image and self-concept can all be assessed from observation during the interview. Physical assessment can also be completed while interviewing the patient. Inspection of the visible skin allows the nurse to assess colour and gives the clue to cardiac perfusion, liver dysfunction or respiratory difficulties. Other diseases and conditions are sometimes readily visible on the face. Observation of personal hygiene,

dress, eye contact, suitability of clothing, make-up and demeanour give insights into the mental status of the patient. Observation and inspection are valuable tools that should be employed from the first moment of patient contact. Utilisation of adequate lighting, exposure of only body areas that require assessment while also maintaining the patient's dignity by covering remaining body areas with a sheet, knowledge of normal variations, comparison of body areas (e.g. strength in each arm) and an unhurried approach with attention to detail will help the nurse to gain information effectively.

Observation and assessment of the patient

Observation of the patient while they are preparing for the head-to-toe physical assessment can provide a great deal of information. For example, their movements as they enter the room or get into the bed will give indications about their ability to balance, the general status of their health, their body build, posture, gait and any obvious deformity or movements, body or breath odour, the range of movement, the level of consciousness and their level of cooperation. Skin and nail assessment can provide valuable cues to underlying systemic pathological conditions.

Observation is used to assess the patient from the 'top' (i.e. head and neurological status) to 'toe' (i.e. toes – movement and peripheral perfusion).

- Assess the patient's cognitive status and general mental state. Identify if the person is orientated to time, person and place plus their normal cognitive status. Patients with dementia may be normally orientated in their home environment but become disorientated and agitated in the hospital setting. Illness may also cause a patient to become disorientated or restless. Assess a patient's general mental health status by assessing their verbal interaction and general appearance. Patients may show levels of anxiety related to their hospital admission or illness. If there are any indications that the patient's mental status requires further assessment, the registered nurse (RN) should be notified as a full mental state assessment may be required.
- Assess the patient's conscious state and neurological functioning. Complete a full neurological assessment if required (see **Skill 2.7**).
- Complete a pain assessment using the relevant facility tool (see **Skill 2.9**).
- Obtain vital signs (see the relevant competencies). The BP, pulse, temperature, oxygen saturation and respiratory status are assessed initially. These provide baseline measurements (see **Skills 2.3**, **2.4** and **2.5**).
- Assess the circulation by reviewing the capillary refill and peripheral perfusion of the patient's limbs (see **Skill 2.8**).
- Assess the respiratory functioning (see **Skill 2.3**).

- Assess the musculoskeletal functioning by assessing motor function – for instance, raising limbs against gravity and resistance, and assessing strength of handgrips bilaterally. Assess range of movement (see **Skill 3.14**). A Falls Risk Assessment must also be carried out by using the relevant Falls Risk Management tool (see **Skill 2.2**).
- Assess skin integrity according to organisational policy. This may encompass pressure injury risk assessment, tattooing, body piercing, infections and other skin problems. The relevant pressure injury assessment scale (e.g. Braden, Norton, Waterlow or Glamorgan Scale) as per hospital policy should be used (see **Skill 3.13** for further information about pressure injury risk assessment).
- Assess bowel function by questioning the patient about the frequency and regularity of their bowel actions and usual type of stool (e.g. Bristol Stool Chart) (see **Skill 3.9**).
- Weight and height are measured to establish the body mass index (BMI). Ask about the patient's regular dietary intake. A malnutrition screening tool may be used and reviewed for at-risk patients.
- Assess the genitourinary functioning by questioning the patient about urinary activity and reproductive and sexual activity. Obtain a clean catch specimen for urinalysis (see **Skill 3.8**). If there are urinary symptoms, these must be reported at once.

Following completion of the head-to-toe physical assessment, the patient should be reassured and asked to relay any further information they think would be of assistance in caring for them.

Ongoing physical assessment
Assessment of the patient does not stop when the head-to-toe assessment and interview are complete. It is an ongoing process that continues to provide data until the patient is discharged.

Perform hand hygiene
Maintain the 5 Moments for Hand Hygiene and perform hand hygiene after touching the patient and the patient's surrounds.

CLEAN, REPLACE OR DISPOSE OF EQUIPMENT
Cleaning and replacing equipment shows respect for other staff members, increases efficiency in the unit and develops good organisational and work habits.

DOCUMENT AND REPORT RELEVANT INFORMATION
Documentation can be extensive. Facilities usually have specific forms for the required information. If no forms exist, document the data that you have gathered in a systematic manner. Use the observation and assessment format described earlier or a systems format to record the information. All vital signs and other relevant data should also be recorded on the observation and response chart (ORC). Respond appropriately to the total score when recording the observations on this chart. The Australian Commission on Safety and Quality in Health Care (ACSQHC, 2019) states that using the ORC correctly promotes accurate and timely recognition of deterioration in a patient's health status, plus prompt action. Any implemented actions should also be documented on the chart in the relevant section. Any other concerns not already identified as needing to be reported can be reported to the RN or shift coordinator.

CASE STUDY

1. Using a nursing history and assessment form from your facility, complete a basic assessment on a family member. Practise the required assessment skills, and collect information about their health history. Follow the processes of professional and effective patient communication when completing this procedure.
2. Evelyn Deer is a 31-year-old woman admitted to your day surgery ward this morning for a right knee arthroscopy procedure. She is athletic and plays team netball, is generally fit and well, and does not have any significant medical history She has been fasting. Her observations are within the normal adult range. Besides completing her vital signs, what other head-to-toe assessments will you perform?

Note: These notes are summaries of the most important points in the assessments/procedures, and are not exhaustive on the subject. The naming of documents or charts may differ from state to state, and facility to facility. In all possible situations the guidelines of the ACSQHC are used when describing national charts or documents (e.g. the ACSQHC Observation and Response Chart is named the Adult Observation and Response Chart in WA, and the Rapid Detection and Response Observation Chart in SA). References of the materials used to compile the information have been supplied. The student is expected to have learned the material surrounding each skill as presented in the references. No single reference is complete on the subject.

REFERENCES

Australian Commission on Safety and Quality in Health Care (ACSQHC). (2019). *Observation and Response Charts*. https://www.safetyandquality.gov.au/our-work/recognising-and-responding-to-clinical-deterioration/observation-and-response-charts

Calleja, P., Theobald, K. & Harvey, T. (2020). *Estes Health Assessment and Physical Examination* (3rd ed.). Singapore: Cengage.

Gray, S., Ferris, L., White, L.E., Duncan, G. & Baumle, W. (2018). *Foundations of Nursing: Enrolled Nurses* (2nd ANZ ed.). Melbourne: Cengage.

Haugh, K.H. (2015). Head-to-toe: Organizing baseline patient physical assessment. *Nursing*, 45(12), p. 58.

North, D. (2017). Promoting direct human contact. *Canadian Nurse*, 113(1), p. 42.

RECOMMENDED READINGS

Australian Commission on Safety and Quality in Health Care (ACSQHC). (2019). *Recognising and Responding to Acute Physiological Deterioration*. http://www.safetyandquality.gov.au/our-work/recognition-and-response-to-clinical-deterioration

Australian Commission on Safety and Quality in Health Care (ACSQHC). (2019). *Comprehensive Care Standard*. https://www.safetyandquality.gov.au/standards/nsqhs-standards/comprehensive-care-standard

Australian Commission on Safety and Quality in Health Care (ACSQHC). (2019). *Recognising and Responding to Acute Deterioration Standard*. https://www.safetyandquality.gov.au/standards/nsqhs-standards/recognising-and-responding-acute-deterioration-standard

Hamilton, D. (2017). Mitigating perceptual error with 'look, listen, feel'. *British Journal of Nursing*, 26(9), p. 507.

Hand Hygiene Australia. (2017). http:www.hha.org.au

ESSENTIAL SKILLS COMPETENCY

Basic Assessment

Demonstrates the ability to effectively carry out a patient's basic assessment as per facility policy

Criteria for skill performance	Y	D
(Numbers indicate *Enrolled Nurse Standards for Practice*, 2016)	(Satisfactory)	(Requires development)
1. Identifies indication (8.3, 8.4)		
2. Gathers equipment (1.2, 1.6, 4.4, 6.4, 8.4, 9.4) and prepares environment: ■ sphygmomanometer, stethoscope, appropriate BP cuff, thermometer, penlight torch and watch ■ height stick and weight scales ■ relevant forms		
3. Performs hand hygiene (1.2, 1.4, 1.8, 3.9, 6.4, 9.4)		
4. Evidence of effective communication with the patient; gives patient a clear explanation of procedure, gains patient consent (2.1, 2.3, 2.4, 2.5, 6.3)		
5. Obtains a thorough nursing history (1.2, 1.4, 2.1, 2.2, 2.3, 2.4, 2.5, 2.6, 2.7, 3.2, 4.1, 4.2, 4.3, 4.4, 5.3, 6.4, 7.1, 7.2, 7.3, 7.5, 8.4, 9.4)		
6. Conducts a systematic assessment of the patient (1.2, 3.2, 4.1, 4.2, 4.3, 4.4, 7.1, 7.2, 7.3, 8.4, 9.4)		
7. Performs hand hygiene (1.2, 1.4, 1.8, 3.9, 6.4, 9.4)		
8. Cleans, replaces and disposes of equipment appropriately (1.2, 1.4, 3.9, 6.5, 9.4)		
9. Documents and reports relevant information (1.2, 1.8, 3.2, 5.3, 6.6, 7.1, 7.2, 7.3, 7.4, 7.5)		
10. Demonstrates ability to link theory to practice (8.3, 8.4, 8.5, 9.4)		

Student:

Clinical facilitator: Date:

CHAPTER 2.2

RISK ASSESSMENT AND RISK MANAGEMENT

INDICATIONS

Whenever a patient is admitted to a healthcare facility or care provider, the goal of every nurse should be to provide safe and appropriate care, avoiding unintentional harm to the patient and achieving the best possible outcome. Health care is an increasingly complex environment, compounded by factors such as a patient's disease process, which place all patients at risk of experiencing an adverse event or clinical incident; that is, an unplanned event that results in or has the potential to harm a patient (NSW Health, 2013). These risks within health care can include clinical and non-clinical risks. Both require management, with most non-clinical risks being managed through workplace health and safety. Clinical risks are those associated with delivering clinical care. They are specific to the patient and can occur any time during the course of patient care. Common incidents that can occur in health care include falls, pressure injuries, medication errors, wrong diagnosis or treatment, hospital-acquired infection or physical assault (WHO, 2018; ACSQHC, 2017).

Clinical risks are identified and managed as part of patient admission, assessment processes and ongoing care. Facility policies to reduce clinical risk include assessment tools and care actions to help reduce the risk of harm to a patient receiving care and also meet the National Safety and Quality Health Service Standards. These standards identify issues such as hospital-acquired infections, falls, pressure injury, safe patient identification, patient handover, use of blood products and patient clinical deterioration. The Comprehensive Care Standard directly states the need that patients at specific risk of harm are identified, and clinicians implement strategies to prevent and manage that harm (ACSQHC, 2019a). This includes pressure injuries, falls and poor nutrition and malnutrition.

As care providers, nurses are required to implement nursing actions to reduce clinical risk for their patients. They need to be actively involved in clinical risk management processes, and embed clinical risk management into their daily routine.

FALLS RISK

The World Health Organization defines a fall as:

> an event which results in a person coming to rest inadvertently on the ground or floor or other lower level.
>
> (WHO, 2021)

A person's risk of falling increases as they age, and the NSW Health Clinical Excellence Commission identified that no:

> other single cause of injury, including road trauma, costs the NSW health system more than falls.
>
> (NSW Health, 2018)

Falls prevention screening and management programs aim to reduce the incidence and severity of falls among hospitalised patients.

All patients are assessed for their falls risk on admission. Anyone who is identified as a high risk is screened to obtain a more in-depth assessment of their risk to then determine actions to be implemented that will reduce the risk of a fall during the admission. The patient's falls risk assessment is then reviewed every 48 to 72 hours (according to facility policy) and when there is any change in the patient's health status. Tools used to assess falls risk are generally recommended by each state/territory health department and are research based.

MALNUTRITION RISK

Malnutrition occurs in approximately 40% of patients in Australian hospitals (ACSQHC, 2018a), with many of the elderly patients at risk. A nutrition screening tool is not specifically a nutrition assessment, but a tool that identifies individuals who are at risk of malnutrition. There are different tools available, and they include questions about current and recent weight loss, body mass index, appetite (poor intake) and existing comorbidities, and assign a numerical score to categorise the risk of malnutrition.

A validated screening tool should be used, and these will vary according to the facility. The Malnutrition Screening Tool (MST) is one of the most frequently used (Department of Health and Human Services, 2015).

GATHER AND PREPARE EQUIPMENT

Collect the required screening tools/documents:
- *Falls Risk Management tool*
- *Pressure Injury Risk Assessment tool* (e.g. Braden Scale or Norton Scale, Glamorgan Scale for children)
- *Malnutrition Screening tool*
- *Cognition Assessment tool* (e.g. mini mental state assessment)

- *further equipment required* for patient assessment (e.g. sphygmomanometer)
- *personal protective equipment (PPE)* – non-sterile gloves and other PPE to reduce infection control risks
- *anti-embolic stockings and/or pneumatic boots and controller*, plus measuring tape for determining correct size.

IMPLEMENT CLINICAL RISK ASSESSMENT AND MANAGEMENT

Perform hand hygiene
Perform hand hygiene before touching the patient or the patient's surrounds and prior to any procedure involving patient contact to reduce the possibility of cross-contamination. Hand hygiene is the most effective method of infection control as it removes transient organisms from the hands of the nurse (see **Skill 1.1**).

Give a clear explanation of the procedure and establish therapeutic communication
Discuss the procedure and gain the patient's consent. Giving a clear explanation is required to gain legal consent and to address policy requirements. It will also assist the patient to cooperate with the procedure, allay anxiety and assist in establishing a therapeutic relationship.

Demonstrate problem-solving abilities
Many clinical risk assessment and management actions are embedded into daily nursing care routines and patient admission procedures. The nurse needs to use the tools that are part of all patient admissions and complete any screening requirements required as part of or within a specific time period of a patient's admission. Many of these actions then require determination of the need for a more comprehensive clinical risk assessment. Refer to facility policies and guidelines when completing these assessments.

The following clinical risk assessment and management actions should be implemented according to the patient's needs.

Clinical communication
Communication within health care is key to safety and reducing patient risk, with correct communication processes and patient identification helping reduce the risk of patient harm. Follow the facility guidelines for clinical handover procedures (see **Skill 7.3**). On admission, two identification bands are placed on all patients (wrist and ankle). Always check the patient's identification band, plus verbally confirm you have the correct patient before administering any nursing care. Further checking and clarification of the patient's identity will occur with specific procedures such as medication administration.

IMPLEMENT A FALLS RISK ASSESSMENT AND MANAGEMENT PLAN

Screening process
Access the facility's falls risk assessment tool, and complete the initial falls risk assessment. This includes assessment of the patient's cognitive status and mobility/balance, and asking if they have suffered any falls in the previous 12 months. If the patient meets any of the criteria identifying them as a risk, move on to the more comprehensive falls risk assessment. Review the patient nursing and health information, plus question and physically assess the patient according to the tool requirements.

This screening process is then repeated according to the patient's health status and facility policy; this can be on a shift-by-shift basis or up to every 72 hours. A falls risk assessment should also be implemented when there is any change in the patient's health status (e.g. post-op, change in level of consciousness) or change in the patient's environment (e.g. being transferred to a new ward).

Implement actions to reduce falls risk
Use the Falls Risk Management tool to determine the required nursing care for the patient. This may be a separate document or a separate part of the risk assessment tool. Basic environmental safety actions or falls risk minimisation actions that should be implemented for all patients are stated on the Falls Risk Management tool. These include the use of bed brakes, lowering the patient's bed to the correct height for the patient, use of bed rails only when it reduces risk of harm, using mobility aids, correct lighting and

access to the patient's call bell. Identify the specific actions listed against the patient's risks. Those relevant to the patient should be identified and also signed as implemented each shift. The nursing actions should also be noted in the nursing care plan, and signed each shift as implemented. Some facilities may have prefilled nursing care plans identifying the minimum interventions for all patients.

Multidisciplinary input

Other allied health professionals such as the physiotherapist or doctor will provide specific information and care actions to reduce a patient's falls risk. Some risk assessment or management tools will have provision for these types of recommendations to be recorded. These instructions should be followed. A risk management action may also include a referral to the physiotherapist or other allied health professional. Follow facility policies to complete this referral process.

Record every fall

All falls should be recorded on a facility incident form (as per facility policy) and in the patient's notes. A fall is classified as an adverse event, even if the patient does not suffer an injury. Following a fall, a new falls risk assessment should be completed.

RECOGNISE AND RESPOND TO PATIENT CLINICAL DETERIORATION

Recognising deterioration of a patient's health status and implementing timely care is a key safety issue (ACSQHC, 2018b). Use of an observation and response chart (ORC) (ACSQHC, 2019b) to monitor and document patients' observations is a key component of a recognition and response system. The chart has been designed to assist nurses in recognising changes in a patient's observations that are early indicators of a patient's deteriorating clinical health status, and then specifying actions to be taken. Use of this ORC has reduced the incidence of medical emergencies as it creates an early warning of patient clinical deterioration and earlier implementation of medical interventions.

As described in Skills 2.3, 2.4 and 2.5, patient observations should be recorded on the observation chart and a score (Adult Deterioration Detection System [ADDS] score) generated from those results. The key on the observation chart is then used to determine the appropriate response to the total ADDS score. This includes an increase in the frequency of the observations and further review by a doctor or senior nurse. The observations chart also includes colour coding in the chart as a guide for identifying observations that are abnormal and that the patient may require further review by a senior nurse or doctor. For example, any observation that is charted in a purple zone will be a medical emergency (i.e. medical emergency team [MET] call unless these parameters

have been adjusted by medical staff within the modification section. The emergency call bell should be pressed to gain immediate assistance.

VENOUS THROMBOEMBOLISM (VTE) RISK

All patients are assessed for their VTE (deep vein thrombosis and pulmonary emboli) risk on admission and when the medication chart is created by the doctor. The nurse should also assess the patient's VTE risk during the admission process and ongoing care by recognising common risk factors, such as age (patients over 50), immobility, surgery and obesity. Appropriate nursing risk management strategies are then implemented, and may include the following.

- Keep all patients as mobile as possible, depending on their health status.
- Encourage active and passive exercises (see **Skill 3.14**).
- Assist the patient to wear anti-embolic stockings (e.g. thrombo-embolic-deterrent stockings – TEDs).
- Pneumatic booties are often used for postoperative patients.
- Administer prophylactic subcutaneous anticoagulant as prescribed by the doctor (see **Skill 5.3** for subcutaneous injection).

Assisting a patient to wear anti-embolic stockings

The patient should be fitted for anti-embolic stockings using a measuring tape and following the manufacturer's instructions to get the correct size. Incorrect sizing can create discomfort and incorrect levels of compression (Jindal et al., 2020). The stockings are applied by placing the stocking over the toes and then fitting the foot and heel correctly. The toes should not stick out. Grasp the stockings with your fingers and then pull them up around the ankle and calf. Continue pulling the stockings up over the remainder of the leg. Smooth out any wrinkles or bunched areas. With full-length stockings, the panel goes towards the inner thigh.

Remove the stockings daily to inspect the patient's skin and allow showering, then put back on as per above.

Apply pneumatic booties

The patient's calf is placed inside the 'bootie'. The velcro tabs are used to help keep the booties closed and in place. Attach the tubing to the tubing system and powered unit as per the manufacturer's instructions, and turn on the power. Adjust settings (if required – some systems have an auto function) according to the patient's needs.

PRESSURE INJURY RISK ASSESSMENT

Pressure injury risk assessment should be completed on every patient within 8 hours of admission to hospital (ACSQHC, 2017). Assessment for a patient's risk of developing a pressure injury must be completed as part of the admission process for all patients, and reassessment for pressure injury risk is required to be completed if there is a change in the patient's condition or level of mobility, a period of immobility (e.g. post-operatively) or at least weekly. Patients with a score showing risk of pressure injury must be reassessed every 24 to 48 hours.

Please refer to **Skill 3.13** for pressure injury assessment.

NUTRITION RISK ASSESSMENT

All patients are weighed upon admission and a basic assessment of their body mass index included in the admission information. An MST is used to assess the patient's nutrition risk as required, depending on the patient's age group (i.e. elderly patients are often routinely screened by many facilities), if they have experienced recent weight loss (without trying), or poor appetite or food intake. Screening should be completed within 24 hours of admission (Department of Health and Human Services, 2015). Patients within certain weight ranges may also be assessed for their nutritional status. Patients are then rescreened weekly in acute care facilities or monthly in long-term facilities. Refer to state/territory health and facility policy for age-group screening requirements and the frequency of the assessment.

To manage the needs of patients with a nutritional risk, complete the relevant referrals and work with other allied health professionals to reduce the patient's risks. The dietitian will prescribe a diet and any required supplements. The doctor will manage health problems. In residential facilities, the dining areas and other social factors should also be reviewed because they can strongly impact on food intake.

REDUCE THE RISK OF HOSPITAL-ACQUIRED INFECTION

Hospital-acquired infections are the most common complication affecting hospitalised patients in Australia, causing pain and prolonging a hospital admission (NHMRC, 2019). Basic principles of infection control to reduce the transmission of infectious agents are used to reduce and manage risk of infection. These principles include the actions of hand hygiene (see **Skill 1.1**) and standard precautions when interacting with patients. Additional precautions (see **Skill 8.13**) are used when a patient's illness creates an increased risk. Other risk management actions include cleaning and decontaminating equipment,

and routine cleaning of the patient environment and other clinical areas.

OTHER SPECIFIC CLINICAL RISK ASSESSMENT ACTIONS

Different procedures and care actions have specific processes used to reduce clinical risks associated with the procedure. These include:

- the use of preoperative and preprocedure checklists (see **Skill 8.2**)
- checking and management of blood products (see **Skill 6.9**)
- medication administration (see **Skills 5.1** to **5.5**).

Pain is a risk associated with hospital treatment. Every patient should be assessed for pain regularly throughout the shift (see **Skill 2.9**) and actions implemented to reduce or manage pain (see **Skill 3.11**).

Age and the presence of disease are two further factors that increase a patient's risk of complications from medical care. A thorough nursing admission assessment (see **Skill 7.4**) will aid in identifying these risk factors.

PERFORM HAND HYGIENE

Maintain the 5 Moments for Hand Hygiene and perform hand hygiene after touching the patient and the patient's surrounds.

CLEAN, REPLACE OR DISPOSE OF EQUIPMENT

Clean and replace used equipment. Wipe any re-useable equipment with the facility disinfecting wipes before replacing in the relevant storage area.

DOCUMENT AND REPORT RELEVANT INFORMATION

Each of the described clinical risk assessment tools will need to be completed and maintained as part of the patient's documentation. Nursing actions will also need to be included in and signed for when completed on the patient's nursing care plan. Information about risk assessment and management strategies should be reported as part of shift handover.

All patient observations should be documented on the ORC immediately after they are measured and the ADDS score totalled. Respond appropriately to the score, reporting to the shift coordinator and implementing the advised strategies. Any responses to patient changes in health status should be shared as part of shift handover.

CASE STUDY

1. Joan Wooley is aged 83. She has had a right cerebrovascular accident, and has a left-sided weakness and needs assistance to be repositioned in bed or in the chair. Joan also requires assistance with eating, hygiene and elimination needs. Her current weight is 51 kg, and staff have noticed that she has a lack of appetite for hospital food. She is continent. Access the Falls Risk Assessment tool relevant to your facility or state health department. Complete this falls risk assessment for Joan.
2. What actions will you implement to reduce the risk of Joan losing further body weight while in hospital?
3. What nursing actions will you implement to reduce Joan's VTE risk?

Note: These notes are summaries of the most important points in the assessments/procedures, and are not exhaustive on the subject. The naming of documents or charts may differ from state to state, and facility to facility. In all possible situations the guidelines of the ACSQHC are used when describing national charts or documents (e.g. the ACSQHC Observation and Response Chart is named the Adult Observation and Response Chart in WA, and the Rapid Detection and Response Observation Chart in SA). References of the materials used to compile the information have been supplied. The student is expected to have learned the material surrounding each skill as presented in the references. No single reference is complete on the subject.

REFERENCES

Australian Commission on Safety and Quality in Health Care (ACSQHC). (2017). *National Safety and Quality Health Service Standards* (2nd ed.). https://www.safetyandquality.gov.au/wp-content/uploads/2017/12/National-Safety-and-Quality-Health-Service-Standards-second-edition.pdf

Australian Commission on Safety and Quality in Health Care (ACSQHC). (2018a). *Hospital-Acquired Complication 13 MALNUTRITION.* https://www.safetyandquality.gov.au/sites/default/files/migrated/SAQ7730_HAC_Malnutrition_LongV2.pdf

Australian Commission on Safety and Quality in Health Care (ACSQHC). (2018b). *Recognising and Responding to Acute Physiological Deterioration.* https://www.safetyandquality.gov.au/our-work/recognising-and-responding-to-clinical-deterioration/

Australian Commission on Safety and Quality in Health Care (ACSQHC). (2019a). *Comprehensive Care Standard.* https://www.safetyandquality.gov.au/standards/nsqhs-standards/comprehensive-care-standard

Australian Commission on Safety and Quality in Health Care (ACSQHC). (2019b). *Observation and Response Charts.* https://www.safetyandquality.gov.au/our-work/recognising-and-responding-to-clinical-deterioration/observation-and-response-charts

Department of Health and Human Services. (2015). *Identifying Nutrition and Hydration Issues.* State Government of Victoria. 5 October. https://www2.health.vic.gov.au/hospitals-and-health-services/patient-care/older-people/nutrition-swallowing/nutrition-and-hydration/nutrition-identifying

Jindal, R., Uhl, J.-F. & Benigni, J. (2020). Sizing of medical below-knee compression stockings in an Indian population: A major risk factor for non-compliance. *Phlebology*, 35(2), 110–114.

National Health and Medical Research Council (NHMRC). (2019). *Australian Guidelines for the Prevention and Control of Infection in Healthcare.* https://www.nhmrc.gov.au/health-advice/public-health/preventing-infection

NSW Health. (2018). *Falls Prevention.* NSW Government. © Clinical Excellence Commission 2018. http://www.cec.health.nsw.gov.au/patient-safety-programs/adult-patient-safety/falls-prevention

NSW Health. (2013). *Clinical Risk Management.* NSW Government. http://www.health.nsw.gov.au/mentalhealth/cg/Pages/mh-risk-management.aspx. © State of New South Wales NSW Ministry of Health. For current information go to www.health.nsw.gov.au

World Health Organization (WHO). (2021). *Falls Fact Sheet.* https://www.who.int/en/news-room/fact-sheets/detail/falls CC BY-NC-SA 3.0 IGO. https://creativecommons.org/licenses/by-nc-sa/3.0/igo/

RECOMMENDED READINGS

Australian Commission on Safety and Quality in Health Care (ACSQHC). (N.D.). *Falls Facts for Nurses. Preventing Falls and Harm From Falls in Older People: Best Practice Guidelines for Australian Residential Aged Care Facilities 2009.* https://www.safetyandquality.gov.au/sites/default/files/migrated/30472-Nurses.pdf

Department of Health and Human Services. (2017). *Falls Risk Assessment Tool (FRAT).* State Government of Victoria. https://www2.health.vic.gov.au/about/publications/policiesandguidelines/falls-risk-assessment-tool

Department of Health and Human Services. (2017). *Clinical Risk Management.* State Government of Victoria. https://www2.health.vic.gov.au/hospitals-and-health-services/quality-safety-service/clinical-risk-management

Department of Health and Human Services. (2017). *Delivering High-Quality Healthcare: Victorian Clinical Governance Framework.* State of Victoria. https://www2.health.vic.gov.au/hospitals-and-health-services/quality-safety-service/clinical-risk-management/clinical-governance-policy

Metro North Hospital and Health Service. (2015). *Malnutrition: Is your Patient at Risk?* Queensland Government. https://www.health.qld.gov.au/__data/assets/pdf_file/0029/148826/hphe_mst_pstr.pdf

SA Health. (2021). *Falls Prevention.* Government of South Australia. https://www.sahealth.sa.gov.au/wps/wcm/connect/public+content/sa+health+internet/clinical+resources/clinical+programs+and+practice+guidelines/older+people/falls+prevention/falls+prevention+for+health+professionals

ESSENTIAL SKILLS ASSESSMENT

Implements clinical risk assessment and management

Demonstrates the ability to complete patient clinical risk assessment and implement relevant risk management nursing care actions

Criteria for skill performance	Y	D
(Numbers indicate *Enrolled Nurse Standards for Practice*, 2016)	(Satisfactory)	(Requires development)
1. Identifies indication (8.3, 8.4)		
2. Evidence of effective communication with the patient; gives patient a clear explanation of procedure, gains consent (2.1, 2.3, 2.4, 2.5, 6.3)		
3. Performs hand hygiene (1.2, 1.4, 1.8, 3.9, 6.4, 9.4)		
4. Demonstrates problem-solving abilities (4.1, 4.2, 8.3, 8.4, 9.4)		
5. Gathers and prepares equipment (1.2, 1.6, 4.4, 6.4, 8.4, 9.4)		
6. Maintains correct clinical communication (e.g. shift handover) and checks patient ID band when implementing nursing care actions (1.2, 1.4, 1.8, 2.1, 2.3, 2.7, 3.2, 3.9, 4.1, 4.2, 4.3, 6.4, 7.1, 7.2, 8.4, 9.4)		
7. Implements a Falls Risk Assessment and Management Plan, including minimal/standard care actions for all patients (1.2, 1.4, 1.8, 2.1, 2.3, 2.7, 3.2, 3.9, 4.1, 4.2, 4.3, 6.4, 7.1, 7.2, 8.4, 9.4)		
8. Charts all patient observations correctly, completing ADDS score; recognises and responds to patient clinical deterioration (1.2, 1.4, 1.8, 2.1, 2.3, 2.7, 3.2, 3.9, 4.1, 4.2, 4.3, 6.4, 7.1, 7.2, 8.4, 9.4)		
9. Recognises venous thromboembolism (VTE) risk, and implements risk reduction care actions according to individual patient needs, including application of TED stockings or pneumatic boots (1.2, 1.4, 1.8, 2.1, 2.3, 2.7, 3.2, 3.9, 4.1, 4.2, 4.3, 6.4, 7.1, 7.2, 8.4, 9.4)		
10. Implements pressure injury risk assessment for all patients (1.2, 1.4, 1.8, 2.1, 2.3, 2.7, 3.2, 3.9, 4.1, 4.2, 4.3, 6.4, 7.1, 7.2, 8.4, 9.4)		
11. Implements nutrition risk assessment for relevant patients (1.2, 1.4, 1.8, 2.1, 2.3, 2.7, 3.2, 3.9, 4.1, 4.2, 4.3, 6.4, 7.1, 7.2, 8.4, 9.4)		
12. Reduces the risk of hospital-acquired infection through using hand hygiene, standard precautions and additional precautions (when required) (1.2, 1.4, 1.8, 2.1, 2.3, 2.7, 3.2, 3.9, 4.1, 4.2, 4.3, 6.4, 7.1, 7.2, 8.4, 9.4)		
13. Implements other specific clinical risk assessment actions, according to patient treatment and needs (e.g. pre-op checklist, medication administration) (1.2, 1.4, 1.8, 2.1, 2.3, 2.7, 3.2, 3.9, 4.1, 4.2, 4.3, 6.4, 7.1, 7.2, 8.4, 9.4)		
14. Performs hand hygiene (1.2, 1.4, 1.8, 3.9, 6.4, 9.4)		
15. Documents and reports relevant information (1.2, 1.3, 1.8, 3.2, 5.3, 6.6, 7.1, 7.2, 7.3, 7.4, 7.5)		
16. Cleans, replaces and disposes of equipment appropriately (1.2, 1.4, 3.9, 6.5, 9.4)		
17. Demonstrates ability to link theory to practice (8.3, 8.4, 8.5, 9.4)		

Student:

Clinical facilitator: Date:

CHAPTER **2.3**

TEMPERATURE, PULSE AND RESPIRATION (TPR) MEASUREMENT

IDENTIFY INDICATIONS FOR OBTAINING TEMPERATURE MEASUREMENTS

Indications for obtaining temperature measurements on patients include:

- establishing a baseline for subsequent comparison
- determining if the temperature changes in response to specific therapies such as antipyretic medication or while administering blood products
- monitoring the temperature of patients at risk for temperature alterations such as infection, hypothermia or hyperthermia, or patients exposed to invasive procedures
- concern that the patient has a temperature outside the normal range.

Normal body temperature is 35.5 to 37.5°C, although exercise, emotional upsets or ovulation can alter the normal range. Consistency in the method of obtaining body temperature readings is important. The observation and response chart (ORC) incorporates a track and trigger system for observations that are outside this range (ACSQHC, 2017).

Assessment is an essential part of the nurse's role and forms part of the nursing process. The nurse must be able to interpret the readings and be aware of normal and abnormal limits, know when to intervene appropriately and offer explanation to the client.

IDENTIFY INDICATIONS FOR ASSESSING PULSE

Indications for assessing pulse include:

- establishing a baseline for subsequent comparison
- determining that the pulse rate, rhythm and volume are within normal limits for the patient
- monitoring the patient's health status, to compare the qualities of peripheral pulses bilaterally
- monitoring patients who are at risk for alterations in their pulse

- prior to the administration of certain medications.

Normal pulse rates for adults range from 60 to 100 beats per minute. The AORC incorporates a track and trigger system for observations that are outside this range (ACSQHC, 2017).

IDENTIFY INDICATIONS FOR ASSESSING RESPIRATION

Indications for assessing respiration include:

- establishing a baseline for subsequent comparison
- determining that the respiratory rate, rhythm, quality and depth are within normal limits for the patient
- monitoring the patient's health status
- assessing respirations prior to and following medication administration (e.g. anaesthesia, morphine, salbutamol)
- monitoring patients who are at risk for alterations in their respiratory status.

Normal respiratory rates for adults range from 14 to 20 breaths per minute. The AORC incorporates a track and trigger system for observations that are outside this range (ACSQHC, 2017).

These vital signs (temperature, pulse and respiration – TPR) are usually nurse-initiated or done according to a prescribed hospital policy. TPR can be monitored any time the nurse feels that the health status of the patient warrants the assessment.

GATHER AND PREPARE EQUIPMENT

Gathering equipment before initiating the procedure creates a positive environment for the successful completion of the procedure. It expedites the completion of the procedure, boosts patient confidence and trust in the nurse, and increases the nurse's self-confidence. Gathering equipment prior to a procedure also provides an opportunity to rehearse the procedure mentally.

- *Electronic thermometers* consist of an electronic machine with a digital readout linked to a thermistor that is covered by a disposable probe cover. The tympanic version or oral probe are commonly used. An alternative type uses an infrared beam, and the instrument does not come in contact with the patient's skin.
- *A watch with a second hand* is necessary to calculate the pulse and respirations per minute.

Thermometer

Electronic thermometers consist of a thermistor rod probe that measures temperature accurately and quickly, a battery-operated electronic pack and disposable probe covers. Probe covers are snapped into place snugly prior to use and disposed of in contaminated waste bins after use. Placing and ejecting probe covers is done according to the manufacturer's instructions. Infrared thermometers emit a small beam onto the patient's forehead, so they do not touch the patient's skin. Each unit has different configurations and the nurse needs to be familiar with the one in use. Follow the manufacturer's instructions. Check the equipment is charged and working correctly and that sufficient probe covers are available if required. Alcohol wipes are also used to clean the equipment after use.

Watch with a second hand

Ensure the watch is visible and easy to read while performing pulse and respiration measurement. Principles of 'bare-below-elbows' should be maintained, so a nurse's fob-style watch is recommended as it is easy to access and see when worn in the upper chest area.

TAKING TEMPERATURE, PULSE AND RESPIRATION MEASUREMENTS

Perform hand hygiene

Perform hand hygiene before touching the patient or the patient's surrounds and prior to any procedure involving patient contact to reduce the possibility of cross-contamination. Hand hygiene is the most effective method of infection control as it removes transient organisms from the hands of the nurse (see **Skill 1.1**).

Give a clear explanation of the procedure and establish therapeutic communication

Discuss the procedure and gain the patient's consent. Giving a clear explanation is required to gain legal consent and to address policy requirements. It will also assist the patient to cooperate with the procedure, allay anxiety and assist in establishing a therapeutic relationship.

Anxiety can alter vital signs, so it is important for the patient to feel relaxed.

Assess the patient

Assess the patient for age, medications, anxiety, general fitness and exercise within the past 20 minutes, as these can all influence the pulse and respiration rate.

The method of taking the temperature will be determined by the patient's mental and physical status. If a tympanic thermometer is to be used, assess the patient's ear for problems such as inflammation, excess wax or redness. If an oral probe is being used, check if the patient has drunk hot fluids (e.g. tea or coffee) in the past 5 to 10 minutes, as this can influence the reading.

Take the patient's temperature

The infrared thermometer is aimed at the patient's forehead and immediately gives a reading. If using the tympanic thermometer, ensure there is a fresh probe cover and the unit is switched on. Insert the probe gently into the external meatus. With your free hand, gently grasp the upper pinna lobe and gently lift it up to straighten the ear canal. An oral probe with an appropriate cover is inserted under the patient's tongue. You may need to hold the probe in place while the reading is taken.

The thermometer will beep to signal completion of registration of temperature. Press the appropriate mechanism to remove the probe cover, then discard it into the contaminated waste bin without contaminating your hands. The temperature will be displayed as a digital readout on the electronic unit.

Measure the patient's pulse

The radial pulse is normally used unless it cannot be accessed (e.g. casts) or if there is a particular reason for assessing another peripheral pulse point (e.g. assessing pedal circulation). The patient is positioned so that the pulse is easily accessed with the forearm beside the body. Resting pulse is usually taken with the patient supine to ensure consistency. Using two middle fingertips (not the thumb, as your own pulse is discernible in the thumb), locate the pulse. Lightly hold your fingers over the pulse so that the pulse is discernible but not occluded and, using the second hand on the watch, count the beat for 1 minute; this allows sufficient time to detect any abnormalities. Assess the rhythm of the pulse by noting the pattern between beats. It is essential to manually feel the patient's pulse to determine rate, rhythm and volume (Gray et al., 2018).

Measure the patient's respirations

Respirations are measured when the patient is unaware of the assessment so that the rate and rhythm are not affected by voluntary control of their respirations. To reduce the patient's awareness of you counting their respirations, it is often easier to count the patient's respirations after having done the pulse rate and continuing to hold your fingers in place but count the respirations instead (Walker, 2016). Watch the patient's shoulders or chest rise and fall. Each inspiration/expiration cycle is counted as one respiration. Use the second hand on the watch to help count the respirations for 1 minute (Walker, 2016). Note any alteration of respirations from a normal rate, rhythm, depth or sound.

- Rate – is it above or below the acceptable limits?
- Rhythm – is it a regular or irregular rhythm?
- Depth – is subjectively measured and recorded as shallow, normal or deep.
- Sound – any audible respiratory sounds need to be reported; identify the type of sound (e.g. wheeze, stridor).

Perform hand hygiene

Maintain the 5 Moments for Hand Hygiene and perform hand hygiene after touching the patient and the patient's surrounds.

CLEAN, REPLACE OR DISPOSE OF EQUIPMENT

Dispose of probe covers correctly as per previous instruction. Clean and store thermometers as per infection control policies. Most institutions use an alcohol wipe to clean the equipment between patients and after use.

DOCUMENT AND REPORT RELEVANT INFORMATION

The temperature, pulse and respirations are documented on the AORC immediately after they are measured so that they will not be forgotten. The Australian Commission on Safety and Quality in Health Care (ACSQHC, 2017) states that using the AORC correctly promotes accurate and timely recognition of deterioration in a patient's health status, plus prompt action. Any implemented actions should also be documented on the chart in the relevant section. Any abnormal readings in temperature, pulse rate or rhythm and respiratory rate or rhythm (and associated symptoms) or trends that may not have a score that requires a response should still be reported to the registered nurse and as part of end-of-shift clinical handover. Vital signs are not assessed in isolation but should be analysed with regard to other signs and symptoms and the patient's ongoing health status.

CASE STUDY

Search for and print an observation and response chart from the ACSQHC website at http://www.safetyandquality.gov.au (try the Adult Deterioration Detection System [ADDS] chart without the blood pressure table).

Patient 1

Sarah Smith is a 45-year-old woman who has been admitted to your ward with a kidney infection. She has no significant past medical history. Her observations are:

- temperature: 38.5°C
- pulse: 104 beats per minute
- respirations: 24 breaths per minute.
  1. Chart these results on the observation and response chart.
  2. What is the ADDS score for this patient (based on TPR only)?
  3. Based on the ADDS score, what nursing interventions are required for this patient?

Note: These notes are summaries of the most important points in the assessments/procedures, and are not exhaustive on the subject. The naming of documents or charts may differ from state to state, and facility to facility. In all possible situations the guidelines of the ACSQHC are used when describing national charts or documents (e.g. the ACSQHC Observation and Response Chart is named the Adult Observation and Response Chart in WA, and the Rapid Detection and Response Observation Chart in SA). References of the materials used to compile the information have been supplied. The student is expected to have learned the material surrounding each skill as presented in the references. No single reference is complete on the subject.

REFERENCES

Australian Commission on Safety and Quality in Health Care (ACSQHC). (2017). *Recognition and Response to Acute Physiological Deterioration.* http://www.safetyandquality.gov.au/our-work/recognition-and-response-to-clinical-deterioration

Gray, S., Ferris, L., White, L.E., Duncan, G. & Baumle, W. (2018). *Foundations of Nursing: Enrolled Nurses* (2nd ANZ ed.). Melbourne: Cengage.

Walker, J. (2016). Assessing respiratory rate and function in the community. *Journal of Community Nursing*, 30(5), pp. 50–4.

RECOMMENDED READINGS

Hamilton, D. (2017). Mitigating perceptual error with 'look, listen, feel'. *British Journal of Nursing*, 26(9), p. 507.

ESSENTIAL SKILLS COMPETENCY

Temperature, Pulse and Respiration (TPR) Measurement
Demonstrates the ability to effectively measure TPR

Criteria for skill performance	Y	D
(Numbers indicate *Enrolled Nurse Standards for Practice*, 2016)	(Satisfactory)	(Requires development)
1. Identifies indication (8.3, 8.4)		
2. Gathers equipment (1.2, 1.6, 4.4, 6.4, 8.4, 9.4): ■ thermometer ■ thermometer (electronic) probe covers ■ watch with a second hand		
3. Prepares the thermometer and watch with second hand (1.2, 3.2, 6.4, 8.4, 9.4)		
4. Performs hand hygiene (1.2, 1.4, 1.8, 3.9, 6.4, 9.4)		
5. Evidence of therapeutic communication with the patient: gives explanation of procedure, gains patient consent (2.1, 2.3, 2.4, 2.5, 6.3)		
6. Positions and prepares patient (1.2, 1.4, 3.2, 8.4, 9.4)		
7. Takes the temperature (1.2, 1.4, 3.2, 4.1, 4.4, 6.4, 8.4, 9.4)		
8. Measures pulse rate, rhythm and volume (1.2, 1.4, 3.2, 4.1, 4.4, 6.4, 8.4, 9.4)		
9. Measures respiratory rate, depth, rhythm and quality (1.2, 1.4, 3.2, 4.1, 4.4, 6.5, 8.4, 9.4)		
10. Performs hand hygiene (1.2, 1.4, 1.8, 3.9, 6.4, 9.4)		
11. Cleans, replaces and disposes of equipment appropriately (1.2, 1.4, 3.9, 6.3, 9.4)		
12. Documents and reports relevant information (1.2, 1.3, 1.8, 3.2, 5.3, 6.6, 7.1, 7.2, 7.3, 7.4, 7.5)		
13. Demonstrates ability to link theory to practice (8.3, 8.4, 8.5, 9.4)		

Student:

Clinical facilitator: Date:

CHAPTER **2.4**

BLOOD PRESSURE MEASUREMENT

IDENTIFY INDICATIONS

The arterial blood pressure (BP) is obtained to assess the haemodynamic health status of the patient, in order to:
- obtain a baseline measure of BP for subsequent comparison
- identify and monitor alterations in BP due to the disease process or medical interventions.

BP measurement may be ordered by the doctor or a senior nurse; can be done as part of regular assessment; meeting hospital policy requirements; or may be nurse initiated. Trends in BP readings over time are more significant than single readings; a single BP reading should never be used in isolation, but as part of an overall clinical assessment.

PREPARE FOR ASSESSMENT

Assessment of blood pressure involves identifying the signs and symptoms of hypertension and hypotension. When completing a blood pressure it is also important to identify factors that affect BP such as activity, emotional stress, medications and recent ingestion of caffeine or nicotine. Other vital signs such as pulse and respirations, previous readings (if available) and current morbidities should also be reviewed. Other factors that are likely to affect BP include renal or cardiovascular diseases, diabetes mellitus, acute pain, postoperative blood/fluid loss, dehydration, increased intracranial pressure and rapid IV infusions.

GATHER EQUIPMENT

Gathering equipment before initiating the procedure creates a positive environment for the successful completion of the procedure. It expedites the completion of the procedure, boosts patient confidence and trust in the nurse, and increases the nurse's self-confidence. Gathering equipment prior to a procedure also provides an opportunity to rehearse the procedure mentally.
- *The sphygmomanometer* consists of a manometer, a cuff containing a bladder, plus a bulb and pressure valve to inflate and deflate the bladder.
- *Aneroid manometers* consist of a calibrated dial that registers variations of pressure within the bladder of the cuff. Pressure alterations in the bladder of the cuff make the needle on the dial move with the pressure variation, and are measured in mmHg. When the cuff is deflated, the needle will slowly drop to lower levels as pressure is released.
- *Automated digital manometers* are frequently used. Dougherty and Lister (2015) and Elliott and Coventry (2012) warn users of automated digital manometers to be aware of the potential for errors in measurement. For example, if there is a weak, thready or irregular pulse; muscular tremors; or there is an abnormally low or high BP reading on the machine, then a manual BP measurement should be performed.
- *Cuffs* are made of materials that don't 'give' when the bladder is inflated, to ensure that the pressure reading is accurate. The chosen cuff should be appropriate to the patient's body size (small to obese sizes are available). The width should be 40% of the circumference, and the bladder encircles 80% of the upper arm (Berman et al., 2021) to prevent inaccurate readings. Thigh cuffs are available for use on the thigh if arms are not suitable.
- *Stethoscopes* consist of: the earpieces, which should fit snugly and comfortably in the nurse's ear; binaurals, which are curved metal tubing that are angled and facing forward to keep the earpieces comfortably in place; rubber or plastic tubing (the shorter it is, within reason, the better the sound; 30 to 40 cm is ideal) to conduct sound; and the chestpiece with a diaphragm and a bell surface. The diaphragm side is the flat surface which is used for checking high-pitched sounds like normal heart sounds and breath sounds, and is thus used for BP measurement. The bell is the conical-shaped side and picks up lower-pitched sounds best, such as heart murmur and bruit sounds.
- Alcohol wipes are used to clean the diaphragm between patients to maintain infection control principles.

BEGIN THE BLOOD PRESSURE MEASUREMENT

Perform hand hygiene

Perform hand hygiene before touching the patient or the patient's surrounds and prior to any procedure involving patient contact to reduce the possibility of cross-contamination. Hand hygiene is the most effective method of infection control as it removes transient organisms from the hands of the nurse (see **Skill 1.1**).

Give a clear explanation of the procedure and establish therapeutic communication

Explain the procedure and gain the patient's consent. Giving a clear explanation is required to gain legal consent and to address policy requirements. It will also assist the patient to cooperate with the procedure, allay anxiety and assist in establishing a therapeutic relationship.

Demonstrate problem-solving abilities

Preparation of the environment is an important problem-solving activity. With many patients, taking a BP involves listening to very faint sounds and sound changes, so the surroundings should be as quiet as possible. Minimising background noise is also important. Asking the patient not to talk to the nurse during the procedure has been demonstrated to prevent significant increase in BP and heart rate (Crisp et al., 2017). BP measurement may be contraindicated in patients who have thrombocytopenia, as it may cause extensive bruising.

Position the patient

Prior to commencing BP measurement, the arm and the patient are assessed for contraindications to BP measurement on that arm such as IV line or cannula; arm/hand injury, local surgery, disease or pain; arteriovenous shunt; current or previous breast, axillary or shoulder surgery; lymphadenopathy; casts or bulky bandages; or known vascular disease in that arm. In such instances the BP measurement should be completed on the opposite arm. Position the patient preferably in a supine position with the forearm extended, palm upward and supported with a pillow. If the patient is sitting, their arm should be supported so the midpoint of the upper arm is at the level of the heart, again with the elbow extended and palm upward. The upper arm is fully exposed so that the cuff can be properly applied. Ensure it is not loose, but firm fitting (Western Nurse, 2018). Sometimes patients require standing BP readings. These are taken immediately after the 'lying' BP, with the patient being assisted to stand and the BP done immediately on standing.

Apply the cuff

Apply the cuff directly over the brachial artery to ensure proper pressure is applied during inflation. Palpate the brachial artery to identify correct placement for the stethoscope. Wrap the fully deflated cuff snugly about 2.5 cm above the antecubital space and secure. Don't apply the cuff over clothing. This applies to using both manual and automatic sphygmomanometers.

MANUAL BLOOD PRESSURE READING

Position the stethoscope

Position the stethoscope in the ears with the earpieces tilting forward – towards your face – so that the earpieces follow the direction of the ear canal and sound is not muffled. Allow the tubing to fall freely from the earpieces to the chestpiece so that friction does not obliterate sound. Turn the chestpiece and use the diaphragm side, and check for sound by gently tapping the diaphragm. Palpate the brachial artery, then place the diaphragm over the brachial artery and hold it there with the thumb and index finger of your non-dominant hand. (See **FIGURE 2.4.1**.)

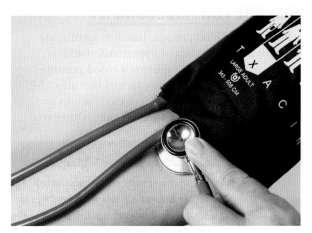

FIGURE 2.4.1 Correct positioning of stethoscope

Auscultate the patient's blood pressure

With the dominant hand, close the pressure valve and pump the bulb until the manometer registers 20 to 30 mmHg above the point where the last auscultatory sound was heard (i.e. listening for the Korotkoff's sounds while slowly pumping the cuff up). These sounds will only be heard once sufficient cuff pressure has been attained. Carefully release the valve on the bulb so that the pressure falls slowly (2 to 3 mmHg/ second) to reduce measurement errors. As the pressure falls, identify the Korotkoff's sounds and the pressure reading on the manometer at which they occur. The first Korotkoff sound that is heard is the systolic reading. The diastolic sound is heard when the tone of the sound changes (i.e. it can become softer or disappear completely). Once identified, deflate the cuff rapidly and completely to decrease patient discomfort. If a repeat is needed to confirm the accuracy of the reading, wait 1 to 2 minutes to promote patient comfort and allow the vessels to normalise.

HOW TO PERFORM A PALPATORY SYSTOLIC DETERMINATION

Palpatory determination of systolic BP may be done when there is difficulty with obtaining an accurate auscultatory systolic BP reading. It can be used in emergency situations, plus some patients may have an auscultatory gap that makes accurate auscultatory measurement difficult. The auscultatory gap is an absence of Korotkoff's sounds for a space of up to 40 mmHg when the cuff pressure is high. This occurs in some people with hypertension.

The radial artery is palpated with the fingertips of the non-dominant hand and the pressure valve is closed. The manometer should be at eye level. The bladder is then inflated by squeezing the bulb repeatedly, until no blood is flowing through the artery and no radial pulse is palpable. Inflate the cuff a further 20 to 30 mmHg. Carefully release the valve on the bulb so that the pressure falls slowly (2 to 3 mmHg/second) to reduce measurement errors. Maintain radial pulse palpation while the pressure falls. When the pulse is first felt, identify the reading on the manometer. The pressure reading on the sphygmomanometer at this point gives an estimate of the systolic BP (i.e. palpatory systolic BP). Deflate the cuff and leave the arm 1 to 2 minutes to allow the blood trapped in the veins to be released and returned to circulation.

AUTOMATIC BLOOD PRESSURE READING

The machine should be turned on prior to application of the cuff. When the cuff has been applied (see earlier), press the start button. The cuff will then automatically inflate, and then deflate slowly. Numbers will display as the cuff deflates, and then a final reading will appear on the screen. If the reading is outside the patient's normal range or if a reading cannot be obtained, a manual BP measurement must be performed immediately.

Remove the cuff

Removing the cuff allows the patient to move the arm and restore circulation.

PERFORM HAND HYGIENE

Maintain the 5 Moments for Hand Hygiene and perform hand hygiene after touching the patient and the patient's surrounds.

CLEAN, REPLACE OR DISPOSE OF EQUIPMENT

Cleaning and returning equipment is important to reduce cross-contamination and to foster efficiency. The sphygmomanometer and cuff are decontaminated as per hospital policy. The stethoscope diaphragm/bell is wiped with an alcohol wipe, between patients, to reduce microorganisms. The earpieces are also wiped with alcohol wipes unless the stethoscope is your personal one, in which case cleaning may not be required.

DOCUMENT AND REPORT RELEVANT INFORMATION

Documentation of the assessment data is done according to the agency policy. BP is recorded on the observation and response chart (ORC). Respond appropriately to the score for the BP and total score for observations when using this chart. Any implemented actions should also be documented on the chart in the relevant section.

Significant change in the BP or Adult Deterioration Detection System (ADDS) scores that do not require reporting should still be discussed with the registered nurse or shift coordinator. The Australian Commission on Safety and Quality in Health Care (ACSQHC, 2017) states that using the ORC correctly promotes accurate and timely recognition of deterioration in a patient's health status, plus prompt action. If the reading was obtained from a site other than the upper arm, indicate where the reading was obtained.

CASE STUDY

Search for and print an observation and response chart from the ACSQHC website at http://www.safetyandquality.gov.au.

Patient 1

You have been looking after Sarah Smith for the previous 3 days on the ward. She has been diagnosed with a kidney infection, and commenced on IV antibiotics. Her observations are:
- temperature: 38.3°C
- pulse: 102 beats per minute

- respirations: 24 breaths per minute
- BP: 170/110 mmHg.
- Chart Sarah's observations on the ORC (based on TPR and BP only).
- What is Sarah's ADDS score?
- What nursing interventions will you implement based on this score?
- What is the medical term used to describe this BP reading?

Note: These notes are summaries of the most important points in the assessments/procedures, and are not exhaustive on the subject. The naming of documents or charts may differ from state to state, and facility to facility. In all possible situations the guidelines of the ACSQHC are used when describing national charts or documents (e.g. the ACSQHC Observation and Response Chart is named the Adult Observation and Response Chart in WA, and the Rapid Detection and Response Observation Chart in SA). References of the materials used to compile the information have been supplied. The student is expected to have learned the material surrounding each skill as presented in the references. No single reference is complete on the subject.

REFERENCES

Australian Commission on Safety and Quality in Health Care (ACSQHC). (2017). *Recognition and Response to Acute Physiological Deterioration.* http://www.safetyandquality.gov.au/our-work/recognition-and-response-to-clinical-deterioration

Berman, A., Snyder, S., Levett-Jones, T., Burton, T. & Harvey, N. (2021). *Skills in Clinical Nursing* (2nd ed.). Melbourne: Pearson.

Crisp, J., Douglas, C., Rebeiro, G. & Waters, D. (2017). *Potter and Perry's Fundamentals of Nursing – Australian version* (5th ed.). Sydney: Elsevier.

Dougherty, L. & Lister, S. (eds). (2015). *The Royal Marsden Hospital Manual of Clinical Nursing Procedures* (9th ed.). Oxford: Wiley-Blackwell.

Elliott, M. & Coventry, A. (2012). Critical care: the eight vital signs of patient monitoring. *British Journal of Nursing*, 21(10), pp. 621–25.

Western Nurse. (2018). Hypertension – back to basics. *Western Nurse.* September–October, pp. 24–5. Perth: Australian Nursing Federation.

RECOMMENDED READINGS

Australian Commission on Safety and Quality in Health Care (ACSQHC). (2019). *Observation and Response Charts.* https://www.safetyandquality.gov.au/our-work/recognising-and-responding-to-clinical-deterioration/observation-and-response-charts

Estes, M.E.Z., Calleja, P., Theobald, K. & Harvey, T. (2020). *Estes Health Assessment and Physical Examination.* (3rd Australian and New Zealand ed.) Melbourne: Cengage.

Gray, S., Ferris, L., White, L.E., Duncan, G. & Baumle, W. (2018). *Foundations of Nursing: Enrolled Nurses* (2nd ANZ ed.). Melbourne: Cengage.

ESSENTIAL SKILLS COMPETENCY

Blood Pressure Measurement
Demonstrates the ability to effectively measure blood pressure

Criteria for skill performance	Y	D
(Numbers indicate *Enrolled Nurse Standards for Practice*, 2016)	(Satisfactory)	(Requires development)
1. Identifies indication (8.3, 8.4)		
2. Gathers equipment (1.2, 1.6, 4.4, 6.4, 8.4, 9.4): ■ sphygmomanometer (aneroid manometer, automated manometer) ■ stethoscope ■ alcohol wipes		
3. Performs hand hygiene (1.2, 1.4, 1.8, 3.9, 6.4, 9.4)		
4. Evidence of therapeutic communication with the patient; gives explanation of procedure, gains patient consent (2.1, 2.3, 2.4, 2.5, 6.3)		
5. Demonstrates problem-solving abilities; e.g. prepares environment (4.1, 4.2, 8.3, 8.4, 9.4)		
6. Positions and prepares patient (1.2, 1.4, 3.2, 8.4, 9.4)		
7. Applies the appropriate cuff (1.2, 1.4, 3.2, 4.4, 6.4, 8.4, 9.4)		
8. Positions the stethoscope appropriately (1.2, 3.2, 4.4, 6.4, 8.4, 9.4)		
9. Auscultates the patient's blood pressure (1.2, 3.2, 4.2, 4.4, 6.4, 8.4, 9.4)		
10. Removes the cuff (1.2, 3.2, 6.4, 9.1)		
11. Performs hand hygiene (1.2, 1.4, 1.8, 3.9, 6.4, 9.4)		
12. Cleans, replaces and disposes of equipment appropriately (1.2, 1.4, 3.9, 6.5, 9.4)		
13. Documents and reports relevant information (1.2, 1.3, 1.8, 3.2, 5.3, 6.6, 7.1, 7.2, 7.3, 7.4, 7.5)		
14. Demonstrates ability to link theory to practice (8.3, 8.4, 8.5, 9.4)		

Student:

Clinical facilitator: Date:

CHAPTER 2.5

PULSE OXIMETRY

IDENTIFY INDICATIONS

The pulse oximeter is a non-invasive device used to measure oxygen saturation (SpO_2) and pulse rate in the peripheral capillary blood. As a non-invasive measurement of peripheral arterial oxygen saturation, it is standard practice to assess a patient's oxygen saturation level on admission and as part of routine observations. It can be used to assess the effectiveness of oxygen therapy or as part of monitoring a patient's overall respiratory status. Pulse oximetry can help identify hypoxaemia before other clinical signs and symptoms (e.g. cyanosis) are evident.

Normal range for oxygen saturation for a healthy adult is 96 to 100%, but can vary according to facility policies. The observation and response chart (ORC) displays the acceptable range of oxygen saturation as 94% and above (ACSQHC, 2019). It incorporates a track and trigger system for observations that are outside this range. The acceptable range of oxygen saturation for patients with chronic obstructive pulmonary disease (COPD) can be lower than this and should be noted as a modification on the chart.

GATHER EQUIPMENT

- A *pulse oximeter* can be a small portable device that includes both the sensor probe and display; or a sensor probe that is attached to electronic observation equipment. The equipment displays the SpO_2, which is the percentage of oxygenated haemoglobin in the arterial blood and the pulse rate. The sensor probe uses two light-emitting diodes (LEDs) to send red and infrared light through the pulsating vascular bed.

A photodetector in the sensor measures the absorption of light as it passes through the vascular tissue. Oxygenated and deoxygenated haemoglobin absorb the light at different rates. From the two rates, the oximeter calculates the percentage of oxygen-carrying haemoglobin (SpO_2).
- *Alcohol wipes* are used to clean the sensor between patients to maintain infection control principles.

OBTAIN THE PATIENT'S PULSE RATE AND OXYGEN SATURATION USING PULSE OXIMETRY

Perform hand hygiene
Perform hand hygiene to reduce cross-contamination and prior to any procedure involving patient contact to reduce the possibility of cross-contamination. Hand hygiene is the most effective method of infection control as it removes transient organisms from the hands of the nurse (see **Skill 1.1**).

Give a clear explanation of the procedure and establish therapeutic communication
Discuss the procedure and gain the patient's consent. Giving a clear explanation is required to gain legal consent and to address policy requirements. It will also assist the patient to cooperate with the procedure, allay anxiety and assist in establishing a therapeutic relationship.

Select and prepare the appropriate site
Probes are commonly placed on a finger, thumb or toe. Alternative types of probes may be applied to the forehead, earlobe or the bridge of the nose if necessary. Select and prepare the appropriate site by checking that the patient has an adequate perfusion in the selected limb and good capillary refill. Check that the skin is clean and intact, and not sweaty, oedematous or cold. Factors that influence the oximeter's degree of error are peripheral temperature, finger thickness or haemoglobin concentration. Skin pigmentation (i.e. melanin concentration), nail polish (Yikar et al., 2019) or artificial nails may also affect the accuracy of the readings.

Demonstrate problem-solving abilities

Pulse oximeters should not be applied to a limb that has an inflated BP cuff as this will affect the blood flow to the extremity and alter the oximetry reading. Cold limbs can alter the reading because of vasoconstriction. Poor peripheral circulation will also interfere with the readings.

Obtain the oxygen saturation reading

Turn on the equipment. Attach the sensor probe to the selected fingertip (or toe). Remind the patient to relax and keep their hand still while the reading is being obtained. The probe can then be removed when the reading is obtained. Compare the pulse reading to the manual radial pulse measurement (see **Skill 2.3**). Evaluate the reading against previous results.

Perform hand hygiene

Maintain the 5 Moments for Hand Hygiene and perform hand hygiene after touching the patient and the patient's surrounds.

CLEAN, REPLACE OR DISPOSE OF EQUIPMENT

Cleaning and returning equipment is important to reduce cross-contamination and to foster efficiency.

Gently wipe the sensor probe with an alcohol wipe, and allow to dry. Return equipment to the relevant storage area. Check and replace any batteries (if required in smaller devices) or plug in to recharge.

DOCUMENT AND REPORT RELEVANT INFORMATION

The SpO_2 is documented on the ORC immediately after it is measured so it will not be forgotten. The Australian Commission on Safety and Quality in Health Care (ACSQHC, 2019) states that using the ORC correctly promotes accurate and timely recognition of deterioration in a patient's health status, as well as prompt action. Respond appropriately to the score for the oxygen saturation and total score for observations, when using this chart. Any implemented actions should also be documented on the chart in the relevant section. Any abnormal oxygen saturation readings or trends that may not have a score necessitating a response should still be reported to the registered nurse and also discussed as part of end-of-shift clinical handover. Oxygen saturation is not assessed in isolation but should be analysed with other vital signs, plus other signs and symptoms and the patient's ongoing health status.

CASE STUDY

Sarah Smith is a 45-year-old woman who has been admitted to your ward with a kidney infection. You are completing the pulse oximetry assessment for Sarah. When completing this reading you note that Sarah has an oxygen saturation of 91% on room air. She does not appear distressed or breathless, but you notice that she has dark purple acrylic false nails and her fingers are quite cool to touch.

1. Will this have any impact on the accuracy of your readings?
2. What action/s would you implement?

Note: These notes are summaries of the most important points in the assessments/procedures, and are not exhaustive on the subject. The naming of documents or charts may differ from state to state, and facility to facility. In all possible situations the guidelines of the ACSQHC are used when describing national charts or documents (e.g. the ACSQHC Observation and Response Chart is named the Adult Observation and Response Chart in WA, and the Rapid Detection and Response Observation Chart in SA). References of the materials used to compile the information have been supplied. The student is expected to have learned the material surrounding each skill as presented in the references. No single reference is complete on the subject.

REFERENCES

Australian Commission on Safety and Quality in Health Care (ACSQHC). (2019) *Observation and Response Charts.* https://www.safetyandquality.gov.au/our-work/recognising-and-responding-to-clinical-deterioration/observation-and-response-charts

Yikar, S.K., Arslan, S. & Nazik, E. (2019). The effect of nail polish on pulseoximeter's measurements in healthy individuals. *International Journal of Caring Sciences.* May–Aug. 12(2), pp. 1–4.

RECOMMENDED READINGS

Calleja, P., Theobald, K. & Harvey, T. (2020). *Estes Health Assessment and Physical Examination* (3rd ed.). Singapore: Cengage.

Dougherty, L. & Lister, S. (eds). (2015). *The Royal Marsden Hospital Manual of Clinical Nursing Procedures* (9th ed.). Oxford: Wiley-Blackwell.

Elliott, M. & Coventry, A. (2012). Critical care: the eight vital signs of patient monitoring. *British Journal of Nursing,* 21(10), pp. 621–5.

Kramer, M., Lobbestael, A., Barten, E., Eian, J. & Rausch, G. (2017). Wearable pulse oximetry measurements on the torso, arms, and legs: A proof of concept. *Military Medicine,* 182, pp. 92–8.

Hamilton, D. (2017). Mitigating perceptual error with 'look, listen, feel'. *British Journal of Nursing,* 26(9), p. 507.

Walker, J. (2016). Assessing respiratory rate and function in the community. *Journal of Community Nursing,* 30(5), pp. 50–4.

PART 2

ESSENTIAL SKILLS COMPETENCY

Pulse Oximetry

Demonstrates the ability to effectively monitor a patient using pulse oximetry

Criteria for skill performance	Y	D
(Numbers indicate *Enrolled Nurse Standards for Practice*, 2016)	(Satisfactory)	(Requires development)
1. Identifies indication (8.3, 8.4)		
2. Gathers equipment (1.2, 1.6, 4.4, 6.4, 8.4, 9.4): ■ pulse oximeter/monitor, or small battery-operated portable unit ■ sensor probe and cord ■ alcohol wipes ■ nail polish remover if necessary		
3. Performs hand hygiene (1.2, 1.4, 1.8, 3.9, 6.4, 9.4)		
4. Evidence of therapeutic communication with the patient; gives explanation of procedure, gains patient consent (2.1, 2.3, 2.4, 2.5, 6.3)		
5. Selects and prepares appropriate site (1.2, 1.4, 3.2, 8.4, 9.4)		
6. Demonstrates problem-solving abilities; e.g. pulse oximeter precautions (4.1, 4.2, 8.3, 8.4, 9.4)		
7. Obtains the oxygen saturation reading (1.2, 1.4, 3.2, 4.4, 8.4, 9.4)		
8. Performs hand hygiene (1.2, 1.4, 1.8, 3.9, 6.4, 9.4)		
9. Cleans, replaces and disposes of equipment appropriately (1.2, 1.4, 3.9, 6.5, 9.4)		
10. Documents and reports relevant information (1.2, 1.3, 1.8, 3.2, 5.3, 6.6, 7.1, 7.2, 7.3, 7.4, 7.5)		
11. Demonstrates ability to link theory to practice (8.3, 8.4, 8.5, 9.4)		

Student:

Clinical facilitator: Date:

CHAPTER 2.6

BLOOD GLUCOSE MEASUREMENT

IDENTIFY INDICATIONS

Blood glucose levels (BGL) may be performed by the nurse for a variety of reasons. These include the following.

- When a patient is initially diagnosed with type I or type II diabetes mellitus or gestational diabetes. In these cases, nurses frequently determine the BGL to assess the effectiveness of the interventions, such as diet, oral medication or insulin (Dunning, 2016). The nurses then teach the patient how to monitor their own BGL. Therefore, the first indication for measuring BGL is to assist the patient in gaining control of their diabetic condition.
- Hospitalisation of a person with unstable diabetes who is at risk for hyperglycaemia or hypoglycaemia. Hospitalisation may disrupt the patient's normal management of their diabetes because of changes in the daily routine. Food in the hospital is often different to that normally consumed by the patient at home.
- Alteration in health status. This usually engenders anxiety, which is a stressor that alters BGLs, along with the stressor of the condition for which they were hospitalised. Hospitalised patients with diabetes usually

require blood glucose readings four times a day (QID) and they may be too ill to perform these themselves. Some patients with unstable BGLs may require these more frequently (e.g. postoperative patients with diabetes, people newly diagnosed with diabetes).

- To determine the cause of loss of consciousness. Patients who are either known to have diabetes, or who have been hospitalised for other reasons and who lose consciousness unexpectedly, should have their BGL measured. A low BGL (below the normal level of 4 mmol/L) may lead to a loss of consciousness. Patients known to have diabetes have their BGL measured so that the doctor can be informed and take appropriate action. Others have their BGL measured so that a low BGL can be ruled out as a causative factor in their loss of consciousness.
- Patients taking medications known to increase BGLs such as steroids, and patients receiving total parenteral nutrition (TPN). These patients are at risk of elevated BGLs and require monitoring.

DEMONSTRATE PROBLEM-SOLVING ABILITIES

Review the doctor's order and hospital policy to determine frequency of glucose monitoring. This procedure is usually performed prior to a meal since ingestion of carbohydrates will increase the glucose level of the blood. Alternatively, a 'postprandial' blood glucose measurement (i.e. 2 hours after meals) may be ordered to assess effectiveness of the patient's diabetes medication management and the clearance of glucose from the blood (Dunning, 2016). Assessment prior to the procedure should include determination of whether the patient is at risk of complications from specific conditions (e.g. bleeding disorders) and an assessment of the site for broken skin, ecchymosis, rashes, lesions or other skin problems. Assessment of the patient's hand can also reveal cold peripheries or impaired circulation that can hamper the collection of

the required blood. The hand may require warming or massaging prior to commencing the procedure.

The normal range for blood glucose reading is 4 to 8 mmol/L, but this normal range can vary for some patients with diabetes. Hyperglycaemia and hypoglycaemia both require patient review. Administration of fast-acting carbohydrate (e.g. glucose drink) is usually required for conscious patients with a low blood glucose reading. The national subcutaneous insulin chart indicates readings below 4 mmol/L require immediate action and notification of the patient's doctor. Always follow facility policy when a low reading has been obtained.

The patient's ability and willingness to learn the procedure should also be assessed as ultimately the patient will need to be able to perform the procedure independently. Blood glucose monitoring can also be conducted as a nurse initiative measure.

GATHER EQUIPMENT

Gather equipment so that the procedure can be completed efficiently.

- *Glucometer.* This is a battery-operated electronic machine that determines the patient's BGL. These machines come in a variety of types and at a range of costs. Some machines also measure ketones. Using the glucometer that the patient will be using at home is the most effective method of teaching the patient to read their own glucose level. Glucometer technology is changing rapidly.
- *Testing strip.* The strips need to be checked for the correct brand that matches the glucometer, expiry date and that the code on the glucometer screen matches the strips. The strip is inserted into the glucometer before blood is placed on the strip.
- *Warm water, flannel and/or cotton swabs.* When possible, patients should be encouraged to wash their hands with warm water prior to the procedure.

This removes food residue and can increase blood flow to the area, allowing for a sufficient sample. Patients may require assistance to wash the selected finger.
- *Cotton balls or gauze swabs.* These are used to provide pressure to stop the bleeding when the peripheral blood has been obtained.
- *Lancet.* This is a single-use disposable device used to puncture the skin to capillary depth.
- *A sharps container.* This is a rigid container used to hold contaminated sharps such as the lancets.
- *Non-sterile gloves.* These protect the nurse from contamination with the patient's blood.
- *National Subcutaneous Insulin Chart.* This is a specific piece of documentation that is used to record BGLs, medications, insulin and urinalysis results. This chart leads to improved management of BGLs in hospitalised patients (ACSQHC, 2019).

PERFORM BLOOD GLUCOSE MEASUREMENT

Perform hand hygiene

Perform hand hygiene before touching the patient or the patient's surrounds and prior to any procedure involving patient contact to reduce the possibility of cross-contamination. Hand hygiene is the most effective method of infection control as it removes transient organisms from the hands of the nurse (see **Skill 1.1**).

Give a clear explanation of the procedure and establish therapeutic communication

Discuss the procedure and gain the patient's consent. Giving a clear explanation is required to gain legal consent and to address policy requirements. It will also assist the patient to cooperate with the procedure, allay anxiety and assist in establishing a therapeutic relationship.

Select the site

The sides of the tip of the fingers of adults are used because there are fewer nerve endings on the sides of the fingers and it is less painful. Ask the patient to keep the hand in a relaxed downward position to slow venous return and thus increase the blood available in the digits. Massage of the area, either by the nurse or the patient, will also increase vasodilation.

Cleanse and prepare the site

Ask the patient which finger they would prefer to use. It is important to rotate sites: (1) to reduce the risk of infection from multiple entry wounds and the risk of the area becoming toughened; and (2) to reduce pain (Dougherty & Lister, 2015). If required, assist blood flow by massaging or milking the finger from the base

of the finger. Wash the patient's selected finger using a warm, wet flannel (or wet cotton swab), and then dry the finger.

Prepare a clean cotton ball for use after obtaining the patient's blood.

Prepare the glucometer

Glucometers should be calibrated daily to ensure accuracy of results. Testing involves calibrating high and low readings using preprepared reagents, and the results are recorded in the logbook. This is often completed by night staff each morning. Check calibration has been completed and recorded according to facility policy before performing routine blood glucose readings. The preparation of the glucometer depends on the machine itself, so always check the manufacturer's instructions.

Check the test strip expiry date, then insert the electrode end of the test strip into the glucometer and ensure that the code displayed on the glucometer matches the test strips (correct code is generally located on the side of the packaging). The glucometer will allow time for collection of the blood on the test strip, or it will automatically turn off. If this occurs, the strip should be carefully removed and reinserted.

Obtain peripheral blood and BGL result

Don non-sterile gloves. Remove lancet cover. Hold the lancet firmly and perpendicular to the side of the fingertip and then press the button (this action may vary depending on the type of lancet used). Pierce the site quickly, to reduce discomfort. Apply a sufficient drop of blood to the strip. Dispose of the lancet into a sharps container and apply the cotton ball onto the puncture site. Hold until bleeding stops.

The glucometer will automatically count down and then display the blood glucose reading on the screen. Follow the prompts from the glucometer, then remove the test strip and dispose of it in the general waste when completed. Remove and discard non-sterile gloves and cotton balls.

Teach the patient

See **Skill 7.5 Health teaching.**

Perform hand hygiene

Maintain the 5 Moments for Hand Hygiene and perform hand hygiene after touching the patient and the patient's surrounds.

CLEAN, REPLACE OR DISPOSE OF EQUIPMENT

The glucometer may be the patient's own and, if so, is stored at their bedside along with the appropriate testing strips. If the glucometer belongs to the ward, it should be cleaned using an alcohol wipe (or according to the facility policy) and returned to its usual storage place.

DOCUMENT AND REPORT RELEVANT INFORMATION

Document relevant information on the National Subcutaneous Insulin Chart. This national chart is used for recording BGLs and the administration of subcutaneous insulin. It is the preferred chart to use. All BGLs are recorded so that patterns can be detected as they emerge. The observation and response chart also has a space for recording a random BGL.

Refer to the guidelines on the National Subcutaneous Insulin Chart for the reading you have obtained and procedures to follow if a BGL is outside of normal range (Dunning, 2016). Facility policy should also be followed, especially for low BGLs. Separately from these guidelines, report any concerns about a patient's BGL to the registered nurse or shift coordinator. It should also be noted on the progress notes. Extremely high or extremely low BGLs should be discussed with the doctor and may require an adjustment in medication.

CASE STUDY

You are working on a surgical ward. Twenty-four-year-old Jonathon Abbott is admitted after a motor vehicle accident (MVA) at 0100 hours. He has a fractured right tibia and fibula post the MVA, and is awaiting theatre in the morning once stable. He has a medical history of type 1 diabetes. On arrival to the emergency department he was drowsy, but is now conscious and slightly confused. You perform a ward BGL on admission, and note the result of 16.4 mmol/L.

1. Give three reasons why Jonathon's BGL is elevated.
2. What nursing actions would you implement based on this result?

Note: These notes are summaries of the most important points in the assessments/procedures, and are not exhaustive on the subject. The naming of documents or charts may differ from state to state, and facility to facility. In all possible situations the guidelines of the ACSQHC are used when describing national charts or documents (e.g. the ACSQHC Observation and Response Chart is named the Adult Observation and Response Chart in WA, and the Rapid Detection and Response Observation Chart in SA). References of the materials used to compile the information have been supplied. The student is expected to have learned the material surrounding each skill as presented in the references. No single reference is complete on the subject.

CRITICAL THINKING

You are going to do a patient's BGL and your colleague mentions that she usually wipes the selected finger with an alcohol wipe prior to obtaining the blood for the glucometer reading. Research the process of obtaining a BGL and the effect of correct preparation of the finger site on a BGL reading.

REFERENCES

Australian Commission on Safety and Quality in Health Care (ACSQHC). (2019). *National Subcutaneous Insulin Charts.* https://www.safetyandquality.gov.au/our-work/medication-safety/medication-charts/national-standard-medication-charts/national-subcutaneous-insulin-chart

Dougherty, L. & Lister, S. (eds). (2015). *The Royal Marsden Hospital Manual of Clinical Nursing Procedures* (9th ed.). Oxford: Wiley-Blackwell.

Dunning, T. (2016). How to monitor blood glucose. *Nursing Standard* (2014+), 30(22), p. 36.

RECOMMENDED READINGS

Gray, S., Ferris, L., White, L.E., Duncan, G. & Baumle, W. (2018). *Foundations of Nursing: Enrolled Nurses* (2nd ANZ ed.). Melbourne: Cengage.

Diabetes Australia. (2020). *Blood Glucose Monitoring.* https://www.diabetesaustralia.com.au/living-with-diabetes/managing-your-diabetes/blood-glucose-monitoring

ESSENTIAL SKILLS COMPETENCY

Blood Glucose Measurement

Demonstrates the ability to effectively assess the blood glucose level of the patient

Criteria for skill performance	Y	D
(Numbers indicate *Enrolled Nurse Standards for Practice*, 2016)	(Satisfactory)	(Requires development)
1. Identifies indication (8.3, 8.4)		
2. Displays problem-solving abilities (4.1, 4.2, 8.3, 8.4, 9.4)		

3. Gathers equipment (1.2, 1.6, 4.4, 6.4, 8.4, 9.4); e.g.:
  ▪ glucometer
  ▪ test strip
  ▪ cotton balls or gauze
  ▪ lancet
  ▪ sharps container, non-sterile gloves
  ▪ diabetic chart		

4. Performs hand hygiene, (1.2, 1.4, 1.8, 3.9, 6.4, 9.4)		
5. Evidence of therapeutic communication with the patient; gives explanation of procedure, gains patient consent (2.1, 2.3, 2.4, 2.5, 6.3)		
6. Selects a site (1.2, 1.4, 3.2, 8.4, 9.4)		
7. Prepares the area (1.2, 1.4, 3.2, 8.4, 9.4)		
8. Prepares the glucometer (1.2, 1.4, 3.2, 4.4, 6.4, 8.4, 9.4)		
9. Dons gloves and obtains peripheral blood (1.2, 1.4, 3.2, 3.9, 8.4, 9.4)		
10. Reads the glucometer (1.2, 1.4, 3.2, 4.4, 6.4, 8.4, 9.4)		
11. Teaches the patient about blood glucose levels and the glucometer (1.2, 6.3, 7.3, 7.5, 8.4, 9.4)		
12. Performs hand hygiene (1.2, 1.4, 1.8, 3.9, 6.4, 9.4)		
13. Cleans, replaces and disposes of equipment appropriately (1.2, 1.4, 3.9, 6.5, 9.4)		
14. Documents and reports relevant information (1.2, 1.3, 1.8, 3.2, 5.3, 6.6, 7.1, 7.2, 7.3, 7.4, 7.5)		
15. Demonstrates ability to link theory to practice (8.3, 8.4, 8.5, 9.4)		

Student:

Clinical facilitator: Date:

CHAPTER **2.7**

NEUROLOGICAL OBSERVATION

IDENTIFY INDICATIONS

Neurological observations assess the functioning of the patient's nervous system. Neurological observations are done on any patient who is in danger of deterioration in central nervous system functioning. The assessment is done frequently (e.g. every 15 minutes to hourly) on patients with an acute neurological condition or whose status may change rapidly. Subtle alterations in the patient's observations can alert the staff to the early onset of neurological complications so that interventions can be implemented. Early detection and intervention

for complications may prevent further deterioration of neurological functioning and irreversible damage such as impaired cognitive function. Neurological assessment can be implemented for conditions such as head trauma, cerebrovascular accidents (stroke), pre- and post-neurological surgery, brain tumours and cerebral infections, as well as in patients whose level of consciousness is diminished for other reasons. They are also implemented whenever a patient experiences a fall.

GATHER EQUIPMENT

This is a time-management strategy as well as a confidence-increasing strategy. The nurse will be able to mentally rehearse the procedure about to be performed. The patient will feel more confident in the nurse if there are no interruptions in the procedure to return to the storage room for forgotten equipment.
- A *sphygmomanometer, BP cuff and stethoscope* are used to assess blood pressure.
- A *thermometer and watch* are used to ascertain body temperature, pulse and respiratory rate.
- A *pulse oximeter* is used to determine the oxygen saturation of the blood and thus the oxygen available to the brain.
- A *penlight torch* is used to determine the size of the pupils and their responsiveness to light.

- A *neurological assessment sheet*. Full neurological observations include the Glasgow Coma Scale (GCS), vital signs and other neurological signs of pupil size and reaction, plus upper and lower limb motor function.
  The GCS was developed for use in detecting slight but significant changes in the patient's brain function. It is a numerical scale whereby a score of 15 indicates the patient is oriented, obeys commands and opens their eyes spontaneously. A score of 7 or less on the GCS indicates coma, and a score of 3 (the lowest possible) indicates the patient is not able to open their eyes, respond to pain or verbalise at all.
  A baseline full neurological assessment is done when the patient experiences changes in their neurological status or if admitted with a neurological condition. Changes are tracked from that time.

PERFORM NEUROLOGICAL OBSERVATION

Perform hand hygiene
Perform hand hygiene before touching the patient or the patient's surrounds and prior to any procedure involving patient contact to reduce the possibility of cross-contamination. Hand hygiene is the most effective method of infection control as it removes

transient organisms from the hands of the nurse (see **Skill 1.1**).

Give a clear explanation of the procedure and establish therapeutic communication
Introduce yourself, and check you have the correct patient. Discuss the procedure and gain the patient's consent. Giving a clear explanation is required to gain legal consent and to address policy requirements. It will also assist the patient to cooperate with the

procedure, allay anxiety and assist in establishing a therapeutic relationship. An explanation that initially tells the patient why the questions are being asked and what you are assessing will allay fears in most patients. If the patient is confused or the level of consciousness is diminished, the explanation may need to be given at each encounter.

Demonstrate problem-solving abilities

Modify the questions asked when assessing the patient to establish orientation with regard to age, culture and existing physical conditions. When dealing with very young children, careful thought will be required about the type of questions that can be used to determine orientation. Recognition of a parent, sibling or a toy will be more telling than their inability to tell the day or place where they are. Elderly patients may have a hearing deficit or dementia that may interfere with completing the assessment. A patient's cultural differences or non-English speaking background may have an impact on a patient's response. These should be recognised and managed appropriately.

There are many issues to be considered when completing these observations, If the patient is blind, eye opening as a response is not reasonable. If the patient has facial trauma and the eyes are affected or swollen shut, pupil response cannot be obtained. If the patient is aphasic, intubated or unable to speak for any reason, orientation cannot be assessed. Opiate use may make the pupils pinpoint, while parasympathetic drugs such as atropine may cause enlarged pupils. Previous cataract surgery will also affect pupil response and size.

Any deterioration from baseline must be reported to the registered nurse (RN) or shift coordinator.

Assess the level of consciousness

The level of consciousness (LOC) indicates brain function, or failure, and is also the most sensitive of the assessments in demonstrating early deterioration of brain function. LOC is assessed by initially observing the patient for awareness and arousal, spontaneous body position and movement, eye opening or verbalisation (assuming they are awake). If no response is noted, the patient is spoken to, at first using a normal volume of speech, then more loudly. Response is opening of the eyes. If there is no response to auditory stimulation, gentle touch is used. Then a mildly painful stimulus such as pressing on a nail may be used. The least amount of pressure is used to minimise trauma or pain, and to not traumatise body tissues.

Assess the orientation of the patient

The patient who is able to respond is asked a series of questions to determine their orientation. They are asked to identify themselves, to say what month, season and year it is and where they are. Some questions are not easily answered, even by patients who have full cognitive ability, after they have been hospitalised for a while, so avoid asking for the day or date. Sometimes patients are able to memorise the right answer, so vary your questions occasionally and ask what their partner's name is (if you know it) or who their employer is. Ask them their home address or the names of their children. Take care to be aware of problems that may interfere with this, as discussed earlier. If the patient is not oriented to person, time and place, ascertain their best verbal response. Scores on the GCS are for confused, inappropriate words, incomprehensible sounds and no response.

Assess motor response

Ask the patient to complete two different actions. Each action should be a single response command that requires a motor response, such as 'touch your nose' or 'wiggle your toes'. Give them some time to comply. Asking the patient to 'grasp my hand' may elicit a response even if the patient is not able to obey commands, since grasping is a reflex. Also ask them to 'let go of my hand', which will determine if they can obey commands. If they are unable to obey commands, apply a painful stimulus (pressing the nail of a finger and toe on each extremity) and watch the response. They may try to localise (i.e. push the stimulus away) or withdraw (i.e. move their hand/ foot away from the pain) or posture. Compare the right and left sides and upper and lower extremities. The *best* response is recorded. Most neurological charts incorporate an assessment of limb movements whereby you are able to document separately the response of each limb if there are differences in the limb movement. Also note any abnormality that indicates altered function in any of the extremities. If the patient is unable to follow commands, watch for movement in each of the limbs for a *localised* response (moves the other hand to the site of the stimulus), *flexion* response (flexes away from the pain), *extension* response (the patient's limb extends from pain) or *flaccid* response (no motor response at all) response to painful stimulus (Dougherty & Lister, 2015).

Assess pupillary activity

Pupil size is controlled by the integration of the sympathetic and parasympathetic nervous systems. Size is assessed in each eye before the light reflex is tested, against a pupil gauge measured in millimetres (see FIGURE 2.7.1). Hold the pupil gauge close to each eye for comparison. Anisocoria (unequal pupil size) occurs in about 17% of the population but should be noted. Pupil shape is determined and noted or drawn to indicate an abnormality.

Pupils

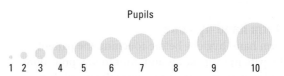

FIGURE 2.7.1 Pupil sizes in millimetres

Pupil reactivity to light is assessed by bringing the light (from the penlight torch) from the lateral side of the patient's head towards the nose. Do not cross the nose with the light. Observe the pupil for constriction (which should be brisk) and repeat, observing the opposite pupil for constriction to indirect light (consensual constriction). Repeat with the other eye. Responses are usually recorded as equal or not, brisk, sluggish or fixed (no response). Do not confuse a prosthetic eye with a fixed pupil. If the patient is photophobic, this procedure may cause discomfort.

Assess muscle strength and tone

Each extremity is tested, unless there is a physical injury or other problem in the limb. The patient is asked to do a series of movements with each limb. Compare the opposite sides. Make sure your instructions are clear and contain only one command. For the upper limbs ask the patient to close their eyes and extend their arms with palms upwards. Observe for weakness and then ask them to push against or pull your hands. The dominant hand is usually stronger. For the lower limbs, ask the patient to flex and then extend their leg while you are providing resistance to their movements. The categories are usually normal, mild weakness, severe weakness, spastic flexion and extension. Changes in motor strength, especially between right and left sides, may indicate neurological changes and are reported immediately to the shift coordinator and medical staff.

Assess vital signs

Vital sign changes are late changes in brain deterioration. Initially, vital signs are monitored every 15 minutes until they are stable, then hourly or as per the facility policy. Temperature alterations may indicate dysfunction of the hypothalamus or of the brain stem. Hyperthermia increases the metabolic rate and thus cerebral metabolism, increasing the brain's need for glucose and oxygen. Hypothermia decreases the metabolic rate, thus decreasing the cerebral blood flow and oxygen concentration to the brain. Central nervous system (CNS) function is affected by alterations in body temperature either above or below the normal.

Pulse rates initially rise as a compensatory mechanism, then slow in instances of increased intracranial pressure due to vagal stimulation from increased BP, and indicate a deterioration of brain function (late).

Respirations alter with the involvement of different areas of the brain. Derbyshire (2018) states that assessment of respiratory function can provide a clear indication of brain function.

The pattern of the respirations should be recorded as well as the rate and depth, since they give clues about damaged areas of the brain. Note Cheyne-Stokes' respiration, rapid, irregular, clustered, gasping or ataxic breathing and, of course, apnoea.

Blood pressure increases, again as a compensatory mechanism. Oedema, haemorrhage, blocked cerebrospinal outflow or lesions (increased intracranial pressure) exert pressure on the vessels in the brain and ischaemia of the tissue results. Blood pressure increases to overcome the pressure on the vessels in an attempt to supply brain tissue with glucose and oxygen. Increased blood pressure or a widening pulse pressure (the difference between systolic and diastolic pressure readings) is a late sign of increased intracranial pressure. Again, watch for small changes over time – trends.

Ensure accurate reporting of any changes identified.

Perform hand hygiene

Maintain the 5 Moments for Hand Hygiene and perform hand hygiene after touching the patient and the patient's surrounds.

CLEAN, REPLACE OR DISPOSE OF EQUIPMENT

If a patient requires regular 'neuro obs', the equipment will remain at the bedside.

DOCUMENT AND REPORT RELEVANT INFORMATION

The information gathered is recorded on the neurological observation chart, where there are places for each of the observations. Respond appropriately to the score for the GCS and other neurological observations. Any alterations in patient condition or concerns should be promptly reported to the RN or shift coordinator. The patient's vital signs should also be recorded in the patient observation and response chart.

CASE STUDY

You are working on a surgical ward. Twenty-four-year old Jonathon Abbott is admitted after a motor vehicle accident at 0100 hours. He has a fractured right tibia and fibula post the MVA, and is awaiting theatre in the morning once stable. He has a medical history of type 1 diabetes. On arrival to the emergency department he was drowsy, but is now conscious and slightly confused.

He is on hourly full neurological observations (FNO).

1.   Access a FNO chart and document the following:

   a.   temperature 36.5°C, pulse 104 beats per minute, respirations 20 breaths per minute, BP 140/72 mmHg

   b.   eyes open spontaneously to speech

   c.   verbal – responds to simple questions but speech is slurred

   d.   motor – able to obey commands but slow to respond (note: due to the fracture of the right lower leg, patient will not be asked to move this leg).

2.   What is Jonathon's GCS score?

3.   What actions will you take based on the observations you have recorded?

Note: These notes are summaries of the most important points in the assessments/procedures, and are not exhaustive on the subject. The naming of documents or charts may differ from state to state, and facility to facility. In all possible situations the guidelines of the ACSQHC are used when describing national charts or documents (e.g. the ACSQHC Observation and Response Chart is named the Adult Observation and Response Chart in WA, and the Rapid Detection and Response Observation Chart in SA). References of the materials used to compile the information have been supplied. The student is expected to have learned the material surrounding each skill as presented in the references. No single reference is complete on the subject.

REFERENCES

Derbyshire, J. & Hill, B. (2018). Performing neurological observations. *British Journal of Nursing*. 27(19), pp. 1110–14.

Dougherty, L. & Lister, S. (eds) (2015). *The Royal Marsden Hospital Manual of Clinical Nursing Procedures* (9th ed.). Oxford: Wiley-Blackwell.

Gray, S., Ferris, L., White, L.E., Duncan, G. & Baumle, W. (2018). *Foundations of Nursing: Enrolled Nurses* (2nd ANZ ed.). Melbourne: Cengage.

RECOMMENDED READINGS

Bloch, F. (2016). Is the Glasgow Coma Scale appropriate for the evaluation of elderly patients in long-term care units? *Journal of Evaluation in Clinical Practice*, 22(3), pp. 455–6. doi:10.1111/jep.12489

Carey, R. & Holland, C. (2016). Top of the Charts: Detecting neurological deterioration more efficiently through improved documentation. *Australasian Journal of Neuroscience*, 26(1), pp. 17–20.

Mehta, R. & Chinthapalli, K. (2019). Glasgow coma scale explained. *BMJ: British Medical Journal (Online)*, 365.

ESSENTIAL SKILLS COMPETENCY

Neurological Observation
Demonstrates the ability to effectively assess the neurological status of the patient

Criteria for skill performance	Y	D
(Numbers indicate *Enrolled Nurse Standards for Practice*, 2016)	(Satisfactory)	(Requires development)
1. Identifies indication (8.3, 8.4)		
2. Gathers equipment (1.2, 1.6, 4.4, 6.4, 8.4, 9.4): ■ sphygmomanometer, BP cuff and stethoscope ■ thermometer, watch with a second hand ■ pulse oximeter ■ penlight torch ■ pen ■ neurological observation sheet (e.g. Glasgow Coma Scale)		
3. Performs hand hygiene (1.2, 1.4, 1.8, 3.9, 6.4, 9.4)		
4. Evidence of therapeutic communication with the patient; gives explanation of procedure, gains patient consent (2.1, 2.3, 2.4, 2.5, 6.3)		
5. Demonstrates problem-solving abilities; e.g. modifies questions with regard to age, culture and existing physical conditions, can describe warning postures (4.1, 4.2, 8.3, 8.4, 9.4)		
6. Assesses level of consciousness (1.2, 1.4, 3.2, 4.1, 4.2, 6.6, 7.1, 8.4, 9.4)		
7. Assesses orientation of the patient (1.2, 1.4, 3.2, 4.1, 4.2, 6.6, 7.1, 8.4, 9.4)		
8. Assesses motor response (1.2, 1.4, 3.2, 4.1, 4.2, 6.6, 7.1, 8.4, 9.4)		
9. Assesses pupillary activity (1.2, 1.4, 3.2, 4.1, 4.2, 4.4, 6.4, 6.6, 7.1, 8.4, 9.4)		
10. Assesses muscle strength and tone (1.2, 1.4, 3.2, 4.1, 4.2, 6.3, 6.6, 7.1, 8.4, 9.4)		
11. Assesses vital signs (1.2, 1.4, 3.2, 4.1, 4.2, 4.4, 6.4, 6.6, 7.1, 8.4, 9.4)		
12. Performs hand hygiene (1.2, 1.4, 1.8, 3.9, 6.4, 9.4)		
13. Cleans, replaces and disposes of equipment appropriately (1.2, 1.4, 3.9, 6.5, 9.4)		
14. Documents relevant information (1.2, 1.3, 1.8, 3.2, 5.3, 6.6, 7.1, 7.2, 7.3, 7.4, 7.5)		
15. Demonstrates ability to link theory to practice (8.3, 8.4, 8.5, 9.4)		

Student:

Clinical facilitator: Date:

CHAPTER 2.8

NEUROVASCULAR OBSERVATION

IDENTIFY INDICATIONS

Neurovascular observations are performed to detect any changes in the neurological (sensory and motor function) and vascular integrity of a limb. This allows the nurse to detect any reduction in vascular supply or pressure on the limb potentially causing injury. Any changes, including subtle changes, are important to recognise and report promptly to the shift coordinator and doctor (Schreiber, 2016). Failure to recognise and report any changes, or to reduce pressure-causing changes, can result in physical harm to the patient.

The indications for assessing neurovascular status are to:

- obtain a baseline prior to surgery on a limb
- assess the status of the circulation and nerve supply to a traumatised (musculoskeletal, vascular and nerve injury) or postoperative limb
- assess application of a cast, splint or tight bandage

- assess tissue oedema on a limb
- assess burns.

Complications of prolonged pressure and impaired circulation to a limb include compartment syndrome, nerve injuries, tissue necrosis and loss of a limb (Spruce, 2017).

The recommended frequency of neurovascular assessments is initially every 15 minutes, then progressing to half-hourly, hourly and then 4-hourly on limbs post-surgery and post-trauma, or if a plaster cast or traction has been applied (Schreiber, 2016). According to facility policy, hourly observations may be continued for an extended time, depending on the patient's condition. If a patient is in either skin or skeletal traction, after the initial phase, neurovascular assessment is completed each shift, or daily after the washing and re-bandaging of the limb. Occasionally, the doctor may increase the frequency if there is concern.

GATHER EQUIPMENT

Gathering equipment prior to proceeding with the assessment is a time-management strategy and increases confidence in the nurse.

- The *neurovascular assessment chart* is left at the bedside. Using the same chart over time allows for

accurate inter-staff communication so that changes in condition can be recognised, despite different nurses performing the individual assessments.

- *Vascular Doppler and gel, if required.*

PERFORMING NEUROVASCULAR OBSERVATION

Perform hand hygiene

Perform hand hygiene before touching the patient or the patient's surrounds and prior to any procedure involving patient contact to reduce the possibility of cross-contamination. Hand hygiene is the most effective method of infection control as it removes transient organisms from the hands of the nurse (see **Skill 1.1**).

Give a clear explanation of the procedure and establish therapeutic communication

Introduce yourself, and check you have the correct patient. Explain the procedure and gain the patient's consent. Giving a clear explanation is required to gain legal consent and to address policy requirements. It will also assist the patient to cooperate with the procedure, allay anxiety and assist in establishing a therapeutic relationship. An explanation that initially tells the patient why the questions are being asked and what you are assessing involves the patient as an active participant in their care. If the patient understands the rationale for the assessment, and the assessment criteria, they will be willing and able to identify any changes or deterioration, and will know to alert the nurse to early changes. Informing the patient of repetitive assessments will also reduce anxiety, since they may otherwise believe their condition is deteriorating.

Demonstrate problem-solving abilities

Provision of privacy by closing the door or pulling the curtains permits more complete disclosure of symptoms, fears and worries that the patient may be reluctant to make in a public forum. Areas of the patient's body may be required to be exposed, but this should be limited to only the areas required for assessment.

Make an assessment

The aim of neurovascular observations is the early identification of decreased peripheral tissue perfusion, nerve or muscle damage so that measures preventing complications can be implemented.

The limb is assessed distal to the injury or site of surgery to determine if the trauma/surgery has interfered with vascular or neurological function. Comparing the affected limb with the unaffected limb gives a basis for determining what is normal or abnormal for the individual. A high level of observation is required. Both limbs are assessed for the following.

- *Pain level.* The patient is asked about pain at the site of injury/surgery using either a numerical rating scale or visual analogue scale. This is the earliest and most reliable symptom of changes in neurological or vascular function. Moderate pain that is controllable with analgesia may be normal postoperatively or following an injury. Early recognition of progressive, intense pain that is unrelieved by repositioning, elevation or even by narcotic analgesics is a symptom of possible complications (Schreiber, 2016). Patients who have intense pain, paraesthesia and paralysis of the limb require rapid intervention to prevent permanent damage. Treatment is based on relieving the pressure. After consultation with a doctor, bandages may need to be loosened, casts split or the patient returned to theatre.
- *Pulses.* Pulses should be assessed bilaterally and scored for their strength. Assess the distal pulses that are accessible and parallel (Schreiber, 2016). The pulse of the limb should be at the same rate and volume as that of the unaffected limb. Mark the pulse location with a permanent marker to ensure consistency between nurses. A Doppler can also be used to assist pulse assessment.
- *Capillary refill.* This is assessed by pressing, then releasing on the skin or nailbed of the extremity. Refill time should be less than 3 seconds.
- *Colour.* Skin may need to be cleansed of blood, dirt and cleansing solutions that may stain the skin before assessing colour. Compare the skin colour to the alternate limb. Assess for pallor, redness, cyanosis or shiny and pale skin. Each of these represents different complications that need to be addressed.
- *Temperature (warmth).* The limb should be of a similar temperature to the unaffected limb. Coolness can indicate reduced blood flow or oedema, and excess warmth venous insufficiency.
- *Motor function (movement).* The patient is requested to move the distal joints. Loss of motor function can be a later sign of neurovascular damage.
- *Sensation.* The distal digits are assessed for sensation. Diagrams of assessment sites are available on the reverse of most neurovascular assessment charts. The patient is asked about abnormal sensation, numbness, pressure, tightness, tingling or any other sensation. Numbness, tingling and change in sensation are symptoms of nerve compression and should be investigated immediately.
- *Oedema.* This can commonly occur following an injury or surgery, but can also cause vascular, nerve and muscle damage. Monitor swelling and progressive oedema.

Note: Colour, warmth, movement and sensation (CWMS) is commonly used terminology when assessing neurovascular status.

Perform hand hygiene

Maintain the 5 Moments for Hand Hygiene and perform hand hygiene after touching the patient and the patient's surrounds.

SPECIFIC RESPONSIBILITIES

It is the nurse's responsibility to immediately alert an experienced registered nurse (RN) if abnormal changes are noted. The RN would assess the patient and notify the doctor. To reduce the risk from different complications, dressings, casts or splints may be loosened. Delay in notification of doctor, and resultant delay in treatment, can result in permanent muscle and nerve damage or even necrosis (Schreiber, 2016).

To ensure consistency in assessment, nurses changing between shifts should also complete a neurovascular assessment together as part of shift handover (Schreiber, 2016). This will help reduce the risk of potential errors caused by differences in judgement of elements such as temperature or colour.

DOCUMENT AND REPORT RELEVANT INFORMATION

Documentation of the observations is maintained on the neurovascular observation chart. Neurovascular status should be noted on the clinical notes once per shift, including description of any changes. Prompt verbal communication of any changes in the neurovascular observations is essential to reduce delays in treatment and the risk of complications.

CASE STUDY

You are working on an orthopaedic ward, looking after 24-year-old Jonathon Abbott. Jonathon was involved in a motor vehicle accident yesterday. He has a broken right tibia and fibula and has been to theatre this morning for an open reduction and internal fixation of the broken bones.

Preoperatively, Jonathon's neurovascular observations for both limbs were:

- pain: leg, left leg no pain, right leg some pain present
- colour: left leg pink, right leg slightly paler
- temperature: left leg normal, right leg cooler
- sensation: currently normal both limbs
- pulses: normal on both limbs
- capillary refill: 2 seconds for left leg and 3 seconds for the right leg
- movement: able to move toes on left foot easily, less easy on right foot as more painful.

Jonathon has now returned to the ward. Neurovascular assessment of the right limb is part of his postoperative observations. His left limb is as previous assessment done pre-op:

- right leg pain: dull ache
- sensation: able to feel toes being touched
- colour: pink
- temperature: cooler than the left foot
- pulses: both foot pulses present
- capillary refill: 3 seconds
- movement: slight movement of his right toes.
1. Why is it important to assess the neurovascular status of both limbs (pre and postoperatively)?
2. Using a neurovascular observations chart, document both the pre-op and post-op neurovascular observations.
3. What is your nursing assessment of Jonathon's neurovascular status post-op?

Note: These notes are summaries of the most important points in the assessments/procedures, and are not exhaustive on the subject. The naming of documents or charts may differ from state to state, and facility to facility. In all possible situations the guidelines of the ACSQHC are used when describing national charts or documents (e.g. the ACSQHC Observation and Response Chart is named the Adult Observation and Response Chart in WA, and the Rapid Detection and Response Observation Chart in SA). References of the materials used to compile the information have been supplied. The student is expected to have learned the material surrounding each skill as presented in the references. No single reference is complete on the subject.

REFERENCES

Schreiber, M.L. (2016). Evidence-based practice. Neurovascular assessment: An essential nursing focus. *MEDSURG Nursing*, 25(1), pp. 55–7.

Spruce, L. (2017). Back to basics: Pneumatic tourniquet use. Association of Operating Room Nurses. *AORN Journal*, 106(3), pp. 219–26.

RECOMMENDED READINGS

Dougherty, L. & Lister, S. (eds). (2015). *The Royal Marsden Hospital Manual of Clinical Nursing Procedures* (9th ed.). Oxford: Wiley-Blackwell.

Smith, S., Duell, D.J. & Martin, B.C. (2016). *Clinical Nursing Skills: Basic to Advanced Skills* (9th ed.). Upper Saddle River, NJ: Prentice Hall.

ESSENTIAL SKILLS COMPETENCY

Neurovascular Observation
Demonstrates the ability to assess the neurovascular status of a patient

Criteria for skill performance	Y	D
(Numbers indicate *Enrolled Nurse Standards for Practice*, 2016)	(Satisfactory)	(Requires development)
1. Identifies indication of neurovascular assessment (8.3, 8.4)		
2. Gathers equipment (1.2, 1.6, 4.4, 6.4, 8.4, 9.4): ■ neurovascular assessment chart		
3. Performs hand hygiene (1.2, 1.4, 1.8, 3.9, 6.4, 9.4)		
4. Evidence of therapeutic communication with the patient; gives explanation of procedure, gains patient consent (2.1, 2.3, 2.4, 2.5, 6.3)		
5. Demonstrates problem-solving abilities; e.g. provides privacy, comfort measures (4.1, 4.2, 8.3, 8.4, 9.4)		
6. Assesses the limb distal to the injury/surgery; compares affected limb with unaffected limb; assesses both limbs for the following: pain, pulses, capillary refill, colour, temperature, sensation and motor function. (1.2, 1.4, 2.7, 3.2, 4.1, 4.2, 6.6, 7.1, 8.4, 9.4)		
7. Performs hand hygiene (1.2, 1.4, 1.8, 3.9, 6.4, 9.4)		
8. Recognises specific responsibilities (7.3, 7.5)		
9. Documents relevant information (1.2, 1.3, 1.8, 3.2, 5.3, 6.6, 7.1, 7.2, 7.3, 7.4, 7.5)		
10. Demonstrates ability to link theory to practice (8.3, 8.4, 8.5, 9.4)		

Student:

Clinical facilitator: Date:

CHAPTER 2.9

PAIN ASSESSMENT

IDENTIFY INDICATIONS

Pain is often referred to as the fifth vital sign. Indications of pain range from invisible to blatant. Non-verbal cues (e.g. grimacing, splinting or guarding an area) must be followed up by a thorough pain assessment. Accurate pain assessment is necessary for effective pain management and to determine the response to treatment. Each person who is cared for by a nurse should be asked if they are comfortable. There are many reasons that patients do not volunteer a pain report. For example, some patients may not wish to increase staff workload; they may fear being seen as weak, dependent or addicted; they may fear that if the pain increases, drugs used now will be ineffective; they may worry about the cost of medications; they may dislike the side effects of the analgesia; they may believe that pain is part of the recovery process or part of life; or they may

believe if they deny the pain they can deny the disease. Also be aware that professionals may be biased about pain. They may erroneously believe that the elderly (or newborn, child or cognitively impaired person) are less sensible in regard to pain, that use of opioid drugs carries unacceptable risks or that pain is an inevitable consequence of ageing, surgery or other medical conditions or treatments.

Pain may be chronic and unrelated to the reason the person is hospitalised. Patients who report acute pain require assessment frequently, plus post administration of analgesia. Patients whose pain is stable or chronic should be monitored every 4 hours and post administration of analgesia. A patient's pain description should be in their own words.

GATHER EQUIPMENT

Gathering the required equipment prior to the procedure is a time-management strategy. The tools necessary for assessing pain are minimal, though must be relevant to the patient. The most important factors are the nurse's understanding of pain perception and attitude to pain. The physiology of pain needs to be understood, including structures of pain perception and the roles of pain centres

in the brain. These factors are discussed in most textbooks of medical/surgical nursing. The actual tools that are used range from simple scales such as Visual Analogue Scales (VAS), numerical scales, colour scales and face scales, to more comprehensive tools that assess many facets of pain and take into consideration that the patient may have dementia (e.g. the Abbey Pain Scale).

ASSESSING THE PATIENT FOR PAIN

Perform hand hygiene

Perform hand hygiene before touching the patient or the patient's surrounds and prior to any procedure involving patient contact to reduce the possibility of cross-contamination. Hand hygiene is the most effective method of infection control as it removes transient organisms from the hands of the nurse (see **Skill 1.1**).

Give a clear explanation of the procedure and establish therapeutic communication

Introduce yourself to the patient, and check you have the correct patient. Explain the procedure and gain the patient's consent. Giving a clear explanation will assist the patient to cooperate with the procedure and will allay anxiety, plus assist in gaining the patient's permission and in establishing a therapeutic relationship. Checking the patient and gaining their consent will also ensure that you meet legal and policy requirements before implementing any procedures.

Effective communication relies on the nurse believing the patient's report of pain. This is crucial to establishing trust. If a patient indicates that they are not comfortable, or if they are unable to do effective postoperative exercises, further assessment is indicated. The patient should be made aware of the intention of the nurse to assess their pain because this knowledge fosters trust in the nurse and a positive attitude that the discomfort will be addressed and alleviated. Patients need to be advised that they do not need to wait to be asked if they have pain. They should be encouraged to vocalise their pain and be educated in the benefits of regular pain relief.

Demonstrate problem-solving abilities

Provision of privacy reduces distractions and permits disclosure of intimate information that the patient may otherwise be reluctant to discuss (e.g. if pain is felt in an embarrassing area – anal or perineal). Cultural differences must be considered because the experience and expression of pain is mediated by culture. These differences in pain response can lead to pain management challenges (Gray et al., 2018).

Assess pain

The assessment of pain depends on the situation. Someone in severe acute pain would be asked a minimum of the assessment questions (location, intensity and quality) in order to establish a baseline before interventions begin. Otherwise, the assessment begins with a history. As with any history, the patient needs to be positioned comfortably, and wearing any required aids such as glasses, hearing aids and dentures. The pain history includes questions about the pain experience. The patient should be given time and a sense of the nurse's belief in the pain that they are experiencing so that they can describe it adequately.

Background information will help the nurse to understand the patient's response to pain and affect the management of pain. Questions that should be asked include:

- the effect of pain on the lifestyle of the patient and on their activities of daily living
- how this patient views the pain
- if the patient feels they have control
- what the patient thinks causes the pain.

A good pain history will give clues as to the condition causing the pain and assist in making treatment choices. Difficulties may arise because of communication barriers – non-English-speaking, people with dementia, deaf, aphasic/dysphasic, neonate, infant, paediatric, mentally ill or confused patients and those who are unconscious or sedated all require different assessment approaches.

A range of valid and reliable specialised assessment tools are available to assist in assessing the non-verbal patient. Tools such as the Faces Pain Scale or the FLACC pain assessment scale have proven valid and reliable with many groups (children, elderly, cognitively impaired and people with communication difficulties) (Ramira et al., 2016). Other tools for the elderly such as the PAINAID scale or the Abbey Pain Scale are used for people with dementia who cannot verbalise. For preverbal children, pain assessment tools consist of pain-associated behaviours, as well as (sometimes) the physiological markers of stress (Battaglini, 2014). Determine which tool is used in the facility where you are.

Further description of the pain will include the following.

- The location of pain needs to be determined. Asking the patient to point to the pain often assists to locate it. A body diagram can be marked with the location of the pain.
- If the pain radiates, ask the patient to touch the point of most severity and follow the pain along its path with their finger.
- The intensity of the pain is determined using a VAS or numerical rating scale. The use of a pain rating scale requires careful explanation and teaching geared to the cognitive level of the patient.
- A description of the quality of the pain is often useful in diagnosing the cause. Ask the patient to describe the pain. A list of pain descriptors often assists if the patient has difficulty in naming the quality of the pain.
- Specifically, the patient should be asked to describe the onset of pain – when it began, if there is a discernible pattern, if there is more than one type of pain being experienced.
- The duration of the pain is discussed: is it constant or episodic; is it of sudden or insidious onset and short or long duration?
- Pain should be assessed on movement as well as at rest.

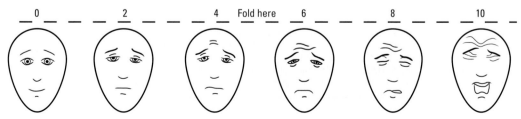

FIGURE 2.9.1 The Faces Pain Scale

In the following instructions, say 'hurt' or 'pain', whichever seems right for a particular child. Score the chosen face 0, 2, 4, 6, 8 or 10, counting left to right so 0 = 'no pain' and 10 = 'very much pain'. Do not use words like 'happy' and 'sad'. This scale is intended to measure how children feel inside, not how their face looks. Show faces only, no numbers.

Finding out any factors that induce the pain or precipitate its occurrence will help the patient avoid these in the future. Similarly, coping strategies and pain control techniques (including medication) that have been used in the past, successfully or not, should be noted. Explore measures the patient uses to relieve the pain such as rest, relaxation, distraction, over-the-counter medications, complementary therapies or any other interventions used. The time of the last dose of any analgesia needs to be recorded. It is important that each pain the patient is experiencing is documented clearly. Patients may be prescribed a variety of pain-relieving medications relevant to a specific category of pain.

Psychological conditions may contribute to the pain experience. Discuss social, emotional and economic problems with the patient. Patients who are unable to verbally report pain (e.g. the cognitively impaired) should be monitored for non-verbal behavioural cues such as restlessness, agitation, withdrawal, tense body language and any repetitive movement (rocking, rubbing). A judgement must be made regarding the presence of pain. There are a variety of tools available (e.g. Abbey Pain Scale) to help the nurse to assess the patient. It is imperative that staff are assessing with the same tool.

The physiological effects of pain need to be observed and recorded. Acute pain often causes tachycardia, a change in blood pressure (usually an increase in systolic pressure), pallor, grimacing, diaphoresis and hyperventilation/tachypnoea. Anxiety and apprehension may accompany acute pain. Chronic pain may not alter the vital signs but be observed by withdrawal, quiet demeanour and unwillingness to communicate, listlessness, fatigue and frustration. Any associated symptoms such as nausea, anorexia, dizziness, visual alterations and shortness of breath need to be determined. The effects on activities of daily living should be explored. Other assessment components include past pain experiences, the meaning of the pain to the patient, coping strategies that were effective in the past and the affective response of the patient.

Perform hand hygiene

Maintain the 5 Moments for Hand Hygiene and perform hand hygiene after touching the patient and the patient's surrounds.

CLEAN, REPLACE OR DISPOSE OF EQUIPMENT

Cleaning and replacing equipment ensures patient safety and efficiency of time use within the nursing unit. Cleaning and returning equipment is also a courtesy to colleagues.

DOCUMENT AND REPORT RELEVANT INFORMATION

Documentation of a pain assessment outlines a baseline against which response to interventions can be monitored. An initial pain assessment also gives healthcare workers clues to the cause of the pain and to its management. Documentation of pain levels and quality (at least) should follow administration of all analgesics. Documentation is completed in the patient progress notes, and on any pain record charts that may be being used (e.g. with patient-controlled analgesia chart or postoperative charts). It should also be recorded on the observation and response chart as part of routine observations.

CASE STUDY

There are many pain tools available to measure a patient's pain.

1. You are working on a busy surgical ward looking after an alert and coherent patient with a possible bowel obstruction, and who is in significant pain. What would be a suitable pain assessment tool to use on this patient?

2. When would the following pain assessment tools be useful and appropriate for patients?
   - Abbey Pain Scale
   - Numerical Pain Scale
   - Faces Pain Scale

3. Can you think of any situations where the assessment tools listed above may not be effective or appropriate?

Note: These notes are summaries of the most important points in the assessments/procedures, and are not exhaustive on the subject. The naming of documents or charts may differ from state to state, and facility to facility. In all possible situations the guidelines of the ACSQHC are used when describing national charts or documents (e.g. the ACSQHC Observation and Response Chart is named the Adult Observation and Response Chart in WA, and the Rapid Detection and Response Observation Chart in SA). References of the materials used to compile the information have been supplied. The student is expected to have learned the material surrounding each skill as presented in the references. No single reference is complete on the subject.

REFERENCES

Battaglini, E. (2014). *Child Pain and Distress: Self-report During Medical Procedures*. Joanna Briggs Institute. http://joannabriggs.org

Gray, S., Ferris, L., White, L.E., Duncan, G. & Baumle, W. (2018). *Foundations of Nursing: Enrolled Nurses* (2nd ANZ ed.). Melbourne: Cengage.

Ramira, M.L., Instone, S. & Clark, M.J. (2016). Pediatric pain management: an evidence-based approach. *Pediatric Nursing*, 42(1), pp. 39–46, 49.

RECOMMENDED READINGS

Burns, M. & McIlfatrick, S. (2015). Palliative care in dementia: Literature review of nurses' knowledge and attitudes towards pain assessment. *International Journal of Palliative Nursing*, 21(8), pp. 400–7.

Claassens, T. (2017). Nursing a patient with acute pain. *Kai Tiaki: Nursing New Zealand*, 23(7), pp. 15–17, 39.

Dougherty, L. & Lister, S. (eds). (2015). *The Royal Marsden Hospital Manual of Clinical Nursing Procedures* (9th ed.). Oxford: Wiley-Blackwell.

Manocha, S. & Taneja, N. (2016). Assessment of paediatric pain: a critical review. *Journal of Basic and Clinical Physiology and Pharmacology*, pp. 323–31.

PART 2

ESSENTIAL SKILLS COMPETENCY

Pain Assessment

Demonstrates the ability to assess a person who is experiencing pain

Criteria for skill performance	Y	D
(Numbers indicate *Enrolled Nurse Standards for Practice*, 2016)	(Satisfactory)	(Requires development)
1. Identifies indication (8.3, 8.4)		
2. Gathers equipment (1.2, 1.6, 4.4, 6.4, 8.4, 9.4): 　■ pain assessment tools		
3. Performs hand hygiene, (1.2, 1.4, 1.8, 3.9, 6.4, 9.4)		
4. Evidence of therapeutic communication with the patient; gives explanation of procedure, gains patient consent (2.1, 2.3, 2.4, 2.5, 6.3)		
5. Demonstrates problem-solving abilities; e.g. provides privacy (4.1, 4.2, 8.3, 8.4, 9.4)		
6. Assesses the patient's pain using the following guidelines (1.2, 1.4, 3.2, 4.1, 4.2, 4.4, 6.3, 6.4, 6.6, 7.1, 8.4, 9.4): 　■ history of present pain 　■ onset and duration 　■ location 　■ quality and character 　■ intensity 　■ aggravating or relieving factors 　■ use of pain assessment tools 　■ associated physical effects		
7. Performs hand hygiene (1.2, 1.4, 1.8, 3.9, 6.4, 9.4)		
8. Cleans, replaces and disposes of equipment appropriately (1.2, 1.4, 3.9, 6.5, 9.4)		
9. Documents relevant information (1.2, 1.3, 1.8, 3.2, 5.3, 6.6, 7.1, 7.2, 7.3, 7.4, 7.5)		
10. Demonstrates ability to link theory to practice (8.3, 8.4, 8.5, 9.4)		

Student:

Clinical facilitator: 　　　　　　　　　　　　　　　　Date:

CHAPTER **2.10**

12-LEAD ECG RECORDING

IDENTIFY INDICATIONS

The 12-lead electrocardiogram (ECG) uses 10 electrode positions to provide 12 different views of the heart's electrical activity, often described as a graphic view of the heart's electrical activity (DeLaune et al., 2016; Garcia, 2015;). Electrical changes that occur when the heart contracts and relaxes are recorded on an ECG via electrodes that are applied to the chest and limbs (Dougherty & Lister, 2015). In a healthy heart, depolarisation is initiated in the sinoatrial node and proceeds through the atria to the atrioventricular node and on through the ventricles. In an unhealthy or damaged heart, the electrical axis will vary as the electrical activity bypasses the area of damage or necrosis.

The indications for obtaining a 12-lead ECG include:

- identification of myocardial infarction (MI), primary conduction disorders and cardiac arrhythmias (Garcia, 2015; Loewe et al., 2015)
- obtaining a baseline ECG for comparison prior to stressful interventions (e.g. surgery, anaesthesia, invasive diagnostic procedures)
- ongoing comparison of the present state of the electrical activity of the heart when a patient has long-term cardiovascular disease.

ECG is an invaluable tool in identifying a patient experiencing a cardiac event, and the subsequent care needs (Garcia, 2015). It is important for the nurse to perform this skill accurately and quickly when a patient may be experiencing chest pain.

GATHER EQUIPMENT

 Gathering the equipment prior to beginning the procedure reduces the time and energy needed to complete the procedure, increases the patient's confidence in the nurse and increases the nurse's self-confidence. Ensuring the availability of the equipment also alerts the nurse to anything that is missing or malfunctioning.

- The *ECG machine* records the electrical activity of the heart muscle and transcribes the waveforms onto a monitor or tracing paper. The ECG machine will include the marked electrodes that should be placed in a specific location for correct readings.
- *ECG paper* comes in sheets, with the types depending on the model of machine used.
- *ECG gel electrode pads* are preprepared and come in a variety of forms, according to the machine being

used, but all contact the patient's skin and pick up the electrical activity. The gel increases the conduction of electrical activity from the skin to the electrode. *Hair clippers* may be required if the patient is hairy, since the electrodes do not conduct electrical impulses unless in direct contact with the skin. Alternatively, a special abrasive strip may be used to increase contact with the skin (Dougherty & Lister, 2015).

- *Alcohol wipes* to remove excess oils from the skin.
- *Tissue or wipes* are used to remove any conduction gel remaining on the skin.

ECG machines can vary between a facility, or ward areas within a facility. To reduce operator error, the nurse should familiarise themselves with the ECG machine in their area (Garcia, 2015). This will also enable prompt response in recording a patient's ECG if they experience chest pain.

PERFORMING A 12-LEAD ECG

Calibrate and prepare the ECG machine according to manufacturer's instructions

Use of the manufacturer's instructions for calibrating and preparing the ECG machine ensures that each reading is as accurate as possible.

Familiarity with the type of machine and its use will increase the accuracy of the recording and decrease patient and nurse stress. Enter relevant information about the patient as prompted by the machine.

Perform hand hygiene

Perform hand hygiene before touching the patient or the patient's surrounds and prior to any procedure involving patient contact to reduce the possibility of cross-contamination. Hand hygiene is the most effective method of infection control as it removes transient organisms from the hands of the nurse (see **Skill 1.1**).

Give a clear explanation of the procedure and establish therapeutic communication

Introduce yourself, and check you have the correct patient. Explain the procedure and gain the patient's consent. Giving a clear explanation is required to gain legal consent and to address policy requirements.

A clear explanation of the procedure will reduce the patient's anxiety and assist the patient to comply with the requirements of the assessment. Some patients fear the electrodes, as they believe they may be shocked. Reassurance that the machine does not create electrical currents but only picks them up through the electrodes should be explained. Explanation regarding lying still is important since muscle movement interferes with the readings by increasing the amount of electrical activity the electrodes pick up. Teaching patients about healthcare facts assists them to make informed decisions and increases their ability to function independently.

Demonstrate problem-solving abilities

Provision of comfort measures will increase the patient's ability to tolerate the requirements of the assessment, which include remaining still and relaxed throughout the recording of the ECG. The patient is positioned in a supine position with all four limbs supported so there is no muscular work required to maintain the position. The head should be supported on one pillow. If the patient has difficulty breathing, they are positioned and well supported in a semi-upright position, again so there is no muscular work required to maintain that position. Muscular effort produces electrical activity that may interfere with the ECG reading.

Prepare the patient

Assist the patient to remove their upper clothing and then into the correct position on their bed. Clothing is removed above the waist to facilitate the location and attachment of leads. Jewellery (including piercings) is removed so there is no electrical interference. Provision of privacy, by drawing the curtains or closing the door, is imperative to preserve patient dignity because the patient's chest will be exposed during the procedure. Excess body hair and diaphoresis can interfere with the attachment of the electrode pads. Assess the patient to determine if hair under the electrode pads requires clipping, and if the skin is dry. Skin areas may also be cleaned with an alcohol wipe to remove oils from the skin, then dried with gauze (Garcia, 2015). Patient preparation will ensure good conduction of the electrical impulses.

Attach the limb electrodes

The limb electrode pads are attached to clean areas on each of the four limbs – the areas chosen should be over fleshy tissue, not bone, and placement should be symmetrical on the arms and legs. The skin needs to be clean to ensure the best conduction of electrical impulses. If necessary, rub the skin surface with the abrasive strip to remove excess hair to ensure adequate contact of the electrodes and gel with the skin. After attaching the electrode pads, identify the relevant marked electrode for each limb (i.e. RL – right leg) and then attach these to the electrode pads.

Attach the chest electrodes

Electrode pads are then attached to the different areas of the patient's chest. Refer to **FIGURE 2.10.1** to identify the location for each of the gelled electrode pads. Care must be taken that the electrodes are accurately placed, since errors in diagnosis can occur if the electrodes are incorrectly placed (Khunti, 2014). Gently use the pads of your fingers to palpate the patient's chest and ribs to locate each of the relevant intercostal spaces. Males may require removal of excess hair in the location of an electrode pad. Electrodes can be placed above or below a woman's breast, although below the breast tissue and against the chest wall is preferred (Garcia, 2015; Wallen, Tunnage & Wells, 2014).

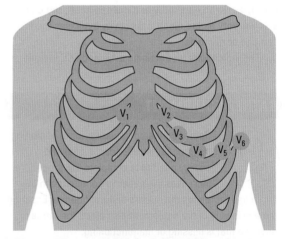

FIGURE 2.10.1 Placement of chest leads (V leads) for a 12-lead electrocardiogram

Correct positioning is achieved by locating the fourth intercostal space for placement of the V_1 and V_2 leads first. Identifying this location correctly will influence the reliability of the final ECG reading (Garcia, 2015; Khunti, 2014). V_4 should be placed on the chest next, in the fifth intercostal space. V_3 is then placed midway between V_2 and V_4. V_5 and V_6 are placed last.

Identify each of the correct chest electrode leads that will be labelled for their specific location. Leads can be colour-coded or identified by lead designations (V_1–V_6) imprinted on the end that attaches to the electrode pad to help with identification.

Chest electrodes are attached to clean sites at:
- V_1 – 4th intercostal space, right sternal border
- V_2 – 4th intercostal space, left sternal border
- V_3 – midway between V_2 and V_4

- V_4 – 5th intercostal space, left midclavicular line
- V_5 – same level as V_4, left anterior axillary line
- V_6 – same level as V_4, left mid-axillary line.

Perform the ECG reading

Ask the patient to relax and refrain from moving, but to breathe normally. As per the machine instructions, commence the ECG recording. If there is an artefact or poor recording (many machines will indicate this when commencing the reading), check the electrodes and connections.

Inform the patient when the reading has been completed, and label the printout with a patient ID label. In addition, the nurse may need to note on the printout if the patient was complaining of chest pain or other symptoms and relevant medical information.

Remove electrodes

For some patients, the electrode pads may need to be left intact for future ECG readings. Otherwise, remove the electrode pads and reposition the patient following the procedure. Although the supine position is generally fairly comfortable, moving to a different position following enforced stillness increases comfort. Excess gel can be removed with tissues.

Perform hand hygiene

Maintain the 5 Moments for Hand Hygiene and perform hand hygiene after touching the patient and the patient's surrounds.

CLEAN, REPLACE OR DISPOSE OF EQUIPMENT

Clean the ECG machine and its leads with disposable wipes according to facility policy. Dispose of used electrode pads and other waste in the general rubbish. Replacing paper and other supplies you have used is a safety measure in case the ECG machine is required in an urgent situation, as well as being a courtesy to other staff.

DOCUMENT AND REPORT RELEVANT INFORMATION

Each ECG reading should be shown to an experienced registered nurse (RN) or to the doctor immediately after it has been recorded. Further documentation of the ECG reading includes the actual recording, noting name, doctor, date and time (if not done by the machine) on the printout. If multiple readings are taken, ECG readings are numbered sequentially. Any signs and symptoms or issues experienced by the patient should be noted on the printout, reported to the RN or doctor and recorded in the progress notes. Some ECG machines may require connection to the internet or computer for the transmission of the ECG.

CASE STUDY

You are an enrolled nurse working on a medical ward. Your patient is Chloe Johnson, who is 28 years of age and has been admitted with anxiety and panic attacks. The registrar has ordered a 12-lead ECG.

1. How will you describe this procedure to Chloe?

2. Chloe asks you why the doctors have requested this procedure. How will you respond?

3. Chloe is very concerned regarding the cleanliness of the machine. How will you alleviate her fears?

4. While doing the ECG, Chloe is a little restless. As her nurse, how will you respond to this?

Note: These notes are summaries of the most important points in the assessments/procedures, and are not exhaustive on the subject. The naming of documents or charts may differ from state to state, and facility to facility. In all possible situations the guidelines of the ACSQHC are used when describing national charts or documents (e.g. the ACSQHC Observation and Response Chart is named the Adult Observation and Response Chart in WA, and the Rapid Detection and Response Observation Chart in SA). References of the materials used to compile the information have been supplied. The student is expected to have learned the material surrounding each skill as presented in the references. No single reference is complete on the subject.

REFERENCES

DeLaune, S.C., Ladner, P.K., McTier, L., Tollefson, J. & Lawrence, J. (2016). *Australian and New Zealand Fundamentals of Nursing*. Melbourne: Cengage.

Dougherty, L. & Lister, S. (eds). (2015). *The Royal Marsden Hospital Manual of Clinical Nursing Procedures* (9th ed.). Oxford: Wiley-Blackwell.

Garcia, T. (2015). Acquiring the 12-lead electrocardiogram: Doing it right every time. *Journal of Emergency Nursing*, 41(6), pp. 474–78.

Khunti, K. (2014). Accurate interpretation of the 12-lead ECG electrode placement: A systematic review. *The Health Education Journal*, 73(5), pp. 610–623.

Loewe, A., Schulze, W. W., Jiang, Y., Wilhelms, M., Luik, A., Dössel, O. & Seemann, G. (2015). ECG-based detection of early myocardial ischemia in a computational model: Impact of additional electrodes, optimal placement, and a new feature for ST deviation. *Biomed Research International*, 2015, pp. 1–11. doi:10.1155/2015/530352.

Wallen, R., Tunnage, B. & Wells, S. (2014). The 12-lead ECG in the emergency medical service setting: How electrode placement and paramedic gender are experienced by women. *Emergency Medicine Journal: EMJ*, 31(10), p. 851.

ESSENTIAL SKILLS COMPETENCY

12-Lead ECG Recording

Demonstrates the ability to obtain a recording from a 12-lead ECG

Criteria for skill performance	Y	D
(Numbers indicate *Enrolled Nurse Standards for Practice*, 2016)	(Satisfactory)	(Requires development)
1. Identifies indication (8.3, 8.4)		
2. Gathers equipment (1.2, 1.6, 4.4, 6.4, 8.4, 9.4): ■ ECG machine with paper ■ pre-gelled electrode pads ■ hair clippers or abrasive strips (if required) ■ alcohol wipes ■ tissues		
3. Calibrates ECG machine according to manufacturer's instructions (1.2, 3.2, 4.4, 6.4, 8.4, 9.4)		
4. Performs hand hygiene, (1.2, 1.4, 1.8, 3.9, 6.4, 9.4)		
5. Evidence of therapeutic communication with the patient; gives explanation of procedure, gains patient consent (2.1, 2.3, 2.4, 2.5, 6.3)		
6. Demonstrates problem-solving abilities; e.g. provides privacy, comfort measures, pain relief; positions patient (4.1, 4.2, 8.3, 8.4, 9.4)		
7. Prepares patient, ensuring privacy and dignity; positions patient correctly (1.2, 1.4, 3.2, 4.4, 6.4, 6.6, 8.4, 9.4)		
8. Attaches electrode pads, then limb leads to clean, hair-free sites on arms and legs (1.2, 1.4, 3.2, 4.4, 6.4, 6.6, 8.4, 9.4)		
9. Determines chest sites and attaches electrode pads to clean, dry, hair-free sites (1.2, 1.4, 3.2, 4.4, 6.4, 6.6, 8.4, 9.4)		
10. Attaches chest leads to electrode pads (1.2, 3.2, 4.4, 6.4, 8.4, 9.4)		
11. Records ECG, checks with RN regarding significance of tracing (1.2, 1.4, 3.2, 3.3, 3.4, 3.5, 4.4, 6.4, 6.6, 8.1, 8.4, 9.4)		
12. Removes ECG leads and when appropriate removes electrode pads and cleanses residual gel off the patient; the patient is left comfortably positioned (1.2, 3.2, 4.4, 6.4, 8.4, 9.4)		
13. Performs hand hygiene (1.2, 1.4, 1.8, 3.9, 6.4, 9.4)		
14. Cleans, replaces and disposes of equipment appropriately (1.2, 1.4, 3.9, 6.5, 9.4)		
15. Documents and reports relevant information (1.2, 1.3, 1.8, 3.2, 5.3, 6.6, 7.1, 7.2, 7.3, 7.4, 7.5)		
16. Demonstrates ability to link theory to practice (8.3, 8.4, 8.5, 9.4)		

Student:

Clinical facilitator: Date:

ACTIVITIES OF DAILY LIVING

Note: These notes are summaries of the most important points in the assessments/procedures and are not exhaustive on the subject. References of the materials used to compile the information have been supplied. The student is expected to have learnt the material surrounding each skill as presented in the references. No single reference is complete on each subject.

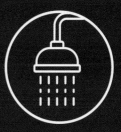

PROFESSIONAL WORKPLACE SKILLS – INCLUDING TIME MANAGEMENT, ROUNDING AND PERSONAL STRESS MANAGEMENT

IDENTIFY INDICATIONS

Time management

Time management skills are essential in being able to prioritise patient care safely and deliver all the required patient care within a shift. They also enable nurses to feel less stressed (Setting Priorities, 2017). The *EN Standards for Practice*, Standard 6 recognises the importance of nursing care being skilled and timely, with indicator 6.5 specifically stating the EN should '*exercise* time management and workload prioritisation' (Nursing and Midwifery Board of Australia [NMBA], 2018). The ability to manage patient care and all other workplace responsibilities will improve as a nurse gains more skills and experience.

Time management includes taking time at the commencement of a shift to identify required patient care, prioritise this care and plan when care will be implemented. A written work plan is used throughout the shift to identify nursing actions completed, those due and others required later in the shift. Taking time to plan is an essential part of time management, as it helps to determine the most effective way of managing (Setting Priorities, 2017). It is also a key part of the nursing process. Time management within a nursing area requires flexibility and adaptability because: a patient's health status may change; an adverse event may occur (e.g. patient fall); patients may use the call bell to request assistance; other health professionals may request care actions or treatments that are not listed in your original work plan; or schedules are interrupted by events such as phone calls, patients being admitted, patients returning from theatre, or an emergency on the floor. These events can then impact on the individual nurse's ability to deliver all the planned care on time. Being flexible and having good time management skills will enable the nurse to adapt and work with these changes that are part of a daily work routine.

Care rounding

Care rounding is a professional skill requiring the nurse to physically interact with every patient in their allocation at least every 1 to 2 hours (depending on facility policy), and can be embedded as part of daily work routines. Many acute hospitals and other care facilities across Australia have implemented policies requiring care rounds by the nursing staff. It is encouraged as part of activities that promote person-centred care and partnering with consumers (ACSQHC, 2019). Rounding should be implemented by all nurses, regardless of policy requirements, making them proactive in the delivery of safe and compassionate nursing care. The questions and actions used in rounding can also be embedded into the settling of a patient when completing all nursing interventions, and before moving on to the next patient. While there is some controversy that rounding can make nursing care task oriented, there is also evidence that it reduces the incidence of falls, reduces pressure injuries, results in less interruption of work routines to answer call bells, improves time management, reduces patient anxiety and improves patient perception of their care, as well as increasing patient and staff satisfaction (ACSQHC, 2019; Bragg et al., 2016; Langley, 2015).

Embedding the questions and actions of care rounding into your routine work schedule and patient interaction will not only increase patient satisfaction for the care being implemented, but improve personal time management and awareness of patients' needs or changes in their health status.

Personal stress management

The World Health Organization (2020) defines work-related stress as:

> the response people have when presented with work demands and pressures that are not matched to their knowledge and abilities and which challenge their ability to cope.

Pressure within the healthcare environment is unavoidable due to the nature of the work, but it can be used to create motivation to complete tasks well and a desire to learn. Excess or unmanageable pressure will create stress that in turn impacts on an employee's performance and personal health. Nurses are described as having some of the highest levels of stress among healthcare professionals (Garcia et al., 2017). The type of work in nursing includes stressful or traumatic situations and events that activate the 'flight or fight response', releasing hormones to enable a physical response, which drains personal emotional reserves. This will in turn reduce personal abilities to cope with the environment and increase personal stress (Fedele, 2017).

While there are many workplace and management factors that will create stress, personal workplace stress can also be increased by poor time management along with a lack of nursing knowledge or skills relevant to the area. There are also personal coping strategies that a nurse can implement within their lifestyle to help reduce and manage stress created by their nursing work (Garcia et al., 2017; Langille, 2017). Failure to manage stress and develop these personal coping strategies can lead to long-term health problems such as headaches, cardiovascular disease, weight gain, impaired memory and concentration, sleep problems, anxiety and depression.

DEMONSTRATE PROBLEM-SOLVING ABILITIES

Assessing, recognising and understanding personal levels of professionalism and workplace personal skills is important. Each nurse should take the time to objectively review their skills, then set realistic goals and strategies to either improve (when there is a need for further development) or consolidate (when skills exist but need refreshing) their abilities. Each of the skills described are developed over time, and will increase in both capability and expectation as a nurse gains more clinical experience and knowledge. Seek to develop honest and appropriate insight to your own ability. Do not create expectations with a timeframe that is too short. Accept feedback from others, and use it constructively. Seek guidance from other mentors and peers when practising these skills, and follow the input from positive role models.

Review the actions for the described professional skills and seek to develop these within your work practice. Descriptions of steps described in other nursing skills such as perform hand hygiene, establish therapeutic communication and documentation have not been noted or described within these skills, as many of the skills mentioned in Part 3 are related to personal professional development, and embedded into routine nursing practice. Care rounding and some components of time management or critical thinking will involve patient contact, or touching of the patient's surrounds. The 5 Moments for Hand Hygiene, therapeutic communication and other principles of a safe healthcare workplace should still be adhered to.

IMPLEMENT TIME MANAGEMENT SKILLS

At the commencement of the shift, nurses are allocated patients or rooms for which they are responsible, and then attend shift handover. During clinical handover, notes should be taken about care and treatment relevant to your allocated patients. After handover is completed, the nurse (or nurses sharing the patients) will then need to review all the charts and nursing care plans relevant to their allocated patients to confirm the nursing actions they are responsible for delivering during that shift. This is the key planning stage of time management, and should not be skipped. Use a time planner or worksheet to outline times throughout the day, and the time when care required for each patient will be performed. A simple grid is commonly used by many facilities (see **FIGURE 3.1.1**), but alternatives can also work just as efficiently. Prioritising the timing of different care actions using the following guidelines may be helpful:

- routine times for actions such as medication, vital signs, blood glucose readings
- specific care requiring completion at or by a specific time (e.g. preparing a patient for theatre or physiotherapy, wound management, patient discharge)
- note charts such as fluid balance or dietary input that need to be recorded after meals or at the scheduled mealtimes
- care actions that are more flexible with time can be included
- mealtimes and tea breaks for the nursing staff should also be included
- when determining a time to implement care actions for patients, allocate sufficient time to each task according to the patient's acuity and the task itself
- schedule less-demanding tasks during meals and tea breaks, as there will be fewer staff on the ward to answer call bells or telephones.

When the care is being shared between a team or some actions are delegated to other care workers, note each person's responsibility on the planning sheet. Liaise with other nurses to plan the appropriate time to complete care that requires two nurses, such as sponging or transferring patients with a hoist.

This time planner can be carried in the nurse's pocket for reference during the shift. If there are multiple people using the same time planner, place it in an accessible area that cannot be seen by patients or others. When working with this time planner, mark off care actions as they are completed and add other care requirements that are added or adjusted during the shift. Refer to it during the shift to check on what has been completed and what is planned next.

Take time to reprioritise and adjust time allocated for care when unplanned situations such as a change in a patient's health status or an adverse event occur. Communicate with the shift coordinator when changes to a patient's status impact your ability to deliver all the required nursing care or a specifically timed nursing action. Other nurses can then assist, or extra staff be requested from management.

PT	0700	0800 (B/FAST)	0900	1000 (M/TEA) 2ND TEA BREAK – 1030	1100	1200 (12.30 lunch)	1300 MY LUNCH	1400 SHIFT HANDOVER
Mr B	730 sh – self	M fbc obs		fbc		fbc		fbc
Mr C		M obs feed		neb	sponge	feed		
Mrs A		M obs			1130 BGL	M		M
Mr VI	insulin	M obs	930 – sh		1130 BGL			
Mrs Br		M 830 – sh		obs				M obs
Mrs P		M fbc obs	Sh – 2 assist	fbc		fbc	woundcare	fbc

FIGURE 3.1.1 Suggested sample planning sheet for six patients

The legal and ethical principles of patient privacy need to be remembered when using and disposing of this time planner. Do not leave it in a public area or in a patient's room. Abbreviations (e.g. RIB – rest in bed, Sh – shower, M – medications) can also be used for identifying care actions and patient names, making it difficult for non-nursing or other healthcare staff to understand. Abbreviations will also help larger amounts of information to be written in a small space. Planning sheets are to be shredded at the end of the shift along with handover notes as they contain patient identification information and notes regarding care.

IMPLEMENT CARE ROUNDING

While planning your work for the shift, schedule time each hour to complete a care round where physical and verbal contact is made with each patient. The first care round can be included as part of planning your workload at the beginning of the shift, while reviewing each patient's care plans and charts. Rounding can also be included while completing other care actions or work tasks, with the questions and actions that are part of rounding being implemented whenever completing a nursing care action, and before moving on to the next patient. Within some facilities, patients are in two- or four-bed rooms, making it easier to see and communicate with the patients while completing your work. Patients in single rooms need to be visited specifically, as there is a higher risk of them being left without any contact from the nurse (or other healthcare workers) for an extended period of time.

A 'care round' requires the nurse to physically visit and interact with the patient each hour (or 2-hourly, according to policy). Any scheduled tasks are implemented, and the patients are asked a series of specific questions to address patient concerns. When entering the patient's bed area or room, introduce yourself and explain why you are there. Use the opportunity to check any charts that may need updating and check the safety and tidiness of the environment (e.g. tripping hazards, bed brakes, excess furniture). Then ask the patient questions to assess their comfort and needs, following the facility's preferred formula. The two common formulas are:

- Five Ps – pain management, personal needs, possessions, position and plugs
- ABCDE – activity, bathroom, comfort, diet and environment (Langley, 2015; Wilson, 2017).

The key concepts of these formulas are to: assess and implement actions for the patient's pain; offer assistance with elimination needs and fluid or dietary intake; ensure the patient is in a comfortable position in the bed or chair; ensure the call bell is in reach; ensure the safety and correct functioning of all equipment being used (e.g. IV pumps and all plugged-in devices); and ensure that personal items are in reach (i.e. water, tissues, TV remote, light switch, waste bag and bedside table). Before leaving, ask the questions, "Is there anything else I can do for you before I leave? I have time now while I am with you." Advise the patient that a member of the nursing team will return in an hour or two to check on them again (Langley, 2015). Then move to the next patient and complete the process again.

IMPLEMENT PERSONAL STRESS MANAGEMENT SKILLS

Personal stress management skills include making adjustments to personal lifestyle, maintaining levels of knowledge relevant to the work area and developing good workplace skills. Within the workplace, consult and work closely with workplace mentors, preceptors and facilitators to receive feedback, identify workplace learning needs and develop these skills. Be self-reflective and realistic about workplace expectations, and accept feedback. Don't take any criticism or guidance as personal. Use your experience and support from facilitators to develop good time management, positive workplace communication and competence in nursing skills. Also be aware of required underlying knowledge. Attend in-service sessions when they are available, and take personal time to study and research.

Developing personal coping skills to help you manage workplace stress, and other stressors in life that can impact on your work, may require making changes in your daily life. Modern life can easily become busy, and sometimes there is a need to slow down or create balance. Identify small actions that can be implemented to make change. Be careful not to attempt making a large number of small changes all at the same time, as this will generate stress itself. The impact of shift work upon regular routines and lifestyle (e.g. sleep patterns, disruption to eating and exercise habits) needs to be managed. The high number of females within the nursing profession also creates stress, often due to them managing family commitments and responsibilities.

The following list of actions are personal skills to help people cope with and manage workplace-generated stress.

- Find value in your work, and put yourself in the right mindset before going to work.
- Arrive at work on time, prepared for shift handover.
- If possible, prepare clothes and good food the night before a shift to reduce rushing before leaving home.

- Establish and maintain a healthy diet (fruit, vegetables, grains and protein), and don't skip meals.
- Relax after work. Take a hot shower, stretch or read a novel, practise meditation, spend time with family and have regular downtime.
- Ensure you have enough sleep each night, and try to maintain a pattern that can help the body establish a sleep routine.
- Exercise regularly.

Assess your current actions and lifestyle patterns, then make a plan of how to maintain or improve on these life skills. Be realistic, and don't attempt to make too many changes at one time. Also be aware of your physical health and act on any health problems such as headaches, cardiovascular disease, weight gain, impaired memory and concentration, sleep problems, anxiety and depression that may be created by ongoing stress. Consult your GP and follow any medical advice they provide.

CASE STUDY

You are an enrolled nurse working on a busy medical ward and have been allocated the care of four patients, all in single rooms (rooms A, B, C and D). Mr Rogers in room A has a left-sided weakness post cerebrovascular accident; Mrs Basil in room B has acute pneumonia and becomes short of breath easily; Mr Roberts in room C has a history of ischaemic heart disease and angina, and tires easily; and Mrs Ingram in room D is frail and has advanced dementia, awaiting placement to an aged care facility.

The patients in rooms A, B and C require a moderate level of assistance with transferring, mobility and meeting their needs for activities of daily living (ADL; i.e. hygiene, grooming and elimination). The patient in room D requires a higher level of assistance with all ADLs and tends to wander out of her room occasionally.

Time management
1. Create a time management plan for the morning shift for these patients.

Care rounding
1. Review the time management plan you have created, and identify when you will complete care rounds during this shift.
2. List the questions you would ask when completing a care round.

Stress management
1. Review the list of personal coping skills. Identify two of these that you could focus on and create a plan of how or what you will do to help you cope with workplace-created stress.

Note: These notes are summaries of the most important points in the assessments/procedures, and are not exhaustive on the subject. The naming of documents or charts may differ from state to state, and facility to facility. In all possible situations the guidelines of the ACSQHC are used when describing national charts or documents (e.g. the ACSQHC Observation and Response Chart is named the Adult Observation and Response Chart in WA, and the Rapid Detection and Response Observation Chart in SA). References of the materials used to compile the information have been supplied. The student is expected to have learned the material surrounding each skill as presented in the references. No single reference is complete on the subject.

REFERENCES

Australian Commission on Safety and Quality in Health Care (ACSQHC). (2019). *FAQ about Partnering with Consumers in the NSQHS Standards* (2nd ed.). http://www.safetyandquality.gov.au/faqs-about-partnering-consumers-nsqhs-standards-second-edition#what-is-partnering-with-consumers?

Bragg, L., Bugajski, A., Marchese, M., Caldwell, R., Houle, L., Thompson, R., Chula, R., Keith, C. & Lengerich, A. (2016). How do patients perceive hourly rounding? *Nursing Management*, 47(11), pp. 11–13.

Fedele, R. (2017). The rise of burnout: An emerging challenge facing nurses and midwives. *Australian Nursing & Midwifery Journal*, 25(5), pp. 18–23.

García-Herrero, S., Lopez-Garcia, J. R., Herrera, S., Fontaneda, I., Báscones, S. M. & Mariscal, M. A. (2017). The influence of recognition and social support on European health professionals' occupational stress: A demands-control-social support-recognition Bayesian network model. *Biomed Research International*, 2017;2017:4673047.

Langley, S. (2015). Effects of rounding on patient care. *Nursing Standard* (2014+), 29(42), p. 51.

Langille, J. (2017). Fight or flight … or fix? Employers must work with employees to address workplace stress. *Canadian Journal of Medical Laboratory Science*, 79(4), pp. 26–9.

Nursing and Midwifery Board of Australia (NMBA). (2018). *Standards for Practice: Enrolled Nurse. NMBA.*

Setting Priorities. (2017). *CNA training advisor: Lesson plans for busy staff trainers*, 15(12), pp. 1–5.

Wilson, L. (2017). *Nursing Staff Responsiveness to Patients and Hourly Rounding.* Wilson Walden University. https://scholarworks.waldenu.edu/cgi/viewcontent. cgi?article=5131&context=dissertations

World Health Organization (WHO). (2020). *Occupational Health: Stress at the Workplace.* https://www.who.int/news-room/q-a-detail/ occupational-health-stress-at-the-workplace

RECOMMENDED READINGS

Department of Health. (2013). *Roll Out of Hourly Patient Rounding at Western Health.* Victoria State Government. https://www2.health. vic.gov.au/about/publications/factsheets/Fact-sheet-11-Patient-rounding

Pignata, S., Boyd, C.M., Winefield, A.H. & Provis, C. (2017). Interventions: Employees' perceptions of what reduces stress. *Biomed Research International*, 2017;2017:3919080.

ESSENTIAL SKILLS COMPETENCY

Professional Workplace Skills
Demonstrates the ability to plan and implement care for the shift

Criteria for skill performance	Y	D
(Numbers indicate *Enrolled Nurse Standards for Practice*, 2016)	(Satisfactory)	(Requires development)
1. Identifies indication (8.3, 8.4)		
2. Demonstrates problem-solving abilities; recognises personal professional skill levels and need for self-development (4.1, 4.2, 8.3, 8.4, 9.4)		

3. Implements time management skills
  a. Gathers relevant patient information from shift handover, plus patient charts and nursing care plans (1.4, 1.5, 2.10, 3.2, 4.2, 6.5)
  b. Takes time to plan and prioritise patient care using a planning sheet; allocates times and actions appropriately (1.4, 1.5, 2.10, 3.2, 6.5, 8.4)
  c. Liaises with other staff (5.2, 7.3)
  d. Revises, reprioritises and updates planning page when unplanned events occur (4.2, 6.5, 8.4)
  e. Keeps planning sheet in location that protects patient privacy (1.1, 1.3)		

4. Implements care rounding
  a. Identifies correct times for care rounding and includes care rounding when completing other nursing care (3.2, 2.10, 6.1, 6.5, 6.6)
  b. Physically visits and interacts with each patient to complete care round (hourly or 2-hourly) (2.1, 2.3, 2.4, 2.5, 3.2, 6.3, 6.5)
  c. Introduces self to patient and explains reason for visit (2.1, 2.3, 2.4, 2.5, 6.3)
  d. Checks patient's charts, personal needs and safety issues; uses a formula to guide questions (i.e. Five Ps or ABCDE) (3.2, 2.10, 6.1, 6.6)
  e. Asks 'Is there anything I can do for you before I leave?'; states time period when another nurse will return before leaving patient's room (2.1, 2.3, 2.4, 2.5, 2.10, 3.2, 6.1, 6.3)		

5. Implements personal stress management
  a. Consults with peers, mentors and facilitator in workplace to gain feedback, plus assesses personal skill and knowledge levels; uses valid self-reflection (8.1, 8.2, 9.1, 10.1, 10.2, 10.3, 10.5)
  b. Develops and uses workplace time management skills (6.5)
  c. Sets realistic goals for workplace self-development (9.1, 10.2, 10.3, 10.5, 10.6)
  d. Assesses own personal lifestyle and needs for adjustment (10.6)
  e. Develops positive workplace attitude (10.6)
  f. Arrives on time, and is prepared for the workplace (6.5, 10.6)
  g. Eats a regular and healthy diet (10.6)
  h. Establishes regular exercise and downtime out of work (10.6)
  i. Gets sufficient sleep, with a regular sleep routine (10.6)
  j. Creates personal goals for any adjustments to personal coping skill (10.6)
  k. Consults others when requiring assistance or other health problems created by stress occur (10.6)		

6. Demonstrates ability to link theory to practice (8.3, 8.4, 8.5, 9.4)		

Student: _____

Clinical facilitator: _____   Date: _____

CHAPTER 3.2

BEDMAKING

IDENTIFY INDICATIONS

Beds are made to promote comfort for the patient, to encourage rest and sleep, and to reduce the risk of pressure injuries. For patients resting in bed, soiled linen can be changed with minimal disruption to the patient. Beds can be made up with the top linen folded into a pack which is quickly spread out across the patient, lessening movement for the patient (e.g. postoperatively), or with the top linen over a bed cradle to keep the bedclothes off the patient.

GATHER EQUIPMENT

Clean linen is collected as necessary. Soiled linen should be changed as required, and other linen changed according to facility policy. Fitted sheets are generally used on the bottom (refer to mattress manufacturers' guidelines for any specific requirements as some will require a flat sheet), and a flat sheet for the top. If there is a risk of incontinence or leakage some care facilities may utilise reusable bed protectors or disposable liners (Koutoukidis et al., 2017).

Extra pillows will help maintain comfort and position. Bed cradles can be used to keep the weight of bedclothes off the patient. Relevant pressure care devices, including pressure-reducing mattresses, will be stated in the patient's care plan. Intravenous poles and drainage carriers may be required, and postoperatively specific instruments may be placed at the bedside. A linen skip, for the soiled linen, should also be collected before the procedure is started (Koutoukidis et al., 2017).

THE BEDMAKING PROCEDURE

Identify safety considerations

Principles of workplace health and safety (WHS) should be maintained with bed brakes applied, the bed height adjusted and the principles of manual handling followed, to reduce the risk of injury to the nurse (WA Department of Commerce, 2020). Become familiar with different types of beds and their functions. Furniture in the area should be moved away from the bed, or the bed wheeled out to enable safe access. If the patient is to be sat out of bed during the process, a suitable chair must be provided. Ensure the bed is at a safe height for them to transfer in and out of bed. Patients who are at risk of falls should have the bed lowered to the lowest height after the bed has been made.

Principles of infection control are also followed. All used linen should be handled with care to avoid the dispersal of microorganisms (NHMRC, 2019). Linen is not shaken nor placed on room furniture or the floor but is placed directly into the linen skip. Check that none of the patient's belongings are caught up in the linen. Ensure you are wearing appropriate personal protective equipment (PPE) when handling linen soiled with body substances and place the soiled linen in a leakproof bag.

Perform hand hygiene

Perform hand hygiene before touching the patient or the patient's surrounds and prior to any procedure involving patient contact to reduce the possibility of cross-contamination. Hand hygiene is the most effective method of infection control as it removes transient organisms from the hands of the nurse (see **Skill 1.1**).

Give a clear explanation of the procedure and establish therapeutic communication

Introduce yourself, and check you have the correct patient. Explain the procedure and gain the patient's consent. Giving a clear explanation is required to gain legal consent and to address policy requirements. It will also assist the patient to cooperate with the procedure, allay anxiety and assist in establishing a therapeutic relationship.

Demonstrate problem-solving abilities

Assess the need for assistance to complete the task. More than one nurse may be needed to make an occupied bed or to transfer the patient from the bed. Use appropriate equipment when moving, transferring or positioning the patient (see **Skills 3.3** and **3.12**). Privacy is maintained by closing the door or pulling the screens. The patient must be covered when sitting out of bed.

Carry out procedure

Make the bed according to the patient's needs. Ensure the bottom sheet is free of wrinkles, as these are uncomfortable and increase the risk of pressure injuries.

Occupied bed

1. Turn on bed brakes, elevate bed to correct working height and then, depending on the patient's condition, flatten the bed as much as possible.
2. Extend the foot of the bed to hold the linen.
3. Loosen the top linen, and leave the top sheet over the patient to maintain their dignity.
4. Fold reusable linen (e.g. blankets) to the foot of the bed.
5. Place any soiled linen in the linen skip.
6. Roll the patient onto their side, ensuring the bed rail is up or a second nurse is on that side.
7. Loosen the bottom sheet, then roll the sheet to the centre of the bed.
8. Roll and tuck the bottom sheet under the patient as much as possible.

9. Place the new bottom sheet/s in position and tuck in on the first nurse's side. If using a flat sheet, mitre the corners.
10. Ensure the sheets are wrinkle free. Roll the remainder of the new sheet to the centre of the bed and tuck under the patient. Additional draw sheets or liners are added following the same principles.
11. Carefully roll patient back onto their other side, facing the first nurse.
12. The second nurse will then pull the used linen through, remove and place in linen skip. Non-sterile gloves and a plastic apron should be worn if there are body fluids. The mattress should be wiped if soiled.
13. The second nurse will then pull clean linen through. Tuck in and ensure sheets are wrinkle free.
14. Roll patient onto their back.
15. Spread a new top sheet over patient (and discard old top sheet). Tuck in the bottom and mitre the corners.
16. Spread and tuck in the blanket and quilt as required, ensuring each is added individually and the corners mitred.
17. Reposition patient as appropriate. Bed rails may be used according to patient safety needs. Leave patient comfortable with call bell and other necessities within reach. Lower bed to appropriate height before leaving patient.

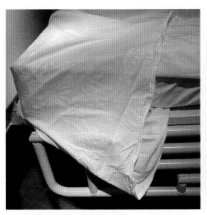 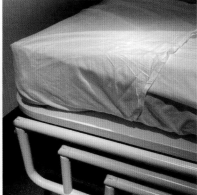 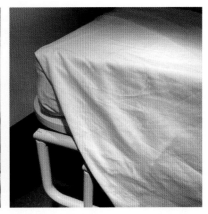

FIGURE 3.2.1 Mitred corners

Unoccupied bed

The same principles are followed, except the patient is out of bed. Remove the pillows from the bed. The bottom sheet is changed first, with the new sheet smoothed out across the bed and tucked in. Add extra draw sheets or liners if required. Add the top sheet and blankets individually, mitring the corners as each one is added. Leave the sheets and blankets loose over the side of the bed, ensure they are even on each side and are not touching the floor.

Return the patient to bed as per **Skills 3.3** and **3.12**. Adjust the bed height and position correctly for the patient. Leave the patient comfortable with the bed handset, call bell and other necessities within reach and lower the bed before leaving the patient.

Perform hand hygiene

Maintain the 5 Moments for Hand Hygiene and perform hand hygiene after touching the patient and the patient's surrounds. Hand hygiene should be implemented between making each bed if several beds are being made at one time.

CLEAN, REPLACE OR DISPOSE OF EQUIPMENT

Soiled linen is placed in the linen carrier. Follow facility policies for different types of linen skips and washing. Ensure linen contaminated with body substances is placed in the correct leakproof bags. Unwanted pillows or other equipment are cleaned as per facility policy and returned to appropriate storage area.

DOCUMENT AND REPORT RELEVANT INFORMATION

This procedure is not usually documented, unless there are unusual circumstances to report.

CRITICAL THINKING

You are working in a four-bed room on an early shift. Two of your patients are self-care and two require being sponged in bed. What important patient care needs should be considered when making an occupied bed?

Note: These notes are summaries of the most important points in the assessments/procedures, and are not exhaustive on the subject. The naming of documents or charts may differ from state to state, and facility to facility. In all possible situations the guidelines of the ACSQHC are used when describing national charts or documents (e.g. the ACSQHC Observation and Response Chart is named the Adult Observation and Response Chart in WA, and the Rapid Detection and Response Observation Chart in SA). References of the materials used to compile the information have been supplied. The student is expected to have learned the material surrounding each skill as presented in the references. No single reference is complete on the subject.

REFERENCES

Koutoukidis, G., Stainton, K. & Hughson, J. (2017). *Tabbner's Nursing Care: Theory and Practice* (6th ed.). Sydney: Elsevier.

National Health and Medical Research Council (NHMRC) (2019) *Australian Guidelines for the Prevention and Control of Infection in Healthcare*. https://www.safetyandquality.gov.au/sites/default/files/2020-03/australian_guidelines_for_the_prevention_and_control_of_infection-in_healthcare_februrary_2020.pdf

WA Department of Commerce. (2020). *Manual Tasks in Healthcare and Social Assistance*. https://www.commerce.wa.gov.au/worksafe/manual-tasks-healthcare-and-social-assistance

ESSENTIAL SKILLS COMPETENCY

Bedmaking
Demonstrates the ability to effectively and safely make a bed, either occupied or unoccupied

Criteria for skill performance	Y	D
(Numbers indicate *Enrolled Nurse Standards for Practice*, 2016)	(Satisfactory)	(Requires development)
1. Identifies indication (8.3, 8.4)		
2. Gathers equipment (1.2, 1.6, 6.4, 8.4, 9.4): ■ linen skip ■ clean linen ■ PPE if required		
3. Identifies safety considerations (1.2, 3.2, 3.9, 6.4, 9.4)		
4. Performs hand hygiene (1.2, 1.4, 1.8, 3.9, 6.4, 9.4)		
5. Evidence of therapeutic communication with the patient; gives explanation of procedure, gains patient consent (2.1, 2.3, 2.4, 2.5)		
6. Demonstrates problem-solving abilities; e.g. assists patient appropriately, provides privacy, provides relevant equipment (4.1, 4.2, 8.3, 8.4)		
7. Carries out procedure following principles of manual handling (1.2, 1.3, 1.4, 1.8, 2.3, 2.7, 3.2, 3.9, 6.1, 6.3, 6.4, 8.4, 9.4)		
8. Assists patient to position of comfort in bed (1.2, 1.4, 1.8, 2.3, 2.7, 3.2, 3.9, 6.1, 6.3, 6.4, 8.4, 9.4)		
9. Performs hand hygiene (1.2, 1.4, 1.8, 3.9, 6.4, 9.4)		
10. Cleans, replaces and disposes of equipment appropriately (1.2, 1.4, 3.9, 6.5, 9.4)		
11. Documents and reports relevant information (1.2, 1.3, 1.4, 3.2, 5.3, 6.6, 7.1, 7.2, 7.3, 7.4, 7.5, 9.4)		
12. Demonstrates ability to link theory to practice (8.3, 8.4, 8.5, 9.4)		

Student:

Clinical facilitator: Date:

CHAPTER 3.3

ASSISTING THE PATIENT TO AMBULATE

IDENTIFY INDICATIONS

Patients require assistance to ambulate for a variety of reasons. These can include cerebrovascular accidents, paralysis, brain damage, an amputation or some musculoskeletal disorders, frail aged and postoperative patients. Assisting the postoperative patient to ambulate is the most effective nursing measure to prevent postoperative complications. Early mobilisation is also beneficial for unwell patients in other settings, including patients who have a high acuity (Klein et al., 2018; Wyatt et al., 2020). This is initially provided by a physiotherapist and then followed up by the nurse. For any patient who has been immobilised, regaining the ability to walk improves the patient's wellbeing.

Prolonged immobility can have severe consequences for the patient. These consequences include the following:

- constipation
- urinary retention
- altered tissue perfusion
- pressure injuries
- hypostatic pneumonia
- osteoporosis
- renal calculi
- deep vein thrombosis/venous thromboemboli.

Early mobilisation can prevent these complications and reduce hospitalisation time). Increasing the mobility of elderly patients through nurse assisted and promoted ambulation helps to maintain independence and improve their health outcomes.

ASSISTING THE PATIENT

Identify safety considerations

Assessment of a patient who has been immobile is required before attempting to assist them to walk. Consult the patient's care plan, falls risk assessment, **Skill 2.2**, mobility chart or physiotherapy chart for individual instructions. Activity tolerance, strength, orthostatic hypotension, pain, coordination and balance should be taken into consideration.

The following are some points to consider.

- Muscle strength and range of motion is determined first, with gradual progression to active range of motion. The physiotherapist will give instructions about relevant exercises for the patient. The patient's sitting balance is encouraged by initially positioning them in an upright position and then assisting them to 'dangle' at the edge of the bed. This is practised until there is no dizziness or swaying noticed or reported.
- Standing balance is encouraged. The patient is assisted to gradually stand at the bedside by pushing up from the bed. Standing balance is attained when the patient is able to keep the trunk still and move their extremities without swaying.

The nurse must remain close to the patient who is ambulating. Rest periods need to be scheduled because ambulation is an increase in activity and the patient may fatigue. Initial exercise and ambulation periods should be short, then gradually increased. Environmental factors also require consideration. The floor must be dry and should be free of clutter, such as electrical cords, scatter rugs, magazines and newspapers. Handrails give the patient a sense of security. The patient should be wearing shoes or slippers that fit well, give good support and have non-skid soles. Anti-embolic stockings (thrombo-embolic-deterrent stockings – TEDs) should not be removed. Medical equipment (IV tubing, urinary catheters, chest drains or wound drains) will require consideration to assist the patient to get out of bed and walk without constraint. IV poles with wheels and hangers to carry urinary catheters or drainage apparatus can be used to increase mobility. Raise the height of the bed so the patient's hips are level with, or higher than, the knees when the feet are on the floor. This reduces the effort of standing for the patient (Dougherty & Lister, 2015). A thorough environmental assessment must be undertaken if the patient is beginning to mobilise in the community setting.

The nurse must also assess their own strength and ability. If unsure, recruit another nurse to assist.

This is a workplace health and safety issue as well as a patient safety measure. Assistive devices (as outlined below) should be available for the patient's use as necessary. Inspect the device to ensure the rubber tips are not worn or showing signs of poor tread, the frame is stable, the hand grips are secure and complete, and the metal tubing is not cracked or damaged (Dougherty & Lister, 2015). If the patient requires specific aids such as crutches or various types of walker, a mobility program should be first completed by a physiotherapist.

Identify assistive devices that may be needed

- *Walkers* provide four points of support, thus giving a wide base, and are the most secure of all of the assistive devices. A range of walkers are available; some have wheels, some have arm supports, some have brakes. The type is determined by the physiotherapist. The top of the standard walker is level with the hands when the elbows are flexed between 25 and 30 degrees. The patient places the walker in front of them and steps forward. Walkers are usually constructed of aluminium since they need to be lightweight.
- *Crutches (underarm and elbow)* are used when single-leg weight-bearing or modified weight-bearing is allowed. The patient needs upper-body strength and arm control to use crutches. The patient's weight is supported by the wrists, hands and shoulders. When using underarm crutches, pressure on the axilla can cause irreversible nerve and tissue damage. Crutches must be measured and fitted by a physiotherapist. Different gaits are used for different types of weight-bearing. The patient requires instruction in the type of gait to be used for their type of disability. The gait pattern is determined by the physician or the physiotherapist and is usually taught to the patient by the physiotherapist.
- *Walking sticks* provide extra stability for patients who have one weak leg but are still able to bear weight on both legs. They also promote a feeling of security. The tip of the stick should have a non-skid rubber surface for safety. The top hand grip is held in line with the hip joint of the unaffected leg, with the patient's elbow slightly flexed. The affected leg and stick are moved forward simultaneously while the unaffected leg bears the weight. The affected leg and stick then take the weight while the unaffected leg is moved forward.

Perform hand hygiene

Perform hand hygiene before touching the patient or the patient's surrounds and prior to any procedure involving patient contact to reduce the possibility of cross-contamination. Hand hygiene is the most effective method of infection control as it removes transient organisms from the hands of the nurse (see **Skill 1.1**).

Give a clear explanation of the procedure and establish therapeutic communication

Establish therapeutic communication; identify your patient and gain the patient's consent. A clear, thorough explanation of the procedure, including distance to be walked, assistance to be expected and instructions to alert the nurse to any fatigue or pain encountered should be given. The patient will then be able to make an informed decision about their strength and ability. Explanation, as always, enlists patient cooperation and helps to alleviate any anxieties they may have. Clarify that the patient has understood the instructions. Most patients are somewhat unsure about leaving the safety of their bed and venturing out on limbs that feel unstable and cause pain. A calm, confident manner, plenty of sincere reassurance and physical support assists the patient to take their first steps.

Workplace health and safety

Ensure principles of workplace health and safety and patient safety needs are met. These include correct bed height, bed brakes on, cooperative patient, a safe environment and use of principles of manual handling, as well as safe and correct equipment (WA Department of Mines, Industry Regulation and Safety, 2020).

Assist the patient to walk

Progressive assistance may be needed. The patient is supported until they gain confidence. Walking with the nurse allows for support of the patient if they lose their balance or feel weak. Assist the weak or dizzy patient to the nearest chair or bed, or if necessary, to the floor.

Perform hand hygiene

Maintain the 5 Moments for Hand Hygiene and perform hand hygiene after touching the patient and the patient's surrounds.

CLEAN, REPLACE OR DISPOSE OF EQUIPMENT

Return a patient's own walking aids to their bed area after use. Common-use equipment should be cleaned with disposable wipes, according to facility policy, after use and returned to the storage area.

DOCUMENT AND REPORT RELEVANT INFORMATION

Documentation of ambulation should include distance walked, assistance required and patient response to ambulation (including any falls and a falls risk assessment). Ensure the nursing care plan and mobility chart is current in stating the patient's mobility needs.

CASE STUDY

Jonathon Abbott, a 24-year-old male patient, was admitted 5 days ago after a motor vehicle accident. He has been to theatre and had surgical repair of the right femur. He is now partially weight-bearing with the aid of elbow crutches. He requires assistance to the bathroom. How will you assist him?

Note: These notes are summaries of the most important points in the assessments/procedures, and are not exhaustive on the subject. The naming of documents or charts may differ from state to state, and facility to facility. In all possible situations the guidelines of the ACSQHC are used when describing national charts or documents (e.g. the ACSQHC Observation and Response Chart is named the Adult Observation and Response Chart in WA, and the Rapid Detection and Response Observation Chart in SA). References of the materials used to compile the information have been supplied. The student is expected to have learned the material surrounding each skill as presented in the references. No single reference is complete on the subject.

CRITICAL THINKING/LIFESPAN

In the following scenarios consider the extra equipment and actions required:
- a 9-month-old child requiring a bath
- a 32-year-old postoperative patient with peripheral intravenous catheter (PIVC), indwelling catheter (IDC), vacuum drain in situ, who is a two-person transfer requiring a shower
- an 83-year-old non-weight-bearing woman who requires a shower on a commode chair.

REFERENCES

Dougherty, L. & Lister, S. (eds). (2015). *The Royal Marsden Hospital Manual of Clinical Nursing Procedures* (9th ed.). Oxford: Wiley-Blackwell.

Klein, K.E., Bena, J.F., Mulkey, M. & Albert, N.M. (2018). Sustainability of a nurse-driven early progressive mobility protocol and patient clinical and psychological health outcomes in a neurological intensive care unit. *Intensive & Critical Care Nursing*, 45 April, 45, pp. 11–17.

WA Department of Mines, Industry Regulation and Safety. (2020). *Manual Tasks in Healthcare and Social Assistance.* Government of Western Australia. https://www.commerce.wa.gov.au/worksafe/manual-tasks-healthcare-and-social-assistance

Wyatt, S., Meacci, K. & Arnold, M. (2020). Integrating safe patient handling and early mobility, *Journal of Nursing Care Quality*, April/June, 35(2), pp. 130–4. doi: 10.1097/NCQ.0000000000000425

RECOMMENDED READINGS

Australian Nursing and Midwifery Federation (ANMF). (2018). *ANMF Policy – Safe Patient Handling.* http://www.anmf.org.au/documents/policies/P_Safe_Patient_Handling.pdf

WorkSafe Victoria. (n.d.). *Safety and Prevention: Your Industry – Aged Care.* Victorian State Government. http://www.worksafe.vic.gov.au/pages/safety-and-prevention/your-industry/aged-care

ESSENTIAL SKILLS COMPETENCY

Assisting the Patient to Ambulate

Demonstrates the ability to effectively and safely assist a patient to ambulate

Criteria for skill performance	Y	D
(Numbers indicate *Enrolled Nurse Standards for Practice*, 2016)	(Satisfactory)	(Requires development)
1. Identifies indication (8.3, 8.4)		
2. Identifies safety considerations (1.2, 1.4, 1.8, 3.2, 3.9, 6.4, 6.6, 8.4, 9.4)		
3. Gathers equipment and mobility aid (1.2, 1.6, 6.4, 8.4, 9.4)		
4. Performs hand hygiene (1.2, 1.4, 1.8, 3.9, 6.4, 9.4)		
5. Evidence of effective therapeutic communication with the patient; gives patient a clear explanation of procedure and confirms patient understanding, gains patient consent (2.1, 2.3, 2.4, 2.5, 6.3)		
6. Assists the patient to walk (1.2, 1.4, 1.8, 2.1, 2.3, 2.7, 3.2, 3.9, 6.1, 6.3, 6.4, 6.6, 8.4, 9.4)		
7. Performs hand hygiene (1.2, 1.4, 1.8, 3.9, 6.4, 9.4)		
8. Cleans, replaces and disposes of equipment appropriately (1.2, 1.4, 3.9, 6.5, 9.4)		
9. Documents and reports relevant information (1.2, 1.3, 1.8, 3.2, 5.3, 6.6, 7.1, 7.2, 7.3, 7.4, 7.5)		
10. Demonstrates ability to link theory to practice (8.3, 8.4, 8.5, 9.4)		

Student:

Clinical facilitator: Date:

CHAPTER 3.4

ASSISTING THE PATIENT WITH EATING AND DRINKING

IDENTIFY INDICATIONS

Fluid and dietary intake are essential components of everyday life. Eating should be an enjoyable experience, but many elderly patients have difficulty swallowing (dysphagia) (Dai et al., 2017; Thompson, 2016). Should there be any doubt about a patient's ability to swallow effectively, a speech therapist would assess the patient and then order a texture-modified diet and thickened fluids. Patients with a variety of neurological and physical impairments may have difficulty feeding themselves, and would require nursing assistance. Respecting individuals and maintaining their dignity while assisting with eating and drinking is an integral part of nursing care.

GATHER EQUIPMENT

A variety of self-help devices such as non-slip placemats or modified cutlery and crockery will be specified on the patient's care plan. Sipper cups or straws may be needed for drinking. Clothing protectors, if needed, must be suitable to a patient's age. Refer to diet charts or the care plan to identify the level of thickened fluids and texture (e.g. soft) for patients with dysphagia. According to facility policy, use pre-prepared thickened fluids, or add fluid-thickening agent as per the manufacturer's instructions.

ASSISTING WITH EATING AND DRINKING

Identify safety considerations

The patient should sit upright to eat and drink, unless their treatment excludes this (e.g. spinal surgery). The temperature of fluids and food should be checked to ensure they are not too hot, particularly drinks, if the patient is using a straw. Trays, plates and glasses should be stable, and unbreakable if the patient could potentially knock them over. Visually impaired people need to have the layout of the food tray or of the table explained to them. Patients with dysphagia should always be monitored when eating (even if feeding themselves), never be rushed and ensure each spoonful is completely swallowed. Dysphagia increases the risk of aspiration pneumonia, malnutrition and dehydration (Dai et al., 2017; Shune & Foster, 2017; Sivertsen et al., 2017).

If the patient experiences any difficulties eating or drinking, cease feeding and report to the registered nurse (RN). It may be necessary to remove food already in the mouth, or even to commence oral suction. Indicators of difficulty with swallowing include coughing, choking or gagging while eating, and taking extended time to eat a meal. Further indicators may occur after a meal, and can include a gurgling voice, sputum coloured with food or fluids, excess drooling or pooling of saliva in the mouth, and regurgitation of food. Patients with these symptoms should be reported to the RN as they may require assessment of their gag reflex by a speech therapist and dietary modification to prevent aspiration of their food and fluids (Thompson, 2016).

Perform hand hygiene

Perform hand hygiene before touching the patient or the patient's surrounds and prior to any procedure involving patient contact to reduce the possibility of cross-contamination. Hand hygiene is the most effective method of infection control as it removes transient organisms from the hands of the nurse (see **Skill 1.1**).

Give a clear explanation of the procedure and establish therapeutic communication

Introduce yourself, and check you have the correct patient. Explain the procedure and gain the patient's consent. Giving a clear explanation is required to gain legal consent and to address policy requirements. It will also assist the patient to cooperate with the procedure, allay anxiety and assist in establishing a therapeutic relationship.

When preparing the patient, explain it is mealtime. This will often facilitate cooperation with activities such as toileting prior to the meal. Patients with dementia may forget to eat their food, so the nurse must explain what is on the plate, and gently remind them to take a mouthful and to swallow it. The actual food and its position on the plate should be described to a visually impaired person. The clock face positioning is the most commonly used method. When feeding patients, the nurse must inform them before offering each spoonful, and describe what is on it. If possible, check that they like what is being offered to them.

Demonstrate problem-solving abilities

Offer toileting facilities 30 minutes prior to the meal, as this will assist patient comfort. Provide hand hygiene opportunities. Check the care plan for mobility assistance. More than one nurse may be needed to transfer the patient or reposition them up the bed into a sitting position. In residential care facilities residents may require prompting and assistance to mobilise to the dining room, especially those with dementia. It is important to encourage residents to use the dining room, as eating is also a social experience that reduces the risk of malnutrition in the elderly (Dijkstra, 2017). Recognise that patient food preferences and dislikes will impact on their motivation to eat or complete their meal (Benigas, 2017). Ensure good oral hygiene is maintained (Thompson, 2016). If the patient has dentures, ensure they are clean and in situ, as this helps make the meal a pleasurable experience. Clear the environment of unnecessary clutter for ease of positioning of the tray or plate. Also remove items that create unpleasant odours, or images that could affect the patient's appetite. Clothing protectors may be required. The care plan would also identify the level of assistance required (e.g. cutting up food or actual feeding).

Assist with eating

Encourage the patient to help themselves as much as possible by assisting them to a sitting position and setting them up with their meal (Thompson, 2016). Whenever possible, encourage patients (including those with dementia who forget) to use or hold their eating utensils, and move the food to their mouth. Prompting patients with dementia to eat or drink using mimicking behaviours has also been found to be successful (Shune & Foster, 2017). Review the diet sheet to ensure the meal is the correct one for

the patient and meets their food preferences. Check the position of the patient, and support with pillows where necessary.

For patients requiring more assistance, the nurse should sit in front or to the side of the patient. Facing the person is a respectful position, and it allows for observation of any problems. Use a smaller sized spoon (e.g. teaspoon) for patients with dysphagia and offer food slowly. Give the patient time to chew and swallow each spoonful before being offered another mouthful. The food should be placed in the unaffected side of the mouth for those with facial paralysis. Check food is not pouching (remaining in the side of the mouth). Wipe the face if there is any food or liquid spilt, to help maintain dignity. As part of the conversation, ask the patient if they like the food. If they don't, try to ascertain their food likes and dislikes, and report this to the dietitian/catering staff. A patient turning their head away when being offered food and fluids is an indication that the diet is not liked or no more food is wanted. Do not try to force-feed the patient, but document and report the intake to the RN. At the completion of the meal, offer mouth care, hand washing and remove clothing protectors. Leave the patient in a comfortable upright position for at least 30 minutes after the meal.

If the patient experiences any difficulties eating or drinking (see safety considerations stated earlier), cease feeding and report to the RN. It may be necessary to remove food already in the mouth, or even to commence oral suction.

Perform hand hygiene

Maintain the 5 Moments for Hand Hygiene and perform hand hygiene after touching the patient and the patient's surrounds.

CLEAN, REPLACE OR DISPOSE OF EQUIPMENT

Remove the finished meal tray/plate and empty glasses as soon as possible. Soiled clothing protectors should be discarded in the linen skip.

DOCUMENT AND REPORT RELEVANT INFORMATION

Record intake on a fluid balance chart or diet chart, if required, and report any discrepancies and difficulties to the RN.

CASE STUDY

An 84-year-Alexander Stopsis has been admitted to the ward post a right-sided cerebrovascular accident. Alexander has been assessed by the speech therapist and ordered level 2 mildly thick fluids and a minced/moist diet.

1. Identify 3 actions you will implement when feeding Alexander.
2. What signs and symptoms will you observe for?

Note: These notes are summaries of the most important points in the assessments/procedures, and are not exhaustive on the subject. The naming of documents or charts may differ from state to state, and facility to facility. In all possible situations the guidelines of the ACSQHC are used when describing national charts or documents (e.g. the ACSQHC Observation and Response Chart is named the Adult Observation and Response Chart in WA, and the Rapid Detection and Response Observation Chart in SA). References of the materials used to compile the information have been supplied. The student is expected to have learned the material surrounding each skill as presented in the references. No single reference is complete on the subject.

CRITICAL THINKING

For each of the following patients with the stated problems or disabilities, describe the type of assistance that may be required with eating and drinking. Include in your answer any safety precautions when relevant.

1. A postoperative patient with IV cannula and IV line inserted in their right hand

2. A patient with dementia

3. An 18-month-old child

4. A visually impaired patient

REFERENCES

Benigas, J. (2017). Optimizing eating and swallowing for people with dementia. *ASHA Leader*, 22(8), pp. 93–5.

Dai, P., Murry, T., Wong, M.M., Yiu, E.L. & Chana, K.K. (2017). Indicators of dysphagia in aged care facilities. *Journal of Speech, Language & Hearing Research*, 60(9), pp. 2416–2426.

Dijkstra, A. (2017). Using the Care Dependency Scale for identifying patients at risk for malnutrition. *BMC Nursing*, 168. doi:10.1186/s12912–017-0218–2

Shune, S.E. & Foster, K.A. (2017). Goal-directed drinking behaviors can be modified through behavioral mimicry. *Journal of Speech, Language and Hearing Research (Online)*, 60(6), pp. 1535–44.

Sivertsen, J., Graverholt, B. & Espehaug, B. (2017). Dysphagia screening after acute stroke: a quality improvement project using criteria-based clinical audit. *BMC Nursing*, 16, pp. 1–8.

Thompson, R. (2016). Identifying and managing dysphagia in the community. *Journal of Community Nursing*, 30(6), pp. 42–7.

RECOMMENDED READINGS

Crisp, J., Douglas, C., Rebeiro, G. & Waters, D. (2017). *Potter and Perry's Fundamentals of Nursing – Australian version* (5th ed.). Sydney: Elsevier.

Dougherty, L. & Lister, S. (eds). (2015). *The Royal Marsden Hospital Manual of Clinical Nursing Procedures* (9th ed.). Oxford: Wiley-Blackwell.

ESSENTIAL SKILLS COMPETENCY

Assisting the Patient With eating and Drinking

Demonstrates the ability to effectively and safely assist the patient who has difficulties eating and drinking

Criteria for skill performance	Y	D
(Numbers indicate *Enrolled Nurse Standards for Practice*, 2016)	(Satisfactory)	(Requires development)
1. Identifies indication (8.3, 8.4)		
2. Gathers equipment (1.2, 1.6, 6.4, 8.4, 9.4)		
3. Identifies safety considerations (1.2, 1.4, 1.8, 3.2, 3.9, 6.6, 8.4, 9.4)		
4. Performs hand hygiene (1.2, 1.4, 1.8, 3.9, 6.4, 9.4)		
5. Evidence of therapeutic communication with the patient; gives explanation of procedure, gains patient consent (2.1, 2.3, 2.4, 2.5, 6.3)		
6. Demonstrates problem-solving abilities; e.g. assists patient appropriately, recognises risk of swallowing difficulties, provides privacy, provides relevant equipment (4.1, 4.2, 8.3, 8.4, 9.4)		
7. Assists with feeding (1.2, 1.4, 1.8, 2.1, 2.10, 3.2, 3.9, 6.3, 6.6, 8.4, 9.4)		
8. Performs hand hygiene (1.2, 1.4, 1.8, 3.9, 6.4, 9.4)		
9. Cleans, replaces and disposes of equipment appropriately (1.2, 1.4, 3.9, 6.5, 9.4)		
10. Documents and reports relevant information (1.2, 1.3, 1.8, 3.2, 5.3, 6.6, 7.1, 7.2, 7.3, 7.5, 9.4)		
11. Demonstrates ability to link theory to practice (8.3, 8.4, 8.5, 9.4)		

Student:

Clinical facilitator: Date:

CHAPTER 3.5

ASSISTING THE PATIENT TO MAINTAIN PERSONAL HYGIENE AND GROOMING NEEDS – SPONGE (BED BATH) WITH ORAL HYGIENE, HAIR WASH IN BED, EYE AND NASAL CARE

IDENTIFY INDICATIONS

Helping a patient to meet their personal hygiene and grooming needs promotes a positive self-image, relaxation and a feeling of wellbeing along with promoting healthy skin and maintaining the body's first line of defence against disease (Gray et al., 2018). Assisting patients to meet their personal hygiene and grooming requirements is a basic human need and a core nursing skill, as most patients require some level of assistance, even if it is only for a brief period of time (Hørdam et al., 2018; Nøddeskou et al.. 2015). The level of assistance required to help a patient meet these activities of daily living is based on the patient's own self-care ability, or limitations created by their treatment (e.g. post-op, rest-in-bed restrictions). Assisting patients to meet their personal hygiene needs also creates an excellent opportunity to assess the patient's general physical status, complete routine daily skin assessments and encourage rehabilitation of the patient's self-care skills. It is also an opportunity for personal interaction and establishing a therapeutic relationship.

Sponging removes perspiration, excess skin oils and dead cells, and minimises body odour. A sponge is implemented when the patient is unconscious or physically unable to get out of bed, or when treatment precludes the possibility of the patient getting up to the shower (e.g. some post-op situations or traction). Consequently, a sponge can range from a full sponge, implemented by the nurse, to an assisted sponge, where the patient is able to partially wash themselves when provided with the equipment and minimal assistance is given by the nurse. Patients who require sponging will also require assistance with their other personal hygiene or grooming needs, which should be included as part of the sponge. These include oral hygiene, hair care, eye care, nasal care to remove dried secretions, shaving for males and dressing (i.e. putting on clothing). Oral hygiene is an essential part of a patient's care needs, and includes the care of a patient's dentures. Dental health is important for an individual's wellbeing, self-esteem and quality of life, as well as contributing to social inclusion, health and general nutrition (Daly & Smith, 2015; Red & O'Neal, 2020). It is important to assess and maintain the integrity of the oral mucosa, teeth and gums. Many patients can usually maintain their oral hygiene with some assistance.

PLAN THE PATIENT'S SPONGE

Assessment of the patient and reviewing their nursing care plan prior to implementing a sponge is important to prevent contravening other care requirements, or assuming a higher level of patient mobility or self-care than is relevant to their physical health status. Review the patient's nursing care plan for personal preferences, other treatment times, mobility needs and any care actions specific to the patient's hygiene. Prior to implementing the sponge, assess the patient for any pain, and administer pain relief if required. Based on the patient's mobility, ensure the correct manual handling equipment is available to reduce the risk of the patient or the nurse sustaining an injury while completing the sponge (Bartnik & Rice, 2013). Refer to **Skill 3.12** for repositioning a patient. The patient's bed linen will also require changing; refer to **Skill 3.2** for information about making an occupied bed.

An individual's choices or preferences for personal hygiene are affected by their social and cultural background. Nurses should not impose their own standards of personal hygiene on the patient or even assume these will be the same as the patient's. Ask the patient about any personal hygiene or grooming preferences such as toiletries, clothing choices or cultural needs if they are not already included on the nursing care plan. The nurse must respect these preferences while maintaining the patient's privacy and dignity at all times.

Social, cultural and religious factors need consideration when attending to hair care. Some religions do not allow for hair washing or brushing (e.g. some Hindi women use combing, brushing and scented oils to cleanse the hair), while others require the hair to be covered (e.g. some Muslim, Orthodox Jewish and Sikh women, and some Sikh men cover their hair with a turban) (Ebrahim et al., 2011). Similarly, in some cultures facial hair is significant

and is never removed without the patient's/relatives' consent.

Active and passive exercises are often implemented while completing a patient's sponge. Please refer to **Skill 3.14**.

GATHER EQUIPMENT

- *Trolley* for carrying equipment.
- *Sponge:* sponge bowl with warm (43 to 45°C) water, soap or patient's preferred cleanser, towels, washcloth and disposable washcloth. Alternatively, a prepackaged bag with moistened washcloths may be used, according to the facility policy. Clean clothing and additional items such as preferred emollient creams or deodorant.
- *Sponge blanket/* (if available) to partially cover patient and provide privacy during procedure.
- *For changing the bed linen:* clean bed linen and a linen skip.
- *Manual handling equipment:* slide sheets and hoist if required.
- *Oral hygiene:* towel, toothpaste, soft bristle toothbrush, small bowl, cup with water, mouthwash, dental floss.
- *For dentures:* denture cup, denture toothpaste (or gentle soap) and soft-bristle toothbrush. For unconscious

patient, or patients with an impaired gag reflex, suction apparatus will be required.
- *Hair care:* patient's hairbrush or comb. If a bed shampoo is required, add a jug with warm water, bucket, bed trough and a plastic sheet for protecting the bed and extra towels. Brush and/or comb for everyday care.
- *Shaving:* an electric razor is preferable. A small bowl with warm water, towel, razor and shaving cream is required if the patient does not use an electric razor.
- *Eye care:* the eyes are cleansed with a washcloth during the sponging procedure. Eye toilets are discussed in **Skill 5.2**.
- *Nasal care:* tissues, rubbish bag, washcloth or gauze swabs if required.
- *Personal protective equipment (PPE):* plastic apron and non-sterile gloves.

IMPLEMENT THE PATIENT'S SPONGE

Give a clear explanation of the procedure and establish therapeutic communication

Introduce yourself, and check you have the correct patient. Discuss the procedure and gain the patient's consent. Giving a clear explanation is required to gain legal consent and to address policy requirements. It will also assist the patient to cooperate with the procedure, allay anxiety and assist in establishing a therapeutic relationship.

Discuss the patient's personal hygiene and grooming needs or preferences with them. A sponge is an excellent opportunity to become better acquainted with the patient. Effective communication and sensitivity to the patient's emotional wellbeing when assisting a patient with their hygiene and grooming needs is vital (Russell et al., 2017). Patients require privacy, dignity and recognition of their cultural needs.

Perform hand hygiene

Perform hand hygiene before touching the patient or the patient's surrounds and prior to any procedure involving patient contact to reduce the possibility of cross-contamination. Hand hygiene is the most effective method of infection control as it removes transient organisms from the hands of the nurse (see **Skill 1.1**).

Don PPE, if required

Use of plastic aprons and non-sterile gloves may be required when sponging a patient to prevent wetting

and soiling of the nurse's uniform and to reduce infection control risks. Gloves are used during the sponge when there will be contact with body fluids, including saliva. PPE requirements will vary according to the care being delivered and the patient's health status.

Demonstrate problem-solving abilities

Personal hygiene and grooming needs are considered private by people in most cultures because of exposure of body areas and the intimate nature of the routines. Close doors and curtains while completing the sponge. Offer the patient a bedpan or urinal before beginning the sponge to reduce interruptions and to increase patient comfort. Maintain principles of workplace health and safety (WHS) and manual handling by adjusting the bed height to reduce strain on the nurse's back. Ensure the patient is positioned in the supine position for the sponge, and slide sheets are available for moving the patient during the procedure. Attend to environmental temperature and draughts as the patient will have areas of their body exposed and may feel the cold. A partial sponge of the lower back, groin and anal area may be performed when a patient has been incontinent.

If a prepacked disposable sponging system is being used, the bowl, washcloth, towels and soap are not required, but the same procedure is followed (Nøddeskou et al., 2015).

Sponge the patient

Sponging is implemented by two nurses, with one standing on each side of the bed. Arrange the equipment on the trolley with the sponge bowl and soap on top. Other items (including deodorants, oral hygiene equipment, fresh linen and clothing) are kept on the lower shelf until needed. Lower the bed rails and position the patient in a supine position. Remove the blankets and quilt, leaving the top sheet covering the patient. It will be used to cover the patient during the sponge to help maintain their privacy and dignity, if a sponge blanket is not being used. Loosen the sheet at the bottom. The bed linen is folded for re-use, or disposed of in the linen skip.

Undressing/dressing: Fold back the sheet and remove the patient's pyjamas or gown. Remove the top half first, leaving the legs covered with the sheet.

- If the patient has a disability in one arm, remove the sleeve from the unaffected arm first and then the affected side. This gives the person more flexibility in manoeuvring out of the clothing.
- If the patient has an IV in situ, the gown is removed from the arm without the IV first. Refer to **Skill 6.3** for further information about changing clothing for a patient with an IV.
- Replace the sheet to cover the exposed areas of the patient.
- Remove pyjama bottoms and underwear by rolling an unconscious or immobile patient onto their side (see **Skill 3.12**). Remove the patient's clothing from the upper leg by moving the pants partially down past the patient's buttocks, then roll to the patient's other side and repeat the same action. Roll the patient onto their back. The clothing can now be fully removed.
- Place the dirty clothing into a laundry bag (patient's own) or linen skip (hospital clothing). Dress the patient in the reverse order when the sponge is completed.

Sponging the patient: Use a towel under limbs while washing each body part. Cover exposed areas of the patient's body with the sponge blanket or top sheet. The bottom sheet and linen will often become wet during a sponge, but will be changed at the end of the procedure. Wet the washcloth enough to ensure thorough washing and rinsing, and then add soap to the washcloth. The soap is not left in the water, to stop it from becoming too soapy. Rinse the washcloth after washing and then rinse the skin before drying the body area. For patients with the ability to wash some of their own body areas, give them a moistened washcloth or towel and assist as required.

A disposable sponging 'bag bath' can be used instead of the traditional bed bath (Nøddeskou et al., 2015). The bag bath kit contains a number of disposable moistened washcloths that are warmed in the microwave according to the manufacturer's instructions and brought to the bedside. The nurse uses a fresh washcloth for each area being cleansed. The skin dries in a few seconds without towelling so the benefits of the emollient are maximised.

Use long, firm but gentle strokes to wash the patient, removing any dirt, oil and bacteria. This is more relaxing and comfortable than short light strokes. Gently dry each area after it is washed. Expose, wash, rinse and thoroughly dry one body part at a time to prevent chilling and maintain privacy. The two nurses work together to wash the body area or limb on their side of the bed, plus assist each other with drying and moving the patient. Pay particular attention to skin folds and other areas where skin touches skin (i.e. axilla, under breasts, abdominal folds, buttock folds and groin) as these areas can become excoriated if left damp. Support large joints (elbows, knees) when the limb is flexed and moved for washing, rinsing and drying.

Body areas are washed in the following sequence, but may require adaptation to individual needs.

- Eyes, from the inner to outer canthus, and face are washed first. With no soap used on these body parts. Some patients may prefer to wash their own face.
- The neck and ears are then cleaned, followed by the arms and hands. Move the sponge bowl onto the bed, and soak each hand as it is washed.
- The chest, axillae and abdomen are washed before covering the patient's top half of the body and then washing the legs and feet. Again, move the sponge bowl onto the bed to soak each foot as it is washed.
- Empty the bowl and change the water.
- Don non-sterile gloves and wash the patient's groin area and genitals. Do not reach towards the perineum or anal area. Maintain the patient's dignity by encouraging conscious patients to perform this themselves, by giving them the wet washcloth. Use a disposable washcloth if there is any risk of contamination from body fluids, and dispose of after use. Remove and dispose of the gloves after washing and drying.
- The water should be changed before washing the patient's back. Prepare the bed linen for changing (as per **Skill 3.2**).
- Use the slide sheets and the procedure for repositioning a patient onto their side (see **Skill 3.12**) to roll the patient and then wash their back. One towel is left in place, similar to the sheets, to protect the patient and fresh linen from becoming soiled.
- Don non-sterile gloves, then wash the anal and perineal area. Use a disposable washcloth to reduce infection control risks.
- Roll the patient onto their other side to remove the soiled sheet, pull through the clean sheet and then tuck it in.
- Clean underwear and pants will need to be put on after the area is washed and dried, following a similar process for removing underwear.

After the wash is completed, apply deodorant, moisturisers and any other creams according to patient preference or the nursing care plan. Dress the patient in clean pyjamas, gown or clothing. Male patients will require shaving each day (see **Skill 3.6**). Oral hygiene and further grooming will also be required as described in the next section.

Reposition the patient and ensure that the call bell is within reach. Replace the top sheet and add other linen as required (as per **Skill 3.2**).

Implement oral hygiene

Oral hygiene can be completed by the patient with assistance or by the nurse, and should be completed as a routine part of every sponge.

- *Conscious patients. Conscious patients* are positioned upright and a towel is positioned over the chest and shoulders to protect the clothing from splashes and dribbles. The patient can hold a disposable cup or small bowl to spit into.

  Don non-sterile gloves to reduce infection control risk. If there is a splashing risk, wear goggles. To reduce this splashing risk, stand behind or next to the patient (if possible), when brushing their teeth. A soft toothbrush is wet with water and a small amount of toothpaste is applied. The patient is asked to keep the mouth open, and the toothbrush, held at a 45-degree angle, is used to cleanse every surface of the teeth. Small, circular movements of the toothbrush are applied, starting at the junction of the teeth and gums and working towards the crown. Light pressure is used to avoid injury. The inside, outside and flat surfaces of both upper and lower teeth are cleansed. The patient spits out the excess toothpaste solution into the bowl. Ask the patient to take a sip of water to rinse the mouth after brushing to remove any remaining debris and leave the mouth feeling refreshed (Lewis & Fricker, 2009; SA Health, 2020). Flossing (unless contraindicated, e.g. thrombocytopenia) should also be encouraged as part of dental hygiene, as it helps to remove debris and plaque that the toothbrush is unable to reach. Assess the patient's teeth, tongue, gums and mucous membranes as part of completing oral hygiene.

- *Conscious patient with an impaired gag reflex.* Follow the same procedure, ensuring suction is available to remove the toothpaste from the patient's mouth. If the patient is unable to tolerate water, refer to facility guidelines and patient care plan for level of thickened water to be used for rinsing the mouth. Suction the patient mouth, removing all fluid after brushing and spitting out the toothpaste (see **Skill 8.8**).

- *Unconscious patient.* The patient remains in a supine (slightly elevated) or side position while oral hygiene is complete. Suction apparatus should also be available. A soft toothbrush (some commercially modified toothbrushes have suction ability) with toothpaste is also used in a similar process to the one described above, using a minimum of toothpaste and water on the toothbrush. Any rinsing of the mouth is performed using the rinsed toothbrush or a jumbo mouth swab. Excess fluid and toothpaste are removed with the suction (see **Skill 8.8**).

- *Denture care.* Dental plates or bridges are removed by either the patient or, if unable, by the nurse. Don non-sterile gloves. Remove the lower denture first by holding the front base of the denture between the thumb and fingers to lift it out. The upper denture is removed by grasping the upper plate at the front teeth with the thumb and second finger. Moving the plate up and down slightly releases the suction securing the plate. Then lift the upper plate and turn it slightly, so one side is lower than the other, to remove the denture from the mouth. To avoid damage or breakage to a partial denture, do not hold the clasps but apply equal pressure on the border of each side of the denture. Dentures can be cleaned in a small bowl or at a clean patient sink. Use a soft toothbrush and mild liquid soap (or denture toothpaste) under the running water to remove any debris and plaque from the dentures. Regular toothpaste is not recommended as it can abrade the surface of the denture. The denture is then thoroughly rinsed and returned to the patient (Lewis & Fricker, 2009). Some patients prefer to soak their dentures in a cleaning agent overnight. The denture should still be cleansed first with a soft toothbrush. The cleaning agent is placed in the denture cup and dissolved in tepid water.

Implement hair care

The patient's hair should be brushed (or combed) and made tidy as part of a routine sponge. Follow the patient's preferred grooming and styling for hair care.

- *Hair wash in bed.* It is preferable to wash the patient's hair in the shower, or as part of a trolley bath. If this is not possible, a bed shampoo can be completed. This entails using a trough designed for bed shampoos, or constructing a trough out of plastic sheets and towels. The head of the bed is removed, or the patient may be assisted up the bed so the trough and towels can be placed under the head and neck. The tail of the trough runs off the bed and empties into a bucket so that used water is not spilled. A small pillow, protected with a waterproof sheet, is placed under the patient's shoulders to increase comfort. A jug with warm (40°C) water is used to wet the hair. The hair is shampooed using the patient's preferred shampoo and the balls of the fingers to massage the scalp to increase circulation. The hair is rinsed, paying particular attention to the nape of the neck where it is difficult to rinse. Add conditioner and rinse well, if the patient requires this. Wrap the hair in a towel and gently dry it using short patting movements to prevent damage to the hair shaft. Remove the bed trough. It is usually necessary to then change the patient's bed linen.

  When the patient's hair is towelled dry, style it according to the patient's preference, taking into consideration the patient's ability to care for their hair. For example, long hair is less likely to matt and tangle in a bed-bound patient if it is braided. Alternatively, dry shampoo may be available for use.

Implement eye care

The eyes are cleansed with a clean disposable washcloth. Place a clean towel under the patient's face/neck. Don non-sterile gloves and use a wet washcloth to wipe the inner eye outwards and remove any secretions. Use a fresh or rinsed washcloth to clean the other eye. For eyes with excess secretions, implement an eye toilet as per **Skill 5.2**.

Implement nasal care

Encourage a conscious patient to blow their nose, using tissues. Don non-sterile gloves to hold the tissue and assist (including wiping the nose) if necessary.

To remove dried secretions and blood, put on non-sterile gloves. Moisten a disposable washcloth or non-sterile gauze with normal tap water and gently wipe the base of the nares. If there is a large area of crusted secretions, sodium chloride 0.9% for irrigation can be used to moisten gauze and wipe the area clean.

Doff PPE

Remove the PPE that was donned in the following sequence: non-sterile gloves, hand hygiene, eyewear/face shield, plastic apron/gown, mask and then hand hygiene (ACSQHC, 2020). Dispose of in the rubbish bag.

Perform hand hygiene

Maintain the 5 Moments for Hand Hygiene and perform hand hygiene after touching the patient and the patient's surrounds.

CLEAN, REPLACE OR DISPOSE OF EQUIPMENT

Clean, replace and dispose of equipment appropriately to leave equipment in useable condition for the next nurse. This is both a time-management strategy and a courtesy to other staff. Slide sheets are returned to the patient locker. Sponge water is tipped out in the dirty utility area. Non-disposable sponge bowls are cleaned (according to facility guidelines) and returned to the relevant area (i.e. the patient's locker or a utility room). Disposable sponge bowls are placed in the macerator, and other disposable items placed in the general waste. Trolleys and other equipment are cleaned with facility disinfecting wipes and returned to their storage area.

Personal toiletries (soap, deodorant, toothpaste, shampoo and conditioner) and equipment (toothbrush, etc.) are dried and returned to the patient's locker for future use. These are personal property and should be treated as such. Denture cups (if not disposable) remain at the patient's bedside, empty when not in use. All soiled hospital linen is placed in the linen skip for laundering. Patient's personal clothing is placed in their laundry bag for the family to collect and wash.

DOCUMENT AND REPORT RELEVANT INFORMATION

Completion of the patient personal hygiene and grooming needs should be signed in the patient's nursing care plan. If active and passive exercises were implemented, these should also be documented in the patient's nursing care plan. Any relevant information or other assessment completed during the sponge should be recorded in the appropriate charts and nursing notes, plus handed over verbally.

CASE STUDY

An 84-year-old woman has been admitted to the ward post right-sided cerebrovascular accident. Currently she is non-weight-bearing and requires a full sponge in bed.

1. What safety measures will you implement when completing this procedure?
2. Other than sponging your patient, what hygiene measures will you perform?

Note: These notes are summaries of the most important points in the assessments/procedures, and are not exhaustive on the subject. The naming of documents or charts may differ from state to state, and facility to facility. In all possible situations the guidelines of the ACSQHC are used when describing national charts or documents (e.g. the ACSQHC Observation and Response Chart is named the Adult Observation and Response Chart in WA, and the Rapid Detection and Response Observation Chart in SA). References of the materials used to compile the information have been supplied. The student is expected to have learned the material surrounding each skill as presented in the references. No single reference is complete on the subject.

REFERENCES

Australian Commission on Safety and Quality in Health Care (ACSQHC). (2020). *Sequence for Putting on and Removing PPE.* https://www.safetyandquality.gov.au/sites/default/files/2020-03/putting_on_and_removing_ppe_diagram_-_march_2020.pdf

Bartnik, L. & Rice, M. (2013). Workplace health and safety. *Medical Sciences, Nurses and Nursing,* 61(9), pp. 393–400.

Daly, B. & Smith, K. (2015). Promoting good dental health in older people: role of the community nurse. *British Journal of Community Nursing,* 20(9), pp. 431–6.

Ebrahim, S., Bance, S. & Bowman, K. (2011). Sikh perspectives towards death and end of life care. *Journal of Palliative Care,* 27(2), pp. 170–4.

Gray, S., Ferris, L., White, L.E., Duncan, G. & Baumle, W. (2018). *Foundations of Nursing: Enrolled Nurses* (2nd ANZ ed.). Melbourne: Cengage.

Hørdam, B., Brandsen, R.V., Frandsen, T.K., Bing, A., Stuhaug, H.N. & Petersen, K. (2018). Nurse-assisted personal hygiene to older adults 65+ in home care setting. *Journal of Nursing Education and Practice*, 8(2). https://www.researchgate.net/profile/Britta_Hordam/publication/320308484_Nurse-assisted_personal_hygiene_to_older_adults_65_in_home_care_setting/links/59df0fda0f7e9bcfab35eccf/Nurse-assisted-personal-hygiene-to-older-adults-65-in-home-care-setting.pdf

Lewis, A. & Fricker, A. (2009). Better oral health in residential care. *Staff Portfolio, Education and Training Program*. http://www.sahealth.sa.gov.au/wps/wcm/connect/774e660047d747529e6d9ffc651ee2b2/BOHRC_Staff_Portfolio_Module_2%5B1%5D.pdf?MOD=AJPERES&CACHEID=ROOTWORKSPACE-774e660047d747529e6d9ffc651ee2b2-IDS.pik

Nøddeskou, L.H., Hemmingsen, L.E. & Hørdam, B. (2015). Elderly patients' and nurses' assessment of traditional bed bath compared to prepacked single units – randomised controlled trial. *Scandinavian Journal of Caring Sciences*, 29(2), pp. 347–52.

Red, A. & O'Neal, P.V. (2020). Implementation of an evidence-based oral care protocol to improve the delivery of mouth care in nursing home residents. *Journal of Gerontological Nursing*, 46(5), pp. 33–9.

Russell, B., Buswell, M., Norton, C., Malone, J.R., Harari, D., Harwood, R., Roe, B., Fader, M., Drennan, V.M., Bunn, F. & Goodman, C. (2017). Supporting people living with dementia and faecal incontinence. *British Journal of Community Nursing*, 22(3), pp. 110–14.

SA Health. (2020). *Oral Health Care Domain – Care of Older People Toolkit*. Government of South Australia. https://www.sahealth.sa.gov.au/wps/wcm/connect/public+content/sa+health+internet/clinical+resources/clinical+programs+and+practice+guidelines/older+people/care+of+older+people+toolkit/oral+health+care+domain+-+care+of+older+people+toolkit

RECOMMENDED READINGS

Dougherty, L. & Lister, S. (eds). (2015). *The Royal Marsden Hospital Manual of Clinical Nursing Procedures* (9th ed.). Oxford: Wiley-Blackwell.

WA Department of Mines, Industry Regulation and Safety. (2020). *Manual tasks in Healthcare and Social Assistance*. 12 November. https://www.commerce.wa.gov.au/worksafe/manual-tasks-healthcare-and-social-assistance

WorkSafe Victorian. (n.d.). *Safety and Prevention: Your Industry – Aged Care*. Victoria State Government. http://www.worksafe.vic.gov.au/pages/safety-and-prevention/your-industry/aged-care

ESSENTIAL SKILLS COMPETENCY

Assisting the Patient to Maintain Personal Hygiene and Grooming – Sponge, Undressing/ Dressing, Oral Hygiene, Eye Care, Nasal Care and Hair Care

Demonstrates the ability to effectively maintain personal hygiene in a dependent patient

Criteria for skill performance	Y	D
(Numbers indicate *Enrolled Nurse Standards for Practice*, 2016)	(Satisfactory)	(Requires development)
1. Identifies indication (8.3, 8.4)		
2. Assesses patient for ability, and need for assistance with hygiene and grooming (7.1, 7.2, 8.1, 8.2, 8.3, 8.4)		
3. Identifies safety considerations and follows WHS principles (1.2, 1.4, 1.8, 3.2, 3.9, 6.4, 6.6, 8.4, 9.4)		
4. Gathers equipment, as relevant to skill being performed (1.2, 1.6, 6.4, 8.4, 9.4)		
5. Evidence of effective therapeutic communication with the patient; gives patient a clear explanation of procedure and confirms patient understanding, gains patient consent (2.1, 2.3, 2.4, 2.5, 6.3)		
6. Performs hand hygiene (1.2, 1.4, 1.8, 3.9, 6.4, 9.4)		
7. Dons PPE as required (1.2, 1.4, 1.8, 2.1, 3.2, 3.9, 8.4, 9.4)		
8. Demonstrates problem-solving abilities; e.g. maintains patient privacy and dignity, alters bed height, attends to environmental temperature, positions patient (4.1, 4.2, 8.3, 8.4, 9.4)		
9. Completes patient sponge (1.2, 1.4, 1.8, 2.1, 2.3, 2.4, 2.7, 3.2, 3.9, 6.1, 6.3, 6.6, 8.4, 9.4): ■ undresses and dresses patient safely ■ sponges and dries patient correctly		
10. Implements or assists patient with oral hygiene (1.2, 1.4, 1.8, 2.1, 2.3, 2.4, 2.7, 3.2, 3.9, 6.1, 6.3, 6.6, 8.4, 9.4)		
11. Assesses skin and oral mucosa (4.1, 4.2, 7.1, 7.2, 7.5, 8.4, 9.4)		
12. Implements or assists patient with other grooming requirements (1.2, 1.4, 1.8, 2.1, 2.3, 2.4, 2.7, 3.2, 3.9, 6.1, 6.3, 6.6, 8.4, 9.4): ■ hair care ■ shaves male patient ■ eye and nasal care		
13. Doffs PPE and performs hand hygiene (1.2, 1.4, 1.8, 3.9, 6.4, 9.4)		
14. Cleans, replaces and disposes of equipment appropriately (1.2, 1.4, 3.9, 6.5, 9.4)		
15. Documents and reports relevant information (1.2, 1.3, 1.8, 3.2, 5.3, 6.6, 7.1, 7.2, 7.3, 7.4, 7.5)		
16. Demonstrates ability to link theory to practice (8.3, 8.4, 8.5, 9.4)		

Student:

Clinical facilitator: Date:

CHAPTER 3.6

ASSISTING THE PATIENT TO MAINTAIN PERSONAL HYGIENE AND GROOMING – ASSISTED SHOWER (CHAIR OR TROLLEY), UNDRESSING/DRESSING, SHAVING, HAIR AND NAIL CARE

IDENTIFY INDICATIONS

Helping a patient to meet their personal hygiene and grooming needs promotes a positive self-image, relaxation and a feeling of wellbeing, along with promoting healthy skin and maintaining the body's first line of defence against disease (Gray et al., 2018). Assisting patients to meet their personal hygiene and grooming requirements is a basic human need and a core nursing skill, as most patients require some level of assistance, even if it is only for a brief period of time (Nøddeskou et al., 2015). The level of assistance required to help a patient meet these activities of daily living is based on the patient's own self-care ability, or limitations created by their treatment (e.g. post-op, rest-in-bed restrictions). Assisting patients to meet their personal hygiene needs also creates an excellent opportunity to assess the patient's general physical status, complete routine daily skin assessments and encourage rehabilitation of the patient's self-care skills. It is also an opportunity for personal interaction and establishing a therapeutic relationship.

Showering is usually the preferred nursing action to help a patient meet their personal hygiene needs. Showering removes perspiration, excess skin oils, dead cells and minimises body odour. An assisted shower occurs when the patient is showered on a chair or on a shower trolley. Showering can range from a simple 'set-up' shower to a fully assisted chair shower or trolley shower. Patients will require assistance with their other personal hygiene and grooming needs, including dressing and undressing, oral hygiene, hair care and shaving, as part of their shower. Oral hygiene should be implemented as a routine care action for all patients having a shower. As stated in Daly and Smith, 'Good dental health is important for a person's sense of wellbeing, self-esteem and quality of life, as well as contributing to social inclusion and general nutrition' (2015).

PLAN THE PATIENT'S SHOWER

Assessment of the patient and reviewing their nursing care plan prior to implementing a shower is important to prevent contravening other care requirements or assuming a higher level of patient mobility or self-care than is relevant to their physical health status. Review the patient's nursing care plan for personal preferences, other treatment requirements (e.g. wound care post-shower or physiotherapy), mobility needs and any care actions specific to the patient's hygiene. Prior to implementing the shower, assess the patient for any pain and administer pain relief if required. Based on the patient's mobility, ensure the correct manual handling equipment is available to reduce the risk to the patient or the nurse when transferring the patient out of bed for the shower (refer to **Skill 3.12** for repositioning a patient and **Skill 3.3** for assisting a patient to ambulate) and ensure the principles of workplace health and safety (WHS) are maintained throughout the procedure.

An individual's choices or preferences for personal hygiene are affected by their social and cultural background. Nurses should not impose their own standards of personal hygiene on the patient or even assume these will be the same as the patient's. Ask the patient about any personal hygiene or grooming preferences such as toiletries, clothing choices or cultural needs, if they are not already included on the nursing care plan. The nurse must respect these preferences while maintaining the patient's privacy and dignity at all times.

Social, cultural and religious factors need consideration when attending to hair care. Some religions do not allow for hair washing or brushing (e.g. some Hindi women use combing, brushing and scented oils to cleanse the hair), while others require the hair to be covered (e.g. some Muslim, Orthodox

Jewish and Sikh women, and some Sikh men cover their hair with a turban) (Ebrahim et al., 2011). Similarly, in some cultures facial hair is significant and is never removed without the patient's/relatives' consent.

GATHER EQUIPMENT

For showering
- *Shower chair (mobile chair/commode or standard shower chair) or shower trolley*
- *Manual handling equipment* (e.g. hoist and slide sheets) as required
- *Shower with handheld shower nozzle*
- *Personal toiletries* such as soap or shower gel, moisturisers and deodorants, hair shampoo and conditioner if required
- *Washcloths and disposable washcloths* for washing groin and anal areas, two towels, towelling floor mat, clean clothing
- *Disposable pre-taped plastic covering* to protect wounds, intravenous (IV) or central venous catheter (CVC) sites, splints, bandaged areas and plaster of Paris/fibreglass splints
- *Personal protective equipment (PPE)*; that is, disposable plastic aprons, disposable shoe covers to reduce infection control risk and to protect the nurse's clothing and shoes, non-sterile gloves

For oral hygiene
- *For brushing teeth:* towel, toothpaste, soft bristle toothbrush, small bowl, cup with water, mouthwash, dental floss

- *For dentures:* denture cup, denture toothpaste (or gentle soap) and soft bristle toothbrush
- *PPE:* non-sterile gloves; goggles if there is a splashing risk

For hair care
- *Brush and/or comb for everyday care, preferred shampoo, conditioner and towels if required*

For shaving
- *An electric razor* is safer, and generally preferred by most facilities. Some patients do have a personal preference for a traditional razor, and will require a *towel, razor and shaving cream.* Check the patient's chart regarding medications or disease, which would exclude the use of a traditional razor (e.g. anticoagulants, thrombocytopenia, depression, confusion, oxygen administration).

For nail care
- *Nail file or emery board, towel, basin with warm water*

IMPLEMENT THE PATIENT'S SHOWER

Perform hand hygiene

Perform hand hygiene before touching the patient or the patient's surrounds and prior to any procedure involving patient contact to reduce the possibility of cross-contamination. Hand hygiene is the most effective method of infection control as it removes transient organisms from the hands of the nurse (see **Skill 1.1**).

Give a clear explanation of the procedure and establish therapeutic communication

Introduce yourself, and check you have the correct patient. Discuss the procedure and gain the patient's consent. Giving a clear explanation is required to gain legal consent and to address policy requirements. It will also assist the patient to cooperate with the procedure, allay anxiety and assist in establishing a therapeutic relationship.

Discuss the patient's personal hygiene and grooming needs or preferences with them. An assisted shower is an excellent opportunity to become better acquainted with the patient. Effective communication and sensitivity to the patient's emotional wellbeing when assisting a patient with their hygiene and grooming needs is vital (Russell et al., 2017). Patients require privacy, dignity and recognition of their cultural needs.

Don PPE

Use of plastic aprons and disposable shoe covers in the shower prevents wetting and soiling of the nurse's uniform and shoes, reducing infection risks. Non-sterile gloves are used when there is a high risk of exposure to body fluids. Review the facility policy as some facilities' policies require the nurse to wear gloves throughout the shower procedure, while others prefer gloves to be worn only when in contact with body fluids. They should always be worn when cleaning the patient's genital, groin, perineal and anal areas. PPE requirements will vary according to the care being delivered and the patient's health status.

Demonstrate problem-solving abilities

Personal hygiene and grooming needs are considered private by people in most cultures because of exposure of body areas and the intimate nature of the routines. Close doors and curtains while completing the shower. Take the patient to the toilet on the way to the shower. Maintain principles of WHS and manual handling throughout the procedure to reduce strain on the nurse's back and reduce the risk of injury to the patient. Most hospitalised and unwell patients are at a high risk of falls when showering and should be showered while sitting on a shower chair, even if they are minimally dependent. Medications, drainage tubes, impaired physical health or reduced mobility increase their risk of falling while in hospital.

Some assessments of the patient's physical ability, progress towards self-care and skin assessments are undertaken while the patient is showering. Review the nursing care plan to identify assessments that should be completed. Rehabilitation patients should be following alternative routines or processes and using specific aids as advised by the occupational therapist and physiotherapist. The nurse needs to be aware of these, along with prompting or encouraging the patient to follow these treatment routines.

Shower the patient

Prepare the shower area by ensuring communal areas are free. Take the patient's toiletries, towels and clothing into the shower cubicle so the shower can be completed without interruption, reducing chilling and tiring of the patient.

Cover the patient's wounds, incisions, splints or peripheral intravenous catheter (PIVC) sites with the disposable waterproof covering to prevent contamination of the site during the shower. Remove the protective strip and ensure the tape seals the covering to the skin area. Some wounds may be left open during the shower, and others may be irrigated as part of the showering process (see **Skill 4.3**). Refer to the wound management plan for the correct actions. The patient is then transferred (refer to **Skill 3.12**) as per their mobility chart from the bed to the mobile shower chair or shower trolley, covered and then transported to the shower. If the patient is ambulant, assist with any drains or IV poles and help them to walk to the shower (see **Skill 3.3**). All patients are showered in at least a shower chair, and assisted to use the handrails to provide support when standing or moving. The shower or bathroom doors should be closed and the curtains drawn to ensure patient privacy. An 'Occupied' sign may be placed on the door. The water temperature is initially regulated to a comfortable temperature without running the water over the patient, to prevent injury. Ensure the temperature is tested with gloveless hands.

Undressing and dressing

Remove the patient's pyjamas or gown, and place the dirty pyjamas into a laundry bag (patient's own) or linen skip (hospital clothing).

- If the patient has a disability (i.e. physical, or surgically limited by bandaging or splints) in one arm, remove the sleeve from the unaffected arm first and then the affected side. This gives the person more flexibility in manoeuvring their clothing. Assist the patient to stand using the rails, to remove their trousers and underwear. Patients who are unable to stand should have their underwear and pants lowered, as described for shower trolley later in this skill, prior to transferring them from the bed to the commode chair.
- If the patient has an IV in situ, the gown is removed from the arm without the IV first. Refer to **Skill 6.3** for further information about changing clothing for a patient with an IV.
- For patients in a shower trolley, remove pyjama bottoms and underwear by rolling the patient onto their side (see **Skill 3.12**). Remove the patient's clothing from the upper leg by moving the pants partially down past the patient's buttocks, then roll to the patient's other side and repeat the same action. Roll the patient onto their back. The clothing can now be fully removed.

Dress the patient using a similar process, after the shower is completed. Use the reverse order for arms or legs with a disability.

Set-up or supervised shower

For patients who do not require assistance, ensure they are set-up and safely sitting on the shower chair. Some patients may still require assistance to remove some clothing. Allow the patient the privacy to wash themselves. Leave them positioned so that they can safely reach the call bell, and then close the door. Supervise the patient indirectly by remaining close by and checking on them. Complete other smaller nursing tasks nearby (e.g. bedmaking) while the patient is showering.

An assisted shower

The level of assistance required will vary according to the patient's health status and mobility. Some patients may only require assistance with their back, legs and feet. Others will need to be fully washed by the nurse.

When showering a patient, use the following guidelines.

- Use the handheld shower to direct the water across the patient and down their body. To avoid getting wet, the nurse should hold the shower nozzle.
- Use a wet washcloth with no soap to wash the patient's face. Wash the eyes first, then face, neck and ears. Most patients will be able to wash their own face when prompted. Do not run the shower across the patient's face unless the patient requests it. If the patient requests a spray of water on their face, direct the spray downward so that water is not forced up the nostrils or into the eyes.
- Then proceed to wash from the neck downward, washing the patient's abdomen, underarms and then their back. Keep the water running on the patient while washing with the washcloth to help maintain warmth for the patient.
- Wash the legs. Squat down to wash the patient's feet.
- Put on non-sterile gloves, and then wash the perineal and groin area. If possible, the patient should stand to wash their perineal, groin and anal areas. Encourage the patient to complete this themselves. Some shower chairs have a large hole to enable washing the patient's buttocks. Use fresh washcloths if they become soiled.
- Rinse the patient thoroughly to prevent irritation from residual soap.

Dry the patient rapidly, using two towels, since the entire body surface is wet and exposed, leading to chilling by convection. A non-slip mat is placed on the floor of the shower after the patient has been washed (so the nurse will not slip while helping the patient or, if the patient is able to assist themselves, so they will not slip). Place one towel across the back and shoulders while drying other body areas. Follow a sequence similar to washing, starting with the face. Take particular care to dry between body folds (e.g. between toes, fingers, under breasts and axillae, inside skin folds) to prevent excoriation and reduce pressure injury risk from moisture (see **Skill 3.13**). Ask the patient to hold the rails, then lean forward to dry their back. To dry the buttocks and upper legs, the patient will need to stand (if able) using the shower rails. A towel can be left on the chair to keep the patient (and then their clothing) dry. Dry the legs and feet first, and ensure the patient is standing on a dry mat. Patients who are unable to stand will require their buttocks and upper legs to be dried when they are transferred back to bed or into their chair. Place their underwear and pants on, up to the patient's knees so they can easily be moved up later.

Assisted shower trolley/trolley bath

Two nurses are required to complete this procedure safely, with one nurse standing on either side of the trolley and assisting each other with the procedure. Insert the plug, and then wash the patient in a similar process to assisted shower, rolling the patient onto their side (see **Skill 3.12**) to wash (and also to dry) their back, anal area and buttocks. Remove the plug and drain the residual water away. Dry the patient rapidly and cover their body with towels while drying to prevent them becoming chilled. Dry and then dress the patient by rolling them, and leave a dry towel under the back to keep the clothing dry.

Further grooming

Apply deodorants, moisturisers as preferred by the patient and assist them to dress in clean pyjamas and underwear as described above. Place a dry chair next to the hand basin, and then assist the patient to complete their oral hygiene (as described in sponging, see **Skill 3.5**), brush or comb and style the hair as the patient prefers and help with shaving for males. Some patients may request assistance with applying make-up or jewellery, especially in the community and residential care facilities. Assist patients to clean and then insert their hearing aid or put on glasses (if required). Completing all of the further grooming actions should be part of the regular shower routine.

Return the patient to their bed or room, and assist to a position of comfort.

Hair wash

This can be incorporated into a shower. Ask the patient to tip their head backwards and direct the water stream from the front of the hair backwards to prevent water running over the face. Wet hair thoroughly and, using the patient's preferred shampoo, lather well using the balls of your fingers to massage the scalp and increase circulation. Rinse well, again from the forehead backwards with the head tipped back. Remove all traces of shampoo to prevent irritation. Add conditioner and again rinse well. Wrap the hair in a towel and gently dry it using short patting movements to prevent damage to the hair shaft.

Shaving

Shaving promotes comfort and contributes to self-confidence and self-worth. Male patients should be shaved each day after their shower. Patients with beards or moustaches are asked if they want it trimmed, washed or brushed, especially if unable to carry out this care themselves.

Shaving can be done by the patient with assistance, or entirely by the nurse. Observe the face for lesions, raised moles and birthmarks so these can be avoided during shaving and thus prevent injury. Place a towel under the patient's neck. An electric razor is preferred in most facilities and patients will usually supply their own. Hold the skin taut with the non-dominant hand and, using short strokes or a circular motion, shave in the direction of the hair growth. Start at the top of hair growth and work down to the neck. Be careful not to shave an established moustache, beard or sideburns. Ask the patient to extend his neck to increase tautness of skin and facilitate hair removal. For the safety razor, check there are no contraindications (i.e. medications or risk of bleeding) before using a safety razor. Lather the face with the preferred shaving cream, then follow a similar pattern for shaving. Rinse the razor between each stroke to keep the cutting edge clean. After shaving, rinse the area to remove excess lather and hair and prevent irritation.

Fingernail care

Nail care does not need to be completed in the bathroom, and can be done by the patient with assistance or entirely by the nurse. Nail care and hand massage is often completed by therapy assistants in residential care facilities. Toenails are not cut or filed by the nurse. Patients requiring toenail care should be referred to a podiatrist. Many patients have medical conditions (e.g. peripheral vascular disease and diabetes mellitus) that require a podiatrist to manage their toenails and reduce the risk of infection and slow healing if cut incorrectly.

The nail edges may just require smoothing with a nail file or emery board – feel each one with your index finger and use the nail file to remove any jagged edges that may catch on clothing, linen or skin. If the nails are long, and the patient agrees, file the nail straight across, removing a small amount of nail at a time. Then smooth and shape the edges with the nail file. Take care that the nail is not filed too short. Apply moisturiser to keep the skin soft and supple.

Doffs PPE

Remove PPE in the following sequence: non-sterile gloves, hand hygiene, eyewear/face shield, plastic apron/gown, mask and then hand hygiene (ACSQHC, 2020). Dispose of in the rubbish bag.

Perform hand hygiene

Maintain the 5 Moments for Hand Hygiene and perform hand hygiene after touching the patient and the patient's surrounds.

CLEAN, REPLACE OR DISPOSE OF EQUIPMENT

Clean, replace and dispose of equipment appropriately to leave equipment in useable condition for the next nurse. This is both a time-management strategy and a courtesy to other staff. Clean the shower area by rinsing the area with the shower hose after finishing. Place any rubbish or disposable items in the general waste. Shower chairs and other equipment should be rinsed and then wiped over using the facility disinfecting wipes and then returned to the storage area. Towels, the mat and facility linen are placed in the linen skip. Return the patient's personal items to their locker. Patient's personal clothing is placed in a laundry bag for the family to collect and wash at home.

Electric razors should be opened and brushed out (over a paper towel) with the brush supplied. The brushings are then folded into the paper and disposed of in the general waste. Disposable razors are disposed of in the sharps container. Communal nail care equipment should be decontaminated according to facility policy (i.e. wiped with disinfecting wipes) before being stored.

DOCUMENT AND REPORT RELEVANT INFORMATION

Completion of patient personal hygiene and grooming needs should be signed in the patient's nursing care plan. Any relevant information or other assessment (e.g. skin assessment, self-care ability) completed during the shower should be recorded in the appropriate charts and nursing notes, plus handed over verbally.

CASE STUDY

Case study 1

Joan Wooley is an 83-year-old woman admitted to the ward. Her carer found her unresponsive at home 4 days ago. Joan has been assessed by the physiotherapist and is a one nurse assist at all times with transfers as she has a mild weakness on her left side. She is not yet walking independently and uses a wheelie commode for elimination and showering.

She requires a shower this morning.
1. Identify the type of shower and how much assistance Joan will require.
2. Outline the actions you will take to maintain her safety while she is in the shower.

Case study 2

Sue Little is a 26-year-old woman who has required surgery for her fractured left tibia and fibula following a motor vehicle accident. Her leg is currently immobilised in a splint, and is bandaged. She has a PIVC in her left hand. She is able to safely weight bear on her right leg when standing or transferring. Sue is active within her limitations post-op.
1. What preparation will you need to do to help Sue have a shower?
2. Identify the type of shower and how much assistance Sue will require.

Note: These notes are summaries of the most important points in the assessments/procedures, and are not exhaustive on the subject. The naming of documents or charts may differ from state to state, and facility to facility. In all possible situations the guidelines of the ACSQHC are used when describing national charts or documents (e.g. the ACSQHC Observation and Response Chart is named the Adult Observation and Response Chart in WA, and the Rapid Detection and Response Observation Chart in SA). References of the materials used to compile the information have been supplied. The student is expected to have learned the material surrounding each skill as presented in the references. No single reference is complete on the subject.

REFERENCES

Australian Commission on Safety and Quality in Health Care (ACSQHC). (2020). *Sequence for Putting on and Removing PPE.* https://www.safetyandquality.gov.au/sites/default/files/2020-03/putting_on_and_removing_ppe_diagram_-_march_2020.pdf

Daly, B. & Smith, K. (2015). Promoting good dental health in older people: role of the community nurse. *British Journal of Community Nursing,* 20(9), pp. 431–6.

Ebrahim, S., Bance, S. & Bowman, K. (2011). Sikh perspectives towards death and end of life care. *Journal of Palliative Care,* 27(2), pp. 170–4.

Gray, S., Ferris, L., White, L.E., Duncan, G. & Baumle, W. (2018). *Foundations of Nursing: Enrolled Nurses* (2nd ANZ ed.). Melbourne: Cengage.

Nøddeskou, L.H., Hemmingsen, L.E. & Hørdam, B. (2015). Elderly patients' and nurses' assessment of traditional bed bath compared to prepacked single units – randomised controlled trial. *Scandinavian Journal of Caring Sciences,* 29(2), pp. 347–52.

Russell, B., Buswell, M., Norton, C., Malone, J.R., Harari, D., Harwood, R., Roe, B., Fader, M., Drennan, V.M., Bunn, F. & Goodman, C. (2017). Supporting people living with dementia and faecal incontinence. *British Journal of Community Nursing,* 22(3), pp. 110–14.

RECOMMENDED READINGS

Australian Nursing and Midwifery Federation (ANMF). (2015). *ANMF Policy – Safe Patient Handling*. http://www.anmf.org.au/documents/policies/P_Safe_Patient_Handling.pdf

Department of Health. (2015). *Post-Fall Management Guidelines: Supplementary Discipline Specific Guidelines*. Perth: Health Strategy and Networks, Department of Health, Western Australia.

Dougherty, L. & Lister, S. (eds). (2015). *The Royal Marsden Hospital Manual of Clinical Nursing Procedures* (9th ed.). Oxford: Wiley-Blackwell.

Lewis, A. & Fricker, A. (2009). Better oral health in residential care. *Staff Portfolio, Education and Training Program*. https://www.sahealth.sa.gov.au/wps/wcm/connect/09fa99004358886a979df72835153af6/BOHRC_Staff_Portfolio_Full_Version%5B1%5D.pdf?MOD=AJPERES&CACHEID=ROOTWORKSPACE-09fa99004358886a979df72835153af6-nwKfcMd

SA Health. (2020). *Oral Health Care Domain – Care of Older People Toolkit*. Government of South Australia. https://www.sahealth.sa.gov.au/wps/wcm/connect/public+content/sa+health+internet/clinical+resources/clinical+programs+and+practice+guidelines/older+people/care+of+older+people+toolkit/oral+health+care+domain+-+care+of+older+people+toolkit

WA Department of Mines, Industry Regulation and Safety. (2014). *Manual Tasks in Healthcare and Social Assistance*. Government of Western Australia. https://www.commerce.wa.gov.au/worksafe/manual-tasks-healthcare-and-social-assistance

WorkSafe Victoria. (n.d.). *Safety and Prevention: Your Industry – Aged Care*. Victorian State Government. http://www.worksafe.vic.gov.au/pages/safety-and-prevention/your-industry/aged-care

ESSENTIAL SKILLS COMPETENCY

Assisting the Patient to Maintain Personal Hygiene – Shower, Undressing/Dressing, Oral Hygiene, Personal Grooming (Including Shaving, Hair and Nail Care)

Demonstrates the ability to effectively maintain personal hygiene in a dependent patient

Criteria for skill performance (Numbers indicate *Enrolled Nurse Standards for Practice*, 2016)	Y (Satisfactory)	D (Requires development)
1. Identifies indication (8.3, 8.4)		
2. Assesses patient for ability, and need for assistance with hygiene and grooming (7.1, 7.2, 8.1, 8.2, 8.3, 8.4)		
3. Identifies safety considerations and follows WHS principles (1.2, 1.4, 1.8, 3.2, 3.9, 6.4, 6.6, 8.4, 9.4)		
4. Gathers equipment as relevant to the skill being performed (1.2, 1.6, 6.4, 8.4, 9.4)		
5. Performs hand hygiene (1.2, 1.4, 1.8, 3.9, 6.4, 9.4)		
6. Evidence of effective therapeutic communication with the patient; gives patient a clear explanation of procedure and confirms patient understanding, gains patient consent (2.1, 2.3, 2.4, 2.5, 6.3)		
7. Dons PPE as required (1.2, 1.4, 1.8, 2.1, 3.2, 3.9, 8.4, 9.4)		
8. Demonstrates problem-solving abilities; e.g. maintains patient dignity and privacy, adjusts water temperature and prepares shower area, attends to environmental temperature (4.1, 4.2, 8.3, 8.4, 9.4)		
9. Assists patient to meet hygiene and grooming needs, according to patient ability (1.2, 1.4, 1.8, 2.1, 2.3, 2.4, 2.7, 3.2, 3.9, 6.1, 6.3, 6.6, 8.4, 9.4): ■ undressing and dressing ■ assisted shower (set-up, assisted or trolley) ■ washes and dries patient safely and correctly		
10. Implements or assists patient with oral hygiene (1.2, 1.4, 1.8, 2.1, 2.3, 2.4, 2.7, 3.2, 3.9, 6.1, 6.3, 6.6, 8.4, 9.4)		
11. Assesses skin and oral mucosa (4.1, 4.2, 7.1, 7.2, 7.5, 8.4, 9.4)		
12. Implements or assists patient with other grooming requirements (1.2, 1.4, 1.8, 2.1, 2.3, 2.4, 2.7, 3.2, 3.9, 6.1, 6.3, 6.6, 8.4, 9.4): ■ hair care ■ shaves male patient ■ other grooming as requested by patient ■ nail care		
13. Doffs PPE and performs hand hygiene (1.2, 1.4, 1.8, 3.9, 6.4, 9.4)		
14. Cleans, replaces and disposes of equipment appropriately (1.2, 1.4, 3.9, 6.5, 9.4)		
15. Documents and reports relevant information (1.2, 1.3, 1.8, 3.2, 5.3, 6.6, 7.1, 7.2, 7.3, 7.4, 7.5)		
16. Demonstrates ability to link theory to practice (8.3, 8.4, 8.5, 9.4)		

Student:

Clinical facilitator: Date:

CHAPTER 3.7

ASSISTING THE PATIENT WITH ELIMINATION – URINARY AND BOWEL ELIMINATION

IDENTIFY INDICATIONS

The management of a patient's continence by supporting and assisting them in their urinary and bowel elimination needs is a vital component of personal care needs and forms part of a nurse's everyday work routine. Relevant nursing actions should be regarded as valued and important care, and more than just a series of required tasks (Russell et al., 2017). Patients may require assistance with meeting their elimination needs for a variety of reasons. These include varied physical or cognitive impairment and medical restrictions (e.g. bed rest with toilet privileges,

postoperative pain). Doctors may order the patient to be maintained on 'bed rest with toilet privileges' in which case the patient can use the toilet with as much assistance as necessary. 'Bed rest' usually means the use of a urinal or bedpan for elimination. Nurses can initiate the use of elimination and continence aids for the patient. Commodes, urinals, bedpans and continence aids provide a receptacle for elimination of patient waste, a means of obtaining a specimen of waste for analysis and a means to obtain an accurate measurement of the patient's output.

ASSESS PATIENT'S ABILITY TO BE INDEPENDENT

Assessing a patient's ability to be independent influences the choice of nursing assistance and elimination aids. Review the patient's mobility chart to determine their level of mobility and required assistance. If the patient is able to ambulate with assistance, taking them to the toilet would be the best option as it is less psychologically unsettling than having to stay in bed, or the bed area, to meet this core personal care need. If the patient is able to transfer but unable to mobilise, a wheelie commode

can transfer them to the toilet or a bedside commode can be used. A commode is similar to a toilet and is less distressing than a bed pan for patients to use. The use of rails in the toilet and over-toilet frames assist patients to access the toilet safely and easily. Urinals and bedpans are usually used in the bed, although some male patients are able to stand at the bedside to use the urinal. Incontinence aids vary, with many enabling patients to avoid embarrassment from episodes of incontinence during their normal daily activities. Actively supporting a patient to maintain their continence needs promotes emotional wellbeing (Yates, 2017).

GATHER EQUIPMENT

Gathering equipment is a time-management strategy. The efficient accomplishment of this procedure reduces the patient's discomfort and embarrassment.

- A *bedside commode* is a chair with a toilet seat and a removable commode bowl below the seat for collection of urine and faeces. They may also have a second plain seat that is closed to transform the commode into a chair.
- A *'wheelie' commode* is a chair on wheels that is designed to be wheeled over a toilet, so the patient is seated on the commode and wheeled to the toilet. Wheelie commodes have locks on their wheels to promote patient safety while the patient is over the

toilet, and when transferring the patient on or off the commode.
- *Over-toilet seat* (elevated toilet seat) is a frame with a toilet seat. It promotes patient safety by reducing the distance to sit down and making the action of sitting on the toilet easier.
- *Toilet rails* are fixed permanently to the walls of the toilet area for patients to use when sitting down, and standing.
- *Bedpans* are commonly available in two types: the regular pan and the fracture or slipper pan, which is smaller and flatter for those patients who have physical limitations or are unable to lift their buttocks onto the regular bedpan. Bedpans are used by female patients

for elimination (urinal and faecal) and are used by male patients for faecal elimination.
- *Urinals* are deep, narrow bottles used by male patients for urinary elimination.
- *Toilet paper* must be available for cleansing the perineum, anal area or penial area after urinary or faecal elimination.
- *Covers* for the bedpan, urinal and commode bowl are used during transport of the used bedpan/urinal to the utility room for disposal. They are more aesthetically pleasing than an open pan or urinal and also help maintain principles of infection control.
- *'Bluey'* is placed under the bedpan to catch any inadvertent spills so the linen is not soiled.
- *Handwashing equipment* should be available: a wet, warm disposable washcloth and towel or hand wipes for cleansing hands following elimination.

- *An air freshener* eliminates odours to reduce embarrassment.
- *Continence aids* include continence pads of various sizes and volume, urinary sheaths and absorbent bed sheets or chair pads. All of these are available in a range of shapes and sizes and are chosen according to the patient's needs. Pads hold varying volumes of fluid and most have the ability to draw the urine away from the skin. Patients using continence pads may also use specific underwear. A urinary sheath will also require a collection bag.
- *Relevant personal protective equipment (PPE)* is gathered for each procedure and standard precautions are followed to handle body secretions and excretions. Non-sterile gloves should be used when there is contact with body fluids, plus a waterproof apron and goggles if there is a risk of splashes.

ASSISTING WITH ELIMINATION NEEDS

Perform hand hygiene
Perform hand hygiene before touching the patient or the patient's surrounds and prior to any procedure involving patient contact to reduce the possibility of cross-contamination. Hand hygiene is the most effective method of infection control as it removes transient organisms from the hands of the nurse (see **Skill 1.1**).

Give a clear explanation of the procedure and establish therapeutic communication
Introduce yourself, and check you have the correct patient. Explain the procedure and gain the patient's consent. Giving a clear explanation is required to gain legal consent and to address policy requirements. It will also assist the patient to cooperate with the procedure, allay anxiety and assist in establishing a therapeutic relationship.

Effective communication and sensitivity to the patient's emotional wellbeing when assisting a patient with their elimination needs is vital (Russell et al., 2017). Patients require privacy, dignity and recognition of their cultural needs. Prompt response to a patient's request for assistance with elimination will reduce a patient's anxiety and reduce the risk of patient injury from falls, skin irritation, pressure injury and poor emotional wellbeing (Yates, 2017). Socially, adults are expected to meet their own elimination needs without assistance and may feel like they are regressing when help is needed. Constipation may be a complication from suppression of the urge to defecate or self-limiting their fluid intake to reduce the need to pass urine. Clear explanation of the reasons why a bedpan or urinal is necessary will help to reduce feelings of inadequacy. Tact and consideration are needed so the patient's embarrassment about sights, sounds and odours is not heightened.

Recognising the non-verbal cues of patients with limited communication skill or dementia is also an important part of the communication process, and will reduce their risk of incontinence (Shih et al., 2015).

Demonstrate problem-solving abilities
Displaying problem-solving abilities to give patients maximum comfort during elimination usually means positioning them as close to the usual anatomical position assumed for toileting as possible. The patient's condition and restrictions will determine this. Use of a commode is preferred, and promotes normal position if the use of a toilet is not possible. If using a bedpan, ensure the bedpan is correctly positioned under the patient.

Take care that the contents of the elimination aid are not spilled during removal. Toilet paper, air freshener and handwashing equipment should be available. Wear non-sterile disposable gloves, plastic apron and goggles for protection against body fluids, especially in removal of elimination aids.

Assist the patient to use a bedside and wheelie commode
The patient is assisted out of bed and onto the commode, according to their mobility chart. Assist the patient to pull down their pants and clothing as required. Ensure the patient's dignity is maintained (i.e. cover all exposed body parts) and wheel the commode chair over the toilet. Ensure the scrotum and genitalia of a male patient does not become trapped between the toilet and the commode chair. If using a bedside commode, the patient can remain in the bed area. If the patient is safe, pull the curtains or close the door and leave them in privacy, with the call bell in their hands. Stand outside the area waiting for the patient to finish. Other patients will require constant supervision.

The patient may or may not need assistance to clean the perineal, anus or penial area. If assistance is needed, help the patient to stand. Use toilet paper in your gloved hand to wipe the perineal area from the pubic area backwards to the anal area in women, so that faecal material is not brought forward to the urinary (or vaginal) meatus, and from behind the scrotum in men. Use one stroke per each piece of paper. If needed, use a wet disposable washcloth to clean the anal area. Assist the patient to pull up their clothing when standing or transferring back to their bed. Provide the patient with handwashing equipment to prevent the spread of microorganisms. Use air freshener if there are no contraindications (patients with respiratory difficulties may react adversely to the aerosolised particles; the perfume in some fresheners is offensive to some patients) to eliminate embarrassing odours. Remove the commode from the room for cleaning.

Give and receive a urinal

Assist the patient to stand at the bedside if mobility permits, or sit in a semi-upright position. Most patients are able to position the urinal independently. If not, place the urinal between the patient's legs with the handle upward. The penis may need to be placed in the urinal neck. Leave the patient in privacy and with the call bell within easy reach. Return when called. Wearing non-sterile gloves, remove the urinal. If required, wipe the tip of the penis to remove any urine. Offer handwashing equipment. Take the covered urinal to the pan room.

Give and receive a bedpan

Place the bedpan on the end of the bed or on an adjacent chair. Fold the covers down to expose the hip and adjust the gown/pyjamas to prevent any soiling. Assist the patient to raise their buttocks off the bed. The supine patient should flex their knees and, resting their weight on heels and back, raise the buttocks. The nurse assists by raising the back of the bed, and assisting the patient to sit up comfortably (if not contraindicated). Place a bluey (waterproof sheet) and the bedpan, with the open end towards the feet, under the buttocks of the patient. If the patient is unable to lift their bottom, follow the principles of manual handling to roll the patient onto their side, insert the bedpan under their buttocks and then roll them back. Make sure the smooth round end of the bedpan is in contact with the buttocks to prevent both abrasion of the skin and spillage of the contents of the pan. A slipper pan is placed with the flat end under the patient's buttocks. Cover the patient, and leave them in privacy with the call bell in reach. Leave the toilet paper within reach. When the patient is finished, remove the cover and ask the patient to raise their buttocks. Remove the bedpan, leaving the waterproof sheet. If the patient requires assistance to clean their perineal area, use a gloved hand to wipe the perineal area from pubic area backwards to anal area in women, and from behind the scrotum in men so that faecal material is not brought forward to the

urinary (or vaginal) meatus. Use one stroke per each piece of paper. Turn the patient on their side and spread the buttocks to clean the anal area in the same manner. Soiled toilet paper is placed in the bedpan. If needed, use a wet disposable washcloth to clean the anal area. Remove the bluey. Provide the patient with handwashing equipment to clean their hands to prevent the spread of microorganisms. If required use air freshener provided there are no contraindications (patients with respiratory difficulties may react adversely to the aerosolised particles; the perfume in some fresheners is offensive to some patients) to eliminate embarrassing odours. Take the covered bedpan to the pan room.

Continence aids

Ensure patients are using a continence aid as recommended by the continence adviser. Pads should be changed when soiled or full. They should be checked when the patient goes to the toilet, repositioned or when washed. Many pads will have a colour strip on the outside or underneath that changes colour to indicate the volume of urine already absorbed. Wear non-sterile gloves and plastic apron to change the pad and place in paper bag.

Continence sheets and chair pads are used with a plastic sheet underneath to protect the bed linen or chair. They are changed when no longer able to absorb the moisture away from the patient. External urinary sheaths are applied to the penile shaft using the supplied adhesive. Ensure no pubic hair is trapped. Attach the open end of the sheath to the tubing from the urinary collection bag. The urinary sheath is checked on a regular basis (for looseness, leakage or tightness) and changed as per facility policy.

Dispose of excreta

Urine and faecal waste (excreta) is disposed of in the toilet or in the dirty utility area. The elimination aid is covered during transport to the dirty utility area as an aesthetic measure and to maintain principles of infection control. Clean gloves are worn for protection against bodily fluids and a plastic apron may be required. Bedpan covers, blueys, soiled pads and urinary sheaths are disposed of in the normal rubbish in the dirty utility room. Liquids are measured (if necessary), observed for characteristics and flushed down the toilet or pan sluice. Pads, urinals and bedpans can be weighed on scales in the dirty utility room to determine the urine volume. Refer to the manufacturer's product guide to help determine the correct volume. Faeces are observed for colour, consistency and amount, and then flushed down the toilet or sluice. See **Skill 3.9**.

Perform hand hygiene

Maintain the 5 Moments for Hand Hygiene and perform hand hygiene after touching the patient and the patient's surrounds.

CLEAN, REPLACE OR DISPOSE OF EQUIPMENT

Clean and then return toileting aids to storage areas. Check the stock levels of disposable equipment and restock if necessary.

Non-disposable pans and urinals are cleaned and disinfected (according to facility guidelines) and returned to the rack. Alternatively, facilities may use a macerator that pulps and disposes of disposable pans or urinals and excreta. Absorbent sheets and chair pads are sent to the laundry for washing. Ensure they are placed in a leakproof bag, according to infection control guidelines for linen. Commodes are cleaned with disposable wipes as per facility policy, then returned to their usual position.

DOCUMENT AND REPORT RELEVANT INFORMATION

Documentation of bowel action is on the patient observation and response chart for all patients and a bowel chart, if being used. The documentation of all output is required for some patients and a fluid balance chart or output chart is used. In this case, all urine will need to be measured (or weighed if using an incontinence pad). Some areas may also require the weighing of liquid faecal excreta to determine the volume.

CASE STUDY

Joan Wooley is an 83-year-old woman admitted to the ward. Four days ago, her carer found her at home lying on the floor. She was initially unresponsive but is now conscious and able to communicate. She has a mild weakness on her left side.

Joan has called for assistance. She would like to have her bowels open, but does not feel steady enough to walk to the toilet.

1. What assessments will you do to decide if you will assist her onto the bedside commode or bed pan?
2. Outline the steps you will take for assisting Joan to use each of the above.

Note: These notes are summaries of the most important points in the assessments/procedures, and are not exhaustive on the subject. The naming of documents or charts may differ from state to state, and facility to facility. In all possible situations the guidelines of the ACSQHC are used when describing national charts or documents (e.g. the ACSQHC Observation and Response Chart is named the Adult Observation and Response Chart in WA, and the Rapid Detection and Response Observation Chart in SA). References of the materials used to compile the information have been supplied. The student is expected to have learned the material surrounding each skill as presented in the references. No single reference is complete on the subject.

REFERENCES

Russell, B., Buswell, M., Norton, C., Malone, J.R., Harari, D., Harwood, R., Roe, B., Fader, M., Drennan, V.M., Bunn, F. & Goodman, C. (2017). Supporting people living with dementia and faecal incontinence. *British Journal of Community Nursing*, 22(3), pp. 110–14.

Shih, Y., Wang, C., Sue, E. & Wang, J. (2015). Behavioral characteristics of bowel movement and urination needs in patients with dementia in Taiwan. *Journal of Gerontological Nursing*, 41(6), pp. 22–9.

Yates, A. (2017). Urinary continence care for older people in the acute setting. *British Journal of Nursing*, 26(9), S28–S29.

RECOMMENDED READINGS

CNA Training Advisor. (2015). *Toileting*, 13(10), 1–5.

Dougherty, L. & Lister, S. (eds). (2015). *The Royal Marsden Hospital Manual of Clinical Nursing Procedures* (9th ed.). Oxford: Wiley-Blackwell.

ESSENTIAL SKILLS COMPETENCY

Assisting the Patient with Elimination

Demonstrates the ability to effectively and safely assist patients with their elimination needs

Criteria for skill performance	Y	D
(Numbers indicate *Enrolled Nurse Standards for Practice*, 2016)	(Satisfactory)	(Requires development)
1. Identifies indication (8.3, 8.4)		
2. Assesses patient's ability to be independent (1.2, 1.8, 7.1, 7.2, 8.4, 9.4)		
3. Gathers equipment (1.2, 1.6, 4.4, 6.4, 8.4, 9.4): ■ commode, bedpan, urinal as required ■ coversheets, PPE as required ■ toilet paper, bluey, air freshener ■ hand hygiene equipment ■ relevant personal protective equipment ■ continence aids (if required)		
4. Performs hand hygiene (1.2, 1.4, 1.8, 3.9, 6.4, 9.4)		
5. Evidence of therapeutic communication with the patient; gives explanation of procedure, gains patient consent (2.1, 2.3, 2.4, 2.5, 6.3)		
6. Demonstrates problem-solving abilities (4.1, 4.2, 8.3, 8.4, 9.4)		
7. Assists the patient to use the commode (1.2, 1.4, 1.8, 2.1, 2.3, 2.4, 2.7, 3.2, 3.9, 6.1, 6.3, 6.6, 9.4)		
8. Gives and removes a urinal (1.2, 1.4, 2.1, 2.3, 2.4, 2.7, 3.2, 3.9, 6.1, 6.3, 9.4)		
9. Gives and removes a bedpan (1.2, 1.4, 1.8, 2.1, 2.3, 2.4, 2.7, 3.2, 3.9, 6.1, 6.3, 6.6, 9.4)		
10. Leaves patient comfortable and safe (1.2, 1.4, 1.8, 2.3, 2.4, 2.7, 3.2, 3.9, 6.1, 6.9, 9.4)		
11. Disposes of excreta (1.2, 1.4, 1.8, 3.2, 3.9, 6.4, 8.4, 9.4)		
12. Performs hand hygiene (1.2, 1.4, 1.8, 3.9, 6.4, 9.4)		
13. Cleans, replaces and disposes of equipment appropriately (1.2, 1.4, 3.9, 6.5, 9.4)		
14. Documents and reports relevant information (1.2, 1.3, 1.8, 3.2, 5.3, 6.6, 7.1, 7.2, 7.3, 7.4, 7.5)		
15. Demonstrates ability to link theory to practice (8.3, 8.4, 8.5, 9.4)		

Student:

Clinical facilitator: Date:

CHAPTER 3.8

URINE SPECIMEN COLLECTION AND URINALYSIS

IDENTIFY INDICATIONS

Urinalysis is the analysis of the patient's urine which contributes to the assessment of a patient's health status. Many medical conditions and fluid volume alterations manifest in the urine and a simple urinalysis may reveal many abnormalities, including a possible urinary tract infection (Collins, 2019; Malmartel et al., 2017; Shimoni et al., 2017). Urinalysis may be completed as part of a patient's admission, preoperatively, if the urine is offensive and the nurse suspects a possible infection, and as part of the management of some medical conditions.

Urine specimens are also collected for laboratory testing (microbiology and biochemistry testing are the most common). These are always ordered by a doctor or a nurse practitioner. The nurse needs to be aware of any ordered test to ensure they can be collected and sent to the laboratory as soon as possible.

GATHER AND PREPARE EQUIPMENT

Gathering equipment before commencing the procedure creates a positive environment for successfully completing the skill. It is also a time-management strategy that provides an opportunity to rehearse the procedure mentally, as well as boosting patient confidence and trust in the nurse and increasing the nurse's self-confidence. Planning and efficiency by the nurse will help to reduce the patient's discomfort and embarrassment when collecting specimens.

Please refer to **Skill 3.7** for specific information about equipment used to assist a patient with their elimination needs.

Equipment specific for the collection of a urine specimen for ward urinalysis or a laboratory specimen is as follows.
- *Commode* with bowl, bedpan, urinal or disposable cup to pass urine in.
- *Urine-testing equipment.* Urine-testing reagent strips or automated electronic urine-testing machine, paper towel and gloves.

- *Personal protective equipment (PPE).* Relevant PPE is gathered for each procedure and standard precautions are followed to handle body secretions and excretions. Non-sterile gloves, plastic apron and googles are worn for personal protection during possible contact with bodily fluids. Notepaper and pen for recording the results before recording on the patient observation chart which cannot be taken into the dirty utility room.
- *Watch (or clock) with second hand* for timing the procedure.
- *Urine specimen collection container, request form and biohazard bag.* The sterile container must be labelled correctly; a biohazard bag in which to place the container should be available. Check for correct specimen container according to the specimen required.
- *Patient ID label* for labelling the specimen container.
- *A 20 mL 'Luer slip' tipped syringe* for catheter specimen of urine.

PERFORM URINALYSIS AND SPECIMEN COLLECTION

Perform hand hygiene
Perform hand hygiene before touching the patient or the patient's surrounds and prior to any procedure involving patient contact to reduce the possibility of cross-contamination. Hand hygiene is the most effective method of infection control as it removes transient organisms from the hands of the nurse (see **Skill 1.1**).

Give a clear explanation of the procedure and establish therapeutic communication
Introduce yourself, and check you have the correct patient. Explain the procedure and gain the patient's consent. Giving a clear explanation is required to gain

legal consent and to address policy requirements. It will also assist the patient to cooperate with the procedure, allay anxiety and assist in establishing a therapeutic relationship.

Effective communication for these nursing procedures is very important. Tact and consideration are needed when dealing with a patient's urine, so that potential embarrassment about sights, sounds and odours is not heightened.

Demonstrate problem-solving abilities

A patient's condition and mobility restrictions will determine if they are positioned on a toilet, bedpan, commode or urinal used for collection of a specimen for urinalysis or the laboratory. Displaying problem-solving abilities to give patients maximum comfort during elimination and collection of the specimen usually means positioning them as close to the usual anatomical position assumed for toileting as possible. The patient's condition and restrictions will determine this. Refer to **Skill 3.7** for guidelines on assisting a patient with their elimination needs.

Perform urinalysis

Collect a clean urine specimen for ward urinalysis using a clean, non-contaminated bedpan, urinal, commode bowl or disposable cup. The nurse may need to assist the patient when collecting the specimen. Mobile patients can provide the specimen independently. Urinalysis is a ward routine, and a fresh specimen of urine is always used. The collection receptacle should be clean to prevent any changes in test results due to contamination.

The ward urinalysis testing is completed in the dirty utility room. Non-sterile gloves, plastic apron and goggles are worn during the testing procedure. Ensure the easy ability to view a watch or clock without contaminating personal clothing during the procedure. If the facility has an automated electronic urinalysis machine, the facility instructions for using this device correctly should be followed and then the printout obtained for attaching to the patient's notes/charts. The urine is initially observed. Characteristics of the urine are determined by observing the amount, colour (lemon, amber, blood stained), clarity (clear or cloudy) and odour of the urine specimen. The urine is then tested using the facility reagent/test strip. Keep a small piece of notepaper on which to write your results that are later recorded on the patient's chart. Any abnormalities should be reported.

A reagent strip is used to test the urine. These strips vary between manufacturers, but the key points listed here are standard inclusions. Check the reagent strips used in the facility for the manufacturer's instructions. Also check the expiry date to ensure the strips are not out of date. Using your gloved fingers, remove one reagent strip from the bottle and recap the bottle tightly. The strip is immersed to ensure all test areas on the strip are in the urine sample, and then withdrawn. Gently blot the back of the strip against a paper towel placed flat on the bench and use a watch or clock on the pan

room wall to note the time the strip is dipped. Hold the test strip as close to the container and the results guide as possible without touching, as this will contaminate the container. Using the guide on the container, read the test areas as their reaction time is reached. The usual result is negative (other than the pH and SG) since none of the components should be in the urine of a healthy person.

- *Specific gravity* (SG) is the degree of concentration of the urine compared with that of an equal volume of distilled water (standard). Normal range is 1005 to 1020. pH determines the acidity:alkalinity of the urine. Normal range is 4.5 to 8.0 (Gray et al., 2018). All urine is tested for these readings. Abnormalities in the reading give information about a patient's health status.
- *Glucose, ketone bodies, protein, bilirubin, blood, nitrites and leucocytes* are abnormalities. Depending on the results, it can indicate medical problems such as changes in kidney function, urinary tract infection or unstable diabetes. Any abnormalities should be reported. Please refer to Joustra and Moloney (2019, p. 160) for more specific information.

Dispose of the collected urine in the sluice or macerator as per the facility protocol. Dispose of the reagent strip, non-sterile gloves, disposable apron and any other items in the general rubbish.

Record the characteristics of the *urine, SG, pH and any abnormal test results* on the patient observation and response chart (ORC) and other relevant documents.

Collection of a urine specimen for the laboratory

Laboratory urine specimens may be collected when a patient voids naturally or from a catheter. Place a patient label onto a sterile specimen container. Before transporting to the laboratory, all specimens will need to be placed in a laboratory biohazard bag and sealed. The request form is placed in the separated outside sleeve that is part of the biohazard bag to prevent contamination of the form by the specimen or specimen container.

- *Catheter specimen.* Urine should not be collected directly from the urine drainage bag, as it will be contaminated. The correct procedure is to first clamp the catheter below the collecting port for approximately 30 minutes. Wearing non-sterile gloves, plastic apron and goggles, swab the aspiration/collecting port. Wait 60 seconds for the alcohol to evaporate. Insert a sterile, 20 mL 'Luer slip' tipped syringe into the port and withdraw urine volume as required (Bardsley, 2015). Some gentle aspiration may be required. Remove the syringe, then remove the clamp. Transfer urine collected into a pre-labelled sterile specimen container, taking care not to contaminate the inside of the container. Place in the laboratory biohazard bag.
- *Midstream urine (MSU) or other specimens.* Wearing non-sterile gloves, plastic apron and goggles, clean patient genitalia with water. Allow the patient to commence voiding and then place the sterile labelled

container under the urine stream to collect a small amount of the midstream urine (Bardsley, 2015; Holm & Aabenhus, 2016). Remove the container, replace the lid and put it in a laboratory biohazard bag. If the patient is orientated and able, they may be able to collect this specimen without assistance.

■ *Twenty-four-hour urine.* Obtain the specific 24-hour collection bottle from the laboratory. At commencement, ask the patient to void and then discard this urine. Note the commencement time on the chart and also note it on the collection bottle. Wearing non-sterile gloves, plastic apron and goggles, all urine voided into a clean receptacle over the next 24 hours is collected and placed in a specific collection container. Exactly at the end of the 24 hours, the patient voids and this final specimen is placed in the container. Note: If any urine specimen is missed, spilt or contaminated, a new container is obtained and the process must start again.

Perform hand hygiene

Maintain the 5 Moments for Hand Hygiene and perform hand hygiene after touching the patient and the patient's surrounds.

CLEAN, REPLACE OR DISPOSE OF EQUIPMENT

Clean the work area where the specimen has been assessed/specimen collected for the laboratory. Dispose any excreta in the sluice, avoiding any splashing or spills. PPE can then be removed and disposed of in the appropriate waste bin. Clean or dispose of goggles according to facility policy. Clean and then return toileting aids to storage areas. Check the stock levels of reagent strips for urinalysis and sterile urine containers for urine specimens, and restock if necessary.

DOCUMENT AND REPORT RELEVANT INFORMATION

Urinalysis is documented on the patient ORC. SG, pH, colour and clarity are always noted, and any other abnormal findings are recorded and reported. Specimen collection is recorded appropriately in the patient's notes and nursing care plan and the patient ORC.

CASE STUDY

Joan Wooley is an 83-year-old woman admitted to the ward. Two days ago, her carer found her at home lying on the floor. She was initially unresponsive but is now conscious and able to communicate. She has a mild weakness on her left side.

Joan has been admitted to the ward and requires a routine ward urinalysis.

1. Explain the procedure for conducting a urinalysis.
2. You note Joan's urine has a pH of 7 and SG of 1010. What is your assessment of these results?
3. Where will you record these results?

Note: These notes are summaries of the most important points in the assessments/procedures, and are not exhaustive on the subject. The naming of documents or charts may differ from state to state, and facility to facility. In all possible situations the guidelines of the ACSQHC are used when describing national charts or documents (e.g. the ACSQHC Observation and Response Chart is named the Adult Observation and Response Chart in WA, and the Rapid Detection and Response Observation Chart in SA). References of the materials used to compile the information have been supplied. The student is expected to have learned the material surrounding each skill as presented in the references. No single reference is complete on the subject.

REFERENCES

Bardsley, A. (2015). How to perform a urinalysis. *Nursing Standard* (2015), 30(2), p. 34.

Collins, L. (2019). Diagnosis and management of a urinary tract infection. *British Journal of Nursing*, 28(2), pp. 84–8.

Gray, S., Ferris, L., White, L.E., Duncan, G. & Baumle, W. (2018). *Foundations of Nursing: Enrolled Nurses* (2nd ANZ ed.). Melbourne: Cengage.

Holm, A. & Aabenhus, R. (2016). Urine sampling techniques in symptomatic primary-care patients: a diagnostic accuracy review. *BMC Family Practice*, 17(72). https://doi.org/10.1186/s12875-016-0465-4

Joustra, C. & Moloney, A. (2019). *Clinical Placement Manual* (1st ed.). Melbourne: Cengage.

Malmartel, A., Dutron, M. & Ghasarossian, C. (2017). Tracking unnecessary negative urinalyses to reduce healthcare costs: A transversal study. *European Journal of Clinical Microbiology and Infectious Diseases*, 36(9), pp. 1559–63.

Shimoni, Z., Glick, J., Hermush, V. & Froom, P. (2017). Sensitivity of the dipstick in detecting bacteremic urinary tract infections in elderly hospitalized patients. *PLoS One*, 12(10).

RECOMMENDED READINGS

Davis, C. (2019). Catheter-associated urinary tract infection: signs, diagnosis, prevention. *British Journal of Nursing*, 28(2), pp. 96–100.

Dougherty, L. & Lister, S. (eds). (2015). *The Royal Marsden Hospital Manual of Clinical Nursing Procedures* (9th ed.). Oxford: Wiley-Blackwell.

National Health and Medical Research Council (NHMRC). (2019). *Australian Guidelines for the Prevention and Control of Infection in Healthcare.* https://www.nhmrc.gov.au/health-advice/public-health/preventing-infection

ESSENTIAL SKILLS COMPETENCY

Urinalysis and Urine Specimen Collection

Demonstrates the ability to effectively and safely assist patients with their elimination needs

Criteria for skill performance	Y	D
(Numbers indicate *Enrolled Nurse Standards for Practice*, 2016)	(Satisfactory)	(Requires development)
1. Identifies indication (8.3, 8.4)		
2. Gathers equipment (1.2, 1.6, 4.4, 6.4, 8.4, 9.4): ■ commode, bedpan as required ■ non-sterile gloves, plastic apron and goggles ■ specimen collection container ■ urine testing equipment ■ clock or watch with second hand ■ further equipment as per required laboratory specimen		
3. Performs hand hygiene (1.2, 1.4, 1.8, 3.9, 6.4, 9.4)		
4. Evidence of therapeutic communication with the patient; gives explanation of procedure, gains patient consent (2.1, 2.3, 2.4, 2.5, 6.3)		
5. Demonstrates problem-solving abilities (4.1, 4.2, 8.3, 8.4, 9.4)		
6. Performs routine urinalysis; collects laboratory urine specimen as required (1.2, 1.4, 4.2, 4.4, 9.4)		
7. Leaves patient comfortable and safe (1.2, 1.4, 1.8, 2.3, 2.4, 2.7, 3.2, 3.9, 6.1, 6.9, 9.4)		
8. Disposes of excreta (1.2, 1.4, 1.8, 3.2, 3.9, 6.4, 8.4, 9.4)		
9. Performs hand hygiene (1.2, 1.4, 1.8, 3.9, 6.4, 9.4)		
10. Cleans, replaces and disposes of equipment appropriately (1.2, 1.4, 3.9, 6.5, 9.4)		
11. Documents and reports relevant information (1.2, 1.3, 1.8, 3.2, 5.3, 6.6, 7.1, 7.2, 7.3, 7.4, 7.5)		
12. Demonstrates ability to link theory to practice (8.3, 8.4, 8.5, 9.4)		

Student:

Clinical facilitator: Date:

CHAPTER 3.9

FAECES ASSESSMENT AND SPECIMEN COLLECTION

IDENTIFY INDICATIONS

Monitoring the regularity of a patient's bowel actions and the type of faeces excreted provides information about a patient's health status. All patients should be asked if they have opened their bowels and the results recorded on the observation and response chart (ORC) each shift. The changes caused by illness or hospital treatment such as pain medication, reduced mobility, reduced fluid intake or dietary change can cause changes in regular bowel actions, especially constipation. Additional assessment of the faeces can provide information that is an important indicator of the patient's health status, as well as reduce the potential for constipation.

Faeces can be assessed for colour and consistency. The Bristol Stool Chart identifies seven different types of faeces (Continence Foundation of Australia, 2020) and provides an aid to accurate and descriptive recording which ensures consistency between members of the clinical team. Changes in a patient's diet or medication can affect the colour and consistency of faeces and alterations in a patient's pattern of defecation, and may also indicate a potential health problem (e.g. a melaena stool is an indication of upper gastrointestinal tract bleeding). Laboratory faeces specimens may be collected to confirm or identify the presence of blood in the faeces or to identify an infectious organism causing diarrhoea.

GATHER AND PREPARE EQUIPMENT

Gathering equipment before commencing the procedure creates a positive environment for successfully completing the skill. It is also a time-management strategy that provides an opportunity to rehearse the procedure mentally, as well as boosting patient confidence and trust in the nurse and increasing the nurse's self-confidence. Planning and efficiency by the nurse will help to reduce the patient's discomfort and embarrassment when collecting specimens.

Please refer to **Skill 3.7** for specific information about equipment used to assist a patient with their elimination needs.

Equipment specific for the collection of a faeces sample for a laboratory specimen is as follows.

- *Commode* with bowl or bedpan for the patient to pass faeces in.
- *Personal protective equipment (PPE)*. Relevant PPE is gathered for each procedure and standard precautions are followed to handle body secretions and excretions. Non-sterile gloves, plastic apron and goggles are worn.
- *Faeces specimen container, request form and biohazard bag*. This container is usually non-transparent and has a built-in scoop in the lid. The container must be labelled correctly; a biohazard bag in which to place the container should be available. Check the correct specimen container according to the specimen required.
- *Patient ID label* for labelling the specimen container.

PERFORM FAECES ASSESSMENT AND COLLECT SPECIMEN

Perform hand hygiene

Perform hand hygiene before touching the patient or the patient's surrounds and prior to any procedure involving patient contact to reduce the possibility of cross-contamination. Hand hygiene is the most effective method of infection control as it removes transient organisms from the hands of the nurse (see **Skill 1.1**).

Give a clear explanation of the procedure and establish therapeutic communication

Introduce yourself, and check you have the correct patient. Discuss the procedure and gain the patient's consent. Giving a clear explanation is required to gain legal consent and to address policy requirements. It will also assist the patient to cooperate with the procedure, allay anxiety and assist in establishing a therapeutic relationship.

Effective communication for these nursing procedures is very important. Tact and consideration are needed when dealing with a patient's faeces, so that potential embarrassment about sights, sounds and odours is not heightened.

Demonstrate problem-solving abilities

A patient's condition and mobility restrictions will determine if they are positioned on a toilet, bedpan or commode to open their bowels, and then enable the nurse to assess the patient's faeces or collect a faeces specimen for the laboratory. Refer to **Skill 3.7** for guidelines on assisting a patient with their elimination needs.

Faeces assessment

Assist the patient with their elimination needs (as per **Skill 3.7**) and collect a specimen in either a bedpan or toilet (using a commode bowl). While continuing to wear gloves, plastic apron and goggles, take the faeces specimen to the designated dirty area to complete a full assessment or to collect a specimen. Assess the faeces to determine the colour, size (volume) and consistency. Refer to the Bristol Stool Chart, which is often left in a visible location in the pan room, to assist with the description of the faeces (Continence Foundation of Australia, 2020). Record the results on the appropriate charts.

Collection of a faeces specimen for the laboratory

Place a patient label onto the sterile specimen container prior to collecting the specimen. If possible, ask the patient to avoid passing urine or leaving toilet paper in the same receptacle as the faeces. Wear non-sterile gloves, plastic apron and goggles when collecting the specimen. Use the small scoop inside the specimen container lid to obtain a spoon-sized specimen from the faeces. Place the specimen in the container and tighten the lid without contaminating the outside of the container (laboratory staff may

refuse to process a specimen if the outer area is contaminated).

After disposing of the waste and performing hand hygiene, check the correct date and time is on the specimen and the request form. Place the specimen in the press seal section of the biohazard bag for transporting to the laboratory. The request form is placed in the separated outside sleeve that is part of the biohazard bag, to prevent contamination of the form by the specimen or specimen container.

Perform hand hygiene

Maintain the 5 Moments for Hand Hygiene and perform hand hygiene after touching the patient and the patient's surrounds.

CLEAN, REPLACE OR DISPOSE OF EQUIPMENT

Clean the work area where the specimen has been assessed/specimen collected for the laboratory. Dispose of any excreta in the sluice, avoiding any splashing or spills. PPE can then be removed and disposed of in the appropriate waste bin. Clean and then return toileting aids to storage areas. Check the stock levels of faeces specimen containers and restock if necessary.

DOCUMENT AND REPORT RELEVANT INFORMATION

Bowel actions are recorded for every patient each shift on the ORC in acute areas, or bowel books in community-based care agencies. Bowel actions should also be recorded on the fluid balance chart if it is used. If the patient is on a bowel chart, refer to the Bristol Stool Chart to describe the faeces. Any abnormalities or specimens sent to the laboratory should be noted in the nursing notes. Specimen collections may also be recorded on the nursing care plan. Changes in the patient's bowel habit should be reported during shift handover, with any sudden changes reported to the shift coordinator and medical team.

CASE STUDY

Joan Wooley is an 83-year-old woman admitted to the ward. Two days ago, her carer found her at home lying on the floor. She was initially unresponsive but is now conscious and able to communicate. She has a mild weakness on her left side.

In the past 24 hours, Joan has had five loose bowel actions.
1. What chart would you use to record and monitor her frequent bowel actions? You are required to collect a stool specimen for sending to the laboratory.
2. Outline the steps you follow to collect the sample.

Note: These notes are summaries of the most important points in the assessments/procedures, and are not exhaustive on the subject. The naming of documents or charts may differ from state to state, and facility to facility. In all possible situations the guidelines of the ACSQHC are used when describing national charts or documents (e.g. the ACSQHC Observation and Response Chart is named the Adult Observation and Response Chart in WA, and the Rapid Detection and Response Observation Chart in SA). References of the materials used to compile the information have been supplied. The student is expected to have learned the material surrounding each skill as presented in the references. No single reference is complete on the subject.

REFERENCES

Continence Foundation of Australia, (2020). *Faecal Continence: Bristol Stool Chart*. https://www.continence.org.au/pages/bristol-stool-chart.html

RECOMMENDED READINGS

Dougherty, L. & Lister, S. (eds). (2015). *The Royal Marsden Hospital Manual of Clinical Nursing Procedures* (9th ed.). Oxford: Wiley-Blackwell.

PART 3

ESSENTIAL SKILLS COMPETENCY

Faeces Assessment

Demonstrates the ability to effectively and safely assist patients with their elimination needs

Criteria for skill performance	Y	D
(Numbers indicate *Enrolled Nurse Standards for Practice*, 2016)	(Satisfactory)	(Requires development)
1. Identifies indication (8.3, 8.4)		
2. Gathers equipment (1.2, 1.6, 4.4, 6.4, 8.4, 9.4): ■ commode, bedpan as required ■ non-sterile gloves, plastic apron and goggles ■ specimen collection equipment and further equipment as per required laboratory specimen		
3. Performs hand hygiene (1.2, 1.4, 1.8, 3.9, 6.4, 9.4)		
4. Evidence of therapeutic communication with the patient; gives explanation of procedure, gains patient consent (2.1, 2.3, 2.4, 2.5, 6.3)		
5. Demonstrates problem-solving abilities (4.1, 4.2, 8.3, 8.4, 9.4)		
6. Assesses faeces and collects faeces specimen as required (1.2, 1.4, 1.8, 2.1, 2.3, 2.4, 2.7, 3.2, 3.9, 6.1, 6.3, 6.6, 9.4)		
7. Leaves patient comfortable and safe (1.2, 1.4, 1.8, 2.3, 2.4, 2.7, 3.2, 3.9, 6.1, 6.9, 9.4)		
8. Disposes of excreta (1.2, 1.4, 1.8, 3.2, 3.9, 6.4, 8.4, 9.4)		
9. Performs hand hygiene (1.2, 1.4, 1.8, 3.9, 6.4, 9.4)		
10. Cleans, replaces and disposes of equipment appropriately (1.2, 1.4, 3.9, 6.5, 9.4)		
11. Documents and reports relevant information (1.2, 1.3, 1.8, 3.2, 5.3, 6.6, 7.1, 7.2, 7.3, 7.4, 7.5)		
12. Demonstrates ability to link theory to practice (8.3, 8.4, 8.5, 9.4)		

Student:

Clinical facilitator: Date:

CHAPTER 3.10

ASSISTING THE PATIENT WITH COLOSTOMY CARE

IDENTIFY INDICATIONS

An artificial opening (stoma) is created on the abdominal wall after a segment of the bowel is surgically removed and a section of the bowel is brought to the surface of the abdominal wall (Australian Council of Stoma Associations [ACSA], 2021a). It is used to treat specific bowel disease (e.g. colon cancer), and can be temporary or permanent. The section of the bowel involved determines the name of the stoma, and also determines the consistency of the faeces (e.g. formed, soft or liquid) excreted through the stoma. Types include an ileostomy which involves the ileum and colostomy which involves the colon. Colostomy is the most common type (Burch, 2017). A pouch is applied to the stoma to collect the faeces.

The stoma therapy nurse will work with all patients who have a stoma to provide support, as well as assist in determining the correct type of appliance (pouch and barrier system) that suits their individual needs. Nurses caring for patients with a stoma should continue to maintain this liaison when assisting patients with the care of a stoma.

GATHER EQUIPMENT

Gathering equipment is a time-management strategy. The efficient accomplishment of this procedure reduces the patient's discomfort and embarrassment.

- *Non-sterile gloves and a plastic apron* are worn for personal protection during possible contact with bodily fluids. *Goggles* may also be worn if there is a splash risk.
- *Washcloth*, plus a *bowl of warm water* to clean the stoma site.
- *New/clean appliance*; that is, a two-piece system with a stoma pouch and barrier (wafer and backplate) or a one-piece system where the barrier and pouch are in one piece (ACSA, 2021b).
- *Template and sharp scissors* for cutting a hole in the wafer to correct size. Some precut systems are available.
- *Other stoma products as preferred by the patient (e.g. stoma paste, protective powders and deodorant).*
- *Paper bag* for disposal of the used bag before placing in the clinical waste.

ASSISTING WITH STOMA CARE

Perform hand hygiene
Perform hand hygiene before touching the patient or the patient's surrounds and prior to any procedure involving patient contact to reduce the possibility of cross-contamination. Hand hygiene is the most effective method of infection control as it removes transient organisms from the hands of the nurse (see **Skill 1.1**).

Give a clear explanation of the procedure and establish therapeutic communication
Introduce yourself, and check you have the correct patient. Explain the procedure and gain the patient's consent. Giving a clear explanation is required to gain legal consent and to address policy requirements. It will also assist the patient to cooperate with the procedure, allay anxiety and assist in establishing a therapeutic relationship.

As with any care that assists patients with their elimination needs, respecting a patient's privacy and preventing embarrassment is important. Patients with a colostomy also require psychological or emotional support in managing their colostomy and accepting the impact it has on their psychosocial wellbeing (Black, 2017). Clear explanations along with support from the nurse can assist the patient in managing the changes to their quality of life (Burch, 2017; Howson, 2019).

Demonstrate problem-solving abilities

Problem-solving abilities to assist with a stoma include recognising a patient's level of ability to be independent with changing a stoma pouch as well as recognising when a stoma pouch has become overinflated with gas or faeces. Be aware of patients with limitations in their hand movement or function, as this will impact on their ability to manage their stoma. Allow them time to adapt and self-manage as much as possible (Black, 2017).

In contrast to long-term stoma management, patients with a newly formed stoma will require more specific interventions as part of their postoperative management. Specific facility policies and surgeon's orders should be followed as part of this process, which includes managing the newly formed stoma site as part of the postoperative wound.

Carry out stoma care

- *Stoma appliances.* Pouches and barriers are designed to absorb odours and gas, as well as protect the skin. Closed pouches are used when solid waste is excreted; drainable ones are used for liquid or semi-solid wastes.
- *Frequency for pouch change.* This is usually 1 to 3 times per day for a colostomy, depending on the patient's frequency and amount of output. A colostomy pouch should be emptied when it is one-third to half-full and at bedtime (Blevins, 2019). Drainable pouches can be left for up to 3 days but need to have the outlet rinsed at each emptying. If the pouch is the drainable type, patients can sit over the toilet, remove the flange and empty the contents into the toilet. These pouches should be emptied before changing. Pouches that have a separate barrier system are changed as required, but the barrier is changed less frequently. Remove the stoma pouch by gently pulling the removal tab downwards to loosen the adhesive while applying light pressure on the skin with your other hand. Adhesive removers can be used to ease the removal of the stoma adhesive and any residue to prevent skin damage (Black, 2017). It is important to check that the stoma pouch of more dependent patients does not become overinflated with flatus or faeces, as they will easily leak or burst when a patient moves.
- *Stoma assessment.* When a pouch is changed, the skin is inspected for redness, irritation and excoriation. Observe the condition of the stoma, the edges and the surrounding skin. A healthy stoma is pinkish-red in colour and has no sensation. It will protrude slightly above the abdominal surface. Check the surrounding skin for any irritation or possible skin breakdown. Management and protection of the surrounding (peristomal) skin is essential in stoma care (Black, 2017). The base plate of the stoma pouch should also be checked for any erosion or presence of faeces. An eroded baseplate may indicate incorrect fitting or the need to change the appliance more frequently (Coloplast, n.d.).
- *Cleaning the stoma.* The stoma is generally cleaned each day in the shower, as part of the patient's regular hygiene care. The area is washed gently and patted dry, and a new barrier applied (if required). A washcloth with warm water can be used at other times to cleanse the area.
- *Replacing the stoma pouch.* Stoma systems will have a barrier that adheres directly to the patient's skin. Each patient will have a personal template for cutting a hole in the centre of the adhesive area that will fit snugly over the stoma. Prior to cleaning or removing the old barrier, trace the template outline onto the new barrier and use small sharp scissors to cut out the shape. The adhesive backing on the new stoma barrier is removed and the adhesive part of the appliance is then placed over the stoma and directly onto the skin. Position the pouch at an angle to allow movement and collection of faeces without the risk of leakage, and make sure it is securely in position.

Immediate postoperative stoma site care

- For the first 48 hours postoperatively, the colour of the stoma should be observed for signs of an effective blood supply and type and quantity of output and when the stoma is first active (Burch, 2017; Dougherty & Lister, 2015). Any signs of active bleeding or the stoma becoming pale, dark or dusky in colour may indicate a reduced blood supply and must be immediately reported to the RN and stoma therapy nurse (Burch, 2017).
- The stoma therapy nurse/therapist should be available to discuss the issues of physical and psychological stress with the patient. The therapist will also provide advice on acquiring appropriate equipment for self-care on discharge. The dietitian will provide dietary advice for reducing flatus, excess odours or sudden 'overfilling' of the pouch.
- An aseptic dressing technique may be used when the pouch is changed during the immediate postoperative period. As the stoma site heals and sutures are removed/dissolve, normal stoma management should be implemented.
- The initial output for a colostomy is usually after 2 days, with flatus followed by soft faeces (Burch, 2017).

Perform hand hygiene

Maintain the 5 Moments for Hand Hygiene and perform hand hygiene after touching the patient and the patient's surrounds.

CLEAN, REPLACE OR DISPOSE OF EQUIPMENT

Excreta is usually disposed of in the toilet or in a pan sluice in the dirty utility area of the unit, avoiding any splashing or spills and wearing non-sterile gloves, disposable apron and goggles for protection against bodily fluids. Loose faeces are easily emptied into the toilet or sluice. Formed and semi-formed faeces may be disposed of with the pouch in the clinical waste, according to the facility's policies.

Use facility wipes to clean and then return any equipment to storage areas. Restock the patient's personal stoma supplies as required.

DOCUMENT AND REPORT RELEVANT INFORMATION

Documentation of bowel action is on the patient observation and response chart in acute areas or a bowel book/record in long-term care areas. Some patients may require recording of bowel actions on a bowel chart or fluid balance chart, if being used. The condition of the colostomy site and type of excreta may also need to be documented in the nursing notes, especially if the patient has a newly formed stoma.

CASE STUDY

Antonio Richards is aged 68 and has a colostomy bag that uses a wafer system. His colostomy produces formed/semi-formed faeces. He usually manages the colostomy himself at home, but is currently unwell and unable to change the colostomy bag.

1. When would you know to change the colostomy bag, and how frequently to complete this action?
2. What actions or observations would you take to assist in managing flatus that can be in the colostomy bag?
3. Outline the steps you will take to change the colostomy bag.

Note: These notes are summaries of the most important points in the assessments/procedures, and are not exhaustive on the subject. The naming of documents or charts may differ from state to state, and facility to facility. In all possible situations the guidelines of the ACSQHC are used when describing national charts or documents (e.g. the ACSQHC Observation and Response Chart is named the Adult Observation and Response Chart in WA, and the Rapid Detection and Response Observation Chart in SA). References of the materials used to compile the information have been supplied. The student is expected to have learned the material surrounding each skill as presented in the references. No single reference is complete on the subject.

REFERENCES

Australian Council of Stoma Associations (ASCA). (2021a). *What is a Stoma?* https://australianstoma.com.au/about-stoma/what-is-a-stoma/

Australian Council of Stoma Associations (ASCA). (2021b). *Stoma Product Guide.* https://australianstoma.com.au/about-stoma/stoma-product-guide/

Black, P. (2017). Supporting patient care with appropriate accessories. *British Journal of Nursing*, 26(17), pp. S20–2.

Blevins, S. (2019). Colostomy care. *MEDSURG Nursing*, 28(2), pp. 125–6.

Burch, J. (2017). Care of patients undergoing stoma formation: What the nurse needs to know. *Nursing Standard*, 31(41), p. 40.

Coloplast. (n.d.). *Keeping Peristomal Skin Healthy.* https://www.coloplast.com.au/global/ostomy/ostomy-self-assessment-tools/arc/apply/

Dougherty, L. & Lister, S. (eds). (2015). *The Royal Marsden Hospital Manual of Clinical Nursing Procedures* (9th ed.). Oxford: Wiley-Blackwell.

Howson, R. (2019). Stoma education for the older person is about keeping it as simple as 1, 2, 3. *Journal of Stomal Therapy Australia*, 39(3), pp. 20–2.

RECOMMENDED READING

O'Flynn, S.K. (2019). Peristomal skin damage: assessment, prevention and treatment. *British Journal of Nursing*, 28(5), pp. S6–12.

ESSENTIAL SKILLS COMPETENCY

Assisting the Patient with Stoma (colostomy) Care

Demonstrates the ability to effectively and safely assist patients with their elimination needs

Criteria for skill performance	Y	D
(Numbers indicate *Enrolled Nurse Standards for Practice*, 2016)	(Satisfactory)	(Requires development)
1. Identifies indication (8.3, 8.4)		
2. Gathers equipment (1.2, 1.6, 4.4, 6.4, 8.4, 9.4): ■ non-sterile gloves, disposable apron and goggles ■ washcloth, plus a bowl of warm water ■ new/clean appliance ■ template and sharp scissors ■ paper bag ■ other patient-preferred items		
3. Performs hand hygiene (1.2, 1.4, 1.8, 3.9, 6.4, 9.4)		
4. Evidence of therapeutic communication with the patient; gives explanation of procedure, gains patient consent (2.1, 2.3, 2.4, 2.5, 6.3)		
5. Demonstrates problem-solving abilities (4.1, 4.2, 8.3, 8.4, 9.4)		
6. Carries out ostomy care (1.2, 1.4, 1.8, 2.1, 2.3, 2.4, 2.7, 3.2, 3.9, 6.1, 6.3, 6.6, 9.4)		
7. Leaves patient comfortable and safe (1.2, 1.4, 1.8, 2.3, 2.4, 2.7, 3.2, 3.9, 6.1, 6.9, 9.4)		
8. Disposes of excreta (1.2, 1.4, 1.8, 3.2, 3.9, 6.4, 8.4, 9.4)		
9. Performs hand hygiene (1.2, 1.4, 1.8, 3.9, 6.4, 9.4)		
10. Cleans, replaces and disposes of equipment appropriately (1.2, 1.4, 3.9, 6.5, 9.4)		
11. Documents and reports relevant information (1.2, 1.3, 1.8, 3.2, 5.3, 6.6, 7.1, 7.2, 7.3, 7.4, 7.5)		
12. Demonstrates ability to link theory to practice (8.3, 8.4, 8.5, 9.4)		

Student:

Clinical facilitator: Date:

CHAPTER **3.11**

PATIENT COMFORT – PAIN MANAGEMENT (NON-PHARMACOLOGICAL INTERVENTIONS – HEAT AND COLD)

IDENTIFY INDICATIONS

Pain is a complex phenomenon that is both a physical and emotional experience. Managing pain should include both pharmacological and non-pharmacological strategies, as pain is rarely managed with just one method, and strategies should be tailored to each patient (Claassens, 2017). Non-pharmacological pain management strategies include: massage; relaxation techniques; reduction of patient stress and anxiety; distraction; mentholated ointments and lotions; music therapy; and hot or cold therapies. Some facilities may also use other non-pharmacological methods such as transcutaneous electrical nerve stimulation (TENS) and acupuncture. Simple comfort measures such as careful repositioning or supporting a painful limb on a pillow are also important.

Indications for use of heat or cold treatment for pain vary. Pain is the major indicator; however, the origin and history of the pain will determine which of these treatments is required or is most effective. The patient's preference should also be considered, as some patients find cold distressing. The doctor or physiotherapist may also order the type, location and duration of heat or cold applications.

Heat is used to increase circulation and thus oxygen and nutrient flow to an area by:
- vasodilation of the arterioles
- reduced viscosity of synovial fluid in the joints
- increased capillary permeability within the painful area.

The vasodilation created by heat therapy assists in reducing inflammation and ischaemia. Heat also reduces muscle spasm and induces muscle relaxation, and has been described as reducing the production of prostaglandins that stimulate muscle contraction (Dineen, 2016). Heat therapy can also stimulate thermoreceptors in the area and block the sensitivity to pain.

Cold is used to promote vasoconstriction and thus decreases oedema and bleeding in an area, and can often be recommended for acute pain (Dineen, 2016). Cold reduces the inflammatory process and decreases contractility of muscles and cellular metabolism. The applications of heat or cold provide cutaneous stimulation, which is an effective pain-relieving technique.

Assessment of pain is the initial step to determine both the suitability of heat or cold, and the location of the application. Assessment of the patient is completed to determine if they are suitable candidates for heat or cold therapy. Age is an important consideration as the very young and very old tolerate heat poorly. Level of consciousness, neurosensory impairment and debility need to be established – the patient must be capable of recognising and appropriately responding to applied heat or cold. The area to be treated is determined, then assessed for intact skin (broken skin has increased sensitivity to heat and cold). Altered circulation in patients with congestive cardiac failure, diabetes mellitus and peripheral vascular diseases cause reduced circulatory function and the application of hot or cold therapy should be reviewed first with the doctor (Dineen, 2016). Heat cannot be dissipated, resulting in local tissue damage; cold is contraindicated because of vasoconstriction.

VERIFY CONTRAINDICATIONS

Always review local facility policies before applying any heat or cold therapy. Some facilities limit the use of heat therapies or types of heat therapy such as wheat packs due to patient safety needs.

Contraindications for the use of *heat therapy* are:
- a traumatic injury (within the first 24 hours) because of vasodilation increasing swelling
- active haemorrhage (or suspected; i.e., internal or recent surgery) because of vasodilation
- non-inflammatory oedema because heat increases capillary permeability
- acute inflammation (e.g. appendicitis) because of increased oedema
- localised malignant tumour because heat accelerates cell metabolism and cell growth and increases circulation
- skin disorders, since heat can further damage compromised skin
- areas receiving radiation therapy
- history of impaired circulation in the area.

Contraindications for the use of *cold therapy* are:
- open wounds, since cold decreases blood supply to the area and tissue damage or delayed healing could occur

- impaired circulation and patients with peripheral vascular disease, since vasoconstriction further impairs nourishment of the tissues; clients with Raynaud's disease will have increased arterial spasms

- cold allergy or hypersensitivity, which could cause hives, erythema, muscle spasm, joint stiffness or severe hypertension
- shivering, which can cause increased metabolic rate and a raised temperature
- areas having radiation therapy.

GATHER EQUIPMENT

Gathering the equipment prior to the procedure is a time-management strategy to eliminate trips back for forgotten equipment. It also helps the nurse to 'rehearse' the procedure before going to the patient's room, thus increasing confidence. Having all of the equipment on hand increases the patient's confidence in the nurse, and the nurse's self-confidence since they will not suffer the embarrassment of leaving the procedure and returning with a forgotten item.

- *A hot or cold pack* is needed to provide the heat or cold therapy. Blue gel heat/cold packs are often used.
- *Protective wrapping and tape* is used to wrap the pack. A 'bluey', small towel or pillowcase may be used to wrap the pack.
- *Pillows* to keep the pack in position, particularly on a limb.

PAIN MANAGEMENT USING HOT OR COLD THERAPY

Perform hand hygiene

Perform hand hygiene before touching the patient or the patient's surrounds and prior to any procedure involving patient contact to reduce the possibility of cross-contamination. Hand hygiene is the most effective method of infection control as it removes transient organisms from the hands of the nurse (see **Skill 1.1**).

Give a clear explanation of the procedure and establish therapeutic communication

Introduce yourself to the patient, and check you have the correct patient. Explain the procedure and gain the patient's consent. Giving a clear explanation will assist the patient to relax, maximising the effect of the procedure and gaining the patient's cooperation, thus reducing the time required to initiate the procedure, as well as assisting in gaining the patient's permission and in establishing a therapeutic relationship. Checking the patient and gaining their consent will also ensure that you meet legal and policy requirements before implementing any procedures.

The nurse should:

- outline preparation – skin inspection, pain assessment, application of heat or cold
- outline indication – that is, that heat or cold may or may not completely eliminate the pain, but it will modify the pain so that the patient can rest or carry out normal activities of daily living (ADLs)
- give a brief explanation of the theory behind the use of the treatment (if the patient wants this information, or is able to understand it).

Demonstrate problem-solving abilities

The nurse should act as a patient advocate when determining pain relief strategies. Problem-solving abilities in assessing pain and selecting appropriate interventions should be focused on the primary concern of patient comfort. Patients who are experiencing pain may or may not manifest the objective symptoms of pain. The nurse must ascertain the level of pain and decide whether to administer pharmacological pain relief as well as this treatment to bring comfort to the patient. Other comfort measures need attention as well. These include, but are not limited to, proper positioning, adequate support of a limb or painful area, offering a bedpan or toilet assistance, attention to associated symptoms such as nausea, provision of privacy and folding bedclothes down to expose area for treatment. Each situation will be individual and excellent nursing care will encompass a broad range of comfort measures.

Heat therapy can also include a warm shower or bath and warm blankets. Cold therapies can include crushed ice or cold wraps.

Prepare the hot or cold pack

Preparation of the hot or cold pack consists of warming or cooling the pack to an appropriate temperature. Thermal receptor stimulation declines rapidly in the initial period of treatment. Adaptation of the tissues to the new temperature causes the patient to feel that the treatment is ineffective and they may request, or get for themselves, hotter/colder packs. Some areas of the body are more sensitive to heat (and cold); for example, the axillae, neck and perineal areas. Care must be taken that a pack intended for these areas is of a more moderate temperature. Hot packs can be warmed in hot water as long as the temperature is checked prior to application. Commercially prepared hot packs are also available. These are re-useable, provide a consistent heat for a long period of time and are easily 'triggered' to produce a safe level of heat by chemical reaction. Follow the manufacturer's instructions for their use. Cold packs are usually kept in a refrigerator or freezer.

Wrap the pack in a protective cover

The pack is wrapped in a protective disposable cover or a pillowcase to increase patient comfort and safety. The cover is taped in place. The wrapped pack is placed on the body part. Pillows may be used to support it in the appropriate position.

Time the treatment

Timing of a treatment is an important aspect of both efficacy and safety. If a hot treatment is continued past the maximal time of effectiveness, the patient is at risk of burns. This time is 20 to 30 minutes or as specified by the health practitioner (i.e. doctor, physiotherapist).

Monitor the treatment site

The treatment site is monitored 5 minutes after application to assess skin condition and comfort. With cold treatment, pallor and mottled skin is considered a reaction; with heat treatment, pain, burning, excessive redness and swelling indicate that the treatment should be stopped. The monitoring may be necessary as often as every 5 to 10 minutes, depending on the ability of the patient to report untoward effects or their previous response to this treatment. Ensure the call bell is within reach of the patient in case of a reaction.

Assess the pain

Assess the patient's pain level and the skin underlying the application following the treatment.

Perform hand hygiene

Maintain the 5 Moments for Hand Hygiene and perform hand hygiene after touching the patient and the patient's surrounds.

CLEAN, REPLACE OR DISPOSE OF EQUIPMENT

Cleaning the plastic packs with decontaminating wipes and returning them to storage (cold packs in the refrigerator or freezer) reduces cross-contamination. Dispose of the protective cover in the general waste, or place the pillowslip in the linen skip for cleaning. Replacing the equipment is a time-management strategy, as well as a courtesy to colleagues. Some facilities may use disposable packs, or each patient may have their own pack for their exclusive use.

DOCUMENT AND REPORT RELEVANT INFORMATION

Documentation of time, date and type of treatment, location and effectiveness of the therapy should be completed.

CASE STUDY

Joan Wooley is an 83-year-old woman admitted to the ward. Two days ago, her carer found her at home lying on the floor. She was initially unresponsive but is now conscious and able to communicate. She has a mild weakness on her left side.

Joan is feeling very uncomfortable and has complained to you about left-sided leg pain with a pain score of 2/10. She has had her routine paracetamol.

1. List three non-pharmacological measures you could implement to help reduce and manage her pain.

Note: These notes are summaries of the most important points in the assessments/procedures, and are not exhaustive on the subject. The naming of documents or charts may differ from state to state, and facility to facility. In all possible situations the guidelines of the ACSQHC are used when describing national charts or documents (e.g. the ACSQHC Observation and Response Chart is named the Adult Observation and Response Chart in WA, and the Rapid Detection and Response Observation Chart in SA). References of the materials used to compile the information have been supplied. The student is expected to have learned the material surrounding each skill as presented in the references. No single reference is complete on the subject.

REFERENCES

Claassens, T. (2017). Nursing a patient with acute pain. *Kai Tiaki: Nursing New Zealand*, 23(7), pp. 15–17, 39.

Dineen, C.W. (2016). Heat or ice? *Health*, 30(10), pp. 65–71.

RECOMMENDED READINGS

Aciksoz, S., Akyuz, A. & Tunay, S. (2017). The effect of self-administered superficial local hot and cold application methods on pain, functional status and quality of life in primary knee osteoarthritis patients. *Journal of Clinical Nursing*, 26(23–24), pp. 5179–90.

PART 3

ESSENTIAL SKILLS COMPETENCY

Patient Comfort – Pain management (Non-Pharmacological Interventions – Heat and Cold)
Demonstrates the ability to provide heat and cold therapy

Criteria for skill performance	Y	D
(Numbers indicate *Enrolled Nurse Standards for Practice*, 2016)	(Satisfactory)	(Requires development)
1. Identifies indication (8.3, 8.4)		
2. Verifies there are no contraindications (1.2, 4.1)		
3. Gathers/prepares equipment (1.2, 1.6, 4.4, 6.4, 8.4, 9.4): ■ hot/cold pack ■ protective wrapping ■ pillows, if required		
4. Performs hand hygiene (1.2, 1.4, 1.8, 3.9, 6.4, 9.4)		
5. Evidence of therapeutic communication with the patient; gives explanation of procedure, gains patient consent (2.1, 2.3, 2.4, 2.5, 6.3)		
6. Demonstrates problem-solving abilities; e.g. provides privacy, comfort measures, pharmacological pain relief as ordered (2.7, 4.1, 4.2, 8.3, 8.4, 9.4)		
7. Selects hot or cold therapy, according to doctor's (or therapist's) orders, or patient needs (1.2, 1.4, 1.8, 3.2, 8.4)		
8. Prepares the hot or cold pack according to manufacturer's direction (1.2, 1.4, 1.8, 3.2, 8.4)		
9. Wraps the pack in a protective cover (1.2, 1.4, 1.8, 3.2, 3.9, 8.4, 9.4)		
10. Places the covered pack on the treatment site (1.2, 1.4, 1.8, 3.2, 3.9, 4.1, 6.1, 8.4, 9.4)		
11. Times the treatment (1.2, 1.4, 1.8, 3.2, 3.9, 8.4, 9.4)		
12. Assesses the treatment site after five minutes for untoward effects (1.2, 1.4, 1.8, 3.2, 3.9, 4.1, 6.1, 7.1, 8.4, 9.4)		
13. Completes the prescribed treatment and assesses pain post treatment (1.2, 1.4, 1.8, 3.2, 4.1, 7.1, 8.4, 9.4)		
14. Performs hand hygiene (1.2, 1.4, 1.8, 3.9, 6.4, 9.4)		
15. Cleans, replaces and disposes of equipment appropriately (1.2, 1.4, 3.9, 6.5, 9.4)		
16. Documents and reports relevant information (1.2, 1.3, 1.8, 3.2, 5.3, 6.6, 7.1, 7.2, 7.3, 7.4, 7.5)		
17. Demonstrates ability to link theory to practice (8.3, 8.4, 8.5, 9.4)		

Student:

Clinical facilitator: Date:

CHAPTER 3.12

POSITIONING OF A DEPENDENT PATIENT

IDENTIFY INDICATIONS

Moving and turning a patient correctly is important to prevent injury to the nurse and to the patient (Warren, 2016). Positioning is often the starting point to maximise the benefits of other interventions (e.g. range of motion or breathing exercises), optimal rest and rehabilitation to facilitate recovery. Correct positioning in bed promotes comfort, hygiene, dignity and functional ability. It also provides proper body alignment and prevents complications of immobility, especially pressure injuries (Hanna et al., 2016; Pickenbrock et al., 2017).

Scheduled repositioning of bed- or chair-bound patients is required to reduce the occurrence of pressure injuries (Van Etten, 2020). An inactive patient may only get exercise during position changes. Position changes for the immobile or inactive patient should occur every 2 to 4 hours to prevent circulatory damage and contractures. A thorough

skin assessment using the relevant skin assessment tool (according to facility policy) should be carried out each time the patient is moved and pressure area care provided (Australian Wound Management Association [AWMA], 2012). Any breaks in skin integrity must be reported and documented.

Lifting is hazardous to the nurse's health (Warren, 2016). A safe patient handling policy is always used to reduce the number of nurse and patient injuries (Mongahan, 2020). Patient-handling equipment (e.g. hoists, sliding sheets, adjustable height beds) is provided to promote patient and nurse safety. Always follow the facility's policies and use the provided equipment in regard to this skill. Workplace health and safety guidelines must be followed. Manual handling techniques are not detailed here, as there are various techniques and they need to be specifically explained.

GATHER EQUIPMENT

- *Clean linen* if necessary.
- *Pillows/positioning aids* are used to:
  (1) provide padding in front of the headboard to protect the head during moves;
  (2) provide support for various body parts during the move; and (3) support the patient in the new position so that muscles can relax.

- *Safe patient handling devices* are available for use with patients. These include slide sheets and hoists. Use these devices according to workplace health and safety risk management assessment to prevent injury to the patient, to you and to the other nursing staff. The appropriate equipment is determined by the facility risk management guidelines and safe patient handling policy.

POSITION THE DEPENDENT PATIENT

Perform hand hygiene

Perform hand hygiene before touching the patient or the patient's surrounds and prior to any procedure involving patient contact to reduce the possibility of cross-contamination. Hand hygiene is the most effective method of infection control as it removes transient organisms from the hands of the nurse (see **Skill 1.1**).

Give a clear explanation of the procedure and establish therapeutic communication

Introduce yourself, and check you have the correct patient. Discuss the procedure and gain the patient's consent. Giving a clear explanation is required to gain legal consent and to address policy requirements. It will also assist the patient to cooperate with the procedure, allay anxiety and assist in establishing a therapeutic relationship. Include an explanation of the nurse's actions, the patient's expected or desired behaviour and any signals that will be used to synchronise the nurses working together.

Demonstrate problem-solving abilities

Determine the need for assistance by referring to the patient's care plan, manual handling documentation and risk assessment for information on the patient's needs and the assistance required for repositioning. Some patients are able to assist a great deal, others are totally dependent. Bariatric patients may require an extra nurse to assist and complete this action safely (Hanna et al., 2016). Assess each situation to minimise risk and exertion, and maximise effectiveness. Do not hesitate to obtain assistance if there is doubt about your ability to move a patient safely. Safe patient handling policies are always followed as they reduce the risk to the nurse and the patient (Australian Nursing and Midwifery Federation [ANMF], 2015). Utilise available equipment as per facility policy and patient requirements.

Ensure privacy by closing the door or drawing the curtains around the bed. Raise the bed to an appropriate and comfortable height for repositioning the patient and lock the bed brakes to prevent the bed from moving during the procedure. Both nurses lower the side-rail nearest to them so that reaching over side-rails will not result in strained muscles. These are safety actions for both nurse and patient. Safely move tubing, drains and drainage apparatus to facilitate changes in position.

Check the environment and complete a risk assessment. Ensure sufficient work space, removal of clutter and trip hazards, and that the floors are non-slip.

Position the patient

Positioning should facilitate the patient's physical, physiological and psychological wellbeing, taking into account the patient's condition and individual characteristics. Check the care plan for specific positioning requirements.

Characteristics such as age, reason for admission, pain, weight and level of dependency will influence the patient's need for assistance and positioning. Some medical conditions and diseases (e.g. fractures, paralysis, lung disease, congestive cardiac failure or hemiparesis) preclude moving patients into some positions. Avoid positioning a patient on a skin area with bony prominences and non-blanchable erythema. Tubes, incisions, drains and intravenous lines will also alter the turning/positioning procedure. The patient's level of consciousness and ability to comply with instructions will affect positioning. For example, an unconscious patient would not be positioned in an upright position because they could not maintain that position and it could potentially obstruct their airway. The preferred positioning for an unconscious patient is the recovery position, but the patient's specific medical condition will determine this. A minimum of two staff would be needed to move an unconscious patient.

Move and position patient appropriately

Pillows or specific positioning aids are placed to support the patient effectively. The body must be supported to maintain its natural contours, symmetry and alignment. More natural body positions also reduce pressure injury risk (Pickenbrock et al., 2017).

Slide sheets help to reduce shearing forces when repositioning the patient, as well as reducing the risk to the nurse from the manual handling task. The head of the bed should be flat/level, as tolerated by the patient. Prepare the slide sheet and place under the patient, with the opening in the direction of the planned movement. The nurse on each side of the patient rolls the top layer of the folded slide sheet close to the patient, and then grasps the rolled sheet (Department for Communities and Social Inclusion [DCSI], 2017). Using the correct posture, the nurses then use good body mechanics to slide the patient gently towards the head of the bed, ensuring no friction or shearing occurs. Return the bed head to the required position for patient comfort.

For more in-depth guidelines, refer to institutional guidelines.

Utilise principles of good body mechanics

Utilise principles of good body mechanics to avoid causing injury to yourself, to the patient and to other staff (ANMF, 2015; Warren, 2016). Avoid twisting the body, maintain a stable centre of gravity and have the feet positioned at shoulder-distance apart to create a stable base of support when positioning a patient. Have the bed at the correct height (the knuckles of clenched hands should be touching the bed). These instructions are outlined in current nursing and workplace health and safety references, and are relevant to any form of manual handling. Organisational policies are very specific about safe patient handling.

Perform hand hygiene

Maintain the 5 Moments for Hand Hygiene and perform hand hygiene after touching the patient and the patient's surrounds.

CLEAN, REPLACE OR DISPOSE OF EQUIPMENT

Clean and replace used equipment for use next time. Slide sheets and hoist slings are patient specific, and replaced when soiled or when the patient is discharged. Follow institution procedure for recharging of hoists and other electrical equipment. This is a time-management strategy and a courtesy to fellow nursing staff.

DOCUMENT AND REPORT RELEVANT INFORMATION

Document relevant information to include time and date, procedure, response and any areas of skin breakdown. Some hospitals do not require that movement and turning be recorded on the nursing notes, but the preferred risk assessment tool must be completed. Follow the hospital policy. Any relevant information obtained during the move should be passed on, either verbally or in writing, so that the healthcare team remains informed.

CASE STUDY

Joan Wooley is an 83-year-old woman admitted to the ward. Two days ago, her carer found her at home lying on the floor. She was initially unresponsive but is now conscious and able to communicate. She has a mild weakness on her left side.

You are required to reposition Joan onto her right side while she is resting in bed.

1. Based on Joan's current medical history, why should she be repositioned onto her right side or her back?
2. How many nurses would be required to implement this nursing care action?
3. What equipment will you require to reposition Joan safely and correctly?

Note: These notes are summaries of the most important points in the assessments/procedures, and are not exhaustive on the subject. The naming of documents or charts may differ from state to state, and facility to facility. In all possible situations the guidelines of the ACSQHC are used when describing national charts or documents (e.g. the ACSQHC Observation and Response Chart is named the Adult Observation and Response Chart in WA, and the Rapid Detection and Response Observation Chart in SA). References of the materials used to compile the information have been supplied. The student is expected to have learned the material surrounding each skill as presented in the references. No single reference is complete on the subject.

REFERENCES

Australian Nursing and Midwifery Federation (ANMF). (2015). *ANMF Policy – Safe Patient Handling.* http://www.anmf.org.au/documents/policies/P_Safe_Patient_Handling.pdf

Australian Wound Management Association (AWMA). (2012). *Pan Pacific Clinical Practice Guideline for the Prevention and Management of Pressure Injury.* Osborne Park, WA: Cambridge Media.

Department for Communities and Social Inclusion (DCSI). (2017). *Safe Work Instructions (SWIs).* Government of South Australia. http://www.dcsi.sa.gov.au/services/disability-services/safe-work-instructions

Hanna, D.R., Paraszczuk, A.M., Duffy, M.M. & DiFiore, L.A. (2016). Learning about turning: Report of a mailed survey of nurses' work to reposition patients. *MEDSURG Nursing,* 25(4), pp. 219–23.

Monaghan, H.M. (2020). The challenge of change: why are staff resistant to using safe patient handling equipment? *International Journal of Safe Patient Handling & Mobility (SPHM),* 10(1), pp. 7–12.

Pickenbrock, H., Ludwig, V.U. & Zapf, A. (2017). Support pressure distribution for positioning in neutral versus conventional positioning in the prevention of decubitus ulcers: a pilot study in healthy participants. *BMC Nursing,* 16(1).

Van Etten, M. (2020). Repositioning for pressure ulcer prevention in the seated individual. *Wounds International,* 11(1), pp. 18–21.

Warren, G. (2016). Moving and handling: Reducing risk through assessment. *Nursing Standard,* 30(40), p. 49.

ESSENTIAL SKILLS COMPETENCY

Positioning of a Dependent Patient

Demonstrates the ability to effectively provide pressure area care, and to safely move a patient in bed

Criteria for skill performance	Y	D
(Numbers indicate *Enrolled Nurse Standards for Practice*, 2016)	(Satisfactory)	(Requires development)
1. Identifies indication (8.3, 8.4)		
2. Gathers equipment (1.2, 1.6, 6.4, 8.4, 9.4): ■ safe patient handling aids (e.g. slide sheet, hoist and hoist slings) ■ clean linen ■ extra pillows		
3. Performs hand hygiene (1.2, 1.4, 1.8, 3.9, 6.4, 9.4)		
4. Evidence of therapeutic communication with the patient; gives explanation of procedure, gains patient consent (2.1, 2.3, 2.4, 2.5, 6.3)		
5. Demonstrates problem-solving abilities; e.g. determines the need for assistance, secures the bed, identifies positions available to use for the patient (4.1, 4.2, 8.3, 8.4, 9.4)		
6. Maintains personal and patient safety; utilises principles of safe body mechanics and safe patient handling policies (3.9, 6.4, 8.3, 8.4, 9.4)		
7. Moves and positions the patient appropriately in bed (1.2, 1.4, 1.8, 2.3, 2.4, 2.7, 3.2, 3.9, 4.4, 6.1, 6.3, 6.4, 8.4, 9.4)		
8. Performs hand hygiene (1.2, 1.4, 1.8, 3.9, 6.4, 9.4)		
9. Cleans, replaces and disposes of equipment appropriately (1.2, 1.4, 3.9, 6.5, 9.4)		
10. Documents and reports relevant information (1.2, 1.3, 1.8, 3.2, 5.3, 6.6, 7.1, 7.2, 7.3, 7.4, 7.5)		
11. Demonstrates ability to link theory to practice (8.3, 8.4, 8.5, 9.4)		

Student:

Clinical facilitator: Date:

CHAPTER **3.13**

PREVENTING AND MANAGING PRESSURE INJURIES

IDENTIFY INDICATIONS

Pressure injuries occur when the skin and underlying tissues are damaged due to pressure, shear or friction. They are a key concern within health care and preventable in most situations. Pressure injuries can occur in a patient, with any of the risk factors. The Comprehensive Care Standard of the National Safety and Quality Health Service Standards includes requirements for preventing and managing pressure injuries. Appropriate pressure injury prevention and management strategies should be applied to all patients in all clinical settings.

Pressure injuries develop when prolonged pressure is placed on the skin, particularly over bony prominences such as heels, knees, buttocks, hips, sacrum, spine, elbows, ears and back of the head. Pressure interferes with circulation, leading to hypoxia, tissue damage and tissue death. Among those at risk are patients who are very thin or obese, malnourished, immobile, incontinent or have poor peripheral circulation. Skin damage by shearing and friction can also lead to pressure injuries, and can easily occur when a patient slides down the bed or is being repositioned. Moisture can macerate the skin and increase the risk of pressure injury.

Risk assessment tools such as Braden, Norton or Waterlow Scales are used to identify patients at risk. The Glamorgan Scale is used for paediatric patients. According to national risk management guidelines, all patients should have a skin assessment and be assessed for risk of pressure injury on admission to hospital. Refer to local facility and state/territory health department policies for specific guidelines on risk assessment tool/s and reporting and management of pressure injuries.

GATHER EQUIPMENT

- *Sponging equipment* if the area is to be washed, pH-appropriate skin cleanser and water-based moisturisers (e.g. sorbolene) as ordered.
- *Pressure-relieving equipment.* The different devices used to prevent or relieve pressure are described as a 'support surface', and classified according to the following descriptions.
  - *Active (alternating pressure) support surfaces.* Produce alternate pressure mechanically. It is usually created by alternating pressure within air cells in a cyclic process and usually available as a mattress.
  - *Reactive (constant low pressure) support surfaces.* These have the ability to respond to pressure and will mould to the patient's shape to redistribute body weight. Includes mattresses, mattress overlays, foam cushions and wedges, gel pads/cushions, and pads filled with polyester fibre with a two-way stretch cover.
  - *Seating support cushions.* These include foam slabs to air-filled cushions.
  - *Heel devices.* Different devices are available. These include pillows or devices that elevate the patient's heels off the bed, 'hydrocellular' heel dressing, air cushions or boots lined with cushioning fleece or egg crate foam. These should be used with caution in restless or falls-risk patients who might get out of bed unsupervised.

IMPLEMENTING PRESSURE AREA CARE

Perform hand hygiene
Perform hand hygiene before touching the patient or the patient's surrounds and prior to any procedure involving patient contact to reduce the possibility of cross-contamination. Hand hygiene is the most effective method of infection control as it removes transient organisms from the hands of the nurse (see **Skill 1.1**).

Give a clear explanation of the procedure and establish therapeutic communication

Introduce yourself, and check you have the correct patient. Discuss the procedure and gain the patient's consent. Giving a clear explanation is required to gain legal consent and to address policy requirements. It will also assist the patient to cooperate with the procedure, allay anxiety and assist in establishing a therapeutic relationship.

Demonstrate problem-solving abilities

Standardised use of the facility's skin assessment and pressure injury risk assessment tools creates reliable and consistent assessments of patients, recognition of at-risk patients and actions for preventing pressure injuries. Refer to the patient's care plan and pressure injury risk assessment tool for information on the patient's needs and the assistance required for pressure area care. The care plan or relevant assessment tool will also identify when the patient requires routine reassessment.

Problem-solving actions include completing a skin assessment as part of routine care actions and identifying a potential pressure injury or actual skin tear. The site will then require assessment to determine the stage/classification of pressure injury, appropriate wound management strategies, pain management and other interventions to assist in the management of the pressure injury.

Provide pressure area care

Pressure area care includes the actions of repositioning a patient using correct manual handling techniques, providing appropriate support surfaces and position, inspecting and protecting the skin and ensuring the patient has adequate nutrition.

Performs pressure injury risk assessment and skin care

Use the facility's skin assessment and pressure injury risk assessment tools to assess the patient. All patients must have a skin assessment and be assessed for risk of pressure injury on admission to hospital and on an ongoing basis (AWMA, 2012). Assessment for a patient's risk of developing a pressure injury must be completed as part of the admission process for all patients, and reassessment for pressure injury risk is required to be completed if there is a change in the patient's condition or level of mobility, a period of immobility (e.g. postoperatively), or at least weekly. Patients with a score showing risk of pressure injury must be reassessed every 24 to 48 hours.

Skin assessment will be completed at least daily as part of regular care actions, each time a patient is repositioned, preoperatively and postoperatively, on discharge and on transfer between facility areas. The patient's skin should be kept dry from moisture, including continence management and microclimate control to reduce sweating. Do not rub or vigorously massage skin that is at risk of pressure injury as this will cause friction and increase pain. A barrier cream can be used to further protect skin from excess moisture. A skin moisturiser can help to rehydrate the patient's skin).

All actual pressure injuries must be assessed using a validated pressure injury assessment scale (AWMA, 2012), with the description and level of injury stated in the relevant documentation.

Nutrition

All patients should have a nutrition screen on admission, using a reliable nutrition screening tool. Also review the patient's ability to feed themselves. A dietitian may be consulted to adjust the patient's nutritional management, and to help ensure the patient has sufficient energy and protein intake along with adequate hydration. A balanced diet will reduce the risk of pressure injury, as well as assist in the management of an existing injury.

Move and position patient appropriately

Repositioning of patients at risk of pressure injuries must be completed 2- to 4-hourly. The area may be washed and dried thoroughly, and moisturisers applied to keep the skin supple. Linen is changed as required. The patient must not be left in a wet bed; this can occur not only with incontinence but with excessive sweating or spilled fluids. The patient is repositioned comfortably, using the appropriate positioning devices (i.e. pressure-distributing chair cushions, mattress and other cushions or wedges). Areas of particular concern are bony prominences, the buttocks, sacral areas and heels, as these are subject to high levels of pressure.

When making choices for mattresses, chair cushions and positioning devices, refer to facility and state/territory health policies that provide specific guidelines on the selection of correct and safe devices.

Please refer to the guidelines in **Skill 3.12** for repositioning a patient as part of pressure care management. Avoid the creation of shearing forces when repositioning a patient. Silk-like fabrics will reduce shear.

Patients who are positioned at a 30 degrees lateral position and alternated from side to side, or a 30 degrees recumbent position, are at a reduced risk of pressure injury. The position of a patient's heels and bony prominences should always be checked when repositioning a patient.

Pressure is relieved by ensuring the patient is placed in different positions, according to the specific turning regimen. Pillows or positioning devices are placed to support the patient effectively and to distribute pressure. The body must be supported to maintain its natural contours, symmetry and alignment. Prevention of injury to the heels is maintained by the use of heel suspension devices and having the knees in slight flexion. The choice of a pressure-distributing mattress should be based on the individual needs, and considering such issues as the patient's level of mobility, size and weight, risk for pressure injury and the need for shear reduction.

Perform hand hygiene

Maintain the 5 Moments for Hand Hygiene and perform hand hygiene after touching the patient and the patient's surrounds.

CLEAN, REPLACE OR DISPOSE OF EQUIPMENT

Clean and replace used equipment. This is a time-management strategy and a courtesy to fellow nursing staff. Some equipment such as foam wedges or cushions and booties are disposable. Pressure mattresses/cushions and gel pads should be cleaned according to the manufacturer's instructions and facility policy.

DOCUMENT AND REPORT RELEVANT INFORMATION

All relevant information about patient assessments or development of a pressure injury should be documented in the relevant nursing notes, nursing care plan and charts. Risk assessment tools should be filed with the patient's notes and assessment scores recorded in the nursing report and care plan. If a pressure injury or skin tear is noted, many facilities require the completion of a 'Pressure Injury or Skin Tear Alert' sticker that is then placed in the patient's notes and a clinical incident notification must be completed. Follow the hospital policy. Any relevant information should be passed on, both verbally and in writing, so that the healthcare team remains informed.

CASE STUDY

Joan Wooley is aged 83. She has had a right cerebrovascular accident, and has a left-sided weakness and needs assistance to be repositioned in bed or in the chair. Joan also requires assistance with eating, hygiene and elimination needs. She is continent.

1. What support surfaces (in bed and in the chair) would you use to prevent Joan developing a pressure injury?

2. What actions will you use when repositioning Joan to reduce her risk of pressure injuries?
3. How often will you assess Joan's skin?
4. If you identify a new pressure injury, what documentation are you required to complete?

Note: These notes are summaries of the most important points in the assessments/procedures, and are not exhaustive on the subject. The naming of documents or charts may differ from state to state, and facility to facility. In all possible situations the guidelines of the ACSQHC are used when describing national charts or documents (e.g. the ACSQHC Observation and Response Chart is named the Adult Observation and Response Chart in WA, and the Rapid Detection and Response Observation Chart in SA). References of the materials used to compile the information have been supplied. The student is expected to have learned the material surrounding each skill as presented in the references. No single reference is complete on the subject.

REFERENCES

Australian Wound Management Association (AWMA). (2012). *Pan Pacific Clinical Practice Guideline for the Prevention and* *Management of Pressure Injury*. Osborne Park, WA: Cambridge Media.

RECOMMENDED READINGS

Australian Commission on Safety and Quality in Healthcare (ACSQHC). (2019). *Action 5.21 Preventing and Managing Pressure Injuries.* https://www.safetyandquality.gov.au/standards/nsqhs-standards/comprehensive-care-standard/minimising-patient-harm/action-521

Australian Commission on Safety and Quality in Healthcare (ACSQHC). (2020). *Preventing Pressure Injuries and Wound Management.* https://www.safetyandquality.gov.au/sites/default/files/2020-10/fact_sheet_-_preventing_pressure_injuries_and_wound_management_oct_2020.pdf

Hanna, D.R., Paraszczuk, A.M., Duffy, M.M. & DiFiore, L.A. (2016). Learning about turning: Report of a mailed survey of nurses' work to reposition patients. *MEDSURG Nursing*, 25(4), pp. 219–23.

Monaghan, H.M. (2020). The challenge of change: why are staff resistant to using safe patient handling equipment? *International Journal of Safe Patient Handling & Mobility (SPHM)*, 10(1), pp. 7–12.

Pagnamenta, F. (2017). The provision of therapy mattresses for pressure ulcer prevention. *British Journal of Nursing*, 26(6), S28–S33.

Pickenbrock, H., Ludwig, V.U. & Zapf, A. (2017). Support pressure distribution for positioning in neutral versus conventional positioning in the prevention of decubitus ulcers: a pilot study in healthy participants. *BMC Nursing*, 16(1).

Warren, G. (2016). Moving and handling: Reducing risk through assessment. *Nursing Standard*, 30(40), p. 49.

ESSENTIAL SKILLS COMPETENCY

Preventing and Managing Pressure Injuries

Demonstrates the ability to effectively provide pressure area care, and to safely move a patient in bed

Criteria for skill performance	Y	D
(Numbers indicate *Enrolled Nurse Standards for Practice*, 2016)	(Satisfactory)	(Requires development)
1. Identifies indication (8.3, 8.4)		
2. Gathers equipment as relevant to patient health status and needs (1.2, 1.6, 6.4, 8.4, 8.5, 9.4)		
3. Performs hand hygiene (1.2, 1.4, 1.8, 3.9, 6.4, 9.4)		
4. Evidence of therapeutic communication with the patient; gives explanation of procedure, gains patient consent (1.2, 2.1, 2.3, 2.4, 2.5, 6.3)		
5. Demonstrates problem-solving abilities; e.g. recognises need for patient skin assessment and pressure injury risk assessment (4.1, 4.2, 8.3, 8.4, 9.4)		
6. Performs pressure area care and assessment: ▪ completes risk assessment for pressure injury ▪ completes skin assessment and skin care ▪ ensures adequate nutrition and hydration (1.2, 1.4, 1.8, 2.1, 2.3, 2.7, 3.2, 3.9, 4.1, 4.2, 4.3, 6.4, 7.1, 7.2, 8.4, 9.4)		
7. Moves and positions the patient according to repositioning regimen, as required, minimising friction and shear; ensures use of correct support surfaces (1.2, 1.4, 1.8, 2.3, 2.4, 2.7, 3.2, 3.9, 6.1, 6.3, 6.4, 8.4, 9.4)		
8. Performs hand hygiene (1.2, 1.4, 1.8, 3.9, 6.4, 9.4)		
9. Cleans, replaces and disposes of equipment appropriately (1.2, 1.4, 3.9, 6.5, 9.4)		
10. Documents and reports relevant information (1.2, 1.3, 1.8, 3.2, 5.3, 6.6, 7.1, 7.2, 7.3, 7.4, 7.5)		
11. Demonstrates ability to link theory to practice (8.3, 8.4, 8.5, 9.4)		

Student:

Clinical facilitator: Date:

CHAPTER 3.14

ACTIVE AND PASSIVE EXERCISES

IDENTIFY INDICATIONS

Inactive patients do not move their joints through the entire range of motion because of limits to their activity. Over time, reduction in the range of movement of the joints occurs due to shortening of ligaments and tendons. The result can be a non-functional joint and eventually a contracture of that joint. Patients (paediatric to elderly) in acute care settings may spend long time periods in bed and can experience a large loss of function and mobility as a consequence, and benefit from early passive, then active, exercises (Cameron et al., 2015). Impaired physical mobility may be due to an acute illness episode, unconsciousness, a stroke or paralysis, surgery and postoperative discomfort, brain injury, pain or general physical deterioration from chronic illness. Knowledge of the diagnosis helps to determine the exercises needed and those that are contraindicated. When more active mobility is limited, regular exercise of the joints prevents the complications of prolonged bed rest or immobility such as spasticity, muscle wasting and shortening of tendons and ligaments (contracture development). It has also been shown to increase cerebral blood flow, venous return and reduce the risk of deep vein thrombosis (Cameron et al., 2015; Sachiko et al., 2015). Completion of range-of-motion exercises will also increase client comfort and help prepare the patient for ambulation.

UNDERSTAND CONSIDERATIONS FOR IMPLEMENTATION

Range-of-motion exercises should be carried out within the pain-free range. Watch the patient for non-verbal expressions of pain during the exercise: facial grimaces, withdrawal of the limb or tensing of the body indicate pain. If a joint movement is painful, the exercise should be discontinued and the physiotherapist should be consulted. The increased exercise level involved in range-of-motion exercises will cause fatigue for many patients. Do not continue the exercises to the point of exhaustion.

Types of range-of-motion exercises are detailed below.

- *Passive* exercises are when the nurse moves the patient's joint through its range of movement with little or no input from the patient. These exercises maintain joint mobility only. This assumes a level of knowledge on the nurse's part of each joint's range of movement.
- *Active* exercises are when the patient moves their own joints through the range of movement. Patients can be taught to do active range-of-motion exercises on weak or inactive joints. They may use adjacent muscles to move a joint. These exercises maintain/increase muscle strength, endurance and cardiorespiratory function in an immobile person.
- *Active assisted* exercises occur where the patient uses one part of the body to move another joint in their body through its range of motion. An example of this would be the patient who has had a cerebrovascular accident and uses the stronger arm and leg to move the weaker ones through their range of motion.

GATHER AND PREPARE EQUIPMENT

Gathering and adjusting equipment prior to initiation of the procedure increases efficiency. Ensure the brakes on the bed are on. Positioning the bed at the nurse's waist level keeps the activity near the nurse's centre of gravity, thereby minimising stress on the nurse's muscles. This reduces energy expenditure and also reduces friction and shearing forces on the patient's skin.

Small and large pillows need to be handy for use to support the patient in side-lying positions. The pillows remain with the patient throughout their hospitalisation.

Small wrist weights or handheld therapy ball are used as required.

PERFORMING ACTIVE AND PASSIVE EXERCISES WITH A PATIENT

Perform hand hygiene

Perform hand hygiene before touching the patient or the patient's surrounds and prior to any procedure involving patient contact to reduce the possibility of cross-contamination. Hand hygiene is the most effective method of infection control as it removes transient organisms from the hands of the nurse (see **Skill 1.1**).

Give a clear explanation of the procedure and establish therapeutic communication

Introduce yourself, and check you have the correct patient. Discuss the procedure and gain the patient's consent. Giving a clear explanation is required to gain legal consent and to address policy requirements. It will also assist the patient to cooperate with the procedure, allay anxiety and assist in establishing a therapeutic relationship.

Demonstrate problem-solving abilities

Prior to performing active or passive exercises, the patient should be assessed on their ability to perform active range-of-motion exercises themselves. Include current and past medical history (e.g. arthritis) in this assessment. The nurse can assist the patient with passive exercises when the patient cannot initiate the movement. Patient alterations in condition or pain can also influence their ability to move without assistance or to tolerate passive movement. The nurse will need to use problem-solving skills to determine the type of exercises (i.e. passive or active) and the schedule for when to implement these exercises. These exercises should be included as part of other patient care actions such as hygiene.

Assess the joints

Check the care plan and the mobility chart for any specific instructions provided by the physiotherapist. Assess the patient's ability to move each joint. There is no need to do range-of-motion exercises on a joint that is moving adequately and which is moved as part of activities of daily living.

Perform active and passive exercises

If the patient is able, a sitting position for the upper body range-of-motion exercises is most effective. The patient should be well supported in this position. If the patient is unable to sit, they are positioned in the supine position with heels close together and arms resting at the sides.

Encouraging the patient to perform simple daily tasks increases the range of motion of all joints and reduces the need to do range-of-motion exercises. During the exercises, a specific systematic pattern should be adopted so that no joint is overlooked. Start the exercises gradually and work slowly. Movement should be smooth and rhythmic to increase comfort for the patient. Common active and passive exercises include flexion and extension of each limb, rotation of the ankles and wrists, as well as opening and closing of the hands.

During passive exercises, support each joint to prevent over-extension. Move the joint slowly and smoothly and as per the care plan. Exercises are performed on a scheduled basis. Passive exercises can be incorporated into daily hygiene routines. Move each joint to the point of resistance but not pain. Use gentle pressure, not force. Start and finish with each joint in its normal neutral position. Take care to note the patient's facial expressions and other non-verbal expressions for evidence of pain. See **TABLE 3.14.1** for suitable range-of-motion exercises.

TABLE 3.14.1 Types of exercise

JOINT AND MOVEMENT	EXAMPLE

1. Shoulder (ball-and-socket joint)
   a. *Flexion*: raise straight arm forward to a position above the head.
   b. *Extension*: return straight arm forward and down to side of body.	

c. *External rotation*: bent arm lateral, parallel to floor, palm down, rotate shoulder so fingers point up. d. *Internal rotation*: bent arm lateral, parallel to floor, rotate shoulder so fingers point down.	

JOINT AND MOVEMENT	EXAMPLE

2. Elbow (hinge joint)
   a. *Flexion*: bend elbow, move lower arm towards shoulder, palm facing shoulder.
   b. *Extension*: straighten lower arm forward and downward.	

c. *Rotation for supination*: elbow bent, turn hand and forearm so palm is facing upward. d. *Rotation for pronation*: elbow bent, turn hand and forearm so palm is facing downward.	

3. Wrist (condyloid) joint
   a. *Flexion*: bend wrist so fingers move towards inner aspect of forearm.
   b. *Extension*: straighten hand to same plane as arm.	

4. Hand and fingers (condyloid and hinge joints)
   a. *Flexion*: make a fist.
   b. *Extension*: straighten fingers.
   c. *Hyperextension*: bend fingers back as far as possible.	

d. *Abduction*: spread fingers apart. e. *Adduction*: bring fingers together.	

5. Thumb (saddle joint)
   a. *Flexion*: move thumb across palmar surface of hand.
   b. *Extension*: move thumb away from hand.
   c. *Abduction*: move thumb laterally.
   d. *Adduction*: move thumb back to hand.	

e. *Opposition*: touch thumb to tip of each finger of same hand.	

6. Hip (ball-and-socket joint)
   a. *Flexion*: move straight leg forward and upward.
   b. *Extension*: move leg back beside the other leg.	

c. *Abduction*: move leg laterally from midline. d. *Adduction*: move leg back.	

JOINT AND MOVEMENT	EXAMPLE

7. Knee (hinge joint)
   a. *Flexion*: bend knee to bring heel back towards thigh.
   b. *Extension*: Straighten each leg, place foot beside other foot.
	120°

8. Ankle (hinge joint)
   a. *Plantar flexion*: point toes downward.
   b. *Dorsiflexion*: point toes upward.	

9. Foot (gliding joint)
   a. *Eversion*: turn sole of foot laterally.
   b. *Inversion*: turn sole of foot medially.	

SOURCE: DELAUNE, S., LADNER, P.K., McTIER, L., TOLLEFSON, J. & LAWRENCE, J. (2016) *AUSTRALIAN AND NEW ZEALAND FUNDAMENTALS OF NURSING*. SOUTH MELBOURNE: CENGAGE. TABLE 39-3, P. 314.

Teach the patient to do active exercises

The patient needs to know what joint is being exercised, why (to maintain mobility and allow specific activities, especially pleasurable ones, to be done) and how to perform the exercises (use a show-and-tell technique). Encouraging the patient to participate and initiate the exercises will also change the actions from a passive to an active exercise and movement of the joint, which will be more beneficial for the patient. Equipment (e.g. small velcro wrist weights or therapy balls), as advised by the physiotherapist, can be used to assist the patient performing active exercises.

Perform hand hygiene

Maintain the 5 Moments for Hand Hygiene and perform hand hygiene after touching the patient and the patient's surrounds.

CLEAN, REPLACE OR DISPOSE OF EQUIPMENT

Clean and replace used equipment. This is a time-management strategy and a courtesy to fellow nursing staff. Wipe re-useable equipment with decontaminating wipes as per facility policy. Disposable items should be placed in the general waste.

DOCUMENT AND REPORT RELEVANT INFORMATION

Documentation on active and passive exercises includes an initial notation of the joints to be exercised and then daily recording in the nursing care plan that the exercises have been completed along with any changes noted.

CASE STUDY

Kim Burch is a 57-year-old man transferred to the ward following cardiothoracic surgery 2 days ago. He now requires one nurse to assist with his mobility, personal hygiene and elimination.

You are required to include active and passive exercises as part of Kim's nursing care.

1. What is the difference between active exercises and passive exercises?
2. What is the purpose of active and passive exercises?
3. When would you implement active and passive exercises as part of your care delivery to Kim?

Note: These notes are summaries of the most important points in the assessments/procedures, and are not exhaustive on the subject. The naming of documents or charts may differ from state to state, and facility to facility. In all possible situations the guidelines of the ACSQHC are used when describing national charts or documents (e.g. the ACSQHC Observation and Response Chart is named the Adult Observation and Response Chart in WA, and the Rapid Detection and Response Observation Chart in SA). References of the materials used to compile the information have been supplied. The student is expected to have learned the material surrounding each skill as presented in the references. No single reference is complete on the subject.

REFERENCES

Cameron, S., Ball, I., Cepinskas, G., Choong, K., Doherty, T.J., Ellis, C.G., Martin, C.M., Mele, T.S., Sharpe, M., Shoemaker, J.K. & Fraser, D.D. (2015). Early mobilization in the critical care unit: A review of adult and pediatric literature. *Journal of Critical Care*, 30(4), pp. 664–72.

DeLaune, S., Ladner, P.K., McTier, L., Tollefson, J. & Lawrence, J. (2016). *Australian and New Zealand Fundamentals of Nursing*. South Melbourne: Cengage.

Sachiko, N., Hisae, H., Etsuko, F., Naoko, M. & Hiromitsu, K. (2015). Passive ankle movement increases cerebral blood oxygenation in the elderly: an experimental study. *BMC Nursing*, 14(1), pp. 1–7. doi:10.1186/s12912-015-0066-x

ESSENTIAL SKILLS COMPETENCY

Range-of-Motion Exercises

Demonstrates the ability to effectively and safely maintain a patient's joint mobility or teach the patient to do so

Criteria for skill performance	Y	D
(Numbers indicate *Enrolled Nurse Standards for Practice*, 2016)	(Satisfactory)	(Requires development)
1. Identifies indication (8.3, 8.4)		
2. Considerations for implementation are understood (1.2, 8.4)		

3. Gathers equipment (1.2, 1.6, 6.4, 8.4, 9.4):
  ▪ small and large pillows as necessary
  ▪ small wrist weights or handheld therapy ball		

4. Performs hand hygiene (1.2, 1.4, 1.8, 3.9, 6.4, 9.4)		
5. Evidence of therapeutic communication with the patient; gives explanation of procedure, gains patient consent (1.2, 2.1, 2.3, 2.4, 2.5, 6.3)		
6. Demonstrates problem-solving abilities; adjusts exercises according to patient ability (4.1, 4.2, 8.3, 8.4, 9.4)		
7. Assesses all joints (1.2, 1.4, 1.8, 2.1, 2.3, 2.7, 3.2, 3.9, 4.1, 4.2, 8.4, 9.4)		
8. Assists the patient to move each joint through its entire range of motion (1.2, 2.3, 2.7, 3.2, 3.9, 4.1, 4.2, 6.1, 8.4, 9.4)		
9. Teaches the patient to accomplish range-of-motion exercises with minimal assistance (1.2, 2.1, 2.5, 3.2, 6.3)		
10. Performs hand hygiene (1.2, 1.4, 1.8, 3.9, 6.4, 9.4)		
11. Cleans, replaces and disposes of equipment appropriately (1.2, 1.4, 3.9, 6.5, 9.4)		
12. Documents and reports relevant information (1.2, 1.3, 1.8, 3.2, 5.3, 6.6, 7.1, 7.2, 7.3, 7.4, 7.5)		
13. Demonstrates ability to link theory to practice (8.3, 8.4, 8.5, 9.4)		

Student:

Clinical facilitator: Date:

CHAPTER 3.15

DEEP BREATHING AND COUGHING, AND USE OF INCENTIVE SPIROMETER

IDENTIFY INDICATIONS

Deep breathing and coughing (DB&C) exercises are a core nursing skill that help patients to improve their respiratory function and reduce the risk of respiratory complications during the postoperative recovery time, during extended bed rest or reduced mobility and from long-term respiratory illness. Deep breathing exercises are also described as diaphragmatic breathing and abdominal breathing exercises (Pattanshetty & Thapa, 2015). Incentive spirometry promotes deep sustained inhalation, and produces a similar outcome to deep breathing when completed regularly throughout the day (Nidhi & Tamang, 2015). The incentive spirometer is a low tech, and disposable, bedside tool.

Both deep breathing and incentive spirometry have been demonstrated to increase the patient's peak expiratory flow rate, expansion of the alveoli and improvement in gas exchange, exercise tolerance and overall quality of life. Including it as a routine and core nursing care action can prevent pulmonary complications following surgery, in patients with long-term respiratory disease (Adam, 2017). Many patients (e.g. with chronic respiratory disease or pain) have shallow breathing, which increases their risk of

complications. Coughing helps clear mucus and secretions from the lungs. A deep cough clears mucus from further down in the lungs, while a huff cough will clear upper respiratory mucus (Cystic Fibrosis Foundation n.d.).

Although the physiotherapist will implement these exercises as part of their care routine, the nurse needs to remind, teach and encourage patients to complete these exercises regularly throughout the day. The nurse's actions of helping the patient to remember when to perform deep breathing and coughing will require use of health teaching skills (see **Skill 7.5**) to reinforce what has been previously learnt and encourage patient independence for completing this procedure correctly. The nurse should also document the patient's compliance with this procedure.

Patients usually complete either deep breathing and coughing or incentive spirometry. Some may use both. The procedure can be ordered by the physiotherapist or doctor as part of regular care routines. A registered nurse may also order deep breathing and coughing exercises when planning nursing care.

GATHER AND PREPARE EQUIPMENT

Gather and check the required equipment prior to starting the procedure. Organisation increases your own confidence and permits a rehearsal of the procedure. It also increases the patient's confidence in the nursing care and minimises the time needed to accomplish the procedure. Most of the equipment used for deep breathing and coughing with incentive spirometry is usually kept at the patient's bedside area.

- *Tissues* for coughing into.
- *Incentive spirometer*, usually labelled with the patient's name and kept on the patient's locker for frequent use.

A new incentive spirometer can be collected from the storeroom if a patient does not already have one.

- *Alcohol wipes* to clean the mouthpiece of the incentive spirometer.
- *Pillows* to help the patient sit in an upright/semi-upright position.
- *Extra pillow or folded towel* to splint any wounds or incisions.
- *Non-sterile gloves and paper bag* for collecting and disposing of the used tissues.
- *Clean specimen jar with yellow lid*, if sputum specimen is required.

ASSIST THE PATIENT TO COMPLETE DEEP BREATHING AND COUGHING EXERCISES

Perform hand hygiene

Perform hand hygiene before touching the patient or the patient's surrounds and prior to any procedure involving patient contact to reduce the possibility of cross-contamination. Hand hygiene is the most effective method of infection control as it removes transient organisms from the hands of the nurse (see **Skill 1.1**).

Give a clear explanation of the procedure and establish therapeutic communication

Introduce yourself, and check you have the correct patient. Explain (and demonstrate) the procedure and gain the patient's consent. Giving a clear explanation is required to gain legal consent and to address policy requirements. It will also assist the patient to cooperate with the procedure, allay anxiety and assist in establishing a therapeutic relationship.

This will help reinforce information shared as part of teaching the patient how to complete this procedure correctly. Information shared with the patient should not only include how to complete this procedure, but the benefits of deep breathing and coughing or incentive spirometry, and how it minimises risks related to hospital procedures or their illness. Allow an opportunity for the patient to ask questions about this procedure and clarify any of their concerns.

Demonstrate problem-solving abilities

Refer to the physiotherapist's instructions for any specific breathing exercises for the patient. Assess the patient's pain, as deep breathing and coughing exercises can increase or cause pain in the first days, post-op. Pain will reduce the patient's willingness to move or breathe deeply and complete the procedure correctly. Although deep breathing, coughing and incentive spirometry are not invasive, the procedure can cause distress for some patients. Adjustments may need to be made for how long the patient inhales or exhales, depending on their current respiratory function or pain.

Perform deep breathing exercises

Position the patient in bed, sitting in an upright or semi-upright position, using pillows and the bed controls to help them sit comfortably. Alternatively, the patient can sit upright in a chair. The nurse should stand next to the patient to guide the patient through the procedure. Place the patient's hands on their abdomen to help them feel the depth of their respirations. If the patient has an incision or wound, they can use a folded towel or small pillow to splint the incision, reducing pain and the feeling of pressure on the site.

Ask the patient to breathe in slowly and deeply through the nose, feeling their shoulders rise and their abdomen move slightly upwards. They should try to expand and fully inflate their lungs, breathing in for approximately 3 to 4 seconds. The patient then relaxes and exhales slowly through the mouth (or pursed lips), feeling the abdomen contract. Exhalation should last approximately 4 to 5 seconds, emptying the lungs completely before the next inhalation. This process is then repeated three to four times. The patient then needs to relax and breathe normally to prevent hyperventilation. After deep breathing is completed, the patient will complete coughing exercises.

Assist the patient to complete coughing exercises

Hand the patient a tissue and explain the importance of coughing into the tissue to reduce infection risks from airborne droplets. If a sputum specimen is required, the patient can cough into a clean specimen jar. Ensure the patient is still in a semi-upright or upright position.

Ask the patient to again place their hands on their abdomen (or splint incisions as described above), complete another deep relaxed breath in and then hold the breath for 1 to 3 seconds. Force the air out, using the abdominal muscles to cough one to two times, forcing the air from the lower lungs. Avoid a coughing fit by having one to two coughs on the out breath. This should clear secretions from the lower lungs, although it can sometimes become caught in the throat.

A 'huff cough' or huffing can be used to clear secretions from the upper airway and into the mouth. The patient takes in only a medium-sized breath, holds the breath for 2 to 3 seconds, and then completes a forceful but slow cough and exhalation. Repeat the process two further times (Cystic Fibrosis Foundation n.d.).

ASSIST THE PATIENT TO USE THE INCENTIVE SPIROMETER

Use an alcohol wipe to clean the mouthpiece of the patient's incentive spirometer. Position the patient in bed, sitting in an upright or semi-upright position, using pillows and the bed controls to help them sit comfortably. Alternatively, the patient can sit upright in a chair. The nurse should stand next to the patient to guide the patient through the procedure.

Place the mouthpiece of the incentive spirometer in the patient's mouth and ask them to close their lips to form a seal. The patient then inhales through the mouthpiece for 3 to 5 seconds (some patients may be required to inhale for up to 10 seconds). The aim is to make the balls in all three chambers rise and float at the top. A deep and long inhalation will help them to rise and float inside the chambers. The patient then exhales slowly. Repeat the process three to four times.

Remind the patient to repeat these exercises during the day

Deep breathing and coughing, or incentive spirometry, is repeated throughout the day, at hourly intervals or as instructed by the doctor or physiotherapist. The nurse should observe the patient to see if they are completing the procedure or remind them regularly when it is time to be repeated. The incentive spirometer should be placed in easy reach of the patient for them to self-initiate, or to respond to a nurse's prompt that it is time to complete this procedure.

Perform hand hygiene

Maintain the 5 Moments for Hand Hygiene and perform hand hygiene after touching the patient and the patient's surrounds.

CLEAN, REPLACE OR DISPOSE OF EQUIPMENT

Wear non-sterile gloves to collect and dispose of used tissues in the general waste. Replace the extra pillows and the towel to their previous location in the patient's bed area. Wipe the outside of the incentive spirometer with the recommended wipes, and place in the patient's bedside area. The incentive spirometer is disposed of when the patient no longer requires it. If a sputum specimen was collected, record the collection in the relevant part of the observation and response chart or nursing care plan. The specimen should be labelled correctly and sent to the laboratory with the request form as soon as possible.

DOCUMENT AND REPORT RELEVANT INFORMATION

Record the completion of deep breathing and coughing, or incentive spirometry, on the patient's nursing care plan for each shift. The patient's ability and cooperation to complete this procedure may be reported as part of the verbal bedside/shift handover.

CASE STUDY

Kim Burch is a 57-year-old man transferred to the ward following cardiothoracic surgery 2 days ago. He now requires one nurse to assist with his mobility, personal hygiene and elimination. He has a peripheral intravenous catheter (PIVC) in situ and is on oxygen via a nasal cannula.

1. Explain how you will teach Kim to do his deep breathing and coughing exercises.

2. What position should he be placed in when performing these exercises?

3. The physiotherapist has also requested Kim to use an incentive spirometer. What is the purpose of an incentive spirometer?

Note: These notes are summaries of the most important points in the assessments/procedures, and are not exhaustive on the subject. The naming of documents or charts may differ from state to state, and facility to facility. In all possible situations the guidelines of the ACSQHC are used when describing national charts or documents (e.g. the ACSQHC Observation and Response Chart is named the Adult Observation and Response Chart in WA, and the Rapid Detection and Response Observation Chart in SA). References of the materials used to compile the information have been supplied. The student is expected to have learned the material surrounding each skill as presented in the references. No single reference is complete on the subject.

REFERENCES

Adams, D. (2017). Where is the incentive in incentive spirometry? CSRT Annual Education Conference in Halifax, Nova Scotia, on 11–13 May 2017. *Canadian Journal of Respiratory Therapy*, 53(3), p. 50.

Cystic Fibrosis Foundation. (n.d.). *Coughing and Huffing.* https://www.cff.org/Life-With-CF/Treatments-and-Therapies/Airway-Clearance/Coughing-and-Huffing/

Nidhi, Sarkaar, S. & Tamang, E.L. (2015). Effectiveness of deep breathing exercises vs incentive spirometry on pulmonary function among patients with chronic airflow limitation. *International Journal of Nursing Education*, 7(2), pp. 261–8.

Pattanshetty, R.B. & Thapa, S. (2015). Effect of early mobilization programme in addition to diaphragmatic breathing exercise versus incentive spirometry on diaphragmatic excursion and PEFR in patients with abdominal surgery – a RCT. *Indian Journal of Physiotherapy and Occupational Therapy*, 9(2), pp. 28–63.

ESSENTIAL SKILLS COMPETENCY

Deep Breathing and Coughing, and Use of Incentive Spirometer

Demonstrates the ability to effectively and safely guide the patient to perform deep breathing and coughing exercises, plus use the incentive spirometer

Criteria for skill performance	Y	D
(Numbers indicate *Enrolled Nurse Standards for Practice*, 2016)	(Satisfactory)	(Requires development)
1. Identifies indication (8.3, 8.4)		
2. Gathers and prepares equipment (1.2, 1.6, 4.4, 6.4, 8.4, 9.4): ■ tissues ■ incentive spirometer ■ alcohol wipe ■ pillows ■ extra pillow or folded towel ■ non-sterile gloves and paper bag ■ clean specimen jar with yellow lid, if sputum specimen is required		
3. Performs hand hygiene (1.2, 1.4, 1.8, 3.9, 6.4, 9.4)		
4. Evidence of effective communication with the patient; gives explanation and demonstration of procedure, gains patient consent; allays patient's anxiety by adequately explaining the procedure (2.1, 2.3, 2.4, 2.5, 6.3)		
5. Demonstrates problem-solving abilities (4.1, 4.2, 8.3, 8.4, 9.4)		
6. Performs deep breathing exercises (1.2, 1.4, 1.8, 2.1, 2.10, 3.2, 3.9, 6.3, 6.6, 8.4, 9.4)		
7. Assists the patient to complete coughing exercises (1.2, 1.4, 1.8, 2.1, 2.10, 3.2, 3.9, 6.3, 6.6, 8.4, 9.4)		
8. Assists the patient to use the incentive spirometer (1.2, 1.4, 1.8, 2.1, 2.10, 3.2, 3.9, 6.3, 6.6, 8.4, 9.4)		
9. Performs hand hygiene (1.2, 1.4, 1.8, 3.9, 6.4, 9.4)		
10. Cleans, replaces and disposes of equipment appropriately (1.2, 1.4, 3.9, 6.5, 9.4)		
11. Documents and reports relevant information (1.2, 1.3, 1.8, 3.2, 5.3, 6.6, 7.1, 7.2, 7.3, 7.4, 7.5)		
12. Demonstrates ability to link theory to practice (8.3, 8.4, 8.5, 9.4)		

Student:

Clinical facilitator: Date:

PART 4

ASEPSIS AND WOUND CARE

Note: These notes are summaries of the most important points in the assessments/procedures and are not exhaustive on the subject. References of the materials used to compile the information have been supplied. The student is expected to have learnt the material surrounding each skill as presented in the references. No single reference is complete on each subject.

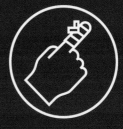

CHAPTER 4.1

ASEPTIC TECHNIQUE – ESTABLISHING A GENERAL OR CRITICAL ASEPTIC FIELD

IDENTIFY INDICATIONS

Aseptic technique is a key component of the National Safety and Quality Health Services (Preventing and Controlling Healthcare-Associated Infection Standard [ACSQHS, 2019]) and is described more specifically in the Australian Guidelines for the prevention and control of infection in healthcare (NHMRC, 2019). It is an essential skill that is applied to many clinical procedures and nursing interventions. The Australian College for Infection Prevention and Control (ACIPC, n.d.) defines it as the 'range of infection control practices which are used to minimise the presence of pathogenic microorganisms during clinical procedures'. Asepsis means 'freedom from infection or infectious (pathogenic) material' (Weller, 1997).

Pathogenic organisms, in sufficient quantity to produce infection, can be introduced to susceptible sites by hands, surfaces and equipment (NHMRC, 2019). The correct use of aseptic technique protects patients during invasive clinical procedures and helps to reduce a patient's risk for hospital-acquired infection (Queensland Health, 2019).

The use of an aseptic technique applies to any nursing intervention that creates a risk of the patient becoming colonised or infected during a clinical procedure (Department of Health and Human Services, 2014). While the use of an aseptic technique is easily recognised as an essential part of wound care, as it minimises the introduction of pathogenic organisms to a wound, the use of an aseptic technique extends to many other regular nursing procedures (Wounds Australia, 2017). These include administering medications, giving an injection, performing blood glucose readings, emptying of indwelling catheter bags and changing IV fluid bags.

TERMINOLOGY AND DEFINITIONS

To implement correct aseptic technique within nursing care actions, it is important to understand the terminology and principles of aseptic technique.

Key sites are breaches in the skin integrity (e.g. IV cannula insertion sites, injection site or a wound) which can be a portal of entry for microorganisms.

Key parts are any parts of or equipment that comes into contact with the patient, or is used as part of a procedure. Contamination of these key parts can transfer microorganisms to the patient (Department of Health and Human Services, 2014). 'Non-touch' of the key part is a vital component of maintaining asepsis, and only key parts come into contact with other key parts or key sites (Wounds Australia, 2017). For example, a key site (incision) can only be touched by a key part (a sterile swab, dampened with sterile normal saline using a sterile forceps).

Non-touch technique is used at all times to maintain asepsis (ACIPC, 2015). This skill requires the nurse's hands not to touch (and contaminate) any key parts or key sites. When sterile gloves are worn, touching of key parts or key sites is kept to a minimum. Examples of a non-touch technique include using sterile forceps or gauze to touch part of a wound, tipping pills into the lid of a medication bottle and then tipping the single pill into the medication cup, or touching only the cap (and not the hub) of a needle.

THE ASEPTIC FIELD

The aseptic field is established either to ensure asepsis or promote asepsis. It is a designated workspace to contain and protect equipment used during procedures from becoming contaminated. The choice of aseptic field depends on the complexity of the procedure being implemented (Wounds Australia, 2017).

General aseptic field promotes asepsis during smaller procedures such as a simple dressing, preparation of IV fluids or the insertion of an IV cannula. A general aseptic field uses a 'non-touch technique'.

Critical aseptic field ensures asepsis and is used when key parts or key sites are unable to be protected from contamination during a procedure (e.g. complex wound care, insertion of a urinary catheter, operating theatre procedures) or when key sites are extensive and a large working area or long duration of contact is required. Sterilised equipment, sterile gloves and other barriers such as gowns are required.

Micro critical aseptic field is a smaller subtype of critical aseptic field, and includes key parts that are protected from contamination by their own sterile cover (e.g. capped syringes, sheathed needles or packaged sterile gauze). A micro critical aseptic field can also be part of a larger general or critical aseptic field.

TYPES OF ASEPTIC TECHNIQUE

The National Health and Medical Research Council (NHMRC) (2019) and ACIPC (2015) outline two types of aseptic technique. The nurse should assess the risks prior to a procedure and determine the correct types of aseptic technique required.

Standard aseptic technique

Clinical procedures managed with standard aseptic technique will be technically simple, short in duration (less than 20 minutes) and involve relatively few and small key sites, and key parts that will also not be touched. Standard aseptic technique requires a general aseptic field, micro critical aseptic field, the use of non-touch technique and non-sterile gloves.

Surgical aseptic technique

This technique is required when procedures are technically complex, involve extended periods of time and large, open key sites or large numerous key parts. To counter these risks, a critical aseptic field and sterile gloves are required, while continuing to maintain a non-touch technique. Often full-barrier precautions are also needed.

FURTHER PRINCIPLES OF ASEPTIC TECHNIQUE AND INFECTION CONTROL

Because aseptic technique aims to prevent the introduction of pathogenic microorganisms via hands, clinical equipment and surfaces, hand hygiene and use of personal protective equipment (PPE), plus the cleaning and drying of surfaces and equipment is an essential part of an aseptic technique (Department of Health and Human Services, 2014). Other core principles include a non-touch technique, glove use and ensuring the asepsis and sterility of equipment. These are explained below.

- *Hand hygiene.* Correct hand hygiene (5 Moments for Hand Hygiene) is the single most important measure to prevent transmission of infection. It protects both the patient and the nurse.
- *Glove use.* Non-sterile gloves are used to protect the nurse from blood or body fluids, when no key sites are being touched. Sterile gloves are used if it is necessary to directly touch any key parts or key sites (NHMRC, 2019). A risk assessment by the healthcare worker determines whether they can perform the procedure and maintain asepsis without touching either the key part or the key site and contaminating it. Longer or more complex procedures may require the use of additional

precautions, including sterile gloves rather than non-sterile gloves.
- *Other PPE.* Based on infection control risk assessment and the principles of standard precautions, PPE such as plastic aprons, face shields or goggles may be required.
- *Cleaning of surfaces and equipment.* Equipment and surfaces are decontaminated prior to a procedure using appropriate solutions or wipes (e.g. decontaminating a trolley). Key parts are made aseptic before a procedure (e.g. using an alcohol wipe to clean an IV bung or the skin surface before an injection). All equipment used during a procedure should also be cleaned and disinfected after use.
- *Environment.* Reduce the risks of contamination of the area where a procedure is to be performed, by adjusting the surrounding environment (National Health and Medical Research Council [NHMRC], 2019). Limit activities such as bed-making, use of commodes by other patients, open windows, cleaning or a confined work area.
- *Sterile equipment.* This is equipment that is free from microorganisms (Weller, 1997). Only sterile items can come into contact with key sites. Sterile items must not come into contact with non-sterile items.

PRINCIPLES OF PRACTICE

Aseptic technique is used when preparing for and undertaking any invasive procedure: that is, one that penetrates the body's natural defence of intact skin and mucous membrane. The principles used in the practice of aseptic technique are (Wounds Australia, 2017; Department of Health and Human Services, 2014):

- sterile objects remain sterile only when touched by another sterile object
- only sterile objects may be placed in an aseptic field
- sterile objects or aseptic fields should be kept in view
- sterile objects/aseptic fields become contaminated by prolonged exposure to air
- a sterile surface that comes in contact with a wet contaminated surface becomes contaminated
- a fluid flows in the direction of gravity or by capillary action
- the edges of an aseptic field are considered contaminated
- skin cannot be made sterile, but washing reduces the number of microorganisms on it
- sterile gloves are used to further prevent transfer of microorganisms
- conversation should be minimised to reduce the spread of droplets
- whatever sterile object is opened for one patient can only be used for that one procedure.

These principles are similar and compatible with the transmission-based precautions recommended by the NHMRC (2019). Conscientiousness, alertness and honesty are essential qualities in maintaining aseptic technique. Unless these principles and guidelines are strictly followed, patient safety is compromised and infection will occur.

ESTABLISHING A GENERAL OR CRITICAL ASEPTIC FIELD FOR A PROCEDURE

The described procedure relates to establishing either a general or critical aseptic field. The principles described can be applied to all procedures that require the use of an aseptic technique. The choice between a general or critical aseptic field will depend on the type of procedure being implemented, the size or number of key site/s and the number of key parts being used. Use a risk assessment process to determine if a general or critical aseptic field is required. A non-touch technique is used for both types of aseptic field.

GATHER AND PREPARE EQUIPMENT

 This step depends on the procedure to be done. All supplies must be available before you proceed to the patient's room, so that the aseptic field, once established, is not left unattended. An aseptic field left unattended is considered contaminated. Any additional items that are needed for the procedure that are not on the trolley will have to be brought and added by a second person.

- *Collect a trolley or clear the working surface* and wipe it down with a disinfecting solution wipe as recommended by the facility to establish a clean (not sterile) work surface. Let the surface dry thoroughly to eliminate the transfer of microorganisms via moisture.
- *A disposable wet-strength bag* for discarded used materials is placed close to the patient so that unsterile material is not brought over the sterile field. The mouth of the bag should be wide enough so that material can be dropped from above into the bag to ensure that sterility of forceps or gloves is not broken.
- *Sterile pack* (e.g. dressing pack) and *other sterile items* as required for the procedure.
- *Alcohol-based hand rub (ABHR)* if not available at the patient's bedside.

Confirm the sterility of the packages by checking the use-by date and whether the package is dry, has tears, water damage, stains or, in the case of a bottle, a broken seal. Out-of-date sterile objects have been on the shelf for an extended period of time and their contents are no longer considered sterile because of the time factor. Tears, punctures, stains and dampness in the packaging indicate that there is a pathway from the exterior to the interior of the package through which microorganisms can gain access. A broken seal on a bottle indicates the bottle's contents have been exposed to the air and are contaminated.

ASEPTIC TECHNIQUE

Perform hand hygiene
Perform hand hygiene before touching the patient or the patient's surrounds and prior to any procedure involving patient contact to reduce the possibility of cross-contamination. Hand hygiene is the most effective method of infection control as it removes transient organisms from the hands of the nurse (see **Skill 1.1**).

Give a clear explanation of the procedure and establish therapeutic communication
Introduce yourself, and check you have the correct patient. Discuss the procedure and gain the patient's consent. Giving a clear explanation is required to gain legal consent and to address policy requirements. It will also assist the patient to cooperate with the procedure, allay anxiety and assist in establishing a therapeutic relationship. Explanation of the positioning and the expectations of the patient will ensure their cooperation and reduce the risk that they will touch and contaminate something sterile.

Demonstrate problem-solving abilities
Ensuring the patient is pain free, position the patient comfortably to eliminate movement during the procedure, which can contaminate sterile items. The patient's position should be considered in relation to the time it is expected they will need to stay still and to the body part that will be exposed, in order to make it accessible for treatment. Maintain privacy to enhance the patient's dignity.

Perform hand hygiene
Perform hand hygiene to remove microorganisms and prevent cross-contamination. ABHR can be used.

Open the package using a non-touch technique
Open the procedure pack (e.g. dressing or catheter pack) by initially removing the outer plastic wrap and drop the inner sterile pack onto the top shelf of the clean trolley or work surface. It is placed flat on the trolley with the initial folded flap facing the nurse. Touch only the outside surface of the wrapper to maintain the sterility of the inner surface. Using thumb and a forefinger, this flap is grasped and pulled out. The remaining corners are carefully folded out to

form the aseptic field. Adjustments to the position of the pack are made from the outside surface or outer edges of the aseptic field. The inside surface of the wrapper has formed a sterile surface, with the object (dressing tray, catheter tray, bowl, etc.) in the centre of the aseptic field. The area inside a border 5 cm from each edge is considered sterile.

Many procedure packs will have dressing forceps tucked into the dressing towel at the top of the contents inside the pack. These forceps (setting-up forceps) are carefully picked up (at the ends that will not come into contact with the wound), using your fingertips. They are used for unpacking and setting up other items on the aseptic field. They are then placed in the lower right-hand (or left-hand) area of the sterile field, where they can be accessed.

Unpack the remaining items in the pack using the setting-up forceps. Place all other forceps in the front lower edge of the field where they can easily be picked up, but within the 5 cm border. Arrange the tray in the middle section (where swabs and other equipment/materials can later be prepared) and other materials to the back third of the field. Maintain this format after adding and arranging extra items.

Add the necessary sterile supplies using a non-touch technique

All packages are opened while standing back from the established aseptic field to avoid contaminants falling from the packaging material onto the field (i.e. do not open packaging over the sterile field).

- *Peeling pouches.* Grasp the opposite edges of the two sides of the wrapper and carefully peel down, fully exposing the item (gauze squares, instruments, catheters, etc.). Without reaching across or touching the aseptic field, drop the item (or lift out with the setting-up forceps) onto the aseptic field from the wrapper, making sure it is within the 5 cm border. Items are dropped from about 15 cm so that the packaging material and your hand do not touch the aseptic field.
- *Opening solution/ampoules.* Add liquids last; ensure there is a container available for the fluid on the aseptic field before you open it, and read the label to ensure you have the correct solution. Open the ampoule/sachet of solution. Twist off the ampoule top and dispose of it in the rubbish bag or tear back the sachet at the marked point and fold back the flap.
- See **FIGURE 4.1.1**. Hold the ampoule/sachet directly over the tray and about 10 cm up to prevent accidentally touching the aseptic field, and pour slowly to prevent splashes, since moisture will contaminate the field by facilitating microorganism movement through the sterile drapes. Ensure you do not contaminate the solution when pouring.

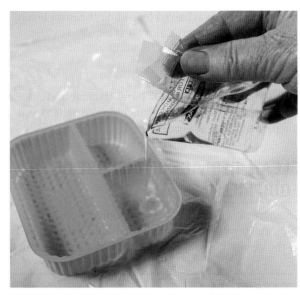

FIGURE 4.1.1 Pouring of fluid from sachet

Perform hand hygiene

After all additional items have been placed on the aseptic field, perform hand hygiene using ABHR to remove microorganisms and prevent cross-contamination.

Manipulating the items using a non-touch technique

Rearranging items on the aseptic field is done with sterile forceps included in commercial prepared packs. These can be different colours and the most easily accessible of the forceps are the setting-up forceps (often yellow). The setting-up forceps and a second set of forceps are carefully picked up, ensuring that nothing else is touched by the nurse's hands or fingers. The forceps are then used to manipulate the items on the field. If the forceps are used for anything wet, keep the tip of the forceps lower than your wrist to prevent liquids from running down the forceps by gravity and then back to the tips to make the forceps unsterile. These setting-up forceps are later used for cleansing and drying of the key site and then discarded.

Perform the required procedure

Perform the required procedure using the principles of the aseptic technique. Ensure all key parts and key sites are protected. Sterile items should only be used once, and then disposed of in the rubbish bag. Only sterile items should come in contact with the key site.

Nurses must assess their patients for risk and choose to use a critical aseptic field as opposed to a general aseptic field if there is an increased chance of infection. If a critical aseptic field is required, don surgical gloves using open gloving as per **Skill 4.9**.

Refer to **Skill 4.2** for further description of basic wound dressing technique. This basic dressing technique (standard aseptic technique) and general aseptic field can be adapted for more complex wounds and procedures (e.g. **Skills 4.3, 4.5 and 4.6**) that require critical aseptic fields and a surgical aseptic technique. This is achieved by adding the extra levels of precaution (e.g. sterile gloves) as required by the specific procedure.

Perform hand hygiene

Maintain the 5 Moments for Hand Hygiene and perform hand hygiene after touching the patient and the patient's surrounds.

CLEAN, REPLACE OR DISPOSE OF EQUIPMENT

Clean, replace and dispose of equipment appropriately. Contaminated disposables are wrapped in the disposable wrapper that has formed the aseptic field, and then placed in the disposable rubbish bag. This material is placed in the contaminated waste bin in the dirty utility room. The trolley or surface is wiped down with the recommended disinfecting solution or wipes. If gross contamination has occurred, facility policy for cleaning should be followed. The trolley is returned to its position in the clean service area of the ward. Sharps, including disposable metal scissors and forceps, are placed in the sharps container.

DOCUMENT AND REPORT RELEVANT INFORMATION

Document in the relevant area, for example, wound care chart.

CASE STUDY

You are an enrolled nurse required to complete different nursing procedures requiring the use of an aseptic technique.

1. List three principles that should be followed to maintain an aseptic technique.
2. Why is it important to close the windows, not make any beds and stop any cleaning while completing a procedure using an aseptic technique?
3. Describe the difference between a standard aseptic technique and a surgical aseptic technique.
4. Define the following terms:
    a. key part
    b. key site
    c. non-touch technique.
5. Identify which of the following is a micro critical aseptic field, general aseptic field or critical aseptic field:
    *   cap covering a new sterile needle
    *   insertion of a urinary catheter
    *   complex wound care
    *   simple dressing
    *   removal of sutures
    *   cap covering the connector end of a new catheter bag
    *   operating theatre.

Note: These notes are summaries of the most important points in the assessments/procedures, and are not exhaustive on the subject. The naming of documents or charts may differ from state to state, and facility to facility. In all possible situations the guidelines of the ACSQHC are used when describing national charts or documents (e.g. the ACSQHC Observation and Response Chart is named the Adult Observation and Response Chart in WA, and the Rapid Detection and Response Observation Chart in SA). References of the materials used to compile the information have been supplied. The student is expected to have learned the material surrounding each skill as presented in the references. No single reference is complete on the subject.

REFERENCES

Australian College for Infection Prevention and Control (ACIPC). (2015). *Aseptic Technique During Invasive Clinical Procedures.* https://www.acipc.org.au/aseptic-technique-resources

Australian Commission on Safety and Quality in Health Care (ACSQHC). (2019). *Preventing and Controlling Healthcare-Associated Infection Standard.* https://www.safetyandquality. gov.au/standards/nsqhs-standards/preventing-and-controlling-healthcare-associated-infection-standard

Department of Health and Human Services. (2014). *Aseptic Technique Standard 3: Preventing and Controlling Healthcare Associated Infections.* Sector Performance, Quality and Rural Health, Department of Health, Victorian State Government. https:// www2.health.vic.gov.au/about/publications/policiesandguidelines/ Standard-3-Aseptic-Technique-Learning-Module-Preventing-and-Controlling-Healthcare-Associated-Infections

National Health and Medical Research Council (NHMRC). (2019). *Australian Guidelines for the Prevention and Control of Infection in Healthcare.* https://www.nhmrc.gov.au/health-advice/public-health/preventing-infection

Queensland Health. (2019). *Aseptic Technique.* Queensland Government. https://www.health.qld.gov.au/clinical-practice/ guidelines-procedures/diseases-infection/infection-prevention/ standard-precautions/aseptic

Weller, B. (Ed.) (1997). *Encyclopaedic Dictionary of Nursing and Health Care.* London: Baillière Tindall: p. 81.

Wounds Australia. (2017) *Application of Aseptic Technique in Wound Dressing Procedure: A Consensus Document.* Osborne Park, WA: Cambridge Media.

ESSENTIAL SKILLS COMPETENCY

Aseptic Technique
Demonstrates the ability to effectively and safely establish and maintain a general or critical aseptic field

Criteria for skill performance	Y	D
(Numbers indicate *Enrolled Nurse Standards for Practice*, 2016)	(Satisfactory)	(Requires development)
1. Identifies indication (8.3, 8.4)		
2. Gathers equipment as relevant to aseptic procedure being performed (1.2, 1.6, 4.4, 6.4, 8.4, 9.4)		
3. Confirms the sterility of the packages (1.2, 1.4, 3.2, 3.9, 9.4)		
4. Evidence of effective communication with patient; gives explanation of procedure, gains patient consent (2.1, 2.3, 2.4, 2.5, 6.3)		
5. Demonstrates problem-solving abilities; e.g. positions patient comfortably (4.1, 4.2, 8.3, 8.4, 9.4)		
6. Performs hand hygiene (1.2, 1.4, 1.8, 3.9, 6.4, 9.4)		
7. Opens the package touching only outer packaging and edges (1.2, 1.4, 3.9, 8.4, 9.4)		
8. Adds necessary sterile supplies using non-touch technique (1.2, 1.4, 3.9, 8.4, 9.4)		
9. Performs hand hygiene again (1.2, 1.4, 1.8, 3.9, 6.4, 9.4)		
10. Uses sterile forceps to handle sterile supplies and arrange aseptic field using non-touch technique (1.2, 1.4, 3.9, 6.4, 9.4): ■ creates either a general or critical aseptic field		
11. Performs required procedure (1.2, 1.4, 2.2, 2.3, 2.4, 2.7, 3.2, 3.9, 4.4, 6.4, 8.4, 9.4): ■ maintains principles of asepsis and uses a non-touch technique throughout procedure ■ uses either standard or surgical aseptic technique, according to the procedure		
12. Performs hand hygiene (1.2, 1.4, 1.8, 3.9, 6.4, 9.4)		
13. Cleans, replaces and disposes of equipment appropriately (1.2, 1.4, 3.9, 6.5, 9.4)		
14. Documents and reports relevant information (1.2, 1.3, 1.8, 3.2, 5.3, 6.6, 7.1, 7.2, 7.3, 7.4, 7.5)		
15. Demonstrates ability to link theory to practice (8.3, 8.4, 8.5, 9.4)		

Student:

Clinical facilitator: Date:

CHAPTER 4.2

SIMPLE DRY DRESSING USING A GENERAL ASEPTIC FIELD

IDENTIFY INDICATIONS

Dry dressings are used most commonly for uncomplicated postoperative incisions and for simple wounds and abrasions. The wound will have little or no drainage. The dressing is protective, reduces the introduction of microorganisms, reduces discomfort or accidental trauma to the site and speeds healing by keeping the wound surface moist. Always check the policy of your organisation regarding the type and preference for dressings to be used.

The principles of establishing a general aseptic field and completing a simple dressing described in this chapter can be extended for completing wound care for complex wounds, and establishing a critical aseptic field, as required for further skills (e.g. **Skills 4.3, 4.5, 4.6, 4.8, 6.8** and **8.6**).

GATHER AND PREPARE EQUIPMENT

Gathering equipment for use during the procedure is a time-management strategy. It allows the nurse to mentally rehearse the steps in the procedure. Having all necessary items available prevents having to seek assistance – leaving a sterile set-up to obtain forgotten items would risk contamination. Being organised creates self-confidence in the nurse and promotes patient confidence. The following items may be required.

- A *dressing trolley* is used to transport materials to and from the bedside; the trolley must be cleaned both before and after the dressing.
- *Dressing packs* are usually commercially supplied and contain a waterproof wrapper that serves as the sterile field when the pack is unwrapped. The inner receptacle containing the gauze swabs is used for the solutions. There are usually sufficient supplies in this for a minimally draining wound. If the wound drainage is more than a small amount, additional supplies of gauze swabs for cleansing and drying will have to be added.
- A *sterile solution* (usually normal saline [NS]) is used to cleanse the wound. The small amount needed may be supplied in plastic ampoules (marked for irrigation) or sachets of 10 to 30 mL. Solutions should be at room temperature, as warm solutions reduce stress reactions in most patients.
- A *wound ruler* is used to assess the wound, although in a simple non-infected incision, the wound ruler is often not necessary.
- *Dressings* are used to protect the wound; for example, a non-adherent dressing that promotes drainage

absorption while minimising adherence of the dressing to the wound by dried exudate. This prevents trauma to the wound during dressing removal. Gauze dressings are also absorbent, but often adhere to a draining wound and can cause trauma and pain when removed. They may be used over the top of the non-adherent dressing for extra bulk. Check the policy and protocol of your facility, or surgeon preferences.

- *Tape* is used to secure the dressing to dry intact skin. Many patients are allergic or sensitive to adhesive tape, so hypoallergenic tape should be used.
- *Gloves* (non-sterile) are used to remove the soiled dressing so that contamination is minimised. A non-touch technique is used for the dressing procedure. Refer to facility policy if non-sterile gloves should be worn throughout the procedure. They will be required if there is a risk of contact with body fluids during the procedure.
- A *waste disposal waterproof bag* is necessary for the disposal of all used and contaminated material to prevent transmission of microorganisms.

Extra items for more complex wounds or risk of exposure to body fluids are:

- *a waterproof apron*, used to prevent/reduce risk from wound exudate
- *goggles* if splashing is anticipated
- *extra forceps* (may be required)
- *masks*, required by some agencies to prevent spray from the nurse's respiratory tract contaminating the wound.

Confirm the sterility of the packages by checking the use-by date and whether the package is dry, has tears, water damage, stains or, in the case of a bottle, a broken seal. Out-of-date sterile objects have been on the shelf for an extended period of time and their contents are no longer considered sterile because of the time factor. Tears, punctures, stains and dampness in the packaging indicate that there is a pathway from the exterior to the interior of the package through which microorganisms can gain access.

All unopened items should be placed on the bottom shelf of the trolley, leaving the top surface as clean as possible for use during the procedure. This includes dressing packs and other sterile items. Take the trolley to the patient's bedside.

APPLY A SIMPLE DRESSING

Give a clear explanation of the procedure and establish therapeutic communication

Introduce yourself, and check you have the correct patient. Discuss the procedure and gain the patient's consent. Giving a clear explanation is required to gain legal consent and to address policy requirements. It will also assist the patient to cooperate with the procedure, allay anxiety and assist in establishing a therapeutic relationship. Explanation of the positioning and the expectations of the patient will ensure their cooperation and reduce the risk that they will touch and contaminate something sterile. Check with your patient regarding pain levels. If giving pain relief, allow time for medication to take effect.

Demonstrate problem-solving abilities

Positioning the patient comfortably will eliminate movement during the procedure, which can contaminate sterile items. The patient's position should be considered in relation to the time that it is expected they will need to stay still for treatment. The wound site should be comfortably accessible to the nurse to eliminate contamination or self-injury from using an awkward position for the treatment. Offering the bedpan or urinal, or assisting the patient to the toilet prior to the procedure will reduce unnecessary interruptions and increase patient comfort. Analgesia given 20 to 30 minutes prior to the procedure (as necessary) will reduce patient discomfort, increase cooperation and help the patient relax. Time the dressing change in consultation with the patient, so that visiting hours or mealtimes are not disrupted.

Prepare the room and environment

Privacy is provided for the patient, to minimise embarrassment, by pulling the curtains around the patient in a shared room or closing the door in a private room. Airflow is restricted by closing windows, reducing vacuuming or bed-making by other staff so that airborne microorganisms are less likely to contaminate the wound. The area of the wound must be well lit to assist with assessment and treatment. A waterproof waste disposal bag is placed near the patient to receive contaminated articles so that transmission of microorganisms is prevented.

Perform hand hygiene

Perform hand hygiene before touching the patient or the patient's surrounds and prior to any procedure involving patient contact to reduce the possibility of cross-contamination. Hand hygiene is the most effective method of infection control as it removes transient organisms from the hands of the nurse (see **Skill 1.1**).

Don personal protective equipment (PPE)

Put on a plastic apron, mask and eye protection, if required. These should not usually be required for a simple dressing as there is limited exposure to body fluids for a simple wound.

Remove the soiled dressing

Tape is removed carefully by supporting the skin around the tape and pulling the tape towards the wound so that stress is not applied to the fresh incision. Use short gentle pulls parallel to the skin to minimise pain and reduce trauma to the wound area. A non-irritating solvent may be used to remove adhesive painlessly. Non-sterile gloves are used when removing the dressing. If the old dressing adheres to the wound, the dressing is moistened with sterile NS and given a few minutes to loosen so that new granulating tissue is not pulled off the healing wound. Remove the dressing with the soiled surface away from the patient to reduce possible distress. Assess for any drainage, noting amount, colour, consistency and odour. The dressing and the gloves are carefully placed in the disposal bag without contaminating the outside of the bag. Some practitioners advocate leaving the complete wound dressing or the primary dressing in place until the sterile field is established, then removing it. This reduces the chance of wound contamination (either by the patient or from the environment) while the nurse is performing hand hygiene and setting up the aseptic field.

Perform hand hygiene

Perform hand hygiene to remove microorganisms and prevent cross-contamination. Alcohol-based hand rub (ABHR) can be used.

Establish a general aseptic field

The choice between a general or critical aseptic field will depend on the type of wound care, the size of the wound (i.e. key site/s) and the number of key parts being used. A simple wound dressing is not complex.

A general aseptic field should be established, and a standard aseptic technique should be used.

Open the dressing pack

Open the dressing pack by initially removing the outer plastic wrap (in prepackaged supplies), and drop the inner sterile tray onto the top shelf of the clean trolley surface. It is placed flat on the trolley with the initial folded flap facing the nurse. Touch only the outside surface of the wrapper to maintain the sterility of the inner surface. Using the thumb and a forefinger, this flap is grasped and pulled out. The remaining flaps are carefully folded out to form the aseptic field. Adjustments to the position of the pack are made from the outside surface or outer edges of the aseptic field. The inside surface of the wrapper has formed a sterile surface, with the object (dressing tray, catheter tray, bowl, etc.) in the centre of the aseptic field. The area inside a border 5 cm from each edge is considered sterile.

There will be a dressing forceps tucked into the dressing towel at the top of the contents inside the pack. These forceps (setting-up forceps) are carefully picked up with the fingertips, at the end that does not touch the patient. They are used for unpacking and setting up other items on the aseptic field. They are then placed in the lower right-hand (or left-hand) area of the sterile field, where they can be accessed.

Unpack the remaining items in the pack using the setting-up forceps. Place all other forceps in the front lower edge of the field where they can easily be picked up, but within the 5 cm border. Arrange the tray in the middle section (where swabs and other equipment/ materials can later be prepared) and other materials to the back third of the field. Maintain this format after adding and arranging extra items.

Add the necessary sterile supplies

All packages are opened while standing back from the established aseptic field to avoid contaminants falling from the packaging material onto the field (i.e. do not open packaging over the sterile field).

- *Peeling pouches.* Grasp the opposite edges of the two sides of the wrapper and carefully peel down, fully exposing the item (gauze squares, instruments, catheters, etc.). Without reaching across or touching the aseptic field, drop the item (or lift out with the setting-up forceps) onto the aseptic field from the wrapper, making sure it is within the 5 cm border. Items are dropped from about 15 cm so that the packaging material and your hand do not touch the aseptic field.
- *Opening solution/ampoules.* Add liquids last; ensure there is a container available for the fluid on the aseptic field before you open it, and read the label to ensure you have the correct solution. Open the sachet/ampoule of solution. Twist off the ampoule top and dispose of it in the rubbish or tear back the sachet at the marked point and fold back the flap. Hold the ampoule/sachet directly over the tray and

about 10 cm up to prevent accidentally touching the aseptic field, and pour slowly to prevent splashes, since moisture will contaminate the field by facilitating microorganism movement through the sterile drapes. Ensure you do not contaminate the solution when pouring.
- *Hand hygiene.* An ABHR or other surgical hand wash is required prior to an aseptic technique as hands have been contaminated by touching the packaging of the items that are put onto the aseptic field. Depending on hospital policy or your own risk assessment, you may need sterile gloves (NHMRC, 2019).

Manipulating the items

Rearranging items on the aseptic field is done with sterile forceps included in commercially prepared packs. These are different colours, and the most easily accessible of the forceps is the setting-up forceps (often yellow). As some sterile packs do not include extra forceps, a pair can be added with the other sterile supplies. After all additional items have been placed on the aseptic field, hand hygiene using ABHR should be completed. The setting-up forceps and a second set of forceps are then carefully picked up, ensuring that nothing else is touched by the nurse. The forceps are then used to manipulate the items on the field. If the forceps are used for anything wet, keep the tip of the forceps lower than your wrist to prevent liquids from running down the forceps by gravity and then back to the tips to make the forceps unsterile. These setting-up forceps are later used for cleansing and drying of the key site and then discarded.

Add all items necessary for the dressing using a standard aseptic technique. Arrange the sterile items within the sterile field using forceps. Add the solution last.

Repeat hand hygiene with ABHR as you have handled packages, tapes, and so on.

Using two pairs of forceps and a non-touch technique, soak the required number of gauze swabs with the cleansing solution, retaining some for drying the wound. Using the forceps, squeeze excess solution from the wet gauze swabs to avoid dripping solution on the wound and skin, as this extra fluid would wash microbes across the skin. Keep the tips of the forceps lower than the handles to prevent their contamination by fluid travelling up the handle and back down. Prepare the final primary and secondary wound dressing as per the wound management plan.

Refer to FIGURE 4.2.1 of an aseptic field.

Apply non-sterile gloves and remove the wound dressing, if it has not already been removed. Dispose of gloves and dressing in the waste disposal bag. Then perform hand hygiene using ABHR.

Cleanse and assess the wound

Use forceps to transfer the sterile drape to your fingertips, holding it at the top edge, and place the sterile drape beside the wound. This extends the

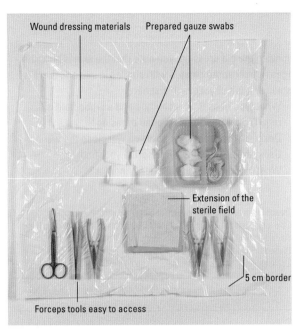

Wound dressing materials   Prepared gauze swabs

Extension of the sterile field

5 cm border

Forceps tools easy to access

FIGURE 4.2.1 An aseptic field

general aseptic field and helps prevent contamination of equipment. Keep the setting-up forceps for cleansing.

Use two sets of forceps and a non-touch technique to clean and dry the wound and peri-wound to remove surface contaminants, bacteria and remnants of previous dressings.

1. A non-touch technique is implemented by picking up a swab with the 'clean' forceps in the aseptic field, then using the forceps to pass the swab to the swabbing forceps. One gauze swab is used for each stroke to cleanse the wound. Place each used swab in the waste disposal bag. Maintain the following principle: clean from the top of the incision to the bottom, since gravity pulls drainage to the bottom of the wound.
2. Use light pressure to reduce trauma to the wound bed when cleansing (Wounds Australia, 2017).
3. Any area that looks infected is cleansed last.

Ensure the peri-wound (surrounding skin) is also cleansed. Using the same principles, dry the cleansed area. The swabbing forceps are then discarded after drying the wound.

During and after cleansing the wound, assess the wound to determine status. Inspect for size, colour, infection or inflammation, wound edges, exudate and the surrounding skin. The wound ruler (held by forceps) can also be used to assess the size of the wound. The acronym TIME (T – tissue; I – infection or inflammation; M – moisture; E – wound edges) helps to guide wound assessment. Measure wound if indicated.

Apply a dry dressing

Dressings are applied to the incision or wound in layers to ensure optimal absorption. Use the two remaining sets of forceps and a non-touch technique.

One set of forceps remains the 'clean' forceps to pick up items from the aseptic field, which are then passed to the other forceps to apply the dressing material. The primary dressing may be a non-stick dressing If more drainage is expected, a thicker secondary dressing is often applied.

Secure the dressing

Once the outer dressing has been put in place, the nurse's hands can touch the outside of the dressing to secure it in place. Secure the dressing with the selected tape (or bandage). Tape strips are applied to all edges of the dressing so that the dressing cannot be folded back to expose the wound. Tape should extend beyond the edge of the dressing so that it will securely adhere to the skin. The patient is assisted to a position of comfort that does not stress the incision or wound.

Doff PPE

Remove PPE in the following sequence: non-sterile gloves, hand hygiene, eyewear/face shield, plastic apron/gown and mask and then perform hand hygiene (ACSQHC, 2020). Dispose of in the rubbish bag.

Perform hand hygiene

Maintain the 5 Moments for Hand Hygiene and perform hand hygiene after touching the patient and the patient's surrounds.

CLEAN, REPLACE OR DISPOSE OF EQUIPMENT

Clean, replace and dispose of equipment appropriately. After securing the wound dressing, contaminated materials are wrapped in the (disposable) wrapper that has formed the aseptic field and placed in the waste disposal bag, which is then placed in the contaminated waste. The trolley is wiped down with the recommended disinfecting solution or wipes. The trolley is returned to its position in the clean service area of the unit.

DOCUMENT AND REPORT RELEVANT INFORMATION

Document relevant information in the wound management plan, care plan and patient notes, including appearance of the wound and drainage, type of dressing applied and the patient's response to the procedure. Note any alteration in comfort levels or changes in the wound condition and report these to the registered nurse.

CASE STUDY

You are required to complete a simple dry dressing for Lei Chung who had a left hip replacement 4 days ago. She has a past medical history of diabetes and hypercholesterolaemia. The current dry dressing is protecting the surgical wound site and requires changing today. A small amount of fresh exudate has been noted on the old dressing. You have been asked by the ward coordinator to assess the wound carefully as Lei has started to complain of wound discomfort and had a slightly elevated temperature that morning. On removing the old dressing, you note that the skin is pink, the edges remain approximated with staples in situ and there is a small amount of yellowish discharge.

1. What type of aseptic technique and aseptic field is required for this simple wound dressing?
2. Describe the process of how you will clean the wound.
3. Using the acronym TIME describe your findings.
4. Where will you document these findings?

Note: These notes are summaries of the most important points in the assessments/procedures, and are not exhaustive on the subject. The naming of documents or charts may differ from state to state, and facility to facility. In all possible situations the guidelines of the ACSQHC are used when describing national charts or documents (e.g. the ACSQHC Observation and Response Chart is named the Adult Observation and Response Chart in WA, and the Rapid Detection and Response Observation Chart in SA). References of the materials used to compile the information have been supplied. The student is expected to have learned the material surrounding each skill as presented in the references. No single reference is complete on the subject.

REFERENCES

Australian Commission on Safety and Quality in Health Care (ACSQHC). (2020). *Sequence for Putting on and Removing PPE.* https://www.safetyandquality.gov.au/sites/default/files/2020-03/putting_on_and_removing_ppe_diagram_-_march_2020.pdf

National Health and Medical Research Council (NHMRC). (2019). *Australian Guidelines for the Prevention and Control of Infection* *in Healthcare.* https://www.nhmrc.gov.au/health-advice/public-health/preventing-infection

Wounds Australia. (2017). *Application of Aseptic Technique in Wound Dressing Procedure: A Consensus Document.* Osborne Park, WA: Cambridge Media.

ESSENTIAL SKILLS COMPETENCY

Dry Dressing Using a General Aseptic Field

Demonstrates the ability to effectively and safely complete a dry (simple) dressing

Criteria for skill performance	Y	D
(Numbers indicate *Enrolled Nurse Standards for Practice*, 2016)	(Satisfactory)	(Requires development)
1. Identifies indication (8.3, 8.4)		
2. Gathers equipment (1.2, 1.6, 4.4, 6.4, 8.4, 9.4): ■ dressing trolley ■ dressing pack ■ non-sterile gloves and other PPE as required ■ sterile solution (usually NS) ■ waste disposal bag ■ dressing, as ordered ■ tape		
3. Evidence of effective communication; gives explanation of procedure, gains patient consent (2.1, 2.3, 2.4, 2.5, 6.3)		
4. Demonstrates problem-solving abilities; e.g. positions patient comfortably, administers analgesia if required (4.1, 4.2, 8.3, 8.4, 9.4)		
5. Prepares room (1.2, 1.4, 1.8, 2.2, 3.2, 8.4, 9.4)		
6. Performs hand hygiene (1.2, 1.4, 1.8, 3.9, 6.4, 9.4)		
7. Dons PPE as required (1.2, 1.4, 1.8, 2.2, 3.2, 3.9, 8.4, 9.4)		
8. Removes soiled dressing (1.2, 1.4, 1.8, 2.7, 3.2, 3.9, 8.4, 9.4)		
9. Performs hand hygiene (1.2, 1.4, 1.8, 3.9, 6.4, 9.4)		
10. Establishes the general aseptic field using a non-touch technique (1.2, 1.4, 3.2, 3.9, 9.4)		
11. Performs hand hygiene (1.2, 1.4, 1.8, 3.9, 6.4, 9.4)		
12. Cleanses wound, assesses wound, using a standard aseptic technique (1.2, 1.4, 2.7, 3.2, 3.9, 4.1, 7.1, 8.4, 9.4)		
13. Applies dry dressing (1.2, 1.4, 2.7, 3.2, 3.9, 8.4, 9.4)		
14. Secures dressing (1.2, 1.4, 2.3, 2.4, 2.7, 3.2, 3.9, 8.4, 9.4)		
15. Removes PPE and performs hand hygiene (1.2, 1.4, 1.8, 3.9, 6.4, 9.4)		
16. Cleans, replaces and disposes of equipment appropriately (1.2, 1.4, 3.9, 6.5, 9.4)		
17. Documents relevant information (1.2, 1.3, 1.8, 3.2, 5.3, 6.6, 7.1, 7.2, 7.3, 7.4, 7.5)		
18. Demonstrates ability to link theory to practice (8.3, 8.4, 8.5, 9.4)		

Student:

Clinical facilitator: Date:

CHAPTER 4.3

WOUND IRRIGATION

IDENTIFY INDICATIONS

Wound irrigations are performed to cleanse a wound of exudate and debris without disturbing new granulating tissue and to facilitate wound healing (Gabriel, 2015). Wounds that require irrigation include cavity wounds, chronic wounds and wounds producing large amounts of exudate. These are wounds healing by secondary intention. Irrigation promotes healing through removal of debris, decreasing the bacterial load in the wound and preventing biofilm activity created by colonising microorganisms, plus loosening and removing dried exudate (Fletcher & Ivins, 2015). A dressing is applied that is protective, reduces the introduction of microorganisms, reduces discomfort or accidental trauma to the site and promotes healing by keeping the wound moist. Current dressing materials can work in combination with wound irrigation, as they assist in

the process of removing debris, absorb different levels of fluid and maintain moisture in a wound.

In most smaller wounds, the irrigation is performed with a syringe, while others may be completed during the patient's daily shower. Wound irrigations in the shower are used frequently in community settings for chronic wounds, but can also be used in acute care settings (Mahoney, 2014). Irrigations for wounds on the sole of the foot should not be completed in the shower (Wounds Australia, 2017). The wound care management plan will identify the correct procedure. Following irrigation of the wound, it would be covered with a sterile disposable drape and the wound dressing completed when the patient has returned to their bed area.

GATHER AND PREPARE EQUIPMENT

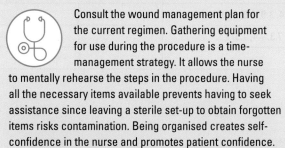

Consult the wound management plan for the current regimen. Gathering equipment for use during the procedure is a time-management strategy. It allows the nurse to mentally rehearse the steps in the procedure. Having all the necessary items available prevents having to seek assistance since leaving a sterile set-up to obtain forgotten items risks contamination. Being organised creates self-confidence in the nurse and promotes patient confidence.

- *Dressing packs* are usually commercially supplied and contain a waterproof wrapper that serves as the aseptic field when the pack is unwrapped. There is a receptacle in the pack that is used for the solution. A sterile drape may also be used to establish an aseptic field on which to work, and maintain a critical aseptic field. Some wound irrigations and the consequent dressing are quite complex procedures requiring larger dressing packs and sterile drapes to maintain the critical aseptic field and follow the principles of a surgical aseptic technique.
- *Sterile normal saline* to cleanse the wound. Normal saline (NS) is isotonic and currently the preferred solution for wound cleansing (Gabriel, 2015), although some hospital policies may recommend other

commercial wound irrigation solutions. The amount needed should be stated on the wound management plan. Warm the solution to body or room temperature to reduce discomfort and promote healing (British Columbia Provincial Nursing Skin & Wound Committee, 2017).
- *A wound ruler* is used to assess the wound and fosters accuracy and consistency.
- *An irrigating syringe* is a 30 to 50 mL syringe that has a longer tip and delivers a steady pressure of solution into the wound to dislodge debris without damaging granulating tissue. A soft catheter may be applied to the tip of a syringe to enable the nurse to direct the solution flow into deep or complex wounds. Commercial irrigation systems with shields and flexible nozzle extensions are available.
- *A kidney dish or bowl* to collect the irrigation fluid as it flows out of the wound and away from the patient.
- *A 'bluey'* is used to prevent soiling of the patient's gown and bed linen. This reduces the potential for additional contamination.
- *Dressings* are used to protect the wound. Refer to the wound management plan for the required wound dressing materials.

- *Tape* is used to secure the dressing to dry intact skin.
- *Non-sterile gloves* are used to remove the soiled dressing so that contamination is minimised.
- *Sterile gloves* are used during the actual procedure as key sites will be touched and contamination of the wound should be minimised. Sterile gloves will also protect the nurse from the patient's body fluids.
- *Eye protection* (goggles) and *plastic apron* are used to reduce exposure to patient body fluids and maintain infection control principles.
- *Masks* may be required by some agencies to prevent droplet spray from the nurse's respiratory tract contaminating the wound.
- A *waterproof bag* is necessary to contain contaminated

material to prevent transmission of microorganisms.

Confirm the sterility of the packages by checking the use-by date and whether the package is dry and whether it has tears, water damage, stains or, in the case of a bottle, a broken seal. Out-of-date sterile objects have been on the shelf for an extended period of time and their contents are no longer considered sterile because of the time factor. Tears, punctures, stains and dampness in the packaging indicate that there is a pathway from the exterior to the interior of the package through which microorganisms can gain access. A broken seal on a bottle indicates the bottle's contents have been exposed to the air and are contaminated.

PREPARE THE ROOM

Privacy is provided for the patient to minimise embarrassment. Airflow is restricted by closing windows and curtains and shutting off fans so that airborne microorganisms are less likely to contaminate the wound. The area must be well lit to assist with assessment and treatment. A waterproof disposal bag is placed near the patient to receive contaminated articles so that transmission of microorganisms is prevented.

PERFORM WOUND IRRIGATION

Perform hand hygiene
Perform hand hygiene before touching the patient or the patient's surrounds and prior to any procedure involving patient contact to reduce the possibility of cross-contamination. Hand hygiene is the most effective method of infection control as it removes transient organisms from the hands of the nurse (see **Skill 1.1**).

Don personal protective equipment (PPE)
A plastic apron and eye protection should be worn as PPE during this procedure.

Give a clear explanation of the procedure and establish therapeutic communication
Introduce yourself, and check you have the correct patient. Discuss the procedure and gain the patient's consent. Giving a clear explanation is required to gain legal consent and to address policy requirements. It will also assist the patient to cooperate with the procedure, allay anxiety and assist in establishing a therapeutic relationship. A clear explanation about the procedure, the patient's position and expectations to the patient will assist with their cooperation and decrease the risk of the patient touching or contaminating sterile equipment.

Demonstrate problem-solving abilities
Position the patient comfortably during the procedure to eliminate movement, which can contaminate sterile items. The patient's position should be considered in relation to the time that it is expected they will need to stay still and the body part that needs to be exposed to make it accessible to irrigation. The patient must also be positioned so that gravitational flow of the irrigating solution permits the solution to flow through the wound from the cleanest area to the dirtiest area and out into the kidney dish. A 'bluey' is placed under the area to be irrigated. The wound site should also be comfortably accessible to the nurse to eliminate contamination or self-injury from using an awkward position for the treatment. Offering to assist the patient to the toilet prior to the procedure will reduce unnecessary interruptions and increase patient comfort. To alleviate pain during wound care, analgesia may be given 30 minutes prior to the procedure.

Remove the soiled dressing
Put on non-sterile gloves, then remove the tape from the previous dressing carefully by supporting the skin around the tape and gently pulling the tape towards the wound so that stress is not applied to the wound bed. If the old dressing (this includes the packing) adheres to the wound, the dressing is moistened with sterile normal saline and given a few minutes to loosen before removal so that new granulating tissue is not damaged. If the wound is being cleansed in the shower, moistening the dressing with water will facilitate the ease of removal. The dressing is assessed for any drainage, noting amount, colour, consistency and odour.

Once the old tape and dressing is removed, the dressing and the gloves are carefully placed in the disposal bag without contaminating the outside of the bag.

Perform hand hygiene
Perform hand hygiene to reduce cross-contamination. An alcohol-based hand rub can be used.

Don sterile gloves using open gloving

Don sterile gloves using an open gloving technique. Refer to **Skill 4.9** for the open gloving technique. Sterile gloves should be used to maintain an aseptic technique, avoid contact with key sites and reduce the risk of exposure to body fluids.

Complete the wound irrigation in either the shower or bedside, according to the wound management plan.

IRRIGATIONS IN THE SHOWER

Prepare the area and equipment

This procedure should not be completed in a shared shower area (Wounds Australia, 2017). Refer to facility policy for guidelines on wounds that should not be irrigated in the shower. Allow the patient to complete their regular shower first, then put on the PPE. Dressings can be moistened or removed during this process if unable to be removed in the initial step. Prepare any sterile equipment that may be required during the cleansing of the wound in the shower.

Tap water has been demonstrated to be safe and effective for many types of wounds and has been found especially effective in chronic wounds (Gabriel, 2015; Simon, 2016; Wounds Australia, 2017). The water temperature should be warm, not hot. Run the water for several minutes to eliminate stagnant water from the tap, before applying it to the wound.

Don sterile gloves using open gloving

Don sterile gloves using an open gloving technique. Refer to **Skill 4.9** for the open gloving technique. Sterile gloves should be used to maintain an aseptic technique, avoid contact with key sites and reduce the risk of exposure to body fluids.

Irrigate the wound

Using a handheld shower nozzle and gentle water pressure, direct warm tap water into the wound opening from approximately 30 cm. Avoid letting the water run over other body areas before it enters the wound area. Some wounds may require extra cleansing with a disposable woven towel (Wounds Australia, 2017).

Cover the wound

After the wound is cleansed, cover the wound with a sterile drape or temporary dressing and enable the patient to dry themselves and return to the bed area where the wound dressing will be completed.

IRRIGATIONS USING SYRINGE

Establish a critical aseptic field

Maintain the principles of an aseptic technique to establish a critical aseptic field. Follow the principles described in **Skills 4.1** and **4.2** respectively. Add all items

necessary for the irrigation and the consequent wound dressing. Add the solution. Place the sterile drape beside the wound; this extends the aseptic field and helps prevent contamination of equipment. Arrange the sterile items for convenience.

Don sterile gloves using open gloving

After establishing the aseptic field, don sterile gloves using an open gloving technique. Refer to **Skill 4.9** for the open gloving technique. Sterile gloves should be used to maintain an aseptic technique, avoid contact with key sites and reduce the risk of exposure to body fluids.

Assess and irrigate the wound

Assess the wound for size (length, width and depth; use a wound ruler if necessary), drainage (amount, colour, consistency, odour) and appearance. Also assess the peri-wound and surrounding skin.

1. To irrigate a wound with a wide opening
    a. Fill syringe with irrigating solution to prepare to irrigate.
    b. Hold syringe tip 2.5 cm above wound edge to prevent contamination of tip (which would necessitate using another syringe).
    c. Applying gentle continuous pressure, flush wound to remove debris and clean wound. Ensure any fibres from dressing materials are removed as part of this process.
    d. Repeat above steps until irrigating solution draining into the kidney dish is clear. This indicates that the wound is clean.
2. To irrigate a deep or irregular wound or one with a small opening
    a. Fill the irrigating syringe.
    b. Attach a small, soft catheter to permit direct flow into hidden areas of the wound.
    c. Insert the moistened tip of the catheter gently into the wound until it touches a surface, then pull back about 1 to 2 cm to remove the tip from the fragile tissue.
    d. Using slow, gentle, continuous pressure and rotation of the tip of the catheter, flush the wound to reach every surface for cleansing.
    e. Pinch off the catheter just below the syringe, keep the catheter tip in the wound and refill the syringe to avoid contamination of the solution.
    f. Repeat steps 2 to 5 until the return flow is clear. The wound will take longer to empty because of the small opening.

Dry the wound using sterile gauze swabs to prevent skin maceration and to increase patient comfort. The facility's protocol should be followed.

Apply a sterile dressing

There may be various wound management protocols and products used at this point. Products are available to debride the wound, maintain moisture and remove exudate. The selection of wound dressing material will depend on the wound. As part of caring for a complex wound, apply fresh sterile gloves and continue to maintain an aseptic technique to complete the required wound dressing. Gloves are removed and discarded when the wound dressing is completed.

Secure the dressing

Secure the dressing with the selected tape. Reposition the patient for comfort.

Doff PPE

Remove PPE in the following sequence: non-sterile gloves, hand hygiene, eyewear/face shield, plastic apron/gown and mask and then perform hand hygiene (ACSQHC, 2020). Dispose of in the rubbish bag.

Perform hand hygiene

Maintain the 5 Moments for Hand Hygiene and perform hand hygiene after touching the patient and the patient's surrounds.

CLEAN, REPLACE OR DISPOSE OF EQUIPMENT

To maintain infection control principles, clean non-sterile gloves and other PPE may be required to reduce exposure to body fluids while disposing of waste. Replace and dispose of equipment appropriately. Contaminated dressing materials are wrapped in the wrapper that has formed the aseptic field and placed in the rubbish bag, which is then placed in the contaminated waste, according to facility policy. While avoiding a splash hazard, the contents of the kidney dish are emptied down the sluice, and the kidney dish disposed of correctly. Clean the trolley with the disinfecting solution or wipes recommended by your facility.

DOCUMENT AND REPORT RELEVANT INFORMATION

Document relevant information in the wound management plan and patient notes. Include the appearance of the wound and drainage, type of dressing applied and the patient's response to the procedure. Note any alteration in comfort levels or changes in the wound condition and report these to the registered nurse.

CASE STUDY

Tama Berryman is a 62-year-old man with 3 chronic leg ulcers on the anterior aspect of the lower left leg.

His wound management plan (WMP) requires the three ulcers to be irrigated in the shower, and then dressed as per the WMP, as part of his wound care.

1. What is the purpose of this wound irrigation?

2. Why should sterile gloves be worn during this procedure?

3. While starting to perform this procedure, you identify that the previous dressing is stuck to his leg. How will you remove the old dressing?

Note: These notes are summaries of the most important points in the assessments/procedures, and are not exhaustive on the subject. The naming of documents or charts may differ from state to state, and facility to facility. In all possible situations the guidelines of the ACSQHC are used when describing national charts or documents (e.g. the ACSQHC Observation and Response Chart is named the Adult Observation and Response Chart in WA, and the Rapid Detection and Response Observation Chart in SA). References of the materials used to compile the information have been supplied. The student is expected to have learned the material surrounding each skill as presented in the references. No single reference is complete on the subject.

REFERENCES

Australian Commission on Safety and Quality in Health Care (ACSQHC). (2020). *Sequence for Putting on and Removing PPE.* https://www.safetyandquality.gov.au/sites/default/files/2020-03/putting_on_and_removing_ppe_diagram_-_march_2020.pdf

British Columbia Provincial Nursing Skin & Wound Committee. (2017). *Procedure: Wound Cleansing.* https://www.clwk.ca/buddydrive/file/procedure-wound-cleansing

Fletcher, J. & Ivins, N. (2015). Is it time to review how we clean leg ulcers? *Wounds UK*, 11(4), pp. 42–8.

Gabriel, A. (2015). Wound irrigation. *Medscape.* https://emedicine.medscape.com/article/1895071-overview

Mahoney, K. (2014). Understanding the basics of wound care in the community setting. *Journal of Community Nursing*, 28(3), pp. 66–75.

Simon, D. (2016). How to improve the community care of leg ulcer patients. *Journal of Community Nursing*, 29(6), pp. 24–8.

Wounds Australia. (2017). *Application of Aseptic Technique in Wound Dressing Procedure: A Consensus Document.* Osborne Park, WA: Cambridge Media.

RECOMMENDED READINGS

Keast, D., Swanson, T., Carville, K., Fletcher, J., Schultz, G. & Black, J. (2014). Ten top tips … Understanding and managing wound biofilm. *Wounds International*, 5(2), pp. 20–4.

ESSENTIAL SKILLS COMPETENCY

Wound Irrigation
Demonstrates the ability to effectively and safely irrigate a wound

Criteria for skill performance	Y	D
(Numbers indicate *Enrolled Nurse Standards for Practice*, 2016)	(Satisfactory)	(Requires development)
1. Identifies indication (8.3, 8.4)		
2. Gathers equipment (1.2, 1.6, 4.4, 6.4, 8.4, 9.4): ■ PPE – non-sterile gloves, apron, eye protection ■ sterile gloves ■ sterile towel/drape For irrigation with syringe: ■ dressing pack, small soft catheter if required ■ irrigating syringe or commercial irrigating pack ■ sterile solution (usually saline 0.9%) ■ waterproof rubbish bag ■ tape ■ kidney dish ■ 'bluey' ■ new wound dressing		
3. Evidence of effective communication with the patient; gives explanation of procedure, gains patient consent (2.1, 2.3, 2.4, 2.5, 6.3)		
4. Demonstrates problem-solving abilities; e.g. positions patient comfortably, administers analgesia if required (4.1, 4.2, 8.3, 8.4, 9.4)		
5. Performs hand hygiene and dons PPE (1.2, 1.4, 1.8, 2.2, 3.2, 3.9, 8.4, 9.4)		
Irrigation in the shower (A)		
6. Prepares room, equipment and water temperature (1.2, 1.4, 1.8, 2.2, 3.2, 8.4, 9.4)		
7. Removes soiled dressing (1.2, 1.4, 1.8, 2.2, 2.7, 3.2, 3.9, 8.4, 9.4)		
8. Performs hand hygiene (1.2, 1.4, 1.8, 3.9, 6.4, 9.4)		
9. Dons sterile gloves using open gloving (1.2, 1.4, 1.8, 2.2, 3.2, 3.9, 8.4, 9.4)		
10. Irrigates and assesses wound (1.2, 1.4, 2.3, 2.4, 2.7, 3.2, 3.9, 4.1, 7.1, 8.4, 9.4)		
11. Applies sterile towel to wound (1.2, 1.4, 2.3, 2.4, 2.7, 3.2, 3.9, 8.4, 9.4)		
Irrigation with a syringe (B)		
12. Establishes the sterile field and maintains aseptic technique (1.2, 1.4, 3.2, 3.9, 9.4)		
13. Performs hand hygiene (1.2, 1.4, 1.8, 3.9, 6.4, 9.4)		
14. Dons sterile gloves using open gloving (1.2, 1.4, 1.8, 2.2, 3.2, 3.9, 8.4, 9.4)		
15. Irrigates and assesses wound (1.2, 1.4, 2.3, 2.4, 2.7, 3.2, 3.9, 4.1, 7.1, 8.4, 9.4)		
16. Applies required wound dressing (1.2, 1.4, 2.3, 2.4, 2.7, 3.2, 3.9, 8.4, 9.4)		
17. Secures dressing (1.2, 1.4, 2.3, 2.4, 2.7, 3.2, 3.9, 8.4, 9.4)		
Both irrigations		
18. Doffs PPE; performs hand hygiene (1.2, 1.4, 1.8, 3.9, 6.4, 9.4)		
19. Cleans, replaces and disposes of equipment appropriately (1.2, 1.4, 3.9, 6.5, 9.4)		
20. Documents and reports relevant information (1.2, 1.3, 1.8, 3.2, 5.3, 6.6, 7.1, 7.2, 7.3, 7.4, 7.5)		
21. Demonstrates ability to link theory to practice (8.3, 8.4, 8.5, 9.4)		

Student:

Clinical facilitator: Date:

CHAPTER 4.4

WOUND SWAB

IDENTIFY INDICATIONS

Wound swabs are collected to identify microorganisms that may be creating a bioburden that could impair wound healing (Bainbridge, 2014). Normal flora commonly colonise a wound without being detrimental to healing, but other bacteria can cause an infection and disrupt wound healing. A wound swab may be ordered to help identify the organism causing infection and antibiotic sensitivity. The doctor or wound nurse specialist will need to complete the pathology request form before collecting a wound swab. If required a wound swab can be collected as part of a regular wound dressing (see **Skill 4.2**).

GATHER AND PREPARE EQUIPMENT

Equipment required for a wound swab is added to the equipment for a wound dressing as described in **Skill 4.2**. Having all the necessary items available prevents having to seek assistance, since leaving a sterile set-up to obtain forgotten items risks contamination. Being organised creates self-confidence in the nurse and promotes patient confidence. Items specific to a wound swab include the following.

- *A sterile normal saline solution*, to cleanse the wound of dead cells and dressing residue prior to collecting the specimen.
- *Non-sterile gloves* as personal protective equipment (PPE) when collecting the specimen.
- *Kidney dish* for holding swab-stick and specimen materials.
- *Swab-stick* for culture and sensitivity (C&S) as per the pathology request and facility policy.

- *Patient ID label.* Complete the label on the swab-stick with patient's details, or use label provided in patient's notes. If the item is sterile, this will need to be completed after the swab has been collected.
- *Biohazard bag and pathology request form* for completion at the end of the procedure.

Confirm the sterility of the packages by checking the use-by date and whether the package is dry, has tears, water damage, stains or, in the case of a bottle, a broken seal. Out-of-date sterile objects have been on the shelf for an extended period of time and their contents are no longer considered sterile because of the time factor. Tears, punctures, stains and dampness in the packaging indicate that there is a pathway from the exterior to the interior of the package through which microorganisms can gain access. A broken seal on a bottle indicates the bottle's contents have been exposed to the air and are contaminated.

COLLECTING THE WOUND SWAB

Give a clear explanation of the procedure and establish therapeutic communication

Introduce yourself, and check you have the correct patient. Discuss the procedure and gain the patient's consent. Giving a clear explanation is required to gain legal consent and to address policy requirements. It will also assist the patient to cooperate with the procedure, allay anxiety and assist in establishing a therapeutic relationship.

Demonstrate problem-solving abilities

If required, ensure pain relief has been administered prior to the procedure. Position the patient comfortably to eliminate movement during the procedure, which can contaminate sterile items. The patient's position should be considered in relation to the expected time they will be required to remain still and to the body part that will be exposed, in order to make it accessible for treatment.

Maintain privacy to enhance the patient's dignity.

Wound swab

If required, a wound swab is collected as part of the regular wound dressing. Please refer to **Skill 4.2** for completing this procedure. The wound swab is collected after the wound has been cleaned with normal saline (Bainbridge, 2014).

The swab-stick should be placed on the lower shelf of the dressing trolley. If the swab-stick is not packaged as a fully sterile item, it cannot be placed onto the sterile field while setting up for the dressing. It should be left on the lower part of the trolley with the biohazard bag.

Perform hand hygiene

Perform hand hygiene before touching the patient or the patient's surrounds and prior to any procedure involving patient contact to reduce the possibility of cross-contamination. Hand hygiene is the most effective method of infection control as it removes transient organisms from the hands of the nurse (see **Skill 1.1**).

Implement procedure for patient's regular wound dressing

Maintaining the principles of an aseptic technique, the wound area is cleansed with normal saline. All excess debris or exudate and dressing product residue should be cleaned from the wound bed. Cleaning the wound reduces the risk of cultivating normal flora (Bainbridge, 2014). Normal saline will clean the area without destroying the bacterial pathogen. Dry the area to remove excess saline and allow 1 to 2 minutes for the microorganisms to rise to the surface of the wound bed.

Don gloves and collect specimen

Don non-sterile gloves. Collect the swab-stick from the bottom of the trolley or sterile field. The Levine technique, rather than a Z-technique, is recommended for collecting the wound swab (Bainbridge, 2014; Keast et al., 2014). The tip of the swab-stick is rotated over a 1 cm^2 area, avoiding the wound edges and peri-wound area, for at least 5 seconds. Use sufficient pressure to express fluid from the wound tissues. The swab-stick may require pre-moistening with sterile normal saline

if the wound is non-exudating. A large wound may require several swabs to be taken from different wound areas, and these swabs are labelled accordingly.

The swab is then placed into the transport medium, taking care not to contaminate the outer area of the container. Place the collected specimen/s in the kidney dish at the bottom of the trolley.

Remove gloves and perform hand hygiene

Remove and dispose of gloves, perform hand hygiene and then continue with the remainder of the regular wound care.

Label specimen and send to laboratory

After the wound care has been completed, the swabs and pathology request form should be labelled, including specimen location, type of wound, collection date and time. Before transporting to the laboratory, all wound swabs will need to be placed in the sealed pocket of the biohazard bag. The request form is placed in the separated outside sleeve that is part of the biohazard bag, to prevent contamination of the form by the wound swab or swab container.

CLEAN, REPLACE OR DISPOSE OF EQUIPMENT

Clean, dispose of waste and restock, as per **Skill 4.2**. Wound swabs can be kept at room temperature, not refrigerated, and should be sent to the laboratory as soon as possible after collection.

DOCUMENT AND REPORT RELEVANT INFORMATION

Document collection of the wound swab in the wound management plan, patient notes and observation and response chart. As part of correct documentation also ensure the pathology form is completed correctly as described earlier. Failure to complete this correctly can result in the wound swab not being processed and returned to the ward area for correction.

CASE STUDY

You are caring for Lei Chung, a 61-year-old woman who had a left hip replacement 5 days ago. She has a past medical history of diabetes and hypercholesterolaemia. The previous day, Lei had complained of some wound discomfort and had a small amount of wound discharge. Her temperature has now increased to 38.2°C, with slightly more discharge evident on the wound dressing in situ.

The wound management nurse has requested a wound swab from Lei's hip wound.
1. What is the purpose of a wound swab?
2. Why would this be ordered for Lei?
3. What is the preferred technique for collecting a wound swab? Explain how you would collect the swab.

Note: These notes are summaries of the most important points in the assessments/procedures, and are not exhaustive on the subject. The naming of documents or charts may differ from state to state, and facility to facility. In all possible situations the guidelines of the ACSQHC are used when describing national charts or documents (e.g. the ACSQHC Observation and Response Chart is named the Adult Observation and Response Chart in WA, and the Rapid Detection and Response Observation Chart in SA). References of the materials used to compile the information have been supplied. The student is expected to have learned the material surrounding each skill as presented in the references. No single reference is complete on the subject.

REFERENCES

Bainbridge, P. (2014). How effective is wound swabbing? A clinimetric assessment of wound swabs. *Wounds UK*, 10(4), pp. 44–9.

Keast, D., Swanson, T., Carville, K., Fletcher, J., Schultz, G. & Black, J. (2014). Ten top tips: Understanding and managing wound biofilm. *Wounds International,* 5(2), pp. 20–4.

RECOMMENDED READINGS

National Health and Medical Research Council (NHMRC). (2019). *Australian Guidelines for the Prevention and Control of Infection in Healthcare.* Australian Government. http://www.nhmrc.gov. au/book/html-australian-guidelines-prevention-and-control-infection-healthcare-2019.

ESSENTIAL SKILLS COMPETENCY

Wound Swabs

Demonstrates the ability to effectively and safely swab a wound

Criteria for skill performance	Y	D
(Numbers indicate *Enrolled Nurse Standards for Practice*, 2016)	(Satisfactory)	(Requires development)
1. Identifies indication (8.3, 8.4)		
2. Gathers equipment (1.2, 1.6, 4.4, 6.4, 8.4, 9.4): ■ kidney dish ■ non-sterile gloves ■ swab-stick for culture and sensitivity ■ sterile normal saline solution ■ biohazard bag, patient ID label and request form ■ other routine wound care materials		
3. Evidence of therapeutic communication with the patient; gives explanation of procedure, gains patient consent (2.1, 2.3, 2.4, 2.5, 6.3)		
4. Demonstrates problem-solving abilities (4.1, 4.2, 8.3, 8.4, 9.4)		
5. Maintains aseptic technique and implements routine wound care prior to collection of wound swab; ensures wound area is cleaned with normal saline (1.2, 1.4, 1.8, 2.2, 3.2, 3.9, 8.4, 9.4)		
6. Dons non-sterile gloves (1.2, 1.4, 1.8, 2.2, 3.2, 3.9, 8.4, 9.4)		
7. Collects swab using Levine technique (1.2, 1.4, 1.8, 2.2, 3.2, 3.9, 8.4, 9.4)		
8. Places swab in transport medium, and specimen in kidney dish before continuing with regular wound care (1.2, 1.4, 1.8, 2.2, 3.2, 3.9, 8.4, 9.4)		
9. Removes gloves and performs hand hygiene (1.2, 1.4, 1.8, 2.2, 3.2, 3.9, 8.4, 9.4)		
10. Continues with wound care dressing (1.2, 1.4, 1.8, 2.2, 3.2, 3.9, 8.4, 9.4)		
11. Performs hand hygiene (1.2, 1.4, 1.8, 2.2, 3.2, 3.9, 8.4, 9.4)		
12. Labels swab and completes information on pathology form before placing in biohazard bag for sending to the laboratory (1.2, 1.4, 3.2, 3.9, 4.2, 8.4, 9.4)		
13. Performs hand hygiene (1.2, 1.4, 1.8, 2.2, 3.2, 3.9, 8.4, 9.4)		
14. Cleans, replaces and disposes of equipment appropriately (1.2, 1.4, 3.9, 6.5, 9.4)		
15. Documents and reports relevant information (1.2, 1.3, 1.8, 3.2, 5.3, 6.6, 7.1, 7.2, 7.3, 7.4, 7.5)		
16. Demonstrates ability to link theory to practice (8.3, 8.4, 8.5, 9.4)		

Student:

Clinical facilitator:

Date:

CHAPTER 4.5

PACKING A WOUND – 'WET-TO-MOIST' DRESSING

IDENTIFY INDICATIONS

Wounds that require packing, or wet-to-moist gauze, are generally deep and narrow cavity-type wounds. Packing the wound with moist gauze can be selected to assist wound healing by maintaining a moist environment, absorbing exudate and preventing the premature closure of the top of the wound before granulation is complete at the base of the wound. These wounds are healing by secondary intention. Wound packing materials include gauze soaked with saline, but other wound materials can be used. The wound management plan will identify the packing required.

Ribbon gauze is soaked in normal saline and then inserted into the wound to absorb exudate, and prevent any dead space or unfilled area of the cavity. Cut gauze edges should not make contact with the wound bed as shed fibres can remain in the wound. Wet-to-moist gauze dressings can dry out easily, and become stuck to the wound (Smith et al., 2015). These dressings can require two to three dressing changes every 24 hours, or access to rehydrate the gauze. They do still have value in some wound care situations.

Wound materials used to manage sinus or cavity wounds should promote a moist environment, assist autolytic debridement, facilitate drainage of exudate, be pain free, not shed fibres and not compromise surrounding skin (Smith et al., 2015). Aside from moist gauze, they can include the following.

- Hydrogels, which provide some absorptive qualities and debride necrotic tissue while also providing a moist healing environment.
- Alginates, which are composed of a material extracted from seaweed. They are applied dry and expand to form a gel as wound exudate is absorbed. They also assist with wound autolysis (Wounds Australia, 2017).
- Polyurethane foams, which are designed to absorb excess exudate, come in different shapes and sizes, and can be cut to a more specific fit if required. They absorb excess exudate while maintaining moisture and protecting the surrounding skin.
- Negative pressure wound therapy (see **Skill 4.6**) is also used.

GATHER EQUIPMENT

The equipment and dressing materials are stated on the wound management plan. Gathering equipment is a time-management technique that increases nurse confidence. A mental rehearsal of the procedure is an excellent action to increase confidence and ensure that no equipment is forgotten. The following is a list of generally used materials for packing a wound. Most wounds that need packing will require use of a surgical aseptic technique within a critical aseptic field, due to the complexity of the procedure.

- *Non-sterile gloves* are used to remove the secondary dressing. A waterproof rubbish bag is placed appropriately to receive used materials so they will not cross a sterile field.
- A *dressing pack* is required. More comprehensive wounds may require further sterile drapes and other materials.
- *Sterile metal forceps* are required to pack the wound.

- *Packing material* – sterile ribbon gauze or other dressing as stated on the wound management plan, for packing the wound.
- *Sterile gloves* to assist in maintaining an aseptic technique as key sites or parts may be touched. There is also exposure to the patient's body fluids.
- *Normal saline* (or other cleansing solutions as ordered) is used to cleanse or irrigate the wound and to soak the gauze packing. Normal saline is the preferred solution.
- *Extra sterile gauze swabs or an irrigation set* (as per hospital policy) are used for cleansing the wound.
- A *wound ruler* is used to estimate the size of the wound.
- *Sterile scissors* are used to cut the required amount of the chosen dressing material from the package supplied. Since wounds vary in size and capacity, less material than the amount supplied is often sufficient to completely fill the cavity, and excess dressing material should not be allowed to sit on intact skin, as the moisture would eventually macerate the skin.

- A *sterile secondary dressing* (as stated in the wound management plan) is taped over the wound. A specific dressing will be ordered to help prevent drying out of the gauze and keep the wound moist.
- *Tape* as ordered.
- *Personal protective equipment (PPE) (plastic apron, eye protection and mask)* should be used to minimise risk created by exposure to the patient's body fluids. Confirm the sterility of the packages by checking the use-by date and whether the package is dry, has tears, water damage, stains or, in the case of a bottle, a broken seal. Out-of-date sterile objects have been on the shelf for an extended period of time and their contents are no longer considered sterile because of the time factor. Tears, punctures, stains and dampness in the packaging indicate that there is a pathway from the exterior to the interior of the package through which microorganisms can gain access. A broken seal on a bottle indicates the bottle's contents have been exposed to the air and are contaminated.

PACK THE WOUND WITH A 'WET-TO-MOIST' DRESSING

Give a clear explanation of the procedure and establish therapeutic communication

Introduce yourself, and check you have the correct patient. Discuss the procedure and gain the patient's consent. Giving a clear explanation is required to gain legal consent and to address policy requirements. It will also assist the patient to cooperate with the procedure, allay anxiety and assist in establishing a therapeutic relationship. Discussing the procedure with the patient will help determine their level of knowledge, help them understand the healing process and relieve some anxiety associated with the procedure.

Demonstrating problem-solving abilities

Positioning the patient to allow access to the wound and facilitate comfort for the patient is important because the procedure can take 15 to 20 minutes. Positioning should also allow for comfort for the nurse to reduce muscle strain and possible contamination of the wound due to inadequate exposure of the wound. Closing the door or curtains and hanging 'procedure in progress' signs assures privacy. Covering the patient with a blanket will reduce exposure. Providing privacy increases patient trust and reduces embarrassment. Assessing the patient's pain level prior to the procedure and administering analgesia so that peak performance of the drug occurs during the packing reduces the discomfort associated with this procedure. Consulting the wound management plan and other healthcare personnel who have recently completed this procedure will give the nurse the relevant information about the wound and the patient, which will facilitate the procedure and alert the nurse to special requirements such as a need for assistance.

Perform hand hygiene

Perform hand hygiene before touching the patient or the patient's surrounds and prior to any procedure involving patient contact to reduce the possibility of cross-contamination. Hand hygiene is the most effective method of infection control as it removes transient organisms from the hands of the nurse (see **Skill 1.1**).

Don PPE

A plastic apron and eye protection should be worn as PPE during this procedure. Put on non-sterile gloves before removing the wound dressing. PPE requirements will vary according to the care being delivered and the patient's health status.

Remove the dressing

Wearing non-sterile gloves, remove the existing outer secondary dressing by loosening all tapes and easing the old dressing off carefully. Observe this dressing for the amount of exudate, colour, odour and consistency before disposing into the rubbish bag.

If the packing appears dry and is sticking to the wound, moisten it with sterile normal saline by squirting solution directly from the ampoule onto the primary dressing.

Removal of a dried-out primary dressing will cause trauma to the granulating tissue and severe pain, so allow time for absorption of the saline and softening of the dressing before removing this primary dressing/packing.

Remove non-sterile gloves and dispose of in the rubbish bag.

Repeat hand hygiene

Perform hand hygiene again at this stage to reduce the risk of cross-contamination. An alcohol-based hand rub should be used.

Establish a critical aseptic field and don sterile gloves

Establish a critical aseptic field using an aseptic technique as described in **Skills 4.1** and **4.2** respectively. When all packages have been opened and contents placed on the aseptic field, put on the sterile gloves using an open-gloving technique (see **Skill 4.9**) and prepare all of the material. If using ribbon gauze, wet the ribbon gauze with normal saline and squeeze out the excess so the packing is damp. Roll the gauze onto forceps to enable easier packing into the wound and place in a relevant position on the sterile field. Prepare alternate packing material as per manufacturer's instructions. Prepare all other dressing materials ready for when the wound packing is complete.

Remove the primary dressing
Carefully remove the pre-moistened primary dressing and dispose of the dressing and forceps in rubbish bag.

Cleanse the wound
Don sterile gloves using open-gloving technique (see **Skill 4.9**). Cleanse the wound and peri-wound (surrounding skin) using either forceps and gauze swabs or an irrigation set as per the wound management plan (see **Skill 4.3**). Dry the peri-wound and wound bed.

Assess the wound and wound margins
Assess the wound and wound margins to monitor the wound healing and the condition of the surrounding skin. Surrounding skin can easily become macerated with wet-to-moist dressings.

Pack the wound
While continuing to maintain an aseptic technique, pack the wound with the recommended packing material.
- Hydrogel is squeezed into the base of the wound.
- Alginates and foams are cut to size (if required) for the wound, then layered into place.
- Ribbon gauze should come into contact with all wound surfaces, and be applied gently. It should fill all of the wound cavity, but not over-pack or be too tight. Use metal forceps to gently push the ribbon or alginate ropes into the base of the cavity and lay back and forward across the wound, while unwinding the gauze from the other forceps. Do not use force. Take great care not to contaminate the ribbon, and do not allow damp packing material to rest on the intact skin of the wound edge. Always leave a 'tail' visible in the wound to ensure all material is able to be removed with future wound care.

When the cavity has been packed, use the sterile scissors to cut the remaining gauze, leaving a small tail visible at the surface. Ensure the dressing material is within the wound margins and not contacting the surrounding skin.

Apply a dry dressing
Cover the wound with the required secondary dressing while continuing to maintain an aseptic technique. If more drainage is expected or if there is a risk of the gauze wetting the patient's clothing, an absorbent dressing may be applied. When the wound is covered, gloves are removed and discarded.

Secure the secondary dressing
Bandage or secure the dressing with the selected tape. The patient is assisted to a position of comfort that does not stress the incision or wound.

Doff PPE
Remove PPE in the following sequence; non-sterile gloves, hand hygiene, eyewear/face shield, plastic apron/gown and mask and then perform hand hygiene (ACSQHC, 2020). Dispose of in the rubbish bag.

Perform hand hygiene
Maintain the 5 Moments for Hand Hygiene and perform hand hygiene after touching the patient and the patient's surrounds.

CLEAN, REPLACE OR DISPOSE OF EQUIPMENT
Clean, replace and dispose of equipment appropriately. Contaminated materials are wrapped in the wrapper that has formed the aseptic field and placed in the rubbish bag, which is then placed in the contaminated waste. Clean the trolley with disinfecting solution or wipes recommended by your facility. If gross contamination has occurred, facility policy for cleaning should be followed. The trolley is returned to its position in the clean area of the ward. Disposable scissors and forceps are placed in the sharps.

DOCUMENT AND REPORT RELEVANT INFORMATION
Document relevant information in the wound management plan and patient notes, including wound appearance and measurements. Note the colour of the wound and peri-wound, any exudate, type of dressing applied and patient's response to the procedure. This validates care given and provides a progress report of the patient's condition.

CASE STUDY

As an enrolled nurse, you are continuing to care for Lei Chung who had a left hip replacement 7 days ago. She has a past medical history of diabetes and hypercholesterolaemia.

The wound swab collected 2 days ago has confirmed that the wound has bacteria present, and she has been commenced on antibiotics to treat the infection.

She has a small area of dehiscence at the lower end of the incision, which is to be packed with saline-moistened ribbon gauze 4-hourly initially for 24 hours, then reviewed.

1. What type of wound healing does packing a wound promote?
2. Identify all the equipment that you would need to collect to perform the wound dressing.
3. Write up a wound management plan for this dressing.

Note: These notes are summaries of the most important points in the assessments/procedures, and are not exhaustive on the subject. The naming of documents or charts may differ from state to state, and facility to facility. In all possible situations the guidelines of the ACSQHC are used when describing national charts or documents (e.g. the ACSQHC Observation and Response Chart is named the Adult Observation and Response Chart in WA, and the Rapid Detection and Response Observation Chart in SA). References of the materials used to compile the information have been supplied. The student is expected to have learned the material surrounding each skill as presented in the references. No single reference is complete on the subject.

REFERENCES

Australian Commission on Safety and Quality in Health Care (ACSQHC). (2020). *Sequence for Putting on and Removing PPE.* https://www.safetyandquality.gov.au/sites/default/files/2020-03/putting_on_and_removing_ppe_diagram_-_march_2020.pdf

Smith, N., Overland, J. & Greenwood, J. (2015). Local management of deep cavity wounds – current and emerging therapies. *Chronic Wound Care Management and Research,* 2015:2, pp. 159–170. https://doi.org/10.2147/CWCMR.S62553

Wounds Australia. (2017). *Application of Aseptic Technique in Wound Dressing Procedure: A Consensus Document.* Osborne Park, WA: Cambridge Media.

RECOMMENDED READINGS

British Columbia Provincial Nursing Skin & Wound Committee (BCPN). (2017). *Procedure: Wound Packing.* https://www.clwk.ca/buddydrive/file/procedure-wound-packing/

National Health and Medical Research Council (NHMRC). (2019). *Australian Guidelines for the Prevention and Control of Infection in Healthcare.* Australian Government. https://www.nhmrc.gov.au/health-advice/public-health/preventing-infection

Souliotis, K., Kalemikerakis, I., Saridi, M., Papageorgiou, M. & Kalokerinou, A. (2016). A cost and clinical effectiveness analysis among moist wound healing dressings versus traditional methods in home care patients with pressure ulcers. *Wound Repair & Regeneration,* 24(3), pp. 596–601.

ESSENTIAL SKILLS COMPETENCY

Packing a Wound – Wet-to-Moist Dressing
Demonstrates the ability to effectively and safely pack a wound

Criteria for skill performance	Y	D
(Numbers indicate *Enrolled Nurse Standards for Practice*, 2016)	(Satisfactory)	(Requires development)
1. Identifies indication (8.3, 8.4)		
2. Gathers equipment (1.2, 1.6, 4.4, 6.4, 8.4, 9.4): ■ non-sterile gloves, sterile gloves, plastic apron and further PPE as required ■ waterproof rubbish bag ■ dressing pack and dressing materials ■ extra gauze swabs or irrigation set ■ 0.9% saline or other cleansing solution ■ primary dressing – sterile ribbon gauze or packing material as ordered ■ sterile forceps ■ sterile scissors ■ secondary dressing material as ordered ■ tape		
3. Evidence of effective communication; gives explanation of procedure, gains patient consent (2.1, 2.3, 2.4, 2.5, 6.3)		
4. Demonstrates problem-solving abilities; e.g. administers analgesia, provides privacy, positions patient appropriately (4.1, 4.2, 8.3, 8.4, 9.4)		
5. Performs hand hygiene and dons PPE as required (1.2, 1.4, 1.8, 2.2, 3.2, 3.9, 6.4, 8.4, 9.4)		
6. Removes soiled secondary dressing (1.2, 1.4, 1.8, 2.2, 2.7, 3.2, 3.9, 8.4, 9.4)		
7. Performs hand hygiene (1.2, 1.4, 1.8, 2.2, 3.2, 3.9, 6.4, 9.4)		
8. Establishes the critical aseptic field, dons sterile gloves, removes moistened primary dressing and cleanses wound (1.2, 1.4, 3.2, 3.9, 9.4)		
9. Assesses wound and surrounding tissue (1.2, 1.4, 2.3, 2.4, 2.7, 3.2, 3.9, 4.1, 7.1, 8.4, 9.4)		
10. Packs wound (1.2, 1.4, 1.6, 1.7, 2.3, 2.4, 2.7, 3.2, 4.1, 8.4, 9.4)		
11. Applies secondary dressing and secures (1.2, 1.4, 2.3, 2.4, 2.7, 3.2, 3.9, 8.4, 9.4)		
12. Doffs PPE and performs hand hygiene (1.2, 1.4, 1.8, 3.9, 6.4, 9.4)		
13. Cleans, replaces and disposes of equipment appropriately (1.2, 1.4, 3.9, 6.5, 9.4)		
14. Documents relevant information (1.2, 1.3, 1.8, 3.2, 5.3, 6.6, 7.1, 7.2, 7.3, 7.4, 7.5)		
15. Demonstrates ability to link theory to practice (8.3, 8.4, 8.5, 9.4)		

Student:

Clinical facilitator: Date:

CHAPTER 4.6

NEGATIVE PRESSURE WOUND THERAPY (NPWT) DRESSING

IDENTIFY INDICATIONS

Negative pressure wound therapy (NPWT) is a wound management technique that uses a sealed wound dressing attached to a vacuum pump which creates continuous or intermittent subatmospheric pressure to the wound. The negative pressure (i.e. suction) is applied to the wound through an open cell foam dressing that is cut to size and packed or laid into the wound (Wound Care Centres, 2020). NPWT can be used to promote wound healing in both acute and chronic wounds. This includes traumatic wounds, partial thickness burns, flaps, skin grafts, dehisced wounds, pressure injuries, diabetic ulcers and venous ulcers (Ranaweera, 2013). NPWT increases blood flow, reduces local tissue swelling, removes excess fluid from the wound and decreases the level of bacteria with the application of continuous or intermittent negative pressure to a wound surface. NPWT is also described as assisting tissue granulation and wound healing (Gleeson & Bond, 2015; Ranaweera, 2013).

In wounds not deep enough to accommodate the open cell foam, different types of NPWT dressings (open-weave gauze or other honeycomb dressing textile) are available. The dressing requires less frequent dressing changes, and can remain intact for 3 to 7 days, or change as needed. NPWT can use a lightweight portable system for minimal to moderately exudating wounds. This may help to reduce pain and enable the patient to be mobile, while also being able to maintain a positive quality of life. Sometimes patients can be treated at home with a visiting healthcare nurse.

DEMONSTRATING PROBLEM-SOLVING ABILITIES

Patients using NPWT need to be assessed for the position of the wound and the ability to maintain a seal, their falls risk (drainage tubing creates a further falls risk), their cognitive ability (reduces the risk of pulling on the tube) and their willingness to adhere to the therapy. If a patient is being managed in the community, they need to maintain the pump while a nurse will complete the required dressing changes.

Positioning the patient to allow access to the wound and facilitate comfort for the patient is important because the procedure can take 15 to 20 minutes. Positioning should also allow for comfort for the nurse to reduce muscle strain and possible contamination of the wound due to inadequate exposure of the wound. Closing the door or curtains and hanging 'procedure in progress' signs assures privacy. Covering the patient with a blanket will reduce exposure. Providing privacy increases patient trust and reduces embarrassment. Assessing the patient's pain level and administering analgesia so that peak performance of the drug occurs during the packing reduces the discomfort associated with this procedure. Consulting the wound management plan and other healthcare personnel who have recently completed this procedure will give the nurse the relevant information about the wound and the patient, which will facilitate the procedure and alert the nurse to special requirements such as a need for assistance.

GATHER EQUIPMENT

The equipment and dressing materials are stated on the wound management plan. Gathering equipment is a time-management technique that increases nurse confidence. A mental rehearsal of the procedure is an excellent action to increase confidence and ensure that no equipment is forgotten. The following is a list of generally used materials for a NPWT dressing. This wound care requires the use of a surgical aseptic technique within a critical aseptic field, due to the complexity of the procedure.

- *Non-sterile gloves* are used to remove the dressing before the wound is cleansed.

- *A waterproof rubbish bag* is placed appropriately to receive used materials so they will not cross a sterile field.
- *A dressing pack* is required. More comprehensive wounds may require further sterile drapes and other materials.
- *Sterile gloves* assist in maintaining an aseptic technique as key sites or parts may be touched. There is also exposure to the patient's body fluids.
- *Normal saline* (or other cleansing solutions as ordered) is used to cleanse or irrigate the wound, and to soak the dressing/packing. Normal saline is the preferred solution.
- *Sterile scissors* are used to cut the foam.
- *Vac dressing (foam) and negative-pressure unit.* If the dressing is simply being changed, then the existing unit will continue to be used.
- *Adhesive transparent tape*, big enough to cover the dressing foam and the first part of the drainage tube.

- *Tape* is used to reinforce or support the sealed dressing and drain tube, if required.
- *Personal protective equipment (PPE) (plastic apron, eye protection and mask)* should be used to minimise risk created by exposure to the patient's body fluids.
- *Alcohol-based hand rub (ABHR).*

Confirm the sterility of the packages by checking the use-by date and whether the package is dry, has tears, water damage, stains or, in the case of a bottle, a broken seal. Out-of-date sterile objects have been on the shelf for an extended period of time and their contents are no longer considered sterile because of the time factor. Tears, punctures, stains and dampness in the packaging indicate that there is a pathway from the exterior to the interior of the package through which micro-organisms can gain access. A broken seal on a bottle indicates the bottle's contents have been exposed to the air and are contaminated.

APPLY THE NPWT DRESSING

Perform hand hygiene
Perform hand hygiene before touching the patient or the patient's surrounds and prior to any procedure involving patient contact to reduce the possibility of cross-contamination. Hand hygiene is the most effective method of infection control as it removes transient organisms from the hands of the nurse (see **Skill 1.1**).

Don PPE
A plastic apron and eye protection should be worn as PPE during this procedure. PPE requirements will vary according to the care being delivered and the patient's health status.

Give a clear explanation of the procedure and establish therapeutic communication
Introduce yourself, and check you have the correct patient. Discuss the procedure and gain the patient's consent. Giving a clear explanation is required to gain legal consent and to address policy requirements. It will also assist the patient to cooperate with the procedure, allay anxiety and assist in establishing a therapeutic relationship. Discussing the procedure with the patient will help determine their level of knowledge, and help them understand the healing process and relieve some anxiety associated with the procedure.

Turn off pump
Before commencing the dressing change, turn off the pump and close the clamp on the drainage tube. Remove and change the canister in the drainage unit, as required.

Remove the dressing
Removal of the dressing is accomplished by loosening all tapes and easing the old dressing off carefully. Non-sterile gloves and sterile forceps can be used. Observe the dressing for amount of exudate, colour, odour and consistency before disposing of the dressing, packing, forceps and gloves in the rubbish bag.

Perform hand hygiene
Perform hand hygiene using ABHR.

Establish a critical aseptic field
Establish a critical aseptic field using an aseptic technique as described in **Skills 4.1** and **4.2**. When all packages have been opened and contents placed on the aseptic field, put on the sterile gloves using an open-gloving technique (see **Skill 4.9**) and prepare all of the material. Prepare the wound material as per the manufacturer's instructions.

Cleanse the wound
Cleanse the wound and peri-wound using forceps and gauze swabs as per **Skill 4.2** (simple dressing). Remove any debris from the dressing material that may be on the wound bed. Dry the peri-wound and surrounding skin. Prepare the wound edges with a skin protectant if required.

Assess the wound and wound margins
Assess the wound and wound margins to monitor the wound healing and the condition of the surrounding skin.

Apply the foam dressing
Use the sterile scissors to cut the foam dressing to the approximate size of the wound. Use forceps to then place the foam gently over the wound. Use enough foam to fill the wound, so when the vacuum

is applied, the height of the foam is close to the top of the wound margin. Steady the dressing with the forceps or a gloved hand (sterile gloves) and then place the end of the drain tube either in or over the foam, according to the manufacturer's instructions.

Apply a transparent adhesive dressing

Continue to steady the foam and drain tube with your forceps or gloved hand. Cover the foam dressing, the first few inches of the drainage tube and the surrounding area of healthy skin with adhesive transparent tape. Alternatively, the wound system may require the cutting of a hole in the transparent tape and then adding and sealing the drain tube to the dressing. Ensure there is a sufficient margin (approximately 2 to 3 cm) around the edge of the foam dressing to remain intact when the negative pressure is applied. Also ensure the seal around where the drain tube is leaving the transparent tape is intact. Reinforce this area if necessary.

Connect the end of the drain tube to the pressure unit

The remaining end of the drain is then connected to tubing from the negative-pressure unit, which is then switched on and programmed to produce the required level of pressure. Once the unit is switched on, the air is sucked out of the foam dressing, causing it to collapse inwards and draw in the edges of the wound. Fluid within the wound will be taken up by the foam and transported into the disposable canister within the main negative-pressure unit.

Secure the dressing

Ensure patient comfort and mobility by securing the drain tube with the selected tape, if required. The patient is then assisted to a position of comfort that does not stress the incision or wound.

Doff PPE

Remove PPE in the following sequence: non-sterile gloves, hand hygiene, eyewear/face shield, plastic apron/gown and mask, and then perform hand hygiene (ACSQHC, 2020). Dispose of in the rubbish bag.

Perform hand hygiene

Maintain the 5 Moments for Hand Hygiene and perform hand hygiene after touching the patient and the patient's surrounds.

CLEAN, REPLACE OR DISPOSE OF EQUIPMENT

Clean, replace and dispose of equipment appropriately. Contaminated materials are wrapped in the wrapper that has formed the aseptic field and placed in the rubbish bag, which is then placed in the contaminated waste. Clean the trolley with disinfecting solution or wipes, as recommended by your facility. If gross contamination has occurred, the facility's policy for cleaning should be followed. The trolley is returned to its position in the clean area of the ward. Disposable scissors and forceps are placed in the sharps.

DOCUMENT AND REPORT RELEVANT INFORMATION

Note the number of foam pieces used in the dressing in the wound management plan. This is to ensure all foam pieces are removed during the next dressing as cavity wounds may make it difficult to see all pieces of the dressing material. Document relevant information about the wound, dressing materials and wound assessment in the wound management plan and patient notes. Note the colour of the wound and peri-wound, any exudate, type of dressing applied and the patient's response to the procedure. This validates care given and provides a progress report of the patient's condition.

CASE STUDY

You are an enrolled nurse working within an acute ward area. Your patient, Benjamin Foster, a 20-year-old student, has recently had a moderately sized wound to his right lower leg surgically debrided following a traumatic motorbike injury. The surgeon has now ordered negative pressure wound therapy to manage the wound.

1. What is negative pressure wound therapy?

2. What type of aseptic technique is required for this wound dressing?

3. Benjamin is keen to be discharged from hospital so that he can continue his university studies in the comfort of his own home. As his nurse, what will you need to consider when planning his return home with the NPWT in situ?

Note: These notes are summaries of the most important points in the assessments/procedures, and are not exhaustive on the subject. The naming of documents or charts may differ from state to state, and facility to facility. In all possible situations the guidelines of the ACSQHC are used when describing national charts or documents (e.g. the ACSQHC Observation and Response Chart is named the Adult Observation and Response Chart in WA, and the Rapid Detection and Response Observation Chart in SA). References of the materials used to compile the information have been supplied. The student is expected to have learned the material surrounding each skill as presented in the references. No single reference is complete on the subject.

REFERENCES

Australian Commission on Safety and Quality in Health Care (ACSQHC). (2020). *Sequence for Putting on and Removing PPE.* https://www.safetyandquality.gov.au/sites/default/files/2020-03/putting_on_and_removing_ppe_diagram_-_march_2020.pdf

Gleeson, L. & Bond, M. (2015). Using a portable, multi-week single-patient use negative pressure wound therapy device to facilitate faster discharge. *Wounds UK,* 11(2) pp. 104–111.

Ranaweera, A. (2013). *What is Negative Wound Therapy?* DermNet NZ. https://www.dermnetnz.org/topics/negative-pressure-wound-therapy

Wound Care Centres. (2020). *Negative Pressure Wound Therapy.* https://www.woundcarecenters.org/article/wound-therapies/negative-pressure-wound-therapy

RECOMMENDED READINGS

Ren, Y., Chang, P. & Sheridan, R.L. (2017). Negative wound pressure therapy is safe and useful in pediatric burn patients. *International Journal of Burns and Trauma,* 7(2), 12–16.

Royal Children's Hospital Melbourne (RCHM). (2020). *Surgical Drains (Non-Cardiac). Clinical Guidelines (Nursing).* March. https://www.rch.org.au/rchcpg/hospital_clinical_guideline_index/Surgical_Drains_(Non_Cardiac)/

ESSENTIAL SKILLS COMPETENCY

Negative Pressure Wound Therapy Dressing

Demonstrates the ability to effectively and safely change the dressing for a negative wound pressure therapy dressing

Criteria for skill performance	Y	D
(Numbers indicate *Enrolled Nurse Standards for Practice*, 2016)	(Satisfactory)	(Requires development)
1. Identifies indication (8.3, 8.4)		
2. Demonstrates problem-solving abilities; e.g. administers analgesia, provides privacy, positions patient appropriately (4.1, 4.2, 8.3, 8.4, 9.4)		
3. Gathers equipment (1.2, 1.6, 4.4, 6.4, 8.4, 9.4) ■ non-sterile gloves ■ dressing tray ■ sterile gloves ■ 0.9% saline or other cleansing solution ■ vac dressing (foam) ■ negative-pressure unit ■ adhesive transparent tape ■ tape if required ■ PPE – plastic apron, eye protection and mask ■ alcohol-based hand rub ■ sterile scissors		
4. Performs hand hygiene and dons PPE as required (1.2, 1.4, 1.8, 2.2, 3.2, 3.9, 6.4, 8.4, 9.4)		
5. Evidence of effective communication; e.g. gives patient a clear explanation of procedure, gains patient consent (2.1, 2.3, 2.4, 2.5, 6.3)		
6. Clamps/turns off negative-pressure system (1.2, 1.4, 1.6, 1.7, 2.3, 2.4, 2.7, 3.2, 4.1, 8.4, 9.4)		
7. Removes soiled dressing (1.2, 1.4, 1.8, 2.2, 2.7, 3.2, 3.9, 8.4, 9.4)		
8. Performs hand hygiene (1.2, 1.4, 1.8, 3.2, 3.9, 6.4, 9.4)		
9. Establishes the sterile field, dons sterile gloves and cleanses wound (1.2, 1.4, 3.2, 3.9, 9.4)		
10. Assesses wound and surrounding tissue (1.2, 1.4, 2.3, 2.4, 2.7, 3.2, 3.9, 4.1, 7.1, 8.4, 9.4)		
11. Applies NPWT wound dressing (i.e. foam) (1.2, 1.4, 1.6, 1.7, 2.3, 2.4, 2.7, 3.2, 4.1, 8.4, 9.4)		
12. Applies outer transparent tape and secures drain tube into the dressing (1.2, 1.4, 2.3, 2.4, 2.7, 3.2, 3.9, 8.4, 9.4)		
13. Connects drain tube to negative-pressure unit and turns on negative-pressure unit (1.2, 1.4, 1.6, 1.7, 2.3, 2.4, 2.7, 3.2, 4.1, 8.4, 9.4)		
14. Doffs PPE and performs hand hygiene (1.2, 1.4, 1.8, 3.2, 3.9, 6.4, 8.4, 9.4)		
15. Cleans, replaces and disposes of equipment appropriately (1.2, 1.4, 3.9, 6.5, 9.4)		
16. Documents relevant information (1.2, 1.3, 1.8, 3.2, 5.3, 6.6, 7.1, 7.2, 7.3, 7.4, 7.5)		
17. Demonstrates ability to link theory to practice (8.3, 8.4, 8.5, 9.4)		

Student: _____

Clinical facilitator: _____   Date: _____

CHAPTER 4.7

SUTURE AND STAPLE REMOVAL

IDENTIFY INDICATIONS

To assist the process of primary intention wound healing, wound edges for a surgical incision or a laceration can be held together by sutures, staples, surgical glue/skin adhesive or tape until healing has proceeded to the point where the support is no longer necessary (Bonham, 2016; Mahoney, 2016). Steri-Strips are used if there is minimal tension on the incision line, and usually for superficial incisions. Surgical glue is often used for wounds in emergency settings, but is not suitable for wounds over mobile areas or with high levels of tension on the wound. It provides a waterproof barrier, is non-invasive, is less painful than suturing and has minimal scarring. Larger or deeper incisions require either sutures or skin clips/staples to bring wound edges together and assist the healing process (Bonham, 2016). Since both of these methods are invasive, they provide a focus for inflammation and a point of entry for infection, and need to be removed when the need for mechanical support of the incision is passed. The timing of suture removal is dependent on the type and depth of the incision, and on the part of the body where it is located. Sutures in the facial areas may be removed after 3 to 5 days, while sutures in other areas will remain intact for 7 to 14 days, depending on their anatomical position, possibility of high tension or mobility of the area (Mahoney, 2016). Deeper dissolvable sutures are not removed. They remain in the tissues and are reabsorbed by the body over a short period of time. Sutures that are left in too long or not fully removed

properly can lead to scarring or other complications, such as a stitch abscess, wound infection or foreign body reaction (Bonham, 2016; Mahoney, 2016).

Although most clinical pathways or care plans will state the routine need for suture removal on days 7 to 10 post-op, a doctor's order is required. Check the order for any specific instructions about removal of alternate sutures and specific wound dressing requirements post removal. Assess the wound edges prior to removing any sutures to check for healing of the wound and closure of wound edges. Also assess the sutures to determine the type of suture (interrupted or non-interrupted/continuous), as this will influence the technique for correct removal.

Alternate sutures/staples should be removed initially, the wound checked for any stress or signs of dehiscence and then the remaining sutures/staples removed. Although not always possible, it is preferable for this to happen across 2 days. Sutures are often removed on the day a patient is due for discharge, or when attending a clinic or GP for suture removal. Sometimes, wounds gape when a suture or staple is removed. If this occurs, removing further sutures could cause dehiscence of the wound. Leave all other sutures/staples in place, and report what has happened to the registered nurse and doctor. A Steri-Strip is often applied to re-approximate the wound edges and support the open area of the wound, and further wound management actions are determined by the team.

GATHER EQUIPMENT

Gathering the equipment prior to the procedure creates a positive environment for the successful completion of the procedure. It expedites completion of the procedure, boosts patient confidence and trust in the nurse, increases the nurse's self-confidence and provides an opportunity to mentally rehearse the procedure.

The following equipment is required for suture, clip or staple removal.

- *Non-sterile gloves* are used to remove the soiled dressing, if there is one. If there is risk of exposure to

body fluids (depending on the wound site), gloves should also be worn while removing the sutures (NHMRC, 2019).
- *The dressing pack and solutions* are used to establish a sterile field and cleanse the site.
- *Sterile stitch cutters* are used to remove the sutures (as suitable to the type of closure, and available in the facility).
- *A staple remover* is used to remove staples or clips.
- *A sharps container* is required if a stitch cutter or disposable staple remover is used.
- *The appropriate dressing* may be used to cover the incision site after removing sutures/clips/staples.

- *Steri-Strips* may be applied for extra support.
- *Sterile metal forceps* (if available) are used to grip the suture more securely.
- *A kidney dish* may be used to place sutures/staples in. Confirm the sterility of the packages by checking the use-by date and whether the package is dry, has tears, water damage, stains or, in the case of a bottle, a broken seal. Out-of-date sterile objects have been on the shelf for an extended period of time and their contents are no longer considered sterile because of the time factor. Tears, punctures, stains and dampness in the packaging indicate that there is a pathway from the exterior to the interior of the package through which microorganisms can gain access. A broken seal on a bottle indicates the bottle's contents have been exposed to the air and are contaminated.

REMOVE SUTURES

Perform hand hygiene

Perform hand hygiene before touching the patient or the patient's surrounds and prior to any procedure involving patient contact to reduce the possibility of cross-contamination. Hand hygiene is the most effective method of infection control as it removes transient organisms from the hands of the nurse (see **Skill 1.1**).

Don personal protective equipment (PPE) as required

A plastic apron and eye protection should be worn as PPE during this procedure. PPE requirements will vary according to the care being delivered and the patient's health status.

Give a clear explanation of the procedure and establish therapeutic communication

Introduce yourself, and check you have the correct patient. Discuss the procedure and gain the patient's consent. Giving a clear explanation is required to gain legal consent and to address policy requirements. It will also assist the patient to cooperate with the procedure, allay anxiety and assist in establishing a therapeutic relationship. Suture and staple removal generally causes minimal discomfort, although some patients remain apprehensive.

Demonstrate problem-solving abilities

Provision of privacy ensures the patient's dignity and reduces embarrassment at the exposure of (usually) private areas of the body. Take the patient to the toilet before the procedure to assist in the comfort level of the patient during the procedure. The patient is positioned to expose the area. The position should be one of comfort to facilitate relaxation and stillness throughout the procedure. This reduces the possibility of contamination of the sterile field.

Carry out the procedure

The principles of using an aseptic technique (see **Skill 4.1**) are followed when removing sutures or staples. The wound may be cleansed first (as per **Skill 4.2**), according to facility policy.

Remove sutures

Intermittent sutures

To remove intermittent sutures, grasp the knot with the forceps in your non-dominant hand. Refer to **FIGURE 4.7.1**. Gently put tension on the knot until the suture comes away from the skin. Slip the stitch cutter under the knot (A) or suture area close to the skin on the opposite side (B). Move the suture cutter using a gentle slicing action and cut the suture as close to the skin as possible. This ensures that the least amount of contaminated suture material is pulled through the suture track and under the skin layers, thereby reducing the chances of infection (Bonham, 2016). Ensure the cutting action does not endanger the patient's skin or create a sharps risk to the nurse. Pull the suture through the incision by steadily drawing on the knot with the forceps. Discard the suture into the kidney dish and repeat the same action for the next alternate suture. Always remove alternate sutures first. Inspect the incision line for approximation. If the incision line is well approximated, and the doctor has ordered removal of all sutures, remove the remaining sutures. Count the number of sutures you remove and document accordingly.

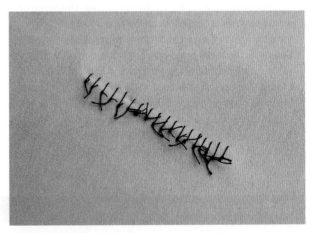

FIGURE 4.7.1 Intermittent sutures

Plain continuous sutures

These are sutures where one thread runs in a series of stitches and is tied only at the beginning and end of the run. Refer to **FIGURE 4.7.2**.

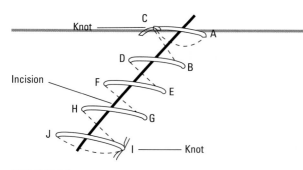

FIGURE 4.7.2 Continuous sutures

Note:

i. Cut the thread of the first suture at (A) opposite the knot (C) then cut the thread of the suture (B) on the same side as (A).

ii. Grasp the knot (C) with the forceps, and gently pull. This completely removes the first stitch as well as the thread beneath the skin which was attached to the stitch (B).

iii. Cut off the visible part of the suture at D, and then remove the top piece.

iv. Grasp the suture at E, and pull through the underlying thread between D and E.

v. Cut the visible part at F, and then remove the top piece.

vi. Grasp the suture at G, and pull through the underlying thread between F and G.

vii. Cut the visible part at H, and then remove the top piece.

viii. Cut the last suture at J, grasp the knot at I, and gently pull through. This completely removes the last suture and the underlying thread between H and I.

Note: For safety reasons, prior to cutting any thread, put gentle traction on it to ensure that the underlying position of the suture is correctly determined).

SUBCUTICULAR SUTURES (DISSOLVABLE/ABSORBABLE OR NON-DISSOLVABLE)

These are a type of continuous suture. First, determine whether the sutures are dissolvable/absorbable or non-dissolvable (check the surgeon's postoperative notes). This *must* be determined *prior* to cutting any sutures.

- *Dissolvable/absorbable.* With forceps, grasp the visible suture (knot) at one end, lift gently and cut under the knot, flush with the skin. Repeat the procedure for the visible suture (knot) at the other end. All external visible signs of suturing are now removed and the underlying (non-visible) sutures are intact. Discard the two knots into the appropriate receptacle.

- *Non-dissolvable.* With forceps, grasp the visible suture (knot) at one end, lift gently and cut under the knot, flush with the skin. Then, grasp the visible knot of the suture at the other end, and gently pull on the knot, removing the underlying suture in its entirety. All the suture is now removed. Discard into the appropriate receptacle.

REMOVE STAPLES

Staple removal is achieved by gently inserting the curved tip of the clip/staple remover under each clip/staple, with the bowl of the curve upward. The staple must sit in the groove of the staple remover. Gently but firmly squeeze the handle of the clip/staple remover fully together. This forces the clip/staple edges out of the skin. When you can see both clip/staple ends, gently rock the staple remover from side to side to loosen the clip/staple ends from the skin, and then lift the clip/staple off the skin and discard it into the kidney dish. Count the number of clips/staples you remove and document accordingly.

Apply Steri-Strips

Steri-Strips may be applied in the intervening spaces between alternate sutures/clips to support the suture line and prevent dehiscence.

Cleanse the incision site

The incision site should be cleansed if any blood or fluid is left on the surface by the removal of the sutures/clips/staples. Asepsis is maintained throughout the procedure to minimise the risk of contamination and subsequent infection.

Doff PPE

Remove PPE in the following sequence: non-sterile gloves, hand hygiene, eyewear/face shield, plastic apron/gown and mask and then perform hand hygiene (ACSQHC, 2020). Dispose of in the rubbish bag.

Perform hand hygiene

Maintain the 5 Moments for Hand Hygiene and perform hand hygiene after touching the patient and the patient's surrounds.

CLEAN, REPLACE OR DISPOSE OF EQUIPMENT

According to hospital policy dispose of used equipment appropriately. The stitch cutter, staple remover, scissors and forceps are disposed of in the sharps container. Clean the trolley with the disinfecting solution or wipes as recommended by your facility and return to its position in the clean area of the ward.

DOCUMENT AND REPORT RELEVANT INFORMATION

The condition of the incision line is documented in the progress notes and wound management plan, noting any dehiscence, gaping, exudate or erythema. Identify when the remaining sutures or staples should be removed. Any Steri-Strips or dressing applied following removal is also noted.

CASE STUDY

You are an enrolled nurse working in a GP practice. You are asked to remove sutures from a patient's abdomen who had surgery appendicectomy 10 days ago. The patient has simple interrupted sutures.

1. Before removing the sutures, how/what will you assess on the suture line?
2. Why is it important to remove alternate sutures first?

3. Where will you cut the suture, before removing it? While completing the suture removal, some of the skin edges start to come apart.
4. What action/s will you implement?
5. What is the potential outcome of the edges of the suture line 'coming apart'?

Note: These notes are summaries of the most important points in the assessments/procedures, and are not exhaustive on the subject. The naming of documents or charts may differ from state to state, and facility to facility. In all possible situations the guidelines of the ACSQHC are used when describing national charts or documents (e.g. the ACSQHC Observation and Response Chart is named the Adult Observation and Response Chart in WA, and the Rapid Detection and Response Observation Chart in SA). References of the materials used to compile the information have been supplied. The student is expected to have learned the material surrounding each skill as presented in the references. No single reference is complete on the subject.

REFERENCES

Australian Commission on Safety and Quality in Health Care (ACSQHC). (2020). *Sequence for Putting on and Removing PPE*. https://www.safetyandquality.gov.au/sites/default/files/2020-03/putting_on_and_removing_ppe_diagram_-_march_2020.pdf

Bonham, J. (2016). Assessment and management of patients with minor traumatic wounds. *Nursing Standard*, 31(8), p. 60.

Mahoney, K. (2016). Managing postsurgical wounds in the patient's home. *Journal of Community Nursing*, 30(5), pp. 16–24.

National Health and Medical Research Council (NHMRC). (2019). *Australian Guidelines for the Prevention and Control of Infection in Healthcare*. https://www.nhmrc.gov.au/health-advice/public-health/preventing-infection

RECOMMENDED READINGS

Marshall, G. (2013). Skin glues for wound closure. *Australian Prescriber*, 36(2) pp. 49–51.

ESSENTIAL SKILLS COMPETENCY

Suture and Staple Removal
Demonstrates the ability to remove sutures, clips or staples correctly

Criteria for skill performance	Y	D
(Numbers indicate *Enrolled Nurse Standards for Practice*, 2016)	(Satisfactory)	(Requires development)
1. Identifies indication (8.3, 8.4)		
2. Verifies written order to remove sutures or staples (1.2, 1.4, 3.2, 9.4)		
3. Gathers equipment (1.2, 1.6, 4.4, 6.4, 8.4, 9.4): ■ non-sterile gloves ■ stitch cutter or staple remover ■ metal forceps ■ sharps container and kidney dish ■ dressing pack and required solution ■ dressing, if required ■ Steri-Strips		
4. Performs hand hygiene and dons PPE if required (1.2, 1.4, 1.8, 3.9, 6.4, 9.4)		
5. Evidence of effective communication; e.g. gives explanation of procedure, gains patient consent (2.1, 2.3, 2.4, 2.5, 6.3)		
6. Demonstrates problem-solving abilities; e.g. provides privacy (4.1, 4.2, 8.3, 8.4, 9.4)		
7. Positions patient (1.2, 1.4, 3.2, 8.4, 9.4)		
8. Performs hand hygiene (1.2, 1.4, 1.8, 3.2, 3.9, 6.4, 9.4)		
9. Sets up dressing tray (1.2, 1.4, 1.8, 3.2, 3.9, 9.4)		
10. Removes alternate sutures/staples (1.2, 1.4, 2.3, 2.4, 2.7, 3.2, 4.1, 8.4, 9.4)		
11. Assesses wound edges, then removes remaining sutures/staples (1.2, 1.4, 2.3, 2.4, 2.7, 3.2, 4.1, 8.4, 9.4)		
12. Cleans wound (and applies new dressing if required) (1.2, 1.4, 3.2, 8.4, 9.4)		
13. Doffs PPE if used and performs hand hygiene (1.2, 1.4, 1.8, 3.9, 6.4, 9.4)		
14. Cleans, replaces and disposes of equipment appropriately (1.2, 1.4, 3.9, 6.5, 9.4)		
15. Documents and reports relevant information (1.2, 1.3, 1.8, 3.2, 5.3, 6.6, 7.1, 7.2, 7.3, 7.4, 7.5)		
16. Demonstrates ability to link theory to practice (8.3, 8.4, 8.5, 9.4)		

Student:

Clinical facilitator: Date:

CHAPTER **4.8**

DRAIN REMOVAL AND SHORTENING

IDENTIFY INDICATIONS

Wound drainage systems are used to remove collections of fluid from around surgical incisions or wounds in order to:

- remove existent fluid collections in the tissues
- prevent the accumulation of fluids, such as blood post-op
- eliminate dead space and promote wound healing
- reduce the risk of post-op wound site infection.

Drain sites are usually situated a short distance from the incision and are dressed separately.

The nurse must understand the type of drain used in order to safely manage the drain post-op and facilitate the correct removal when ordered. There are two basic types of drains:

- passive or gravity drains (e.g. Bore, Pigtail, Penrose or corrugated drains) combine gravity, pressure within the wound and capillary action to drain fluid from the wound
- vacuum drains that exert a low negative pressure on the site to remove exudate.

Drains are removed when there is no further drainage or the drainage is minimal. If left too long, the drain itself becomes a track for the introduction of infective microorganisms into the wound. The drain may or may not be sutured in place. This information will be recorded on the theatre notes.

The doctor orders removal of a drain approximately 48 hours post operation. Vacuum drains left in situ for too long may allow granulation tissue to form at the tip of the drain tube. Some gravity drains are often shortened 2 to 3 days prior to removal, and have a safety pin applied close to the skin to prevent the drain from slipping back into the wound. This drain shortening procedure is similar to drain removal. Orders for drain removal usually include whether the incision dressing is to be changed or left intact and whether vacuum drain suction is to be left on or not. Some facilities and authors advocate breaking suction or clamping the tube before removal; however, some manufacturer's instructions state to leave suction on. It is essential to refer to the surgeon's instructions and the facility's policy prior to drain removal to ensure the correct procedure is followed.

GATHER EQUIPMENT

Gathering the equipment prior to the procedure creates a positive environment for the successful completion of the procedure. It expedites completion of the procedure, boosts patient confidence and trust in the nurse, increases the nurse's self-confidence and provides an opportunity to mentally rehearse the skill.

The following equipment is required for drain removal.

- *Non-sterile gloves* are used to remove the soiled dressing from the drain site.
- *Sterile gloves* should be used to manipulate the sterile items and the drain during removal. Key sites will be touched during the drain removal process.
- *The dressing pack and solutions* (usually normal saline) are used to establish a critical aseptic field and cleanse the site.
- *The appropriate dressing* must be used to cover the drain site.

- *Sterile scissors or stitch cutters* are used to remove the retaining stitch in the drain (if any). *A sharps container* is required if a stitch cutter is used. The scissors are also used to cut the drain if being shortened.
- *A sterile safety pin* is used to anchor the remainder of a shortened drain.
- *A 'bluey'* is used to protect bed linen and the patient during the procedure.
- *Face mask, plastic apron and eye protection* protect the nurse's skin and mucous membranes from body fluid splashes.
- *Alcohol-based hand rub (ABHR)* is placed on the dressing trolley for hand hygiene during the procedure.

Confirm the sterility of the packages by checking the use-by date and whether the package is dry, has tears, water damage, stains or, in the case of a bottle, a broken seal. Out-of-date sterile objects have been on the shelf for an extended period of time and their contents are no longer considered sterile because of the time factor. Tears, punctures, stains and dampness in the packaging indicate that there is a pathway from the exterior to the interior of the package through which microorganisms can gain access. A broken seal on a bottle indicates the bottle's contents have been exposed to the air and are contaminated.

REMOVE THE DRAIN

Perform hand hygiene

Perform hand hygiene before touching the patient or the patient's surrounds and prior to any procedure involving patient contact to reduce the possibility of cross-contamination. Hand hygiene is the most effective method of infection control as it removes transient organisms from the hands of the nurse (see **Skill 1.1**).

Give a clear explanation of the procedure and establish therapeutic communication

Introduce yourself, and check you have the correct patient. Discuss the procedure and gain the patient's consent. Giving a clear explanation is required to gain legal consent and to address policy requirements. It will also assist the patient to cooperate with the procedure, allay anxiety and assist in establishing a therapeutic relationship. Drain removal can be an uncomfortable procedure, especially for vacuum drains. An explanation can help increase their ability to cooperate and tolerate a stressful procedure.

Demonstrate problem-solving abilities

Provision of privacy ensures the patient's dignity and reduces embarrassment at the exposure of (usually) private areas of the body. Take the patient to the toilet before the procedure to assist in the comfort level of the patient during the procedure. Analgesia should be offered 30 minutes prior to the procedure so that when given it has time to minimise discomfort. The patient is positioned to expose the area. The position should be one of comfort to facilitate relaxation and stillness throughout the procedure. This reduces the possibility of contamination of the sterile field.

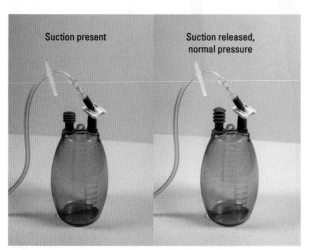

FIGURE 4.8.1 Vacuum drain

Vacuum drains – normalise the suction

To minimise discomfort when removing vacuum drains, the pressure within the drain is normalised prior to removal, according to the drain manufacturer's instructions. This can include clamping the drain or adjusting the pressure dial 5 to 20 minutes prior to the actual removal. If the drain has a pressure dial, the drain tube should then be clamped. The drain system should remain intact (VariVac International Medical Research, 2018).

Pigtail drains – uncoil prior to removal

A Pigtail drain is a long, thin drain with a locking tip. The tip coils to a pigtail shape at the end of the catheter by a thread-like string that can be mistaken for a suture. These drains must be uncoiled prior to removal to prevent tissue trauma and pain for the patient. For most of these drains, the string is cut to release the coil (Royal Children's Hospital Melbourne [RCHM], 2020). Refer to facility policy and manufacturer's instruction for correct uncoiling technique prior to removing this drain. (See **FIGURE 4.8.2**.)

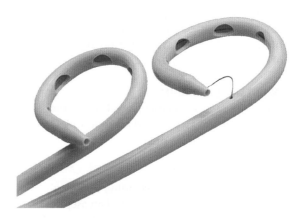

FIGURE 4.8.2 Pigtail drain

Measure the drainage in the bottle

Measure the level of drainage by checking the fluid level on the bottle's pre-marked measuring scale. Ideally this should be done prior to the removal to reduce the risk of exposure to body fluids. Ensure the bottle is placed on a flat surface and your eye is at the same level you are measuring. Note any previously marked drainage amounts (usually timed and dated on the side of the drainage bottle), and subtract the final volume from these amounts. This will determine the level of fluid drained since the previous recording of drainage.

Perform hand hygiene

Maintain the 5 Moments for Hand Hygiene and perform hand hygiene after touching the patient and the patient's surrounds.

Don personal protective equipment (PPE)

Put on the eye protection, plastic apron and face mask (if required). PPE protect the nurse from the patient's body fluids. PPE requirements will vary according to the care being delivered and the patient's health status.

Set up the dressing tray and establish a critical aseptic field

Establish a critical aseptic field using an aseptic technique as described in **Skills 4.1** and **4.2** respectively. The aseptic field also provides a place to put the sterile scissors/stitch cutter for later use. A 'bluey' is placed between the drain site and the dressing trolley to prevent staining of bed linen.

Remove the drain dressing

Don non-sterile gloves, then remove the drain dressing to expose the drain. Non-sterile gloves are used to remove the dressing to prevent contamination of the nurse's hands.

Repeat hand hygiene

Perform hand hygiene again at this stage to reduce the risk of cross-contamination. An ABHR can be used.

Don sterile gloves using open gloving

Don sterile gloves using an open-gloving technique. Refer to **Skill 4.9** for the open-gloving technique. Sterile gloves should be used to maintain an aseptic technique, avoid contact with key sites and reduce the risk of exposure to body fluids.

Carry out the procedure

The principles of using an aseptic technique and working in a critical aseptic field are followed when removing or shortening a drain.

Cleanse the drain site

The wound is cleansed first, according to policy.

Continuing to use the forceps and an aseptic technique, the drain site is cleansed using normal saline.

Cut the retaining suture

Using the sterile stitch cutter, the retaining suture is cut close to the skin so that the drain can be removed. Refer to **Skill 4.7** for guidelines on suture removal.

Remove the drain

Ensure specific pre-removal instructions are followed for vacuum and Pigtail drains.

Supporting the surrounding skin, the drain is gently removed using a continuous motion. Grasp the drainage tube close to the insertion site using your dominant hand. Using a gauze swab, gently support the drain site with your other hand. Rotate the drain tube slightly at the insertion site, then pull gently on the tube. Pull firmly and ease the drain from the wound until all of the drain is removed. Longer drain tubes may require you to move your hand along the tube as it comes out and loop the tube into your hand as you remove the complete length. Check the drain to ensure that the tip is intact. Gentle pressure with a gauze swab over the drain site after removal will reduce bleeding post removal. The patient should be distracted during the procedure to minimise discomfort. Requesting the patient to wriggle the toes is usually an effective distraction.

Discard the removed drain into the rubbish bag. Remove sterile gloves and perform hand hygiene.

Shorten a passive or gravity drain

If shortening of the drain is ordered, cut the retaining suture and remove (see **Skill 4.7**). If the drain has previously been shortened, the safety pin is left in place. Using forceps, the drain is carefully pulled out to the length ordered by the doctor (generally 2 cm each day). Wearing sterile gloves, a new sterile safety pin is carefully reattached to the drain as close to the skin as possible (take care not to pierce the gloves or stab yourself). The excess drain length is then cut off, but only after the new safety pin is in place.

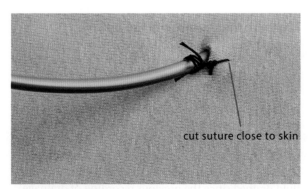

cut suture close to skin

FIGURE 4.8.3 Cut the retaining suture

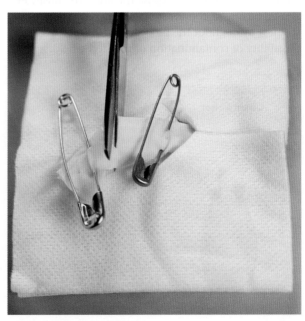

FIGURE 4.8.4 Shortening a drain

Discard the cut-off piece of drain into the rubbish bag. Remove sterile gloves and perform hand hygiene.

Cleanse the drain site and apply dressing
The drain site is cleansed of any blood or fluid left on the surface by the removal or shortening of the drain. A sterile dry dressing is applied to minimise the risk of infection. Some gravity drain sites may use a drainage or stoma bag over the drain site if there is a large amount of exudate. An aseptic technique is maintained throughout the procedure to minimise risk of contamination and subsequent infection. The drain site should be checked for soakage 15 minutes after removal of the drain.

Doff PPE
Remove PPE in the following sequence: non-sterile gloves, hand hygiene, eyewear/face shield, plastic apron/gown and mask and then perform hand hygiene (ACSQHC, 2020). Dispose of in the rubbish bag.

Perform hand hygiene
Maintain the 5 Moments for Hand Hygiene and perform hand hygiene after touching the patient and the patient's surrounds.

CLEAN, REPLACE OR DISPOSE OF EQUIPMENT
Equipment is cleaned or disposed of. The stitch cutter is disposed of in the sharps container. After using the measuring scale on the side of the bottle, vacuum containers with contents are generally placed in the biohazard container – refer to facility biological waste policy for disposal of drains. The drain system should not be opened, but remain intact (VariVac International Medical Research, 2018). Clean the trolley with disinfectant solution or wipes and return to its position in the clean area of the ward.

DOCUMENT AND REPORT RELEVANT INFORMATION
Drainage is measured and recorded on the appropriate fluid balance chart to maintain an accurate record of amount. Ensure the volume in the drain is measured prior to removal or disposal. The removal of the drain is documented in the clinical notes, care plan, wound management chart, and appropriate fluid balance chart. Some facilities require the doctor's order sheet also to be signed. Clinical notes should include the date and time of shortening or removal, signature, amount and type of drainage, the condition of the skin around the drain incision and the patient's reaction to the procedure. The patient should be observed following removal of a drain for any bleeding or excess soakage on the new dressing.

CASE STUDY

You are working in a busy surgical ward. You have two patients with postoperative drains, and both are due for removal today, according to the post-op nursing care plan. Jim Irons has a Pigtail drain and David Everingham has a VariVac vacuum drain.

1. What will you do prior to removing the drains to confirm it is correct to remove the drains this shift?

2. What actions will you implement prior to the drain removal for:
    a. Pigtail drain
    b. VariVac vacuum drain?

3. Where will you document the removal of the drain?

4. What observations will you make of the drain site, post removal?

Note: These notes are summaries of the most important points in the assessments/procedures, and are not exhaustive on the subject. The naming of documents or charts may differ from state to state, and facility to facility. In all possible situations the guidelines of the ACSQHC are used when describing national charts or documents (e.g. the ACSQHC Observation and Response Chart is named the Adult Observation and Response Chart in WA, and the Rapid Detection and Response Observation Chart in SA). References of the materials used to compile the information have been supplied. The student is expected to have learned the material surrounding each skill as presented in the references. No single reference is complete on the subject.

REFERENCES

Australian Commission on Safety and Quality in Health Care (ACSQHC). (2020). *Sequence for Putting on and Removing PPE.* https://www.safetyandquality.gov.au/sites/default/files/2020-03/putting_on_and_removing_ppe_diagram_-_march_2020.pdf

Royal Children's Hospital Melbourne (RCHM). (2020). *Surgical Drains (Non-Cardiac). Clinical Guidelines (Nursing).* March. https://www.rch.org.au/rchcpg/hospital_clinical_guideline_index/Surgical_Drains_(Non_Cardiac)/

VariVac International Medical Research. (2018). *VariVac Canister.* https://varivac.com/products/varivac-canister/

RECOMMENDED READINGS

Kumar, S., Chatterjee, S., Gupta, S., Satpathy, A., Chatterjee, S., & Ray, U. (2017). Role of subcutaneous closed vacuum drain in preventing surgical site infection in emergency surgery for perforative peritonitis: A randomized control study. *Bangladesh Journal of Medical Science*, 16(1), pp. 85–90.

National Health and Medical Research Council (NHMRC). (2019). *Australian Guidelines for the Prevention and Control of Infection in Healthcare.* https://www.nhmrc.gov.au/health-advice/public-health/preventing-infection

Van Straten Medical. (2017). *Van Straten Medical Wound Drains.* https://k2medical.za.com/products/van-straten-medical-wound-drains/#tabs|1

Wounds Australia. (2017). *Application of Aseptic Technique in Wound Dressing Procedure: A Consensus Document.* Osborne Park, WA: Cambridge Media.

ESSENTIAL SKILLS COMPETENCY

Drain Removal and Shortening
Demonstrates the ability to shorten or remove a drain correctly

Criteria for skill performance	Y	D
(Numbers indicate *Enrolled Nurse Standards for Practice*, 2016)	(Satisfactory)	(Requires development)
1. Identifies indication (8.3, 8.4)		
2. Verifies written order to remove or shorten the drain (1.2, 1.4, 3.2, 9.4)		
3. Gathers equipment (1.2, 1.6, 4.4, 6.4, 8.4, 9.4): ■ PPE – plastic apron and goggles ■ non-sterile and sterile gloves ■ stitch remover and fine sharp scissors if required ■ sharps container ■ dressing pack, required dressing materials ■ sterile normal saline for irrigation (cleansing the wound) ■ sterile safety pin if required ■ 'bluey' ■ waterproof rubbish bag ■ alcohol-based hand rub		
4. Performs hand hygiene (1.2, 1.4, 1.8, 3.9, 6.4, 9.4)		
5. Evidence of effective communication; e.g. gives explanation of procedure, gains patient consent (2.1, 2.3, 2.4, 2.5, 6.3)		
6. Demonstrates problem-solving abilities; e.g. provides privacy, pain relief and other comfort measures (4.1, 4.2, 8.3, 8.4, 9.4)		
7. Prepares equipment and releases suction on vacuum drain/releases coil for Pigtail drain (1.2, 1.4, 3.2, 4.4, 6.4, 8.4, 9.4)		
8. Measures and records wound drainage (1.2, 1.4, 3.2, 3.9, 8.4, 9.4)		
9. Positions patient (1.2, 1.4, 3.2, 8.4, 9.4)		
10. Performs hand hygiene and dons PPE as required (1.2, 1.4, 1.8, 2.2, 3.2, 3.9, 8.4, 9.4)		
11. Loosens/removes dressing, disposes of gloves, applies hand gel, cleanses wound site using aseptic technique, removes any sutures (1.2, 1.4, 1.8, 3.2, 3.9, 6.4, 8.4, 9.4)		
12. Applies hand gel and dons sterile gloves (1.2, 1.4, 1.8, 2.2, 3.2, 3.9, 8.4, 9.4)		
13. Shortens/removes drain as ordered (1.2, 1.4, 1.8, 2.7, 3.2, 3.9, 4.1, 8.4, 9.4)		
14. Cleans and dresses wound (1.2, 1.4, 3.2, 3.9, 8.4, 9.4)		
15. Doffs PPE and performs hand hygiene (1.2, 1.4, 1.8, 3.9, 6.4, 9.4)		
16. Cleans, replaces and disposes of equipment appropriately (1.2, 1.4, 3.9, 6.5, 9.4)		
17. Documents and reports relevant information (1.2, 1.3, 1.8, 3.2, 5.3, 6.6, 7.1, 7.2, 7.3, 7.4, 7.5)		
18. Demonstrates ability to link theory to practice (8.3, 8.4, 8.5, 9.4)		

Student:

Clinical facilitator: Date:

CHAPTER 4.9

GOWNING AND GLOVING (OPEN AND CLOSED)

IDENTIFY INDICATIONS

The aim of maintaining a critical aseptic field is to ensure asepsis during a procedure and prevent the transfer of microorganisms to a patient. Sterile gowns and gloves are worn for procedures that require the use of an aseptic technique and a critical aseptic field or use of a surgical aseptic technique. Double gloving (using two layers of surgical gloves) may be required in some circumstances. Open gloving is used for procedures where sterile gloves are required to maintain a critical aseptic field, or if key parts or key sites are being touched during a procedure.

GATHER EQUIPMENT

- A *gown pack* (often commercially prepared and disposable) containing a gown of appropriate size and a sterile towel is placed in an appropriate area prior to starting the surgical scrub. The outer wrapping is opened to produce a sterile field. The sterile towel should be on top of the gown and readily accessible.

- *Sterile gloves* of appropriate size (and within date) are opened and the inner packet containing the gloves is placed on the critical aseptic field using an aseptic technique. Make sure that the gloves are placed so that the towel and the gown are *accessible, as they will be required before the gloves.*

PERFORM SURGICAL SCRUB AND DRY HANDS

Prior to the scrub, apply protective cap, surgical mask and eyewear as per risk management or location requirements. A surgical scrub is carried out for the length of the time required by the agency or by the procedure. Refer to the surgical scrub procedure stated in **Skill 4.10** for correct handwashing and drying procedure. Ensure the hands are thoroughly dried with the sterile towel prior to gowning and gloving to prevent maceration and chapping of the hands, and dampening of the gown. Dry hands are also essential for ease of gloving.

COMPLETE 'OPEN GLOVING' PROCESS

Open gloving is used most frequently outside the operating theatre, and is used without a sterile gown. Sterile gloves are worn when key parts and key sites are being touched during a procedure. They maintain asepsis, protect complicated wounds from contamination and the nurse from body fluid exposure (Victorian Department of Health, 2014).

- Open the inner packet. Make sure the folds are pulled firmly to keep them open and avoid contamination. The gloves should be positioned with the palms up, thumbs to the outside and cuffs at the bottom. Avoid touching the gloves or inner part of the packaging.

- Using your non-dominant hand, pick the glove for the dominant hand out of the packet, touching only the inside of the cuff. Lift it above the packet, away from your body. Keep the thumb of your dominant hand folded against your palm and slide your fingers inside the glove, taking care not to contaminate the outer surface. Do not be concerned about the fit of the glove at this point, even if all of the fingers are not in position, since you can adjust both gloves more easily later. Students may reverse the dominant/non-dominant hand order. This is satisfactory, provided the principles are followed.

- Slip the fingers of your gloved dominant hand under the cuff of the remaining glove. Keep your

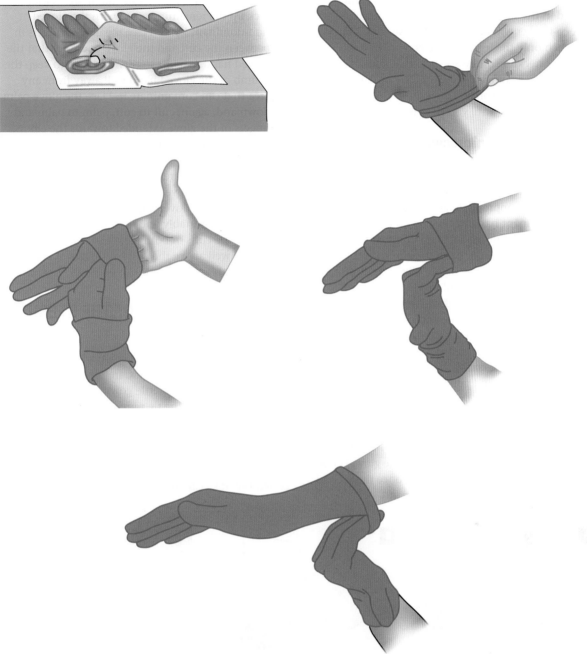

SOURCE: RADIOLOGY KEY, ASEPTIC TECHNIQUES, HTTPS://RADIOLOGYKEY.COM/ASEPTIC-TECHNIQUES-2/

FIGURE 4.9.1 Open gloving – steps for open gloving technique

thumb extended and away from any exposed skin. Keep your wrist straight so there is no chance that the fingers of the second glove can contact exposed skin. Lift the glove away from the packet and slip the fingers of the non-dominant hand into the glove.

- Adjust both gloves, making sure to touch only the sterile, outer surfaces of both gloves.

COMPLETE 'CLOSED GLOVING' PROCESS

Donning sterile gown

Wearing a sterile gown and closed gloving are usually carried out in areas such as an operating theatre where a surgical aseptic technique is being used. A critical

aseptic field is being maintained. Key parts and key sites are also being touched during surgical procedures.

After completing the surgical scrub, pick up the sterile gown in both hands along the inner seam at the neckline using only the thumb and first finger. The gown will be folded inside out. With the remaining three fingers of both hands grasp the bulk of the gown and move back from the table. Maintaining a hold with thumb and forefinger, and with arms at shoulder height, release the remaining three fingers of both hands to let the gown drop to its full length. The gown should not touch anything, so its sterility is maintained. Place one hand inside the shoulder of the gown. Repeat with the other hand and work both hands down the inside of the arms of the gown. Do not move fingers outside of the sleeve or touch any part of the outside of the gown, or the entire gown will become unsterile. Make sure hands do not emerge from the sleeves but remain inside the cuffs and encased in the sleeves. Use the sleeves as mittens.

A co-worker will be required to assist you. They will touch only the inside of the gown. They will adjust the neckline of the gown so that your uniform is entirely covered front and back. The neck ties will be tied by your co-worker. The waist ties remain tied in front of your waist until you have donned the gloves.

The 'closed gloving' process

- Keeping your hands enfolded within the cuffs of the sterile gown, flip open and flatten the sterile packet containing the gloves.
- Position the appropriate glove on the non-dominant hand by picking up the cuff of the glove with the sleeve-enclosed dominant hand and placing it cuff to cuff, palm to palm with the glove fingers pointing towards your elbow, and thumb to thumb (palm to palm and fingers along arm). With your non-dominant hand still inside the sleeves of the sterile gown, grasp the cuff of the glove lying on top of this non-dominant hand.
- Pull on the first sterile glove by grasping the upper, inner edge of the cuff with your sleeve-encased dominant hand and pulling it over the top of your non-dominant hand. The glove cuff should encase the entire hand and cuff of the gown. With the dominant hand holding the cuff of the gown, carefully advance the non-dominant hand into the glove. Do not be concerned if the glove is not properly fitted. It can be adjusted once the second sterile glove is on the dominant hand.

- To position the glove on the dominant hand, pick up the remaining glove with the gloved non-dominant hand. Place the gloved fingers in between the cuff and the glove to ensure that the gloved hand remains sterile. Take care to keep the thumb of the gloved hand well away from any area that can contaminate it. Place the glove palm down and, again, cuff to cuff, palm to palm and fingers of the glove extended towards the elbow.
- Pull on the second sterile glove in a similar manner to the first sterile glove, but using the gloved hand to carefully adjust the cuff of the second sterile glove. Again, carefully advance the hand into the glove. Adjust both gloves so that they fit comfortably and do not impair circulation. Adjust the cuffs of both gloves so that they extend well above the cuffs of the gown and are comfortable as well.

TIE THE WAIST TIES OF THE STERILE GOWN

Tie the waist ties of the sterile gown with the assistance of your co-worker. Carefully untie the waist ties in the front of the sterile gown, making sure that the entire length of the tie remains in your control. To do this, gather the ties into the palms of your hands before you untie the knot. Keep the front tie held in your left hand. Hand the furthest tip of the tie attached to the back of the gown to your sterile gloved co-worker. Take care not to contaminate your glove.

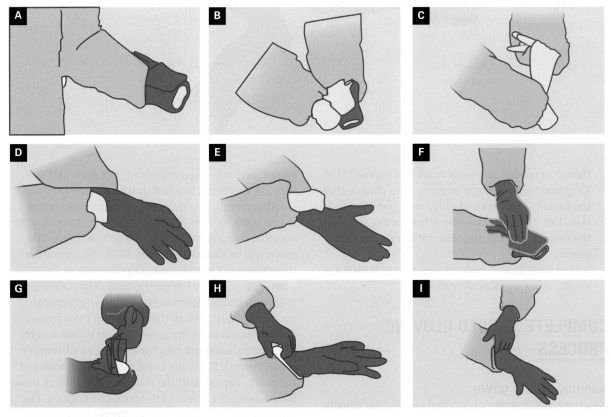

FIGURE 4.9.2 Closed gloving – steps for closed gloving technique

Some facilities prefer that the co-worker uses a sterile artery clip to take the tie. Carefully turn three-quarters of a circle, making sure that no sterile areas are contaminated. Grasp the tie held by your co-worker no further than halfway along its length. Your co-worker will drop the distal end of the tie (or disengage it from the artery clip). Tie the two ties together, making sure that you do not contaminate your hands on the distal portion of the tie.

DEFINE THE STERILE AREAS

The front of the gown is considered sterile to the waist. Arms are considered sterile to 5 cm above the elbows. Any area that is not visible is considered contaminated. All sterile procedures are carried out without extraneous movement since excessive movement increases the risk of contamination and creates air currents that could transmit organisms to the patient or to the sterile field.

CASE STUDY

Review the concepts of aseptic technique and different types of aseptic fields in **Skill 4.1** and further resources about aseptic technique to answer the following questions.

1. List three procedures that would require the use of sterile gloves within the ward area (e.g. they would include a critical aseptic field).

2. Identify two areas within the hospital where staff are required to use closed gloving in their routine procedures.

Note: These notes are summaries of the most important points in the assessments/procedures, and are not exhaustive on the subject. The naming of documents or charts may differ from state to state, and facility to facility. In all possible situations the guidelines of the ACSQHC are used when describing national charts or documents (e.g. the ACSQHC Observation and Response Chart is named the Adult Observation and Response Chart in WA, and the Rapid Detection and Response Observation Chart in SA). References of the materials used to compile the information have been supplied. The student is expected to have learned the material surrounding each skill as presented in the references. No single reference is complete on the subject.

REFERENCES

Victorian Department of Health. (2014). *Scrubbing, Gowning, Gloving and Asepsis Competency Tool*. Sector Performance, Quality and Rural Health, Victorian State Government.

RECOMMENDED READINGS

Australian College for Infection Prevention and Control (ACIPC). (2015). *Aseptic Technique During Invasive Clinical Procedures*. https://www.acipc.org.au/aseptic-technique-resources/

Johnson, J. & Osborne, S. (2016). Surgical hand antisepsis, gowning and gloving – not necessarily the way it has always been done. *ACORN: The Journal of Perioperative Nursing in Australia*, 29(2), 52–4.

ESSENTIAL SKILLS COMPETENCY

Gowning and Gloving (Open and Closed)
Demonstrates the ability to effectively and safely don sterile gown and gloves

Criteria for skill performance	Y	D
(Numbers indicate *Enrolled Nurse Standards for Practice*, 2016)	(Satisfactory)	(Requires development)
Open gloving		
1. Identifies indication (8.3, 8.4)		
2. Gathers equipment (1.2, 1.6, 4.4, 6.4, 8.4, 9.4): ■ gown pack containing a gown of appropriate size and sterile towel ■ sterile gloves of appropriate size		
3. Washes hands using a surgical scrub/handwash and dries hands using a sterile towel (1.2, 1.4, 1.8, 3.9, 6.4, 9.4)		
4. Opens the sterile wrapper containing the gloves (1.2, 1.4, 3.2, 8.4, 9.4)		
5. Removes glove correctly and pulls on the first sterile glove (1.2, 1.4, 1.8, 3.2, 3.9)		
6. Removes second glove correctly and pulls on the second sterile glove (8.4, 9.4)		
7. Defines the sterile areas (1.2, 1.4, 1.8, 3.2, 3.9, 4.1, 8.4, 9.4)		
8. Demonstrates ability to link theory to practice (8.3, 8.4, 8.5, 9.4)		
Closed gloving		
1. Identifies indication (8.3, 8.4)		
2. Gathers equipment (1.2, 1.6, 4.4, 6.4, 8.4, 9.4): ■ gown pack containing a gown of appropriate size and sterile towel ■ sterile gloves of appropriate size		
3. Washes hands using a surgical scrub/handwash and dries hands using a sterile towel (1.2, 1.4, 1.8, 3.9, 6.4, 9.4)		
4. Picks up the gown (1.2, 1.4, 3.2, 8.4, 9.4)		
5. Places hand inside gown shoulder, works the arms down (1.2, 1.4, 3.2, 8.4, 9.4)		
6. Has a co-worker tie the neck ties (1.2, 1.4, 3.2, 8.4, 9.4)		
7. Opens the sterile wrapper containing the gloves (1.2, 1.4, 3.2, 8.4, 9.4)		
8. Positions the glove on the non-dominant hand (1.2, 1.4, 3.2, 8.4, 9.4)		
9. Pulls on the first sterile glove (1.2, 1.4, 3.2, 8.4, 9.4)		
10. Positions the glove on the dominant hand (1.2, 1.4, 3.2, 8.4, 9.4)		
11. Pulls on the second sterile glove (1.2, 1.4, 3.2, 8.4, 9.4)		
12. Attends to waist ties of the sterile gown according to type (1.2, 1.4, 3.2, 8.4, 9.4)		
13. Defines the sterile areas (1.2, 1.4, 1.8, 3.2, 3.9, 4.1, 8.4, 9.4)		
14. Demonstrates ability to link theory to practice (8.3, 8.4, 8.5, 9.4)		

Student:

Clinical facilitator: Date:

CHAPTER 4.10

SURGICAL SCRUB (SURGICAL HAND WASH)

IDENTIFY INDICATIONS

Surgical scrubs are performed to remove resident and transient microorganisms from the arms and hands of the nurse and to leave an antimicrobial residue on the skin that discourages the growth of microorganisms for several hours. They are done prior to procedures in operating theatres, delivery suites and burn treatment units, and before some specific ward-based procedures that require a surgical aseptic technique and a critical aseptic field.

DEMONSTRATE PROBLEM-SOLVING ABILITIES

The initial surgical scrub for the day should be for 5 minutes. Subsequent scrubs are for 3 minutes (SA Health, 2020). Check the facility policy to determine the length of the scrub. Use of chlorhexidine solution as part of the scrub procedure is also required. Some areas may allow the alternative use of an alcohol-based hand rub (ABHR) if there is no evidence of soiling on the hands (NHMRC, 2019), and these should be used according to the manufacturer's instructions for approximately 3 minutes (SA Health, 2020). Research has shown it to be as effective as other handwashing and scrubbing (Liang Qin & Mehigan, 2017; SA Health, 2020). It is of key importance that all areas of the arms and hands have been cleaned, rinsed and dried (Johnson & Osborne, 2016). Each agency has its own protocol for surgical scrubbing so the following is therefore only a guide. Recent research has shown that use of a scrub brush increases the potential for skin damage, so some facilities may no longer use these as part of their scrub routine (Johnson & Osborne, 2016; SA Health, 2020).

GATHER EQUIPMENT

Once the procedure has commenced, touching anything that is not sterile necessitates starting the procedure over again.

- *Scrub sink.* The surgical scrub is done at a scrub sink with running warm water.
- *Antimicrobial scrub solution*, such as chlorhexidine gluconate, is used to remove microbes and leave an antimicrobial residue on the hands for several hours. Staff need to be aware of the potential for allergic responses to such solutions.
- *A sterile sponge/brush (for specialised areas such as operating theatre)* may still be used within some facilities to clean the fingernails (Department of Health, 2015), according to facility policy. They are supplied in a sealed pack that must be opened using aseptic technique. Some sponges are impregnated with a Betadine solution while others have no antimicrobial properties of their own. Others are a combination of sponge and brush for nails and creases, while others are just sponges.
- *A chlorhexidine/alcohol dispenser* with a non-touch operated plunger would be provided.
- *A sterile hand towel* is included in the gown pack and is situated on top of the gown for convenience. If there is no gown pack, a sterile towel pack will be used. Open these aseptically and ensure that the towel is fully exposed so that it can be picked up without contaminating either the hands or the gown underneath it.
- *Alcohol-based scrub solution* where there is an option in the facility.

PREPARE FOR THE SURGICAL SCRUB

Nails should be short, clean and free of polish. Artificial nails and chipped or old nail polish are both sources of microbial contamination because the minute cracks and crevices harbour Gram-negative microorganisms and fungus, so these must be removed before scrubbing (NHMRC, 2019). According to the level of required aseptic technique, aseptic field, patient risk assessment and the hospital area, put on the scrub cap (so that all hair is covered), face mask and eye protector before scrubbing. The top of the face mask has a metal strip embedded in the band. Place the face mask across the bridge of the nose and tie upper ties behind the head. With the bottom of the mask under the chin, tie the lower ties at the nape of the neck or over the top of the head. Pinch the metal strip so it sits snugly over the nose. If glasses are worn, the edge of the mask should be under the glasses to minimise fogging. Avoid talking, laughing and, if possible, sneezing or coughing when wearing a mask, since these activities dampen the mask and force microorganisms through and around the mask.

Once the hands are scrubbed, touching anything that is not sterile causes contamination and the scrub must then be repeated. Open and prepare the gown pack and gloves before scrubbing, so that they can be donned immediately. Place the pack in a convenient position. Open both packs using an aseptic technique relevant to setting up a critical aseptic field, exposing the towel and gown in the gown pack, so that the towel can be used when the scrub is completed.

PERFORM THE SURGICAL SCRUB

Adjust the water temperature

Taps are turned on and left on throughout the scrub so that they are not touched during the procedure. Taps at scrub sinks usually have knee, foot or sensor controls. Water must be warm for facilitating removal of microbes without damage to skin. Cold water is less efficient at removing oils and thus the microbes in them, and hot water can cause damage to the stratum corneum (keratin) layer of the epidermis, which allows microbes to penetrate to the living layers of the skin, so they can colonise.

Open the sponge/brush pack if required

Open the sponge/brush pack using aseptic technique. The pack is checked prior to opening to ensure sterility. The fully opened sponge/brush pack is placed at a convenient location (usually at the back of the sink) so it can be accessed without touching the packaging or the sink.

Wet hands and apply antimicrobial scrub solution

Hands are wet from fingertips to wrist, with fingertips kept higher since the fingertips will become the least contaminated area. Apply about 5 mL of antimicrobial solution. Do not touch the container with your hands. Most containers at scrub sinks will be arranged so that the elbow, feet or sensor controls can be used to access the solution. Work the solution into a lather. The next stages will vary according to policy. Some organisations require nurses to scrub hands before lathering the arms; others prefer them to wet and lather the hands and arms before scrubbing the nails. This gives the antimicrobial substance time to work. The sponge method or hand lathering is done according to the individual facility procedures.

Wash hands and clean beneath fingernails

Thoroughly wash hands using a firm circular motion on the backs and palms of the hands to loosen bacteria. Interlace the fingers and thumbs and rub the hands back and forth. Move each hand in turn down to the wrist and rotate the wrist in the palm of the opposite hand. For the first scrub of the session, while the hands are still lathered, pick up the brush and scrub beneath each nail to clean the debris out from under the nail. Debris is more easily removed from a wet surface.

Scrub hands and arms

All surfaces must be scrubbed – remember the four sides of each finger and thumb, the webs between the fingers, the lateral surfaces of each hand, as well as the back and palm. Be vigilant about scrubbing the creases in the palm, the knuckles and the wrist. Scrub up the forearm, dividing it into the lower, middle and upper forearm that continues to 5 cm above the elbow. Add water as needed to keep a good lather. Keep the fingertips higher than the elbows. When one hand/arm is completed, repeat the sequence for the other hand/arm.

Rinse the hands and arms thoroughly

Rinse the hands and arms thoroughly, keeping the fingertips higher than the elbow, to remove the loosened bacteria and sediment. When all traces of lather are rinsed off, turn the taps off with the foot, elbow or sensor control. If using the taps will contaminate your hands, leave the tap running for someone else to attend to. Keep hands up above the waist, elbows bent and arms extended in front.

Dry the hands and arms thoroughly

Dry the hands and arms thoroughly since moist skin is subject to chapping and breakdown. Carefully pick up the sterile towel from the gown pack by one corner. Use half of the towel to dry one hand/arm from fingertips to above the elbow. Pat and squeeze the skin dry while rotating the arm rather than rubbing. Holding the towel with the still wet hand, pick up the dry end with the dry hand and dry the remaining hand. Be sure the drying is thorough – it is very difficult to put gloves on damp skin. Discard the towel.

Continue with gowning and gloving

Keep the dry, clean hands in front of you and above your waist to prevent accidental contamination. Proceed to gowning and gloving (see **Skill 4.9**).

DOCUMENT AND REPORT RELEVANT INFORMATION

Documentation of this skill is not necessary as it is part of other procedures.

CASE STUDY

1. Locate and read the surgical scrub (surgical hand wash) policy in a facility where you are seconded for clinical practice.

2. Identify two areas within a hospital that would require staff to use a surgical scrub technique as part of their frequent work tasks.

3. Identify two nursing skills that require the use of a surgical aseptic technique and a surgical hand wash.

Note: These notes are summaries of the most important points in the assessments/procedures, and are not exhaustive on the subject. The naming of documents or charts may differ from state to state, and facility to facility. In all possible situations the guidelines of the ACSQHC are used when describing national charts or documents (e.g. the ACSQHC Observation and Response Chart is named the Adult Observation and Response Chart in WA, and the Rapid Detection and Response Observation Chart in SA). References of the materials used to compile the information have been supplied. The student is expected to have learned the material surrounding each skill as presented in the references. No single reference is complete on the subject.

REFERENCES

Department of Health. (2015). *Surgical Skin Disinfection Guideline*. Queensland Government. https://www.health.qld.gov.au/__data/assets/pdf_file/0020/444422/skin-disinfection.pdf

Johnson, J. & Osborne, S. (2016). Surgical hand antisepsis, gowning and gloving – not necessarily the way it has always been done. *ACORN: The Journal of Perioperative Nursing in Australia*, 29(2), pp. 52–4.

Liang Qin, L. & Mehigan, S. (2017). The effects of surgical hand scrubbing protocols on skin integrity and surgical site infection rates: A systematic review. *ACORN: The Journal of Perioperative Nursing in Australia*, 30(2), pp. 21–30.

National Health and Medical Research Council (NHMRC). (2019). *Australian Guidelines for the Prevention and Control of Infection in Healthcare*. https://www.nhmrc.gov.au/health-advice/public-health/preventing-infection

SA Health. (2020). *Hand Hygiene Clinical Guideline: Version 1.4*. Government of South Australia. https://www.sahealth.sa.gov.au/wps/wcm/connect/765d5d0046d2cefe9be0fb2e504170d4/Clinical_Guideline_Hand_Hygiene_v1.4+5.05.2020.pdf?MOD=AJPERES&CACHEID=ROOTWORKSPACE-765d5d0046d2cefe9be0fb2e504170d4-nxyXr3F

RECOMMENDED READINGS

Macinga, D.R., Edmonds, S.L., Campbell, E. & McCormack, R.R. (2014). Comparative efficacy of alcohol-based surgical scrubs: The importance of formulation. *AORN Journal*, 100(6), pp. 641–50.

ESSENTIAL SKILLS COMPETENCY

Surgical scrub

Demonstrates the ability to effectively and safely prepare to assist in a surgical procedure – surgical scrub

Criteria for skill performance	Y	D
(Numbers indicate *Enrolled Nurse Standards for Practice*, 2016)	(Satisfactory)	(Requires development)
1. Identifies indication (8.3, 8.4)		
2. Demonstrates problem-solving abilities; e.g. prepares gown pack and gloves before scrubbing; dons cap, face mask and eye protector before scrubbing (4.1, 4.2, 8.3, 8.4, 9.4)		
3. Gathers equipment to sink with running warm water (1.2, 1.6, 4.4, 6.4, 8.4, 9.4): ■ antiseptic or alcohol based scrub solution ■ sterile sponge/brush (if required by facility) ■ sterile hand towel		
4. Adjusts water temperature, opens sponge/brush pack (1.2, 1.4, 3.2)		
5. Wets hands and applies antiseptic scrub solution (1.2, 1.4, 1.8, 3.2, 3.9, 6.4, 8.4, 9.4)		
6. Washes hands and cleans beneath fingernails (1.2, 1.4, 1.8, 3.2, 3.9, 6.4, 8.4, 9.4)		
7. Scrubs hands and forearms (1.2, 1.4, 1.8, 3.2, 3.9, 6.4, 8.4, 9.4)		
8. Rinses hands (1.2, 1.4, 1.8, 3.2, 3.9, 6.4, 8.4, 9.4)		
9. Dries the hands and arms with sterile towel (1.2, 1.4, 1.8, 3.2, 3.9, 6.4, 8.4, 9.4)		
10. Continues with gowning and gloving (1.2, 1.4, 1.8, 3.2, 3.9, 6.4, 8.4, 9.4)		
11. Demonstrates ability to link theory to practice (8.3, 8.4, 8.5, 9.4)		

Student:

Clinical facilitator: Date:

CHAPTER **4.11**

CHEST DRAINS AND UNDERWATER SEAL DRAINAGE (UWSD) MANAGEMENT

IDENTIFY INDICATIONS

Chest or intrapleural drains are used to remove a collection of air (pneumothorax), fluid, pus (pyothorax) or blood (haemothorax) from the pleural space into a collecting device to restore negative pressure within the pleural cavity and drain fluid or blood (Berman et al., 2020).

This drainage of air or fluid from the pleural space via an intercostal catheter (ICC) (attached to the tubing of the chest drainage unit) allows negative intra-thoracic pressures to be re-established, leading to lung expansion (Royal Children's Hospital Melbourne [RCHM], 2016; Burch, 2020). The underwater seal apparatus (attached to the intercostal catheter) also prevents backflow of air or fluid into the pleural cavity, and prevents mediastinal shift. If the patient has a pneumothorax, a chest drain is inserted in the upper anterior chest. If there is blood or fluid in the chest, they are generally placed mid axillary at the 5th or 6th intercostal space. Chest drains may be inserted routinely in theatre (e.g. post certain thoracic surgeries), intensive care units, emergency departments and ward areas in emergency situations (RCHM, 2016). A chest X-ray is required post procedure to confirm the position is correct after insertion.

REVIEW SAFETY CONSIDERATIONS

Appropriate chest drain management is essential to maintain respiratory function and haemodynamic stability. Caring for patients with intrapleural chest drains requires knowledge and skill to ensure patient safety, avoid complications and prevent respiratory collapse.

Safety considerations include keeping a pair of 17 to 18 cm tubing clamps per drain at the bedside at all times while the chest drain is in situ for use in an emergency only (RCHM, 2016). Other clamping of chest tubes is contraindicated as a tension pneumothorax may develop. Milking the tube can also cause complications, and is only done with written orders from medical staff. Milking drains creates a high negative pressure that can cause pain, tissue trauma and bleeding (RCHM, 2016).

GATHER AND PREPARE EQUIPMENT

This is a time-management strategy as well as a confidence-increasing strategy. The nurse will be able to mentally rehearse the procedure as equipment is gathered. The patient will feel more confident in the nurse (thereby decreasing anxiety and reducing distress) if there are no interruptions in the procedure to return to the storage room for forgotten equipment. The following equipment is required for management of chest drains and UWSD:

- stethoscope
- sphygmomanometer
- thermometer
- pulse oximeter
- watch with second hand

Equipment used in care of a patient with a chest drain

There is a great variety of drainage systems available for use.

The UWSD systems can be sterile disposable underwater seal bottle/s that enable the removal of air and fluid from the pleural cavity that is released below the level of the water in the UWSD system. This system is a closed drainage system which creates a one-way valve between atmospheric pressure and the negative intrapleural pressure. The air and fluid in the intrapleural cavity are forced into and through the chest tube when the patient breathes out. This air/fluid bubbles out of the tubing and into the water (fluid), then out into the atmosphere (air). Since the end of the tube is under water, air cannot be sucked back into the intrapleural cavity and the negative intrapleural pressure caused by inspiration is not strong enough to pull the water all the way up the tubing.

Commercial drainage units are disposable, self-contained, multiple chamber systems, which consist of the drainage chamber, the water seal chamber and the suction chamber.

Dry collection chamber systems with one-way valves have been introduced to replace UWSD systems. As there are many sophisticated collection chambers available commercially, nurses must familiarise themselves with the manufacturer's instructions for products used.

A pair of 17 to 18 cm tubing clamps per drain are required at the bedside at all times while the chest drain is in situ, for use in emergency *only* (check facility policy).

IMPLEMENT ASSESSMENT AND MANAGEMENT OF THE PATIENT AND THE DRAINAGE SYSTEM

Perform hand hygiene

Perform hand hygiene before touching the patient or the patient's surrounds and prior to any procedure involving patient contact to reduce the possibility of cross-contamination. Hand hygiene is the most effective method of infection control as it removes transient organisms from the hands of the nurse (see **Skill 1.1**). This is particularly important for the patient who is vulnerable following surgery or trauma to the chest, or who has had a procedure such as insertion of an intercostal catheter.

Give a clear explanation and communicate effectively with the patient

Conditions that affect breathing and oxygenation are anxiety-producing, and increasing anxiety levels increase the body's need for oxygen. Patients who have chest drains require reassurance and information about the chest drainage system and their condition, which will help to reduce their anxiety. Explain to them that the chest drain is sutured in place. Moving in bed and moving around the room should not cause it to be displaced. Remind them that the tubing is flexible but fairly stiff and that they should not kink the tubing or lie on it because of the resulting obstruction. Explain to the patient that frequent observation of the system and checking of their status will be done. This allays fears that their condition is abnormal or worsening. Tell the patient what to expect in regard to normal drainage. The patient should also be educated that fluctuation of the water level and intermittent bubbling is normal. The patient is informed of the need for effective pain management and about the availability of prescribed analgesia and other pain management strategies. Ask the patient to immediately report any shortness of breath or chest pain.

Start-of-shift checks

At the start of the shift, assess the patient and the chest drain/s, and ensure all safety equipment is available and in working order. A head-to-toe approach is then required to monitor the patient's progress while the drainage is in place. Regular observations are central to maintaining a safe environment.

Assessment of the UWSD drainage system

The assessment of the UWSD should be carried out hourly as follows.

- Check that the underwater seal drainage unit is below the level of the chest so that fluid cannot flow backwards into the pleural cavity. It must be maintained in an upright position so that the end of the tubing remains below the waterline.
- Check that the tubing is securely anchored to the patient's skin to prevent pulling of the drain and prevent accidental dislodgement.
- Check that the tubing is free of kinks, dependent loops or other external obstructions to allow for free drainage.
- Check that all of the connections are secure and report any that are loose. A water seal drainage system must be airtight along the length of tubing between the pleural space and the water seal. Note the amount and colour of drainage. Mark the time and date on a line drawn at the level of the drainage each time the drainage volume is checked. Report any sudden decrease or absence of drainage, or excessive drainage to the registered nurse (RN) or medical officer. Observe the fluctuation of the fluid level in the drainage tube ('swinging'). The water should rise with inspiration and fall with expiration, provided suction is not being used. This fluctuation will stop when the lung is re-expanded, if the tubing is obstructed or if there are loose connections. If the fluctuation stops and the lung has not re-expanded, check the tubing for air leaks or for obstruction and report promptly. If the patient has a pneumothorax, observe for bubbling on expiration in the underwater seal chamber.
- If inserted for other conditions or procedures (e.g. surgery), drainage should decrease gradually and change from bloody to pink to straw colour.
- Observe the occlusive dressing for drainage and intactness. The insertion site should be checked daily, and the dressing around it kept clean and dry. Observe for signs of fluid drainage, inflammation, infection and subcutaneous emphysema (surgical emphysema).

Suction is not usually required. Technically, gravity drainage applies suction to enable any siphon system to work. In some cases, special low-level suction (via a thoracic low suction unit) may be attached to the drainage system if gravity drainage is not sufficient. These orders should be written by the medical staff. Check that the settings remain as ordered (RCHM, 2016). Some collection chambers, such as the dry system, include a suction regulator.

The enrolled nurse (EN) should familiarise themselves with the manufacturer's instructions and report any concerns to the RN/medical officer promptly.

Assess respiratory status

This is carried out every 1 to 2 hours unless the patient's condition warrants more frequent checking. Observe for skin colour, chest movement and quality of respirations as well as rate. Take oxygen saturation levels (see **Skill 2.5**). The EN may also be required to auscultate the chest, according to organisational policy. Report any concerns or alterations in the patient's condition immediately.

Assess vital signs

Following stabilisation, the vital signs (see **Skill 2.3**), including a pain assessment (see **Skill 2.9**), are monitored every 2 to 4 hours unless there are indications to assess more often. As always, follow the facility's policy.

Teach and encourage the patient to do coughing and deep breathing exercises

Coughing and deep respirations force air and fluid out of the intrapleural cavity. This increases the rate at which the lungs re-expand. The exercises should be done hourly, and an incentive spirometer may be used to assist the patient with deep breathing (see **Skill 3.15**).

Referral to the physiotherapist should be done to enhance chest movement and prevent a chest infection.

Assess pain

Effective coughing and deep breathing exercises are difficult, if not impossible, to achieve if the patient is experiencing pain; therefore, effective pain management is essential.

To reduce pain, patients may tend to breathe shallowly, which consequently can increase the risk of a chest infection. Patients should be prescribed effective analgesics (Millar, 2018) to encourage deep breathing and mobility, with pain assessments conducted frequently and documented. Adequate supporting of the intrapleural chest drain tubing may also help.

Change the patient's position frequently

Reposition the patient regularly for comfort as well as to promote drainage (e.g. semi-upright or upright position). Encourage active or passive range-of-movement exercises on the shoulder of the affected side as the patient may limit movement of that side to reduce discomfort at the insertion site (Berman et al., 2020).

Psychological care

Patients with respiratory issues are often breathless and anxious. In addition to supporting these patients with their activities of daily living (ADLs), such as hygiene, nutrition and hydration, the nurse is often required to offer extra attention and reassurance, and repeat explanations of any required procedures.

CLEAN, REPLACE OR DISPOSE OF EQUIPMENT

Replacing used equipment increases efficiency and demonstrates regard for fellow staff members. Drainage units are disposed of fully intact in the biological waste. Put on gloves and other protective equipment as per facility policy.

DOCUMENT AND REPORT RELEVANT INFORMATION

Documentation of care given to a patient with the chest drain must include the results of vital signs and respiratory assessments on the observation and response chart. Other information about the drainage tubes may also be recorded on this chart. Further documentation will include the fluid balance chart for drainage loss, nursing care plan and patient progress notes.

CASE STUDY

Ben Ewart is a thin, tall 24 year-old male patient who suffered a large spontaneous pneumothorax while playing hockey. He had a similar problem about 5 years ago. He has just arrived on your ward, post insertion of an intercostal catheter (attached to UWSD) in the emergency department (ED) of the hospital.

1. Describe the nursing management of the UWSD system as it applies to Ben (i.e. for air and fluid drainage).

   From your observations, Ben appears rather anxious and states that he can see lightly coloured blood-stained fluid and bubbles appearing in the drainage bottle. He has also noticed that the fluid moved 'up and down' (swinging) in the drainage tube. The doctor in the ED had explained the procedure and what to expect after the ICC insertion, but Ben can't remember all that he was told, and the analgesia given in the ED has made him feel a little tired and drowsy.

2. Describe how you will answer his concerns/questions.

   Ben is encouraged to use the incentive spirometer in order to facilitate chest expansion, but is hesitant about using this device due to concerns regarding increasing his pain and discomfort.

3. How will you manage these concerns he has regarding pain?

Note: These notes are summaries of the most important points in the assessments/procedures, and are not exhaustive on the subject. The naming of documents or charts may differ from state to state, and facility to facility. In all possible situations the guidelines of the ACSQHC are used when describing national charts or documents (e.g. the ACSQHC Observation and Response Chart is named the Adult Observation and Response Chart in WA, and the Rapid Detection and Response Observation Chart in SA). References of the materials used to compile the information have been supplied. The student is expected to have learned the material surrounding each skill as presented in the references. No single reference is complete on the subject.

REFERENCES

Burch, A. (2020). Management of the patient with spontaneous pneumothorax. *Medsurg Nursing,* May/Jun 2020, 29(3): , pp. 209–10.

Berman, A., Frandsen, G., Snyder, S., Levett-Jones, T., Burston, A., Dwyer, T., Hales, M., Harvey, N., Moxham, L., Langtree, T., Reid-Searl, K., Rolf, F. & Stanley, D. (2020). *Kozier & Erb's Fundamentals of Nursing, Volumes 1–3.* (5th ed.) Melbourne: Pearson.

Millar, F.R. & Hillman, T. (2018). Managing chest drains on medical wards. *BMJ*, 363, p. k4639.

Royal Children's Hospital Melbourne (RCHM). (2016). *Chest Drain Management. Clinical Guidelines (Nursing).* https://www.rch.org.au/rchcpg/hospital_clinical_guideline_index/Chest_Drain_Management/

ESSENTIAL SKILLS COMPETENCY

Chest Drains and Underwater Seal Drainage Management

Demonstrates the ability to effectively and safely manage a patient who has a chest drain/underwater seal drainage

Criteria for skill performance	Y	D
(Numbers indicate *Enrolled Nurse Standards for Practice*, 2016)	(Satisfactory)	(Requires development)
1. Identifies indication (8.3, 8.4)		
2. Discusses special considerations (1.2, 3.2)		

3. Gathers equipment (1.2, 1.6, 4.4, 6.4, 8.4, 9.4):
  ▪ stethoscope
  ▪ sphygmomanometer
  ▪ thermometer
  ▪ pulse oximeter
  ▪ watch		

4. Performs hand hygiene (1.2, 1.4, 1.8. 3.9, 6.4, 9.4)		
5. Evidence of effective communication with the patient; e.g. gives patient a clear explanation of procedure, reassurance of the patient, gains consent (2.1, 2.3, 2.4, 2.5, 6.3)		
6. Assesses the underwater seal drainage system hourly (1.2, 1.4, 1.8, 3.2, 3.9, 4.1, 4.2, 4.4, 6.4, 6.6, 8.4, 9.4)		
7. Assesses the patient's respiratory status 1- to 2-hourly and assesses vital signs (1.2, 1.4, 1.8, 3.2, 3.9, 4.1, 4.2, 4.4, 6.4, 6.6, 8.4, 9.4)		
8. Assesses pain (1.2, 1.4, 1.8, 2.1, 3.2, 4.1, 4.2, 6.6, 7.1, 8.4)		
9. Teaches and encourages coughing and deep breathing exercises (1.2, 1.4, 3.2, 4.2, 6.3, 7.3, 7.5, 8.4, 9.4)		
10. Assists the patient to change position (1.2, 1.4, 1.8, 2.3, 2.7, 3.2, 3.9, 4.4, 6.1, 6.3, 6.4, 8.4, 9.4)		
11. Cleans, replaces and disposes of equipment appropriately (1.2, 1.4, 3.9, 6.5, 9.4)		
12. Documents and reports relevant information (1.2, 1.3, 1.8, 3.2, 5.3, 6.6, 7.1, 7.2, 7.3, 7.4, 7.5)		
13. Demonstrates ability to link theory to practice (8.3, 8.4, 8.5, 9.4)		

Student:

Clinical facilitator: Date:

MEDICATION

Note: These notes are summaries of the most important points in the assessments/procedures and are not exhaustive on the subject. References of the materials used to compile the information have been supplied. The student is expected to have learnt the material surrounding each skill as presented in the references. No single reference is complete on each subject.

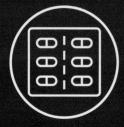

CHAPTER **5.1**

MEDICATION ADMINISTRATION – ORAL, SUBLINGUAL, BUCCAL, TOPICAL AND RECTAL

IDENTIFY INDICATIONS

Oral medication is the most common form of medication, and involves swallowing a medication in some form. It is the least expensive method of medication administration and, generally, the least unpleasant to patients. Drugs have a slower rate of absorption by the oral route because of the time required to digest and absorb them.

Sublingual medications such as glyceryl trinitrate spray are administered under the tongue and are quickly absorbed through the mucous membranes.

Buccal administration involves placing a tablet or lozenge in the cheek cavity and allowing it to dissolve and be absorbed over time.

Topical medications include creams, lotions, powder and ointments, as well as patches and rectally administered medications, such as suppositories. They are absorbed through skin or mucosa and may be ordered in place of oral or parenteral drugs.

VERIFY THE DOCTOR'S ORDER

Verify the doctor's order prior to administering the medication since no medication can be legally administered without a valid, signed order from a qualified healthcare provider (dentists and nurse practitioners are licensed to prescribe a limited number of medications). A valid medication order should be written on the relevant National Inpatient Medication Chart (ACSQHC, 2019a) or the national residential medication chart (ACSQHC, 2019b). A valid order consists of the patient's full name; the time, date, month and year the order is written; the generic drug name (clearly written and correctly spelled); the dose, strength and amount; the route of administration; and the frequency or time of day of administration. The doctor's signature and legible printing of their name must also be documented on this order. Some over-the-counter (OTC) or non-prescription medications can be given without an order. These are usually listed in the facility's policy manual, and must be recorded as a nurse-initiated medication on the medication chart.

Nurses are responsible and accountable for questioning any order that is unclear, incomplete or that seems inappropriate or unreasonable for the patient. To do this, the nurse must also know the patient's diagnosis, the purpose of the medication, its therapeutic effect, any side effects or adverse and toxic effects, the usual dose and any pertinent nursing implications, such as the ability to swallow, as well as the patient factors that mediate response to drugs such as age, weight and psychological factors. So that potentially harmful substances are not administered, the nurse must also ascertain any drug or food allergies that the patient may have by checking the allergies on the medication chart, noting if the patient is wearing an allergy alert ID band and asking the patient if they have any allergies. For oral medications, the patient must be able to take the drug by mouth; that is, the patient does not have an NBM (nil by mouth) or fasting order (determine if some medications are still to be administered when fasting), does not have nausea or vomiting, and is able to swallow. The nurse must observe for signs of irritation or allergy to topical medications. Evidence of effectiveness must also be observed with some medications; for example, the patient reports to be nausea free 30 minutes post administration of an oral anti-emetic, or evacuation has occurred post administration of an evacuant rectal suppository.

ABIDE BY THE GENERAL CONCEPTS OF WORKING WITH THERAPEUTIC SUBSTANCES

Legal responsibilities when working with medications include their secure storage and safe administration. All medications should be kept in a locked medications drawer, cupboard or trolley. Controlled substances (schedule 4R and schedule 8 drugs) are kept in double-locked cabinets attached to a wall to which access is limited by the use of one set of keys. Keys are always in the possession of a registered nurse (RN). A precise inventory of all controlled drugs is kept as they are used, wasted or added to the unit stock. Facility policy will determine the frequency for checking stock of restricted medications.

No medication can be administered without a valid signed order written by the prescribing doctor onto the medication sheet. Verbal orders and telephone orders are acceptable at some facilities, but there will be a protocol for their use. The nurse receiving the order has it and the transcription verified by a second nurse. The doctor responsible must sign the order within 24 hours. Any abbreviation used in a medication order must be approved by the facility, and follow the abbreviations recommended for use in the National Inpatient Medication Chart user guide (ACSQHC, 2016). The enrolled nurse (EN) student can currently administer drugs up to schedule 4 under the supervision of the RN, but this will depend on the relevant legislation and health department policies in each state.

Calculating accurate dosages is an essential skill required to ensure safe administration of medications. A mathematical calculation is used to determine the dose for each patient. One of the common formulae used is:

$$\frac{\text{strength (or stock) required}}{\text{strength (or stock) available}} \times \frac{\text{volume}}{1}$$

Paediatric and geriatric dosage calculations are especially critical because of the physiological differences in the young and very old (relative body size, immature or degenerating organ systems) that make the margin for error smaller, as well as making the response to the drug more unpredictable. These calculations may use a different formula and refer to nomograms to calculate correct dosage. Check any drug calculations with the RN. Ensure that the environment is distraction-free, in order to avoid chance of error.

Drug names and classifications are designed to organise the vast amount of information known about medications. Medications generally have three names. The chemical name reflects the chemical composition of the drug. The generic name is often derived from the chemical name, but is shorter. Drugs are listed in the MIMS under the generic name. This is also the name that should be used when drugs are ordered. The trade name is the name given by the manufacturer for marketing purposes. An example is paracetamol (generic name), which is sold in supermarkets or pharmacies as, among others, Panadol and Dymadon (trade names). Drugs are classified according to the body systems on which they exert their effects (e.g. cardiac, renal, musculoskeletal), the clinical indications (e.g. antihypertensive, diuretic, anti-inflammatory) or the physiologic properties (e.g. beta-blockers, calcium channel blockers).

Responsibility to the patient involves assessment, health teaching and patient advocacy. Assessment of the physiological or psychological function that the drug is expected to affect is required prior to and after administering medications. Examples would be pain assessment prior to administering analgesia, pulse assessment prior to administering Digoxin and BP assessment when administering an antihypertensive. These assessments may indicate that the RN should be notified and the drug may be withheld, or they could provide a baseline for use in evaluating the effectiveness of the drug. The nurse must also assess the patient's medication history (a review of the patient's current and past drugs used – prescribed, OTC or recreational) and history of allergies or adverse reactions to drugs. Some OTC drugs and herbal preparations (including vitamins) may interfere with prescription medications, potentially influencing drug effectiveness, toxicity or adverse reactions. Patient understanding of their medications is of key importance and helps to increase safety in medication administration. Educate the patient and provide printed information about medications, dose of the drug, its frequency, adverse effects and how to minimise these to the patient. They need to know any implications of taking the drug (e.g. if it should be taken with meals or on an empty stomach), and if it should be taken in the morning but not in the evening (e.g. diuretics ordered twice a day are usually given at 0800 hours and 1400 hours so the patient can sleep at night). Maintaining the drug regimen at home is discussed and adaptations of the scheduling of the drugs is made to accommodate the patient's home schedule without compromising the efficacy of the drug. Be alert to any cues the patient or family might give about not continuing to use the drug (i.e. cost, inconvenience, side effects, negative self-concept). Discussion of these may improve the patient's commitment to sustaining the prescribed treatment.

UNDERSTAND SAFETY MECHANISMS OF DRUG ADMINISTRATION

- Understand the facility's system for administering drugs. There are generally two systems in use. The first is the stock supply/individual patient supply, in which stock and labelled patient prescriptions are kept at the patient's bedside in a locked drawer or on a trolley and dispensed as needed from the bulk supplies and the patient's prescriptions. The second system in common use in residential aged care facilities is the unit dose system (e.g. Webster packs, DoseAid sachet packaging). In the system, all drugs (other than controlled/schedule drugs) that the patient will take in a 24-hour period are dispensed by the pharmacy and individually packaged with the drug name, dose and expiration date, as well as the patient name, number and name of the ordering doctor.
- Electronic management and dispensing systems have been implemented in some newer or updated

facilities. Medication is dispensed in a specific dispensing room, using a barcode on a patient's medication chart. Refer to facility policy guidelines.

- Prepare medications in a quiet place without distractions. Avoid interruptions and engaging in conversations so your concentration is focused on preparing the drug. Use a 'Do not disturb' sign to prevent disruptions.
- Use only medications from containers whose labels are complete and clear to avoid mistaking one medication for another.
- Check the expiration date on each medication. Do not give out-of-date medications as their potency may be affected. Do not give medications that are discoloured or are cloudy or have sediment (if liquid) if they should not be so.
- Do not touch the medication with your hand or fingers. It breaches the practice of maintaining an aseptic technique. Minute particles of the drug may irritate or be absorbed by the skin. Maintain a non-touch technique by using the cap of containers to dispense the required number of tablets before you tip them into the medication cup. If touching the medication is required, wear non-sterile gloves to reduce exposure of the nurse to the medication via the skin.
- Do not leave medications unattended or out of your sight since they may be taken or removed by unauthorised individuals.
- If interrupted during medication preparation by a more urgent task, return the medications to the storage area, secure them and repeat safety checks when resuming the medication round. This reduces the errors made by loss of concentration.

- Do not return an unused, unlabelled medication to a container to prevent inadvertent mixing of two medications or placement of a medication in an incorrect container.
- Check the medication chart for an allergy caution, look for an allergy ID band (red) and ask the patient if they have any known allergies.
- Administer only medications that you have dispensed personally.
- Observe that the patient takes their medication to ensure the correct administration of the prescribed drug to the correct patient at the correct time. Never leave a medication on a bedside locker for the patient to take at a later time.
- Ensure skin patches are applied correctly and securely, old patches are removed and the sites are rotated to prevent irritation.
- Some drugs require the special precaution of being double-checked by two RNs because of their potency or to prevent accidental errors in dosage. Check the policy of the facility.
- Listen to the patient. Many, if not most, patients know their medications well and any query by them as to the number or appearance of the medication should be taken seriously before administering the dose. This validates the patient's knowledge and prevents drug administration errors.
- Sign (or initial) the medications sheet as soon as a dose of medication is taken by the patient. This prevents a potential overdose since another nurse might administer a second dose of the medication thinking that it has not been given.

GATHER EQUIPMENT

- *Medications*. In acute areas, medications are kept at the patient's bedside in a locked drawer or a locked cupboard or the locked medication dispensing room. Other areas may use a locked medication trolley. The drawer or trolley is usually stocked with all of the necessary equipment for administering medication, such as pill cutters and a medication crusher.
- *The medication chart* with the signed valid order.
- *Medication cup* for holding the pills as they are dispensed.

- *Equipment to aid preparation and administration*, such as pill cutters or crushers, and oral liquid dispensers will be required according to the medication prescribed or patient needs. Use of specific dispensers with oral liquids is required. Topical medications will require the use of non-sterile gloves for application. Insertion of rectal medications will require non-sterile gloves, a 'bluey', a paper bag, a kidney dish and a lubricant.

PROCESS FOR MEDICATION ADMINISTRATION

Perform hand hygiene

Perform hand hygiene before touching the patient or the patient's surrounds and prior to any procedure involving patient contact to reduce the possibility of cross-contamination. Hand hygiene is the most effective method of infection control as it removes transient organisms from the hands of the nurse

(see **Skill 1.1**). Oral medication administration uses a non-touch technique and hand hygiene to prevent contamination of the medication and reduce the microorganisms that could be transmitted to the alimentary tract of the patient.

Give a clear explanation of the procedure and establish therapeutic communication

Establish therapeutic communication by identifying your patient and gaining the patient's consent. Checking the patient and gaining their consent will also ensure that you meet legal and policy requirements before implementing any procedure. Give the patient a clear explanation of the procedure and name of the drug, and determine the patient's knowledge of it. They should be aware of its name, the dose they take, its expected effects and probable side effects. This gives the patient information on which to base decisions about treatment. If required, refer to the relevant facility medication resource to clarify your knowledge. Ask the patient about any drug or medication allergies. Once the patient has consented to take the medication, the nurse discusses how to maximise the effects and minimise the adverse effects of the medication. Discussing the medication with the patient gives them a sense of control. It also allows the nurse to assess if more teaching is required, and to gauge the patient's understanding of their treatment. Determine the patient's preferred fluid with which to take medication. Cold fluids are preferable as they minimise bitter aftertastes of some medications.

Ensure that patients using transdermal patches are aware that they should not remove the patch themselves, as nursing staff will do this at the appropriate time.

If a rectal suppository is for bowel evacuation, the patient must be given a clear explanation of the expected outcome. The nurse must ensure the call bell is at hand and toilet facilities are easily available.

Demonstrate problem-solving abilities

Position the patient to facilitate the medication administration. Most patients prefer to sit upright to swallow medications. If that position is impossible, the patient should be positioned for safety and comfort; for example, lying on their side rather than supine. Assessing the patient for ability to sit, swallow and follow instructions is important to secure the safety of the patient. Some medications require assessment of the patient prior to administering them. Examples are a respiratory assessment prior to administering a bronchodilator in an asthmatic patient, fluid balance for a patient receiving diuretics, pulse assessment prior to administering digitalis, and respiratory rate and depth before administering a narcotic.

Obtaining an appropriate form of the medication facilitates its administration. A patient may be unable to swallow a tablet, making the liquid form of the medication more effective. Although many tablets can be crushed (with exceptions such as enteric-coated, slow-release and foul-tasting tablets), the safety for crushing a medication should be checked with the pharmacist or area policy before proceeding. Some areas may also require separate crushing and administering of individual tablets to reduce the risk of medication interaction. A clean crushing device prevents contamination of the drug with traces of previous drugs. Mix the crushed tablet with soft food (jam, yoghurt, apple sauce) to assist the patient to swallow it. The medication trolley (if in use) and the original medication chart are taken to the patient's bedside.

Use the 'rights of medication administration'

There are a minimum of eight 'rights of medication administration'. These include the following.

1. *The right time.* There is a scheduled medication administration time for most medications ordered on a regular, set basis (e.g. BD, QID) as an organisational time-management strategy. If using the standard schedule would compromise the drug order, an individual patient's needs or the effectiveness of the drug, the nurse has the discretion to accommodate patient preferences or to maximise drug effectiveness and discuss the prescribed time with the doctor and/or pharmacist. Some drugs, such as insulin given prior to a meal, are required to be given at a specified time. PRN (as needed) drugs are given as required, not to a set time.

2. *The right medication* is chosen, after verifying the validity of the order, from the drugs in the drawer or trolley. The name of the medication on the container label is checked three times against the ordered medication: first when the medication is picked up from the drawer or trolley, second against the medication order when the medication is dispensed out of the container and third when the medication is returned to the drawer or trolley.

3. *Right expiration date.* Ensure the medication has not expired or been opened longer than the recommended time.

4. *Ensure the medication is given via the right route.* The right route must always be followed and is noted from the medication chart (each route is discussed below and in further skills).

5. *The right dose* is imperative to gain a therapeutic level of the medication. Calculate the dose to be given and check your calculations with the RN.

6. *The right patient* receiving the medication is vital. Complete three points of patient identification by asking the patient to give you their name and date of birth, then check their name, date of birth and patient identification number (on the identification band) against the label on the medication chart. It is a safety requirement to check the identification of any patient every time a medication is administered.

7. *The right prescription/documentation* includes a correctly completed medication chart and medication order. The right documentation is completed when the medication has been given and swallowed and the medication chart is signed by the nurse. Initial the slot beside the time the drug was given – this will be beside the individualised medication order which describes the drug name, dose, route, time and prescriber's details. If the drug was not given, note this on the medication sheet using the appropriate code from the 'reason for nurse not administering' box

on the medication chart. Describe the reason and the actions undertaken by the nurse in the patient notes.

8. *Right to refuse.* The patient has the right to refuse to take a medication. Consent for administration of the medication must be obtained. If the medication is refused, note this on the medication sheet using the appropriate code from the 'reason for nurse not administering' box on the medication chart. Describe the reason and the actions undertaken by the nurse in the patient notes.

Other 'rights' to follow include: right reason, right preparation, right identification of allergies, right response and right education.

Facility and health department policy in each state will refer to different numbers of 'rights' for medication administration. *While these variations exist, the actual rights all reflect the same requirement.*

Administer oral medications

Prepare the medication

Tablets or capsules are poured from the container into the lid of the container using an aseptic technique, and then transferred to the medication cup so that the nurse's hands or fingers do not touch the medication. It also enables counting the correct number of tablets. Several different tablets and capsules can be placed in the same medication cup. Keep tablets/capsules that require an assessment prior to administration separate (in an extra cup) so they can be withheld if necessary. Tablets that are pre-scored can be halved by using a pill cutter. Check with the pharmacist for instructions on whether the tablet is safe to be split. Tablets to be crushed (note that some medications cannot be crushed – if in doubt check with the pharmacist) are crushed using a specific pill crusher or in a clean mortar, and ground to a fine powder with the pestle. Each pill is crushed and administered separately – not mixed together (Lohmann et al., 2015). The crushed medication is then mixed with a soft food for administration. Medications that come as a powder are mixed with water or juice at the bedside so there is no time for them to solidify and become difficult to swallow. Effervescent powders/tablets are given quickly after they dissolve as this often improves their palatability.

Liquid medication is shaken if it is a suspension to distribute the drug evenly through the liquid. The cap is removed and placed upside down on a surface to avoid contaminating the inside of the cap. The oral dispenser method is preferred for accuracy in measurement. This includes an enteral syringe with a compatible connector that is attached to the bottle and must be used to reduce risk of administration route errors. They are stored separately from other syringes and should also be labelled as oral dispensers. The tip of this dispenser will not connect to an intravenous (IV) injection site. The enteral syringe is removed from its packaging and the tip connected to the supplied connector. The plunger is slowly withdrawn until the correct dose is obtained.

The enteral syringe is removed from its packaging and the tip connected to the supplied connector. The plunger is slowly withdrawn until the correct dose is obtained.

Prior to the administration of any medications, the eight rights of medication administration must be observed.

Assist the patient to take the medication

In most instances, this is accomplished by handing the patient the medicine cup and a glass of fresh water or beverage of their choice. Tablets or capsules placed on the back of the tongue stimulate the swallowing reflex and are more easily swallowed. Tipping the head slightly forward facilitates swallowing. If the patient cannot hold the medication cup, use the cup (or a teaspoon) to introduce the tablets one at a time into the patient's mouth. Give the patient plenty of time to swallow each medication before introducing another. Liquid medications are dispensed directly from the oral dispenser into the mouth. Oral lozenges should be given last, and the patient advised to suck and not swallow or chew the lozenge.

If the patient has a nasogastric or percutaneous endoscopic gastrostomy (PEG) tube, refer to **Skill 5.5**.

Administer sublingual medication

Sublingual medications are administered onto the mucous membranes under the patient's tongue. Ask the patient to open their mouth and lift their tongue. Place the tablet or spray onto the area at the base of the tongue (Gray et al., 2018). Instruct the patient not to swallow the medication. Ensure all the medication is absorbed under the tongue before drinking or eating any food. Advise the patient to let the medication dissolve and be absorbed by the mucous membranes in the area.

Administer buccal medication

To administer buccal tablets or drops, put on gloves and use fingers to open the side of the patient's mouth. Place the drops or tablet onto the oral mucosa of the cheek, near the molars. Patients should not chew or swallow buccal medication (Gray et al., 2018). Advise the patient to let the medication dissolve and be absorbed by the mucous membranes in the area.

Administer topical medications

Ensure patient privacy and assist the patient into a comfortable/required position. Put on non-sterile gloves. Assess the condition of the patient's skin and then apply the required cream, ointment or topical patch. Cream should be applied as a thin smear over the skin surface. Transdermal patches should be marked with the date and time, sites rotated and old patches removed and discarded appropriately when a new patch is applied.

PART 5

Administer rectal medications, such as suppositories

Suppositories may be ordered as a medication therapy or to facilitate bowel movement. Prepare the patient by having them turn onto the left side and flex the right knee. Ensure privacy is maintained. Place a 'bluey' under the patient's buttocks. Don non-sterile gloves, unwrap the suppository and apply lubricating gel as required. Separate the buttocks and apply a little gel to the anus. Gently insert the suppository approximately 3 to 4 cm into the rectum using your index finger. It may help the patient to take deep breaths at this stage. After the suppository is inserted correctly, gently withdraw your finger. Remove gloves, reposition patient as required and dispose of equipment correctly.

When administering an **enema**, prepare the patient similarly to administering a suppository. Don non-sterile gloves. Prepare the enema by removing the small cap and lubricate the nozzle. Gently separate the buttocks with your non-dominant hand then slowly insert the nozzle of the enema into the patient's rectum, holding the enema by the lower end. Gently progress the enema the full length of the nozzle. Ensure you do not push hard against any resistance you might feel as this may cause damage to the bowel. When the enema is fully inserted into the rectum, grasp the lower end of the enema containing the fluid and squeeze from the base to insert the fluid into the rectum. Do not let go as you squeeze out all of the fluid, otherwise fluid will return from the rectum and back into the enema. Fingers can be moved upwards to assist insertion of all fluid, and the package rolled up if it is a larger sized enema. Maintaining the squeezing of the packaging, remove the enema when all fluid has been administered.

If the suppository or enema is to assist with bowel elimination, ensure the call bell is in reach. Tell the patient to try to remain lying on their left side and retain the suppository/enema for approximately 15 minutes if possible. Assist them to the toilet if required.

Perform hand hygiene

Maintain the 5 Moments for Hand Hygiene and perform hand hygiene after touching the patient and the patient's surrounds.

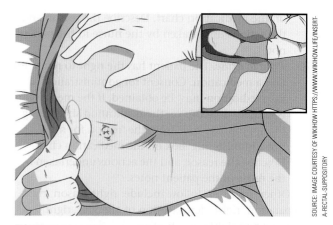

FIGURE 5.1.1 Inserting a suppository

Note: Insert suppository using forefinger

CLEAN, REPLACE OR DISPOSE OF EQUIPMENT

Anything used for the administration of a medication is discarded if disposable or cleaned and returned to the drawer or trolley if non-disposable. Medications are ordered from the pharmacy if they are running low. The medication chart is returned to its designated place for the next medication round. Gloves and 'blueys' are disposed of correctly.

DOCUMENT AND REPORT RELEVANT INFORMATION

Documentation is done on the medication chart and consists of an initial or signature in the appropriate time slot beside the drug order. Only authorised abbreviations should be used. If an assessment was done (e.g. pulse, BP), it is also noted in the designated section on the medication chart. If a patient has refused to take a medication or some other unexpected event occurs, use the relevant code on the medication chart in the appropriate time slot (e.g. if patient is vomiting, mark V in a circle) and then document more fully in the patient's notes. The effects of the medications – expected or unexpected – are assessed 30 minutes to 1 hour after administration and this is documented. Side effects/adverse effects should be reported to the doctor and the remaining doses of the drug withheld.

CASE STUDY

Joseph Martin is a 63-year-old man admitted to your ward for management of his hypertension. He is also a type 2 diabetic. You are completing the 0800 hours medication round on the second day of Joseph's admission, and he has asked you about his medications. He has said there is one more tablet than he normally takes at home, and another tablet is a different colour to his normal breakfast medications. You review the medication chart to identify the medications Joseph brought in when he was admitted, and the medications he is currently prescribed as an inpatient. Your facility dispenses medications from their generic hospital stock, and not the patient's personal supply.

1. The doctor has prescribed one new medication for Joseph, but all the other medications are the same as he took at home. How will you explain this to the patient and respond to his query about his medications?

2. List the eight rights you need to follow when administering medication to a patient.
3. How will you identify the correct patient?
4. What is the correct medication chart that should be used for an inpatient in an acute hospital?
5. What do you need to check to ensure you have a valid medication order?
6. The patient asks you to leave the tablets on his bedside locker and he will take them later. How will you respond to this?
7. When will you sign the medication chart?
8. One of the medication orders requires only half a tablet. How will you give half a tablet?
9. The patient is also prescribed glyceryl trinitrate, sublingual PRN. Describe where and how you will give this medication when it is required.

Note: These notes are summaries of the most important points in the assessments/procedures, and are not exhaustive on the subject. The naming of documents or charts may differ from state to state, and facility to facility. In all possible situations the guidelines of the ACSQHC are used when describing national charts or documents (e.g. the ACSQHC Observation and Response Chart is named the Adult Observation and Response Chart in WA, and the Rapid Detection and Response Observation Chart in SA). References of the materials used to compile the information have been supplied. The student is expected to have learned the material surrounding each skill as presented in the references. No single reference is complete on the subject.

REFERENCES

Australian Commission on Safety and Quality in Health Care (ACSQHC). (2016). *National Inpatient Medication Chart User Guide*. https://www.safetyandquality.gov.au/publications-and-resources/resource-library/national-inpatient-medication-chart-nimc-user-guide

Australian Commission on Safety and Quality in Health Care (ACSQHC). (2019a). *National Standard Medication Charts*. https://www.safetyandquality.gov.au/our-work/medication-safety/medication-charts/national-standard-medication-charts

Australian Commission on Safety and Quality in Health Care (ACSQHC). (2019b). *National Residential Medication Chart*. https://www.safetyandquality.gov.au/our-work/medication-safety/national-residential-medication-chart

Gray, S., Ferris, L., White, L.E., Duncan, G. & Baumle, W. (2018). *Foundations of Nursing: Enrolled Nurses* (2nd ANZ ed.). Melbourne: Cengage.

Lohmann, K., Gartner, D., Kurze, R., Schösler, T., Schwald, M., Störzinger, D., Hoppe-Tichy, T., Haefeli, W.E. & Seidling, H. M. (2015). More than just crushing: a prospective pre-post intervention study to reduce drug preparation errors in patients with feeding tubes. *Journal of Clinical Pharmacy and Therapeutics*, 40(2), pp. 220–5.

RECOMMENDED READINGS

Broyles, B., Reiss, B., Evans, M., McKenzie, G., Pleunik, S. & Page, R. (2020). (3rd ed.). *Pharmacology in Nursing: Australian and New Zealand Edition*. Melbourne: Cengage.

Nursing and Midwifery Board of Australia (NMBA). (2020). *Fact Sheet: Enrolled Nurses and Medicine Administration*. http://www.nursingmidwiferyboard.gov.au/Codes-Guidelines-Statements/FAQ/Enrolled-nurses-and-medicine-administration.aspx

Tiziani, A. (2017). *Harvard's Nursing Guide to Drugs* (10th ed.). Sydney: Mosby Elsevier.

PART 5

ESSENTIAL SKILLS COMPETENCY

Medication Administration – Oral, Sublingual, Buccal, Topical and Rectal

Demonstrates the ability to effectively and safely administer oral (i.e. swallowed orally), sublingual (under the tongue), buccal (into mucous membrane of the inner mouth/cheek), topical (on to the skin) and rectal (e.g. suppositories) medication

Criteria for skill performance	Y	D
(Numbers indicate *Enrolled Nurse Standards for Practice*, 2016)	(Satisfactory)	(Requires development)
1. Identifies indication (8.3, 8.4)		
2. Verifies the validity of the medication order (1.1, 1.2, 1.3, 1.4, 3.1, 3.9, 5.5, 8.4, 9.4)		
3. Gathers equipment (1.2, 1.6, 4.4, 6.4, 8.4, 9.4): ■ medications – in locked drawer by patient's bed or in trolley/cupboard ■ medication chart ■ fresh water and glass for oral medications ■ medication cup ■ pill cutter, pill crusher, oral liquid dispenser as required ■ non-sterile gloves, and other equipment if required		
4. Performs hand hygiene (1.2, 1.4, 1.8, 3.9, 6.4, 9.4)		
5. Evidence of effective communication with the patient; e.g. gives patient a clear explanation of procedure, discusses adverse effects of the medication, gains patient consent (1.2, 2.1, 2.3, 2.4, 2.5, 3.2, 6.3, 7.3, 7.5)		
6. Displays problem-solving abilities; e.g. positions patient, obtains appropriate form of medication, assesses patient, provides privacy (4.1, 4.2, 8.3, 8.4, 9.4)		
7. Abides by the general concepts of working with therapeutic substances when administering medications (1.1, 1.2, 1.3, 1.4, 2.2, 3.1, 3.2, 8.4, 9.4)		
8. Uses the 'rights of medication administration' (1.1, 1.2, 1.3, 1.4, 2.2, 3.1, 3.2, 3.9, 5.5, 8.4, 9.3, 9.4)		
Oral medication		
9a. Prepares the medication (1.1, 1.2, 1.3, 1.4, 1.6, 1.7, 1.8, 2.2, 3.1, 3.2, 3.9, 8.4, 9.4): ■ removes medication from pill bottle or blister/sachet packaging using an aseptic, non-touch technique; or ■ measures liquid medication with an oral liquid dispenser		
9b. Assists the patient to take the medication via oral route; ensures all medication is swallowed safely (1.2, 1.4, 1.8, 2.2, 3.2, 3.9, 6.1, 8.4, 9.4)		
Sublingual medication		
10a. Prepares the medication using an aseptic technique (1.1, 1.2, 1.3, 1.4, 1.6, 1.7, 1.8, 2.2, 3.1, 3.2, 3.9, 8.4, 9.4): ■ removes from pill bottle; or ■ opens spray using aseptic technique		
10b. Assists the patient to take the medication: ensures medication is administered under patient's tongue; ensures it is not swallowed (1.2, 1.4, 1.8, 2.2, 3.2, 3.9, 6.1, 8.4, 9.4)		
Buccal medication		
11a. Prepares the medication: removes from pill bottle/opens spray or drops using aseptic technique (1.1, 1.2, 1.3, 1.4, 1.6, 1.7, 1.8, 2.2, 3.1, 3.2, 3.9, 8.4, 9.4)		
11b. Assists the patient to take the medication: ensures medication is administered into mucosa on the inside of the cheek, near the molars; ensures medication is not swallowed (1.2, 1.4, 1.8, 2.2, 3.2, 3.9, 6.1, 8.4, 9.4)		
Topical medication		
12. Assists patient to apply the correction medication to the skin wearing non-sterile gloves (1.2, 1.4, 1.8, 2.2, 3.2, 3.9, 6.1, 8.4, 9.4)		
Rectal medication		
13a. Prepares the medication: removes medication from packaging using an aseptic, non-touch technique (1.1, 1.2, 1.3, 1.4, 1.6, 1.7, 1.8, 2.2, 3.1, 3.2, 3.9, 8.4, 9.4)		
13b. Correctly positions and administers rectal medication to patient wearing non-sterile gloves (1.2, 1.4, 1.8, 2.2, 3.2, 3.9, 6.1, 8.4, 9.4)		

13c. Removes gloves and performs hand hygiene (1.2, 1.4, 1.8, 3.9, 6.4, 9.4)		
14. Cleans, replaces and disposes of equipment appropriately (1.2, 1.4, 3.9, 6.5, 9.4)		
15. Documents and reports relevant information (1.2, 1.3, 1.8, 3.2, 5.3, 6.6, 7.1, 7.2, 7.3, 7.4, 7.5)		
16. Demonstrates ability to link theory to practice (8.3, 8.4, 8.5, 9.4)		

Student:

Clinical facilitator: Date:

CHAPTER 5.2

MEDICATION ADMINISTRATION – EYE DROPS OR OINTMENT, AND EYE CARE

IDENTIFY INDICATIONS

Identify the indication for the use of eye drops/eye ointment. Eye drops and ointments are used for a variety of reasons. They may be used to keep the eye moist and prevent corneal damage if the patient is unconscious or has reduced production of lacrimal fluid. They may also be used to act locally and reduce inflammation; to fight bacterial, viral or fungal infections; or to constrict or dilate the pupil.

VERIFY WRITTEN ORDERS AND IDENTIFY THE EYE TO BE TREATED

Written orders are necessary for medication administration to ensure that the patient receives the correct medication and dosage (i.e. number of drops) at the right time and in the correct eye. Instillation of eye medication is to be treated the same as any medication procedure – ensure the 'rights' of drug administration (see **Skill 5.1**) are observed. Different medications or different dosages may be ordered for each eye. If more than one medication is ordered for each eye, the timing of administration should be staggered to promote maximum absorption. If eye drops and ointment are both ordered for the same eye, instil the drops first to promote better absorption. Check organisational policy as to which eye drops can be administered by a student enrolled nurse.

GATHER EQUIPMENT

Gathering equipment prior to the procedure is a time-management strategy. It increases the nurse's confidence and the patient's confidence in the nurse. The following materials are brought to the bedside and placed on a clean surface.

- *The medication chart* is used for checking the 'rights of medication administration'. The prescribed medication should be checked for the drug name, to ensure it is an ophthalmological preparation, strength, patient's name, expiration date, opening date, any cloudiness, discolouration and precipitation (some ophthalmic solutions are suspensions and are meant to be cloudy). If you are opening a new bottle of drops, clearly mark it with the patient's name and expiration date (28 days after opening the bottle or tube). Each patient will have an individual bottle of the prescribed medication. To prevent cross-infection, this bottle is not used for anyone else.
- *Non-sterile gloves* are used for the protection of the nurse and the patient.
- *A clean washcloth and warm water* are used to cleanse the eye (adhere to the policies of the hospital in which you are practising) as required prior to administering the medication.
- *Sterile dressing pack and sterile normal saline (NS) for irrigation* are required for specific post-op ophthalmic patients to reduce infections risks (Gwenhure & Shepherd, 2019).
- *Unscented tissues* are used to blot excess drops or secretions that run out of the conjunctival sac. Scented ones can cause irritation to the eyes.

ADMINISTERING EYE DROPS OR OINTMENT

Perform hand hygiene and don gloves
Perform hand hygiene before touching the patient or the patient's surrounds and prior to any procedure involving patient contact to reduce the possibility of cross-contamination. Hand hygiene is the most effective method of infection control as it removes transient organisms from the hands of the nurse (see **Skill 1.1**). Non-sterile gloves protect the nurse from the patient's secretions and reduce the spread of microorganisms.

Give a clear explanation of the procedure and establish therapeutic communication
Introduce yourself, and check you have the correct patient. Explain the procedure and gain the patient's consent. Giving a clear explanation is required to gain

legal consent and to address policy requirements. It will also assist the patient to cooperate with the procedure, allay anxiety and assist in establishing a therapeutic relationship. Patients need to know the expected sensations and effects of the medication.

Demonstrate problem-solving abilities

Ensure adequate lighting to perform the procedure. Provide privacy, comfort measures and pain relief as necessary. Provision of privacy reduces anxiety and feelings of embarrassment. Provision of comfort measures such as toileting, positioning, fluids or pain relief will increase the patient's comfort and minimise disruptions to the procedure. Advise the patient that the instillation of eye drops and ointment may cause transient blurring of vision. Soft or gas-permeable contact lenses should be removed by the patient before instillation and re-inserted at least 15 minutes after the eye drops (Broyles, 2020).

Clean the eye (eye care)

Assess the condition of the external eye structures. As necessary, remove secretions, old medication and any debris from the lids by completing eye care. Always treat the uninfected or uninflamed eye first to reduce the risk of cross-infection.

Use warm water and a clean area of the washcloth to clean the eye. To reduce the risk of damaging the cornea and to remove any crusted discharge, always bathe the lids with the eyes closed first (Gwenhure & Shepherd, 2019). Each stroke is started at the inner canthus and swept towards the outer canthus. If there is a large amount of matter at the inner canthus, this is removed first using a dabbing stroke so that the matter is not moved back across the eye. If there is crusted matter on the lids, gauze swabs soaked in sterile saline (or the warm damp washcloth) can be rested on the closed lids for a short time to soften the crusting and make removal easier. If required, set up the dressing pack to complete the eye care, follow an aseptic technique for setup, then discard the forceps. Forceps are not used for this procedure as they could injure the patient's eye. Similar to an aseptic two-hand technique, pick up the gauze swab using a gloved hand. Wet the swab, and pass to the other hand and wipe the eye as described above. Use a fresh gauze swab for each wipe.

Remove and replace non-sterile gloves. Position the patient. Have the patient tilt their head back (unless there is cervical spine trauma) and roll their eyes upward and away from the nurse. This position provides an area furthest away from the tear duct to place the medication. Any excess will flow away from the tear duct to minimise systemic absorption of the solution. Rolling the eyes upward and away from the nurse moves the cornea away from the lower lid and reduces the risk of corneal damage from the inadvertent touching of the medication container to the cornea or from dropping solution onto the cornea.

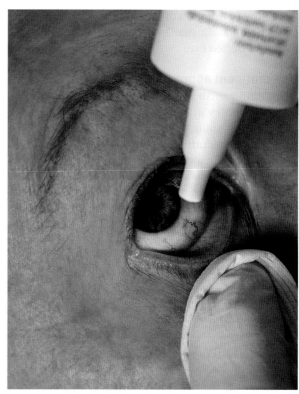

FIGURE 5.2.1 Administration of eye drops

Instil the eye drops

Open the bottle and place the lid securely on a clean surface – either on its side or with the open portion uppermost. If the medication is inadvertently contaminated by touching the tip to anything, it must be discarded.

Steady the nurse's dominant hand against the side of the patient's forehead. This reduces the chance of inadvertently touching or damaging the eye with the container. The administering hand will move with the patient's head if it moves. With a tissue over the fingers of the non-dominant hand, gently pull the lower lid downward to form a sac in the conjunctival fold into which the medication can be placed. The fingers pulling the lower lid gently downward should rest on the bony orbit to minimise the risk of touching the cornea and prevent any pressure being put on the eyeball. This also reduces the patient's ability to squint or to blink.

With the dominant hand remaining on the forehead, approach the eye from the side to reduce the blink reflex. Hold the medication container 1 to 2 cm above the conjunctival sac to minimise chances of accidental contact and therefore injury to the eye or contamination of the medication. Bacterial colonisation of the medication following contamination occurs quickly if the tip is touched to the eye or by the fingers (Gwenhure & Shepherd, 2019). Placing the medication in the outer third of the conjunctival sac will reduce discomfort (i.e. of stimulating the cornea). When the patient blinks, the medication is distributed over the entire eyeball. Blotting with a clean tissue removes excess medication, increasing comfort and reducing the possibility of irritation of skin. If ordered, the eye is taped closed and a sterile eye pad is taped securely over the affected eye.

Use ointment appropriately

Discarding a small amount of ointment prior to administration will remove any ointment that has been contaminated by the lid or inadvertent contamination during use. The ointment is then squeezed in a thin line into and along the conjunctival sac (as above) to ensure the greatest coverage across the eyeball. When the patient rolls their eyes behind closed lids, the ointment melts with body heat and the medication is distributed over the eyeball.

Doff gloves and perform hand hygiene

Remove gloves and discard appropriately and then perform hand hygiene. Maintain the 5 Moments for Hand Hygiene and perform hand hygiene after touching the patient and the patient's surrounds.

CLEAN, REPLACE OR DISPOSE OF EQUIPMENT

Place gloves and soiled tissues (and waste from eye toilet if relevant) into a general waste bin. Return medication to appropriate storage (generally below 25°C and protected from the light).

DOCUMENT AND REPORT RELEVANT INFORMATION

The medication is signed off on the medication chart, ensuring the correct eye is identified and signed on the chart. When relevant, the appearance of the eye should be noted in the patient's notes.

CASE STUDY

You are working in an outpatient diabetic retinopathy clinic. Each patient requires tropicamide one drop to each eye prior to eye photos.

1. Utilising resources available, look up tropicamide eye drops.

2. What is the purpose of this medication?
3. Describe the process of placing eye drops into the eyes.
4. What information will you give the patient prior to inserting the eye drops?

Note: These notes are summaries of the most important points in the assessments/procedures, and are not exhaustive on the subject. The naming of documents or charts may differ from state to state, and facility to facility. In all possible situations the guidelines of the ACSQHC are used when describing national charts or documents (e.g. the ACSQHC Observation and Response Chart is named the Adult Observation and Response Chart in WA, and the Rapid Detection and Response Observation Chart in SA). References of the materials used to compile the information have been supplied. The student is expected to have learned the material surrounding each skill as presented in the references. No single reference is complete on the subject.

REFERENCES

Broyles, B., Reiss, B., Evans, M., McKenzie, G., Pleunik, S. & Page, R. (2020). *Pharmacology in Nursing: Australian and New Zealand Edition* (3rd ed.). Melbourne: Cengage.

Gwenhure, T. & Shepherd, E. (2019). Principles and procedure for eye assessment and cleansing. *Nursing Times* [online],

115(12), pp. 18–20. https://www.nursingtimes.net/clinical-archive/assessment-skills/principles-and-procedure-for-eye-assessment-and-cleansing-28-11-2019/

RECOMMENDED READINGS

Australian Commission on Safety and Quality in Health Care (ACSQHC). (2016). *National Inpatient Medication Chart User Guide*. ACSQHC, Sydney.

Bryant, B., Knights, K., Darroch, S. & Rowland, A. (2019). *Pharmacology for Health Professionals Australia* (5th ed.). Sydney: Elsevier.

Dougherty, L. & Lister, S. (eds). (2015). *The Royal Marsden Hospital Manual of Clinical Nursing Procedures* (9th ed.). Oxford: Wiley-Blackwell.

Gray, S., Ferris, L., White, L.E., Duncan, G. & Baumle, W. (2018). *Foundations of Nursing: Enrolled Nurses* (2nd ANZ ed.). Melbourne: Cengage.

ESSENTIAL SKILLS COMPETENCY

Medication Administration – Eye Drops or Ointment, and Eye Care
Demonstrates the ability to effectively administer ophthalmic medication

Criteria for skill performance	Y	D
(Numbers indicate *Enrolled Nurse Standards for Practice*, 2016)	(Satisfactory)	(Requires development)
1. Identifies indication (8.3, 8.4)		
2. Verifies written order; identifies eye to be treated (1.1, 1.2, 1.3, 1.4, 3.1, 3.9, 5.5, 8.4, 9.4)		
3. Gathers equipment (1.2, 1.6, 4.4, 6.4, 8.4, 9.4) ■ medication chart ■ prescribed eye drops or ointment ■ non-sterile gloves ■ tissues For eye care: ■ non-sterile gloves ■ washcloth ■ sterile dressing pack (if required) ■ sterile normal saline for irrigation ■ rubbish bag (if required)		
4. Performs hand hygiene and dons non-sterile gloves (1.2, 1.4, 1.8, 3.9, 6.4, 9.4)		
5. Evidence of effective communication with the patient; e.g. gives patient a clear explanation of procedure, discusses adverse effects of the medication, gains patient consent (1.2, 2.1, 2.3, 2.4, 2.5, 3.2, 6.3, 7.3, 7.5)		
6. Demonstrates problem-solving abilities; e.g. provides privacy, comfort measures, (4.1, 4.2, 8.3, 8.4, 9.4)		
7. Abides by the general concepts of working with therapeutic substances when administering medications (1.1, 1.2, 1.3, 1.4, 2.2, 3.1, 3.2, 8.4, 9.4)		
8. Uses the 'rights' to administer the medication (1.1, 1.2, 1.3, 1.4, 2.2, 3.1, 3.2, 3.9, 5.5, 8.4, 9.3, 9.4)		
9. Checks the eye and cleanses/performs eye care if required (1.2, 1.4, 1.8, 3.2, 3.9, 8.4, 9.4)		
10. Position patient's head appropriately (1.2, 8.4, 9.4)		
11. Steadies dominant hand on patient's forehead (1.2, 8.4, 9.4)		
12. Pulls lower lid down with non-dominant hand (1.2, 8.4, 9.4)		
Eye drops		
12a. Instils drops into conjunctival sac (1.2, 8.4, 9.4)		
12b. Asks patient to blink (7.3)		
12c. Uses a tissue to blot excess medication off lid/cheek (1.2, 8.4, 9.4)		
Eye ointment		
13a. Ointment: squeezes a little ointment out and discards (1.2, 8.4, 9.4)		
13b. Squeezes a ribbon of ointment into lower conjunctival sac (1.2, 1.4, 3.2, 8.4, 9.4)		
13c. Asks patient to roll their eyes behind closed lids (7.3)		
14. Removes non-sterile gloves and performs hand hygiene (1.2, 1.4, 1.8, 3.9, 6.4, 9.4)		
15. Cleans, replaces or disposes of equipment appropriately (1.2, 1.4, 3.9, 6.5, 9.4)		
16. Documents and reports relevant information (1.2, 1.3, 1.8, 3.2, 5.3, 6.6, 7.1, 7.2, 7.3, 7.4, 7.5)		
17. Demonstrates ability to link theory to practice (8.3, 8.4, 8.5, 9.4)		

Student:

Clinical facilitator: Date:

CHAPTER 5.3

MEDICATION ADMINISTRATION – INJECTIONS

IDENTIFY INDICATIONS

Parenteral medication administration involves the injection of a medication into a body tissue. The following are types of parenteral medication.

1. *Intradermal* (into the dermis layer of the skin) is most commonly used for allergy testing and tuberculosis (TB) screening. Because it is the area of slowest absorption of the parenteral sites, minute volumes of potentially allergy-causing medication can be administered.

2. *Subcutaneous (subcut)* (injection into the subcutaneous tissue) is commonly used to administer insulin or heparin. It is more rapidly absorbed than oral medications, but slower than intramuscular. Only small volumes can be injected.

3. *Intramuscular (IM)* (injection into a muscle mass) is used for narcotic, antiemetic, psychiatric or antibiotic medications. This site can take larger volumes and more irritating solutions than either of the previous sites. The rate of absorption is quicker due to the greater blood supply.

4. *Intravenous (IV)* administration is used for antibiotic, antiemetic or analgesia medication administration (see **Skills 6.5, 6.6** and **6.7** detailing the administration of IV medication).

5. *Epidural, intra-arterial, intra-osseous, intrapleural, intrathecal and intraperitoneal* are also forms of parenteral administration that are generally not performed by enrolled nurses.

Parenteral administration of medication is faster acting than oral administration, since the medication does not go through the digestive process but is absorbed directly from the tissues into the bloodstream, and then to the target tissues. Other indications for parenteral administration of medications are situations in which the oral route is not available (nil by mouth, nausea, oral surgery) or when the medication would be destroyed by digestion, such as heparin or insulin. Because of the rapid effect and the irretrievable nature of injected medications, the patient must be closely monitored for both therapeutic and toxic effects.

VERIFY THAT THE ORDER IS VALID

Verify that the order is valid (see **Skill 5.1**) and check the medication chart for time, route, dose and drug. Nurses are responsible for questioning any order that is unclear, incomplete or that seems inappropriate or unreasonable for the patient. To do this, the nurse *must know* the patient's diagnosis, the purpose of the medication, its therapeutic effect, any adverse effects, the usual dose and any pertinent nursing implications, as well as the patient factors that mediate response to drugs such as age, weight and psychological factors. So that potentially harmful substances are not administered, the nurse must also ascertain any medication or food allergies that the patient may have by checking the allergies on the medication chart, noting if the patient is wearing an allergy alert ID band and asking the patient if they have any allergies. Some medications administered via injection are given as PRN (as needed) medications, which require review of the indication and maximum dose in 24 hours as stated on the medication chart. Insulin and anticoagulants will be noted on the medication chart, with the actual dose prescribed on a separate national subcutaneous insulin chart or anticoagulant medication chart.

GATHER EQUIPMENT

Knowledge of the equipment is essential to be able to choose the correct items for each injection to minimise discomfort.

- *Syringes* are plastic, disposable and come in a range of sizes from 0.5 to 5 mL for injections (and up to 20 mL for intravenous injections). They are sterile and packaged individually. Syringes have three component parts: the calibrated barrel that holds the medication; the plunger that pushes the medication out; and the tip, which connects to the needle. Tips can be Luer slip or Luer lock (most facility policies require use of a Luer lock), which are designed for use with a range of connectors for various purposes as well as for attaching needles. The barrel of the syringe is marked in scales of measurement – both millilitres and tenths of millilitres, or units in an insulin syringe. Insulin syringes come with an attached needle. Some medications (e.g. enoxaparin) use prefilled syringes with a needle already attached.
- *Needles* are also disposable. They are made of stainless steel and come with a plastic cap in a sterile package. There are also three parts to the needle: the hub that connects to the syringe; the cannula, which is the hollow shaft through which the medication flows; and the bevel, which is the slanted part at the tip of the cannula. Needles have three variables.
  1. Short or long bevel. Short bevel is used for IV and intradermal injections so the bevel will not become occluded, and long bevels are used for subcutaneous and IM injections because they are sharper and cause less discomfort.
  2. Length of the cannula. These range from 1 to 5 cm for the purposes of normal injections. Some needles for special purposes can be up to 12 cm in length.
  3. The gauge of the cannula. This varies from #14 (very large bore) to #28 (very fine bore). The smaller

gauges cause less discomfort, but the larger gauge needles may need to be used if the medication is oily or viscous.

Safety needles have been developed to reduce the incidence of needlestick injuries and are the preferred needle to be used. The manufacturer's recommendations must be followed for use.

- *Ampoules* are small, glass or plastic single-dose containers of medication. The medication is sealed into the glass or plastic container, the neck of which must be snapped off to get to the medication. Most glass ampoule necks are pre-scored so they break cleanly.
- *Vials* are single or multi-use glass containers with rubber stoppers. They may contain either liquid medication for immediate use or powdered medication that requires reconstitution. The medication is accessed through the rubber stopper.
- *Filter needles* may be used to reduce the risk of glass or rubber particulate matter being withdrawn with the medication and inadvertently injected into the patient.
- *Non-sterile gloves*.
- *Alcohol wipes* are alcohol-soaked sterile pads that are used to clean vial tops, cleanse the skin of the patient prior to injection (for IM injections) and may be used to wrap around the neck of glass ampoules to prevent injury during snapping off the neck. Check facility procedures as these are not always used.
- *Gauze swabs* are used to tend to the puncture site.
- A *kidney dish or injection tray* is used to transport the filled syringe and needle, the alcohol wipes and the empty ampoule to the bedside.
- *The sharps container* is a rigid plastic container used to protect nursing and domestic staff from accidental needlestick injuries. All used needles, syringes and glass containers are placed in the sharps container as soon as the injection has been given and documented.

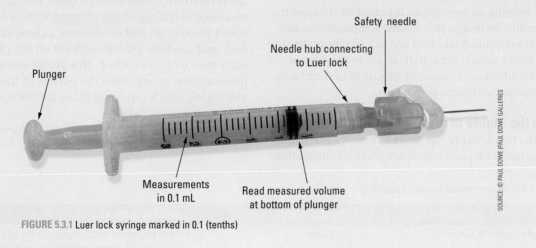

Plunger

Measurements in 0.1 mL

Read measured volume at bottom of plunger

Needle hub connecting to Luer lock

Safety needle

SOURCE: © PAUL DOWE (PAUL DOWE GALLERIES)

FIGURE 5.3.1 Luer lock syringe marked in 0.1 (tenths)

ADMINISTERING INJECTIONS

Perform hand hygiene

Perform hand hygiene before touching the patient or the patient's surrounds and prior to any procedure involving patient contact to reduce the possibility of cross-contamination. Hand hygiene is the most effective method of infection control as it removes transient organisms from the hands of the nurse (see **Skill 1.1**). An aseptic technique is also maintained when administering an injection. Non-sterile gloves are used to reduce infection risk.

Give a clear explanation of the procedure and establish therapeutic communication

Establish therapeutic communication; identify your patient and gain the patient's consent. Checking the patient and gaining their consent will also ensure that you meet legal and policy requirements before implementing any procedure. Having an injection is a source of fear and anxiety to the majority of patients. Listening to fears and concerns, correcting misapprehensions and explaining some of the techniques that you use to minimise discomfort (see later this skill) will help the patient to allay fear and anxiety. Discussing the therapeutic effects and side effects will prepare the patient for the sensations they will feel and, in some cases, potentiate the effects of the drug.

Adhere to the general concepts of therapeutic substances (parenteral)

The concepts are the same as those listed in **Skill 5.1**. The following safety concerns are specific to parenteral medications.

- All injections require an aseptic technique.
- Never recap the needle on a used syringe (i.e. after a medication has been administered to a patient). This is to prevent a needlestick injury. Ampoules, empty vials, needles and used syringes are discarded in sharps containers to reduce the risk of needlestick injuries during disposal. Any needlestick or sharps injury, whether 'clean' (while the needle is sterile) or 'contaminated' (after used on the patient), must be reported.
- Inject only medication solutions that are designated 'for injectable use only'. Parenteral administration of a solution designed for oral or topical use can result in adverse reactions ranging from an abscess to more drastic effects such as a fatal systemic effect.
- Choosing an appropriate injection site reduces the incidence of injection-related complications. Site selection must take into account facility policy, the client's muscle mass, BMI, access to site, ease of site identification, rotation of sites, type of drug being injected and client preferences.

Use the 'rights of medication administration'

For the list of 'rights', see **Skill 5.1** These are even more important with parenteral medication administration

because of the rapid onset of the effects of parenteral medication. This leaves little time to intervene if a mistake occurs.

Draw up the medication

Choose the appropriate equipment. TABLE 5.3.1 indicates the usual equipment for each of the administration modes.

Don non-sterile gloves. Open the syringe and drawing-up needle packages and maintain an aseptic technique. Follow the principles of an aseptic technique, and firmly attach the ends of needle and syringe together, ensuring the ends of the opened needles and syringes are not contaminated in the process (they are 'key parts', or areas within a micro-critical aseptic field that should not be touched or placed on the bench) before placing in a kidney dish. A drawing-up needle should be used when drawing up medications from an ampoule or vial. Air should be removed and the syringe primed to the correct volume. When using a Luer lock, carefully recap the needle to then twist it off using an aseptic technique, and discard in the sharps container.

While continuing to maintain an aseptic technique (i.e. do not place the syringe in the kidney dish while opening the packaging of the new needle), a new giving needle is attached to the syringe.

When drawing up insulin, the attached needle is used for drawing up and administering the medication. Follow manufacturer's instructions when using an 'insulin pen'.

To remove air bubbles and measure the exact amount of medication, hold the syringe vertically with the needle upwards, and tap the barrel to release any air bubbles trapped by the surface tension of the fluid. Carefully push the plunger until all of the air is expelled. Take care not to expel and lose too much of the prescribed medication. Check the level to ensure an accurate dose. The dose is measured at the top of the plunger. If there is excess, invert the syringe and needle over a clean kidney dish and carefully push downward on the plunger until the excess is expelled. This avoids excess medication running down the outside of the needle and barrel, which can cause tissue irritation if it touches the nurse's skin.

Remove the drawing-up needle and discard it in the sharps container, then place the giving needle on

TABLE 5.3.1 Recommended injection equipment

	INTRADERMAL	SUBCUTANEOUS	INTRAMUSCULAR
Needle length	0.7–2 cm	1–2.5 cm	2.5–3 cm (needle length depends on the subcutaneous fat – more fat, longer needle needed to reach muscle)
Needle gauge	25–26 gauge	25–27 gauge	21–23 gauge (select the smallest gauge appropriate for the patient and the medication viscosity for comfort)
Syringe size	1 mL (check that scale is marked in appropriate increments for medication dose)	1–2 mL (insulin syringes must be used when administering insulin)	2–5 mL to accommodate 3 mL of solution and still be easily used
Volume	0.01–0.1 mL	1–1.5 mL maximum	Small muscle: 1 mL maximum; large muscle: 3–5 mL

the filled syringe. Avoid contaminating the exposed ends of the needle and syringe (i.e. 'key parts') during this process.

Medication is prepared from the following.

■ *A vial.* Remove the protective cap from the vial, clean the rubber stopper with an alcohol wipe and allow to air dry, then set the vial on the bench. Now remove the drawing-up needle cap and draw air to equal the amount of medication you require, and carefully penetrate the middle of the rubber stopper of the vial with the needle, maintaining sterility. Keep the needle above the level of the medication to avoid forming bubbles, which decrease the accuracy of measurement, and inject the air into the vial to create positive atmospheric pressure in the vial so the medication flows out easily. Turn the syringe, needle and vial upright so the syringe markings are at eye level (to increase accuracy) and the needle tip is in the medication, and withdraw the required medication. Refer to **FIGURE 5.3.2**. As described above, withdraw the needle, expel the air and measure the exact amount of medication.

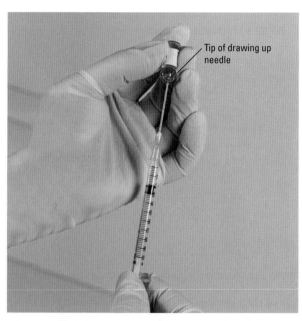

Tip of drawing up needle

FIGURE 5.3.2 Technique to 'draw up' medication

Note: Invert the ampoule, and keep the top of the needle below the fluid level to withdraw medication. Do not squirt fluid back into the ampoule.

■ *Reconstitution of a powder in a vial.* This involves a similar procedure. Initially, remove a quantity of air from the vial containing the powder equal to the amount of diluent to be added by inserting the needle into the vacant space above the powder and withdrawing the air. Draw up the designated diluent from a separate vial or ampoule (see below for ampoule) and, turning the powder vial, needle and syringe upright, inject the diluent into the powder vial. Remove the needle from the vial and rotate the vial until all of the powder is dissolved. Withdraw the medication as described above.

■ *An ampoule.* Select ampoule. If a glass ampoule is being used, remove medication trapped in the neck of the ampoule by moving it in a circular motion to create centrifugal force and overcome the surface tension that is holding the liquid in the neck. Flicking the upper portion of the ampoule with a fingernail also breaks surface tension. Snap off the neck of the ampoule by breaking away from you. The top of a plastic ampoule is twisted off – take care that your fingers don't touch the top of the opening and contaminate the ampoule. Remove the drawing-up needle cap and insert the needle into the ampoule without it touching the rim of the ampoule, thus preventing contamination. With the tip of the needle kept below the level of the fluid, draw back on the plunger until the requisite amount of medication is obtained. It may be necessary to tip the ampoule slightly on its side to obtain all of the medication. Draw back a small amount of air into the barrel to remove all of medication from the drawing-up needle. Remove the needle from the ampoule.

Place the syringe and needle, a fresh alcohol wipe if used, gauze swab or cotton ball and the empty ampoule or vial in a kidney dish or on an injection tray so they can be easily carried to the bedside. Take the medication chart with you. Sharps containers are regularly kept at the foot of the patient's bed or near the hand basin in the patient's room, along with alcohol gel.

Note: Some commercially prepared and prefilled syringes contain an air bubble that must not be removed. Check packaging prior to preparation and administration. They also come with the needle attached.

Demonstrate problem-solving abilities

Position the patient for comfort, access to the injection site and privacy.

Intradermal injections are usually given on the inner aspect of the forearm. The patient should be seated or lying in a comfortable position with the forearm of their non-dominant hand exposed, extended and supported in a position of comfort. The injection is given approximately 10 to 12 cm above the wrist, usually on the non-dominant arm.

Subcutaneous injections are given in many areas of the body that have good circulation. They are rotated around the body to assist absorption and minimise discomfort. The upper, lateral aspect of the arms, lower abdomen or anterior thighs are often used. Anticoagulant injections are generally administered in the abdomen. Insulin injections can be rotated around the upper arms, anterior thighs and abdomen. Subcutaneous injections in the abdominal area should be given at least 3 to 5 cm away from the umbilicus and below the midline. Refer to **FIGURE 5.3.3**.

Intramuscular injections should be given in the thickest part of the muscle, and the volume given will vary with the site. The ventrogluteal muscle is considered the preferred site (Broyles et al., 2020)

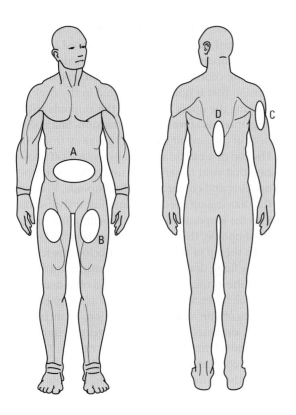

FIGURE 5.3.3 Subcutaneous injection sites

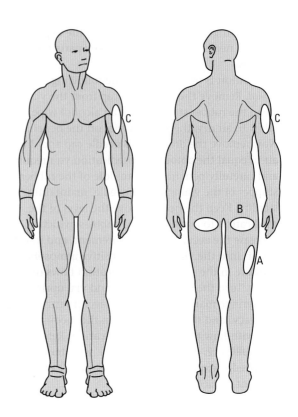

FIGURE 5.3.4 Intramuscular injection sites

and is required by most hospital policies, as these gluteals are not close to major blood vessels and nerves. Research has also shown fewer complications when using this site. Up to 4 mL can be injected. The vastus lateralis muscle in the leg can receive up to 5 mL, and the deltoid in the arm no more than 2 mL (Crisp et al., 2016). The dorsogluteal in the buttocks may be used, but has a lower absorption rate and the risk of hitting the sciatic nerve. Always check the facility policy prior to administration to ensure the preferred site is being used. Also review the age of a child to help identify the preferred site. Some sites, such as the dorsogluteal or ventrogluteal, are not used in infants or children who have not been walking for at least 1 year (Broyle et al., 2020). Refer to **FIGURE 5.3.4**.

The ventrogluteal site is located by having the patient lie on their side, and placing the nurse's heel of the opposite hand (i.e. left hand on right hip) on the hip over the greater trochanter. The index finger is placed over the anterosuperior iliac spine and the middle finger stretched to form a 'V'. The injection site is in the middle of the 'V', no lower than the first knuckle. Refer to **FIGURE 5.3.5**. The vastus lateralis is located by having the patient lie on their back. On the side of the leg, divide the thigh into thirds between the greater trochanter and the knee. Divide the anterior thigh and posterior thigh in half to find the midline. The injection is given within this area (i.e. midline of middle third).

Consider patient privacy, even if the injection to be given is not located in an intimate position or does not require exposing the body. Most patients would prefer to have the door closed or curtains drawn for

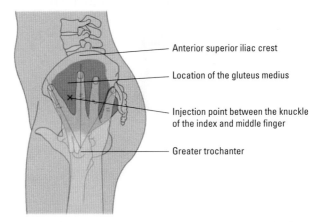

Anterior superior iliac crest

Location of the gluteus medius

Injection point between the knuckle of the index and middle finger

Greater trochanter

FIGURE 5.3.5 Intramuscular injection site – ventrogluteal injection site

fear of their response to the injection causing them embarrassment.

Locate and assess the appropriate site
Perform hand hygiene. Don non-sterile gloves. Assess the site for skin breaks or rashes, lesions, tenderness, inflammation and the amount of subcutaneous fat. Palpate subcutaneous tissue and underlying muscle mass as applicable to determine if there is induration (localised hardening of the soft tissue) or other contraindications. For any parenteral drug administration, the tissue into which the medication is placed must be well perfused for best effect. An alcohol wipe is used to cleanse the skin for intramuscular injections. Allow the site to dry to reduce irritation during the injection as alcohol irritates the tissue and may cause the patient to feel a stinging sensation.

Administer the medication safely and comfortably

- *Intradermal*. As these are used in specific situations, the nurse would be given further education as required.
- *Subcutaneous*. Remove the needle cap and discard it in the kidney dish. Grasp a fold of skin between the thumb and index finger of the non-dominant hand to elevate the subcutaneous tissue and prevent injecting the medication into the muscle. Hold the syringe like a dart between the thumb and fingers of the dominant hand to give control over the movement of the syringe. Stabilise your hand/wrist on the patient's skin so the amount of force and the distance of needle insertion can be controlled.

  Quickly insert the needle at a 45- or 90-degree angle, depending on the amount of subcutaneous tissue, and according to policy. Use a 90-degree angle for insulin. Release the skin held with the non-dominant hand and use that hand to stabilise the syringe by holding the lower end of the syringe. Stabilising the syringe reduces movement of the syringe and needle and reduces discomfort.

  Gently push on the plunger with the thumb or a finger of the dominant hand and slowly inject the medication into the subcutaneous tissue. Medication is injected slowly so tissue is distended slowly, minimising pain.

  Support the skin (but do not apply pressure) around the puncture site and quickly withdraw the needle to minimise pain and flick the safety cover over the needle with your thumb or forefinger.

  Do not massage the site. Immediately place the used needle in the kidney dish, for disposal in the sharps container. Perform hand hygiene. Note: Swabbing of the skin prior to administration of subcutaneous injections is not routinely practised and aspirating to check if the needle has entered a blood vessel is not necessary, but check hospital policy on giving subcutaneous injections.
- *Intramuscular – Z-track* (preferred IM injection technique in many facilities). Always used for solutions that will cause irritation, and staining. Research has shown this method of IM injection also reduces the pain experienced when giving an intramuscular injection (Kara & Yapucu Güneş, 2016). It is now described by many facilities and government health departments as the preferred method for IM injections. Locate the correct site and cleanse with an alcohol wipe. Leave the alcohol wipe on the skin above the site to mark the area, and allow site to dry (30 seconds). Remove the needle cap and discard it in the kidney dish. Using the base or side of the non-dominant hand, the skin and underlying tissue is pulled to one side. Hold the syringe like a dart between the thumb and index fingers of the dominant hand to give control over the

movement of the syringe. Stabilise your hand/wrist on the patient's skin so the amount of force and the distance of needle insertion can be controlled. Quickly insert the needle at a 90-degree angle.

Stabilise the syringe by holding the lower end of the syringe with the fingers, while keeping the skin and underlying tissue pulled to one side with the rest of the hand. Stabilising the syringe reduces movement of the syringe and needle and reduces discomfort. According to facility policy, aspirate the syringe and check for blood (Sisson, 2015; Thomas et al., 2016). With the dominant hand, pull back on the plunger to aspirate. Pulling back on the plunger creates negative pressure in the barrel and if the needle has entered a blood vessel, blood will be drawn into the barrel. If this happens, withdraw the needle and discard the needle, syringe and medication and start again, since injecting medication into a vessel could cause the patient harm.

If no blood appears, push gently on the plunger and slowly inject the medication into the muscle tissue. Medication is injected slowly so tissue is distended slowly, minimising pain.

Quickly withdraw the needle to reduce pain (for iron injections, wait 10 seconds, then withdraw the needle), and flick the safety cover over the needle with your thumb or forefinger, then let the skin return to its normal anatomical position. As the needle is withdrawn, tension on the tissues is released. This helps seal the track and the solution doesn't leak back out into the surface tissues.

Immediately place the used needle in the bedside sharps container or in the kidney dish for disposal in the sharps container. A gauze swab can be held over the injection site to apply gentle pressure. Perform hand hygiene and remove gloves.
- *Intramuscular* (standard technique). Similar principles and actions are followed, as per the Z-track injection. The skin and underlying tissues at the injection site are managed differently. Locate the correct site and cleanse with an alcohol wipe. Leave the alcohol wipe on the skin above the site to mark the area, and allow site to dry (30 seconds). Remove the needle cap and discard it in the kidney dish. Pull the skin over the injection site taut with the forefinger and index finger for the ventrogluteal site, or thumb and index finger for other sites, of the non-dominant hand to make the skin easier to pierce and to lessen discomfort.

  Hold the syringe like a dart between the thumb and index fingers of the dominant hand to give control over the movement of the syringe. Stabilise your hand/wrist on the patient's skin so the amount of force and the distance of needle insertion can be controlled. Quickly insert the needle at a 90-degree angle.

Release the skin with the non-dominant hand and use it to stabilise the syringe by holding the lower end of the syringe. With the dominant hand, pull back on the plunger to aspirate. If blood appears in the syringe, withdraw the needle and discard the needle, syringe and medication and start again, since injecting medication into a vessel could cause the patient harm.

If no blood appears, push gently on the plunger and slowly inject the medication into the muscle tissue. Medication is injected slowly so tissue is distended slowly, minimising pain.

Quickly withdraw the needle to reduce pain and flick the safety cover on the needle with your thumb or forefinger. Immediately place the used needle in the bedside sharps container or in the kidney dish for disposal in the sharps container. A gauze swab can be held over the injection site to apply gentle pressure. Perform hand hygiene and remove gloves.

Injection tips

The following additional nursing measures can assist in reducing patient discomfort.
- Choose the smallest gauge needle for the site and the solution to be administered.
- Take care to keep the outside of the needle free of solution that may irritate tissue.
- Locate the injection site using anatomical landmarks. Do not inject when skin is irritated or broken.
- Alternate injection sites to avoid repeated trauma to one area.
- Use distraction such as conversation or relaxation techniques to reduce patient anxiety.

Tend to the puncture site appropriately

Intradermal injections are not massaged because the medication is supposed to stay in one place to slow absorption and give a focal point for a reaction (allergy, tuberculin testing). No massage or pressure should be applied to subcutaneous sites. Gentle pressure may be applied to intramuscular injection sites, and assists if bleeding occurs due to trauma to

the capillaries during the injection. Administration of parenteral medication to a child requires special consideration.

Doff gloves and perform hand hygiene

Remove gloves, discard appropriately and then perform hand hygiene. Maintain the 5 Moments for Hand Hygiene and perform hand hygiene after touching the patient and the patient's surrounds.

CLEAN, REPLACE OR DISPOSE OF EQUIPMENT

All used syringes, needles, ampoules and empty vials are carefully disposed of in a designated sharps container at the bedside to reduce the risk of needlestick injury to nursing and domestic staff. Alcohol wipes and non-sterile gloves are deposited in the general rubbish. The kidney dish or injection tray is disposed of correctly. All stock is replenished as necessary and medications are ordered from the pharmacy to ensure a ready supply for the next 24 hours.

DOCUMENT AND REPORT RELEVANT INFORMATION

Regularly scheduled medications are initialled on the medication chart next to the appropriate time slot (i.e. anticoagulant medications and insulin are signed on the specific, separate chart). Once-only and PRN medications are charted in the appropriate section of the medication chart. Some injections, such as preoperative sedation or medication, may also require signatures on the theatre sheet and notation in the patient's notes. Controlled substances must be signed out of the drug cupboard by a registered nurse (RN). If the patient is receiving analgesia, a notation about its effectiveness is made in the patient's notes.

CASE STUDY

As the nurse caring for Sarah Phillips (a 68-year-old woman), you are required to administer her daily dose of enoxaparin 40 mg subcutaneously as part of her venous thromboembolism (VTE) prophylaxis. When you go to the relevant cupboard to collect the medication, you identify it comes in a prefilled syringe.

1. What type of medication is enoxaparin and why is it used for VTE prophylaxis?
2. What is the trade name for enoxaparin?
3. The prefilled syringe contains the medication, and a needle is already attached. What other equipment will you require to administer this medication?
4. What is the preferred site for this medication? Draw a diagram to illustrate your answer.
5. When you go to give the medication, what procedure will you follow to check that you have the correct patient?
6. Before giving the medication, you check the administration site and identify several large dark bruises where Sarah has had previous enoxaparin injections. What is the possible cause of these bruises and what action will you implement?

→

Later in the shift, Sarah complains of feeling nauseated. You review her medication chart in the PRN section and note that she is ordered an antiemetic IM. You review this order with the RN, and are going to give her this medication.

7. List two common antiemetic medications, and the dose that can be given intramuscularly.

8. What size syringe and giving needle will you use to administer this medication?

9. What is the preferred site to administer this medication? Explain how you will locate the site correctly.

10. How long will it be before the medication will take effect?

Note: These notes are summaries of the most important points in the assessments/procedures, and are not exhaustive on the subject. The naming of documents or charts may differ from state to state, and facility to facility. In all possible situations the guidelines of the ACSQHC are used when describing national charts or documents (e.g. the ACSQHC Observation and Response Chart is named the Adult Observation and Response Chart in WA, and the Rapid Detection and Response Observation Chart in SA). References of the materials used to compile the information have been supplied. The student is expected to have learned the material surrounding each skill as presented in the references. No single reference is complete on the subject.

REFERENCES

Broyles, B., Reiss, B., Evans, M., McKenzie, G., Pleunik, S. & Page, R. (2020). *Pharmacology in Nursing: Australian and New Zealand Edition* (3rd ed.). Melbourne: Cengage.

Crisp, J., Douglas, C., Rebeiro, G. & Waters, D. (2017). *Potter and Perry's Fundamentals of Nursing – Australian version* (5th ed.). Sydney: Elsevier.

Kara, D. & Yapucu Güneş, Ü. (2016). The effect on pain of three different methods of intramuscular injection: A randomized controlled trial. *International Journal of Nursing Practice*, 22(2), pp. 152–9.

Sisson, H. (2015). Aspirating during the intramuscular injection procedure: a systematic literature review. *Journal of Clinical Nursing*, 24(17–18), pp. 2368–75. doi: 10.1111/jocn.12824.

Thomas, C.M., Mraz, M. & Rajcan, L. (2016). Blood aspiration during IM injection. *Clinical Nursing Research*, 25(5), pp. 549–59. doi: 10.1177/1054773815575074.

RECOMMENDED READINGS

Australian Commission on Safety and Quality in Health Care (ACSQHC). (2016). *National Inpatient Medication Chart User Guide*. ACSQHC, Sydney.

Dougherty, L. & Lister, S. (eds). (2015). *The Royal Marsden Hospital Manual of Clinical Nursing Procedures* (9th ed.). Oxford: Wiley-Blackwell.

Li, Yimei. (2017). *Injections: Intramuscular. Evidence summaries.* Joanna Briggs Institute

Kara, D., Uzelli, D. & Karaman, D. (2015). Using ventrogluteal site in intramuscular injections is a priority or an alternative? *International Journal of Caring Sciences*, 8(2), pp. 507–13.

Reynolds, T., & Saxton, L. (2015). Developing training in intramuscular injections. *Mental Health Practice*, 18(9), p. 14.

ESSENTIAL SKILLS COMPETENCY

Medication Administration – Injections

Demonstrates the ability to effectively and safely administer intramuscular and subcutaneous medications

Criteria for skill performance	Y	D
(Numbers indicate *Enrolled Nurse Standards for Practice*, 2016)	(Satisfactory)	(Requires development)
1. Identifies indication (8.3, 8.4)		
2. Verifies the validity of the medication order (1.1, 1.2, 1.3, 1.4, 3.1, 3.9, 5.5, 8.4, 9.4)		
3. Gathers equipment (1.2, 1.6, 4.4, 6.4, 8.4, 9.4): ■ appropriate syringe, needles ■ alcohol wipes, gauze swab ■ non-sterile gloves ■ kidney dish ■ ordered medication in vial or ampoule ■ sharps container ■ medication chart		
4. Performs hand hygiene (1.2, 1.4, 1.8, 3.9, 6.4, 9.4)		
5. Evidence of therapeutic communication with the patient; gives explanation of procedure, gains patient consent (2.1, 2.3, 2.4, 2.5, 6.3, 7.3, 7.5)		
6. Adheres to the general concepts of working with therapeutic substances (1.1, 1.2, 1.3, 2.2, 3.1, 3.2, 3.9, 8.2, 8.4, 9.4)		
7. Uses the 'rights of medication administration' (1.1, 1.2, 1.3, 1.4, 2.2, 3.1, 3.2, 3.9, 5.5, 8.4, 9.3, 9.4)		
8. Draws up medication using an aseptic technique to prepare medication (1.1, 1.2, 1.3, 1.6, 1.7, 1.8, 2.2, 3.2, 3.9, 8.4, 9.4)		
9. Performs hand hygiene and dons non-sterile gloves (1.2, 1.4, 1.8, 3.9, 6.4, 9.4)		
10. Displays problem-solving abilities; e.g. positions patient, obtains appropriate form of medication, assesses patient if warranted (4.1, 4.2, 8.3, 8.4, 9.4)		
11. Locates and assesses appropriate site (1.2, 1.4, 2.7, 3.2, 8.4, 9.4)		
12. Safely administers medication to maximise effects and minimise discomfort (1.2, 1.4, 2.2, 3.2, 3.9, 8.4, 9.4)		
13. Tends to puncture site appropriately (1.2, 1.4, 3.2, 8.4, 9.4)		
14. Removes gloves and performs hand hygiene (1.2, 1.4, 1.8, 3.9, 6.4, 9.4)		
15. Cleans, replaces or disposes of equipment appropriately (1.2, 1.4, 3.9, 6.5, 9.4)		
16. Documents and reports relevant information (1.2, 1.3, 1.8, 3.2, 5.3, 6.6, 7.1, 7.2, 7.3, 7.4, 7.5)		
17. Demonstrates ability to link theory to practice (8.3, 8.4, 8.5, 9.4)		

Student:

Clinical facilitator: Date:

CHAPTER 5.4

MEDICATION THERAPY – INHALED MEDICATION (METERED-DOSE INHALERS AND NEBULISERS)

IDENTIFY INDICATIONS

Inhaled medications are used to prevent and control symptoms, plus reduce exacerbations for patients with long-term respiratory disease such as asthma and chronic obstructive pulmonary disease (NPS Medicinewise, 2017). The different types of devices include metered-dose inhalers, dry powder inhalers and nebulisers. They contain either a single or combination of medications. The choice of delivery device will be decided by the patient's doctor, and prescribed on the medication chart. While some hospitalised patients may normally self-administer their medications, the nurse administering is responsible to either assist with administration because of the patient's current physical limitations or ensure the patient uses a correct technique.

GATHER AND PREPARE EQUIPMENT

This is a time-management strategy as well as increasing the patient's confidence in the nurse.

- *The medication chart.* This is used for checking the 'rights of medication administration'. The prescribed medication should be checked for dose, patient's name, expiration date and opening date.
- *Prescribed medication.*
- *Medication delivery device.* Most metered-dose inhalers contain the medication within the inhaler. Elderly patients may use a hand-grip device to assist them with holding and actuating their inhaler (National Asthma Council of Australia [NACA], 2017a). Refer to facility policies for preferred delivery devices (e.g. T-piece or face mask) if a nebulised medication is prescribed.

- *Spacer.* This is used with pressurised metered-dose inhalers to assist with delivery technique. A spacer will make it easier to inhale medication from a pressurised inhaler, allowing the patient to also breathe deeply and slowly. The medication will also remain in the spacer until it is all breathed in. Use of a spacer in combination with a metered-dose inhaler is as effective as nebulised medication and is the preferred option (NACA, 2017b; NPS Medicinewise, 2017).

For nebulised medication, the following equipment will be required.

- *Oxygen tubing with connectors*
- *Wall outlet compressed air* (or oxygen in some facilities)
- *Small air compressor*, if no wall outlet air is available

ADMINISTERING THE INHALED MEDICATION

Perform hand hygiene

Perform hand hygiene before touching the patient or the patient's surrounds and prior to any procedure involving patient contact to reduce the possibility of cross-contamination. Hand hygiene is the most effective method of infection control as it removes transient organisms from the hands of the nurse (see **Skill 1.1**). Preparing inhaled medications involves a 'clean technique'.

Give a clear explanation of the procedure and establish therapeutic communication

Difficulty breathing is distressing and increases anxiety. A calm tone of voice while talking to the patient and use of closed questions requiring a brief yes/no answer will assist the patient to relax and become more cooperative. Introduce yourself to the patient, and check you have the correct patient. Explain the procedure and name of the drug, then gain the patient's consent. The patient should be aware of the drug name, dose, its expected effects and probable side effects. This gives the patient information on which to base decisions about treatment. Ask the patient about any drug or medication allergies. Checking the patient and gaining their consent will also ensure that you meet legal and policy requirements before implementing any procedures. Discussing the medication with the patient gives them a sense of control. It also allows the nurse to assess if more teaching is required, and to gauge the patient's understanding of their treatment.

Attend to safety precautions and legal requirements for medication administration

As with all medication administration, the following principles should be maintained.

- Use the 'rights' of medication administration (see **Skill 5.1**).
- Adhere to the general concepts for the use of therapeutic substances (see **Skill 5.1**) and safe medication administration.
- Verify that the order is valid (see **Skill 5.1**) and check the medication chart for time, route, dose and drug.

Demonstrate problem-solving abilities

Patients receiving inhaled medication should be positioned upright or at a minimum of 45% (semi-upright) position. This will allow greater lung expansion and assist with correct delivery of the medication. If the patient is unable to hold the inhaler or spacer, the nurse will need to hold the device while the patient inhales the medication.

Administering medication via metered-dose inhaler

Metered-dose inhalers are used to enable the delivery of a metered volume of the medication as a fine spray. The concentrated dose delivered has a rapid effect. There are four main types of metered-dose inhalers: pressurised, breath-actuated, dry powder and soft mist.

- *Pressurised metered-dose inhalers.* Although these inhalers can be used without a spacer, it is recommended because they make the medication easier to inhale. After ensuring the correct medication is being used, shake the inhaler, then attach to the spacer. The patient places their mouth over the mouthpiece. Press the inhaler to release one dose, and the patient immediately breathes in either one slow deep breath for five seconds or four normal breaths. The inhaler should then be shaken and reattached before repeating the process for the next dose.
- *Breath-actuated inhaler.* The medication is released when the patient uses the mouthpiece and breathes in. Shake the inhaler before use. Ask the patient to exhale, then place their mouth over the mouthpiece and inhale deeply. Do not exhale into the inhaler.
- *Dry pressure inhaler.* The medication can be contained within the device or in a separate capsule. Prime and position the inhaler according to the manufacturer's instructions. The patient exhales, places their mouth over the mouthpiece, then breathes in quickly and deeply.
- *Soft-mist inhaler.* Prime the inhaler. The patient should exhale, then place their mouth over the mouthpiece and inhale while also pressing the dose button. Breathing in can be slower (but longer) than with pressurised metered-dose inhalers. Refer to the pharmacist for supporting advice on how to use individual inhalers. They can vary according to the manufacturer.

Administering medication via nebuliser

Nebulisers create a medication vapour by forcing pressurised air through the liquid to create a fine mist. This is breathed in through a mouthpiece or mask. Prepared nebules containing the prescribed medication are most frequently used. A normal saline neb can also be delivered using sterile saline ampoules following the same procedure for medication delivery.

Unscrew the cap from the nebuliser cup (bottom section). After re-checking the medication is correct, remove the top of the nebule and then squeeze the prescribed nebule into the cup section of the nebuliser. Replace the cap, taking care not to spill or lose any of the liquid. The nebuliser is then attached to the T-piece (or mask) and oxygen tubing, then to the wall supply compressed air/oxygen. The flow rate is adjusted to no less than 8 to 10 L/minute. Ensure the solution is misting before placing the mask or mouthpiece in place. If a compressor is used, place it on a flat surface and plug into the power supply before switching on.

Administration should take no longer than 8 to 10 minutes. Patients will need to seal their lips around the mouthpiece and breathe through their mouth if using a T-piece delivery device. When all the medication has been administered, remove the mask and turn off the air supply. Nebulisers and the T-piece/mask should be cleaned with warm water and left to air dry, ready for the next dose.

Perform hand hygiene

Maintain the 5 Moments for Hand Hygiene and perform hand hygiene after touching the patient and the patient's surrounds.

CLEAN, REPLACE OR DISPOSE OF EQUIPMENT

- *Cleaning a spacer.* Spacers should be cleaned as per facility policy, or more frequently if a patient has a chest infection. Dismantle the spacer and clean in warm water with dishwashing liquid. Allow to air dry, as drying with cloth or paper towel can result in static causing the medication to stick to the sides (NACA, 2017b). The spacer should also be checked for cracks and that the valve is working properly.

■ *Inhalers.* Wipe the outer area of the plastic inhaler, including the mouthpiece, with warm water and detergent. Air dry.

■ Medications are ordered from the pharmacy if they are running low. The medication chart is returned to its designated place for the next medication round.

DOCUMENT AND REPORT RELEVANT INFORMATION

Administration of metered-dose inhalers and nebulisers should be signed in the medication chart. The patient's response to the medication should be reported to the shift coordinator and in the nursing notes, especially when it is being used for urgent symptom relief.

CASE STUDY

You are an enrolled nurse working in a busy general practice. One of your regular clients, Bevan Childs (aged 51 years), has just been commenced on another medication called Seretide Accuhaler 250/50 which he is to use daily for his late-onset asthma. He also uses a Salbutamol puffer (with a spacer) when needed.

1. The patient asks you if he can use the new Accuhaler when he has an asthma attack, instead of the Salbutamol puffer. What is your response? (Check the Seretide information in a suitable pharmacology book or the NPS Medicinewise site.)
2. Give an outline of the correct method for Bevan to use the Accuhaler.

Note: These notes are summaries of the most important points in the assessments/procedures, and are not exhaustive on the subject. The naming of documents or charts may differ from state to state, and facility to facility. In all possible situations the guidelines of the ACSQHC are used when describing national charts or documents (e.g. the ACSQHC Observation and Response Chart is named the Adult Observation and Response Chart in WA, and the Rapid Detection and Response Observation Chart in SA). References of the materials used to compile the information have been supplied. The student is expected to have learned the material surrounding each skill as presented in the references. No single reference is complete on the subject.

REFERENCES

National Asthma Council of Australia. (2017a). *Australian Asthma Handbook.* http://www.asthmahandbook.org.au/management/devices/device-choice

National Asthma Council of Australia. (2017b). *Spacer Use and Care.* https://www.nationalasthma.org.au/living-with-asthma/resources/patients-carers/factsheets/spacer-use-and-care

NPS MedicineWise. (2017). *Inhaler Devices for Respiratory Medicines.* NPS MedicineWise. https://www.nps.org.au/medical-info/consumer-info/inhaler-devices-for-respiratory-medicines

RECOMMENDED READINGS

Australian Commission on Safety and Quality in Health Care (ACSQHC). (2016). *National Inpatient Medication Chart User Guide.* https://www.safetyandquality.gov.au/publications-and-resources/resource-library/national-inpatient-medication-chart-nimc-user-guide

Broyles, B., Reiss, B., Evans, M., McKenzie, G., Pleunik, S. & Page, R. (2020). *Pharmacology in Nursing: Australian and New Zealand Edition* (3rd ed.). Melbourne: Cengage.

Dougherty, L. & Lister, S. (eds). (2015). *The Royal Marsden Hospital Manual of Clinical Nursing Procedures* (9th ed.). Oxford: Wiley-Blackwell.

PART 5

ESSENTIAL SKILLS COMPETENCY

Metered-Dose Inhalers

Demonstrates the ability to effectively and safely administer inhaled medication therapy

Criteria for skill performance	Y	D
(Numbers indicate *Enrolled Nurse Standards for Practice*, 2016)	(Satisfactory)	(Requires development)
1. Identifies indication (8.3, 8.4)		
2. Gathers and prepares equipment (1.2, 1.6, 4.4, 6.4, 8.4, 9.4): ■ medication chart ■ medication ■ metered-dose inhaler (and spacer) ■ nebuliser with oxygen tubing ■ small air compressor if required		
3. Performs hand hygiene (1.2, 1.4, 1.8, 3.9, 6.4, 9.4)		
4. Evidence of therapeutic communication with the patient; e.g. gives explanation of procedure, gains patient consent (2.1, 2.3, 2.4, 2.5, 6.3)		
5. Attends to safety precautions including the 'rights of medication administration' (1.1, 1.2, 1.3, 1.4, 2.2, 3.1, 3.2, 3.9, 5.5, 8.4, 9.3, 9.4)		
6. Demonstrates problem-solving abilities; e.g. positions patient in semi-upright position (4.1, 4.2, 8.3, 8.4, 9.4)		
7. Prepares and administers inhaled medication (1.2, 1.4, 3.2, 3.9, 4.4, 6.4, 8.4, 9.4)		
8. Assists the patient to take the medication (1.2, 1.4, 1.8, 2.2, 3.2, 3.9, 6.1, 8.4, 9.4)		
9. Performs hand hygiene (1.2, 1.4, 1.8, 3.9, 6.4, 9.4)		
10. Cleans, replaces or disposes of equipment appropriately (1.2, 1.4, 3.9, 6.5, 9.4)		
11. Documents and reports relevant information (1.2, 1.3, 1.8, 3.2, 5.3, 6.6, 7.1, 7.2, 7.3, 7.4, 7.5)		
12. Demonstrates ability to link theory to practice (8.3, 8.4, 8.5, 9.4)		

Student:

Clinical facilitator: Date:

CHAPTER 5.5

MEDICATION ADMINISTRATION – VIA AN ENTERAL TUBE

IDENTIFY INDICATIONS

Patients may be administered medication via an enteral tube (NGT – nasogastric tube, PEG – percutaneous endoscopic gastrostomy) if they have swallowing difficulties, are unable to swallow oral medications or have an impaired conscious state. Identify the need to administer medications from the patient's medication chart.

VERIFY WRITTEN ORDERS

Written orders are necessary for medication administration to ensure that the patient receives the medication and dosage at the right time and via the correct route. The pharmacist should have left instruction for each medication about the preparation (e.g. crushing, dissolving, etc.) for enteral administration.

GATHER EQUIPMENT

Gathering equipment before initiating the procedure creates a positive environment for the successful completion of the procedure and provides an opportunity for the nurse to rehearse the procedure mentally.

- *Non-sterile gloves* are worn to comply with standard precautions.
- *Equipment for checking nasogastric tube (NGT) placement* – a 10 or 20 mL enteral (non-Luer) syringe (with purple or orange plunger) to remove a small amount of gastric content to test for pH; small medication cups for testing aspirate in; pH indicator test strips.
- *Equipment for checking gastrostomy (PEG) tube*, as per the brand and type of tube in situ. There are many different commercial types of tubes available (e.g. balloon, button) with their own specific requirements for tube position checking.

- *Kidney dish.*
- *The administration apparatus* – 50 mL enteral (non-Luer) syringe with purple or orange plunger.
- *An adapter* may be required to connect the nasogastric tube to other equipment.
- *Equipment to prepare medication* – mortar and pestle for crushing, extra measuring cups for dissolving, and oral liquid dispenser for measuring liquid medication.
- *Medication chart and medications.*
- *Warm tap water for flushing.*
Note: for safety reasons, equipment and disposable items used for giving nasogastric feeds are identified with purple or orange flanges, plungers, tips, etc. If the tube is inserted as a drain, the tube and other equipment should not have purple or orange colouring.

REVIEW SAFETY CONSIDERATIONS AND DEMONSTRATE PROBLEM-SOLVING ABILITIES

Administering medication via an enteral route is not the same as an oral route, although there can be confusion where it is considered to be the same. Consultation must be made with the pharmacist and doctor to review the order if the route is stated as oral, or the prescription for a patient normally receiving oral medications is changed to an enteral route. The pharmacist should also review the medication chart to confirm the process for preparing the medication for enteral administration. An alternate medication or route may also need to be considered. Crushing of medications can be contrary to medication manufacturer guidelines, making this not suitable for the medication administered. Nurses should also be aware of potential interaction issues:

- medication interaction with the feed or other medications within the tube
- medication interactions with the feed in the stomach

- medication to medication interactions when medications are prepared in non-washed containers, not prepared in separate/individual containers or the tube is not flushed between each individual medication (Richardson, 2016; White & Bradnam, 2015).

As with all medication administration, the principles of safety and the eight Rs, as well as the legal and ethical requirements discussed in **Skill 5.1**, should be followed.

The principles for safety when administering medications via an enteral feed also include the safety principles for enteral feed administrations. Please refer to **Skill 8.12** to review these safety issues. This includes ensuring that the syringe is connected to the correct port (e.g. not the balloon port).

ADMINISTERING MEDICATIONS VIA AN ENTERAL TUBE

Perform hand hygiene and don non-sterile gloves

Perform hand hygiene before touching the patient or the patient's surrounds and prior to any procedure involving patient contact to reduce the possibility of cross-contamination. Hand hygiene is the most effective method of infection control as it removes transient organisms from the hands of the nurse (see **Skill 1.1**). This is a clean procedure. Non-sterile gloves may be used to comply with standard precautions if exposed to body fluids when aspirating the tube, or to follow workplace health and safety (WHS) principles when crushing/preparing the medications.

Give a clear explanation of the procedure and establish therapeutic communication

Introduce yourself, and check you have the correct patient. Discuss the procedure and gain the patient's consent. Giving a clear explanation is required to gain legal consent and to address policy requirements. It will also assist the patient to cooperate with the procedure, allay anxiety and assist in establishing a therapeutic relationship.

Position the patient for medication administration

As with enteral feeds, the patient should be positioned to at least 45 degrees, or to a sitting position, if condition permits prior to and when administering medications. The patient should remain in this position for 30 minutes after the medications have been administered to reduce the risk of vomiting or aspiration of the medications.

Check and then prepare the medication

Review the medication chart for any ordered medications that are due, and follow the principles of medication administration to check the correct medication is being prepared for administration to the correct patient. Medication should be prepared prior to checking the tube placement, and then administered. Each medication is dissolved, measured or crushed separately (Society of Hospital Pharmacists of Australia, 2019; White & Bradnam, 2015). Refer to the pharmacist's guidelines for how individual medications should be prepared, and for any specific requirements for administration, including withholding feeds post medications or sequence for medications to be administered.

- Dissolving. Many granular compounds can be 'suspended' in liquid and others dissolved into individual measuring cups or syringes. Some dissolvable medications can be placed inside a syringe, the plunger returned and water sucked into the syringe.
- Measuring liquid. Liquid is measured into individual enteral syringes by connecting the syringe to the connector on the medication bottle. They may also require further dilution before administration if they are too viscous.
- Crushing. A mortar and pestle or pill crusher is used for medications approved for crushing into a fine powder. Clean equipment between each medication. Do not crush multiple medications at one time. Separate each medication into a medication cup and add a small amount of water.

Check placement of the tube

Nasogastric tubes require confirmation of the tube placement in the stomach prior to administration of medications every time medications are given. Please refer to **Skill 8.12** for a description of how to confirm the placement of a nasogastric tube. Other gastrostomy/PEG tubes require confirmation that the tube has not been dislodged or disconnected. Refer to the manufacturer's instructions regarding the ongoing management of specific brands of gastrostomy/PEG tubes.

Flushing the tube

The enteral tube should be flushed with 30 mL of room temperature (warm) water prior to administering the medications to clear the tube and ensure tube patency. The tube is then flushed after each medication is administered (i.e. between each medication) with 5 to 10 mL of water.

Flushing the tube between feeds and medication administration also reduces the risk of microbial colonisation within the enteral tube (NHMRC, 2020).

Medication administration via enteral feeding tube using gravity method

Continuous feeds should be ceased for 15 minutes prior to administering medications (check facility policy). After medications have been prepared and tube placement confirmed, connect a clean 50 mL nasogastric syringe barrel to the end of the tube. To avoid any air entering the inserted tube, use your fingers to kink the tube when opening the end-cap/spigot and until fluid is placed in the syringe. While keeping the tube kinked, stabilise the syringe with the same hand to prevent spillage when adding fluid into the barrel.

Add the water flush to clear the tube. Move fingers to unkink the tube, and allow the fluid to flow down the tube. To enable a slow gravitational flow, keep the syringe at or above the height of the patient's nose. A syringe plunger must never be used to force fluid down the tube (if the fluid does not flow or the tube is blocked, refer to a registered nurse for further assistance).

Medications are then administered one at a time into the syringe, allowed to flow into the stomach and then flushed with 10 mL of water before adding the next medication. When the water has come to the bottom of the syringe, kink the tube to prevent air entering the tube, then add more liquid. When all the medications have been administered, flush the tube with 30 mL of water. After the final flush, the tube is kinked, the syringe is disconnected and the tube closed.

Doff gloves and perform hand hygiene

Maintain the 5 Moments for Hand Hygiene and perform hand hygiene after touching the patient and the patient's surrounds.

Record fluid intake

After the medication has been administered, the amount of fluid administered is recorded on the fluid balance chart. The medication chart should also be signed for each medication administered.

CLEAN, REPLACE OR DISPOSE OF EQUIPMENT

The pill crusher and mortar and pestle should be washed with warm soap and water and then dried. Dispose of testing aspirate and other disposable items. Tidy the bedside area and reduce clutter. Cleaning the equipment maintains WHS and infection control, and is a courtesy to other staff.

DOCUMENT AND REPORT RELEVANT INFORMATION

A nasogastric chart will record the tube length and pH test when the tube is inserted and at each feed. As discussed earlier, drainage, aspirate and fluid administered are recorded on the relevant charts.

CASE STUDY

You are caring for Samuel Thomas, who is aged 75 and recently suffered a stroke. He has a reduced gag reflex and the doctor has ordered a nasogastric tube to be inserted for nutrition, hydration and the administration of medications. Samuel has a medical history of cardiovascular disease and diabetes, for which he has been taking several medications.
1. When you review the medication chart, you note that the admitting doctor has prescribed the medications to be administered orally. Will this be the same route as crushing or dissolving and administering the medications via the nasogastric tube?

When administering the medications at 0800 hours you follow the pharmacist's instruction to prepare each medication by crushing and dissolving it separately in a small amount of water. Each medication is to be administered separately.
2. What is the reason for doing this?
3. Why is it necessary to position Samuel at a 45-degree angle in the bed prior to and after administering the medication?
4. Why is it necessary to flush the tube before administering the medications, between each medication and after all medications have been administered?

Note: These notes are summaries of the most important points in the assessments/procedures, and are not exhaustive on the subject. The naming of documents or charts may differ from state to state, and facility to facility. In all possible situations the guidelines of the ACSQHC are used when describing national charts or documents (e.g. the ACSQHC Observation and Response Chart is named the Adult Observation and Response Chart in WA, and the Rapid Detection and Response Observation Chart in SA). References of the materials used to compile the information have been supplied. The student is expected to have learned the material surrounding each skill as presented in the references. No single reference is complete on the subject.

CRITICAL THINKING

Thinking of the clinical skills discussed in all the previous skills for Part 5, list three key components you need to consider in each of the following scenarios.
1. A nebuliser to a 12-month-old baby
2. Oral medications to a 4-year-old child
3. An intramuscular injection to an infant or toddler
4. A subcutaneous injection to a teenager
5. Multiple medications at the same time (e.g. 0800 hours) via a nasogastric tube, to an 82-year-old male patient
6. Eye drops to a 78-year-old female patient with dementia
7. When removing a topical Schedule 8 patch, identify issues relating to your scope of practice and disposal of the patch that will influence your actions in this situation
8. When administering medications to paediatric and geriatric patients, identify the dose-related issues you need to check when reading the order on the medication chart

REFERENCES

National Health and Medical Research Council (NHMRC). (2020). B4.2.4 Enteral feeding tubes. *Australian Guidelines for the Prevention and Control of Infection in Healthcare*. NHMRC.

Richardson, T. (2016). *Medication Administration via Enteral Feeding Tubes*. https://www.alfredhealth.org.au/contents/resources/clinical-resources/MedicationAdministration AndDrugInteractions.pdf

Society of Hospital Pharmacists of Australia. (2019). *How to Give Your Medicine by Enteral Tube. Patient Information*. https://www.shpa.org.au/sites/default/files/uploaded-content/website-content/website-content/giving_medicines_into_your_enteral_tube_-_drtc.pdf

White, R. & Bradnam, V. (2015). *Handbook of Drug Administration via Enteral Feeding Tubes* (3rd ed.). London: Pharmaceutical Press.

RECOMMENDED READINGS

Agency for Clinical Innovation (ACI) and the Gastroenterological Nurses College of Australia (GNCA). (2015). *A Clinician's Guide: Caring for People with Gastrostomy Tubes and Devices. From Pre-insertion to Ongoing Care and Removal*. https://www.aci.health.nsw.gov.au/__data/assets/pdf_file/0017/251063/gastrostomy_guide-web.pdf

Australian Commission on Safety and Quality in Health Care (ACSQHC). (2016). *National Inpatient Medication Chart User Guide*. https://www.safetyandquality.gov.au/publications-and-resources/resource-library/national-inpatient-medication-chart-nimc-user-guide

ESSENTIAL SKILLS COMPETENCY

Administration of Enteral Medication
Demonstrates the ability to safely and efficiently administer medications via an enteral tube

Criteria for skill performance (Numbers indicate *Enrolled Nurse Standards for Practice*, 2016)	Y (Satisfactory)	D (Requires development)
1. Identifies indication (4.1, 6.1, 7.1, 8.3, 8.4)		
2. Verifies written order (1.2, 1.4, 3.2, 3.9, 5.5, 9.4)		
3. Gathers equipment (1.2, 1.6, 8.4) ■ medications and medication chart ■ pH indicator strips ■ non-sterile gloves ■ small medication cups, measuring cups, pill crusher, enteral syringe, oral liquid dispenser, enteric syringes for checking placement and administration: 10 mL and 50 mL (and any connectors if required) ■ water for flushing		
4. Evidence of therapeutic communication with the patient; e.g. gives explanation of procedure, gains patient consent (2.1, 2.3, 2.4, 2.5, 3.2, 6.3, 7.3, 7.5)		
5. Demonstrates problem-solving abilities; e.g. provides privacy (4.1, 4.2, 8.3, 8.4, 9.4)		
6. Performs hand hygiene, dons non-sterile gloves (1.2, 1.4, 1.8, 3.2, 3.9, 6.4, 9.4)		
7. Positions patient upright (1.2, 1.4, 3.2, 5.4, 8.4, 9.4)		
8. Confirms placement of NGT or PEG tube (as per manufacturer's instructions) (1.2, 1.4, 3.2, 3.9, 4.4, 5.4, 6.4, 8.4, 9.4)		
9. Uses the 'rights' to administer the medication (1.1, 1.2, 1.3, 1.4, 2.2, 3.1, 3.2, 3.9, 5.5, 8.4, 9.3, 9.4)		
10. Medication is prepared as per pharmacist instructions, then administered safely using gravity flow method; tube is flushed prior, between and after all medications are administered (1.2, 1.4, 3.2, 3.9, 4.4, 5.4, 6.4, 8.4, 9.4)		
11. Removes gloves and performs hand hygiene (1.2, 1.4, 1.8, 3.9, 6.4, 9.4)		
12. Cleans, replaces or disposes of equipment appropriately (1.2, 1.4, 3.9, 6.5, 9.4)		
13. Documents and reports relevant information (1.2, 1.3, 1.8, 3.2, 5.3, 6.6, 7.1, 7.2, 7.3, 7.4, 7.5)		
14. Demonstrates ability to link theory to practice (8.3, 8.4, 8.5, 9.4)		

Student:

Clinical facilitator: Date:

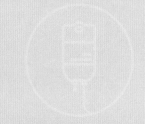

INTRAVENOUS CARE

Note: These notes are summaries of the most important points in the assessments/procedures and are not exhaustive on the subject. References of the materials used to compile the information have been supplied. The student is expected to have learnt the material surrounding each skill as presented in the references. No single reference is complete on each subject.

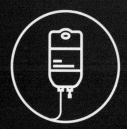

CHAPTER 6.1

VENEPUNCTURE

IDENTIFY INDICATIONS

Venepuncture provides access to the venous system via a needle to obtain blood for diagnostic purposes or to monitor a patient's response to treatment. Blood tests provide valuable information about a patient's general health, biochemical, haematological, metabolic, immune and nutritional status. The medical staff order these blood tests, and they are the most commonly performed invasive procedure in healthcare (Martel, 2017). Accessing the venous system is an invasive procedure and requires a patient's verbal consent after explaining the procedure and the need for the required blood test to be performed.

Most institutions consider venepuncture an advanced skill. If facility policy permits nursing staff to perform this skill, they will complete in-service and competency assessment programs.

OUTLINE SAFETY CONSIDERATIONS

The venous system is a closed system which venepuncture breaches, providing an entry point for microorganisms. It is essential that venepuncture is carried out using an aseptic technique. Workplace health and safety principles should be followed to reduce the risk of needlestick injury or contact with the patient's blood. Various vacuum, non-touch and 'safety-needle' systems are available to assist in meeting these safety needs. Familiarise yourself with the safety devices available at your facility. Standard precautions must be maintained, and well-fitting non-sterile gloves should be worn. Determine the person's identity by asking their full name and date of birth and checking their identification band against the request form to ensure the specimen is obtained from the correct patient. Determine any patient preparation required (e.g. fasting for many tests) and that it has been done.

The medical staff or a nurse practitioner must complete laboratory requisitions for all blood tests. The person collecting the specimen generally provides their name, signature and the time and date of collection.

Knowledge of the patient's medical history, current and recent medications and diagnosis is essential to alert the nurse of any potential clinical risks. Common complications include haematoma, nerve injury or haemolysis of the specimen (Makhumula-Nkhoma et al., 2015; Martel, 2017). Haemolysis of the specimen can occur with incorrect technique, including contamination of the needle with the alcohol wipe. The blood cells break down, causing the specimen to turn bright red. This specimen is unsuitable as the changes will interfere with the test results (Muegge, 2017). If there are bleeding disorders (e.g. pancytopenia, thrombocytopenia purpura) or a recent history of steroid or anticoagulant use, a longer period of pressure needs to be applied to the puncture site after taking the blood.

GATHER EQUIPMENT

Gathering the following equipment prior to the procedure increases efficiency and patient confidence in the nurse.

- The 'bluey' protects bed linen.
- *Non-sterile gloves* uphold standard precautions and maintain an aseptic technique.
- A *tourniquet* impedes venous return, engorging the veins and facilitating access. Tourniquets are a single-use disposable device.
- A *disposable access device with an integrated safety system and a vacuum collection system (as per facility preference)* are used to draw the blood from the venous system. The access device usually has a 21-gauge needle which enables the blood to be withdrawn without excessive discomfort to the patient and prevents damage of the cellular components of the blood (RBC) from crushing (haemolysis). The Vacutainer® system is specialised equipment used for accessing a vein. It consists of the plastic holder into which screws a double-sided needle and stoppered test tube with a vacuum.
- *Appropriate vacuumed test tubes* are needed. These attach to the vacuum collection system and automatically

collect the required amount of blood. The stoppers on the test tubes are colour-coded for various types of diagnostic studies. Refer to the chart available on the unit for a list of the various tests and the appropriate test tube. Some contain preservatives, others anticoagulants or coagulants, and some contain nothing. Collect the blood samples in the organisation's correct order of drawing blood (Muegge, 2017).

- *A sharps container* receives needles following use.
- *Alcohol wipes* cleanse the skin prior to inserting the needle. Alcohol destroys microorganisms on the skin.
- *A gauze swab/low-lint swabs and circular pressure dressing or tape* are used to apply pressure to the puncture site.

PERFORMING VENEPUNCTURE

Perform hand hygiene
Perform hand hygiene before touching the patient or the patient's surrounds and prior to any procedure involving patient contact to reduce the possibility of cross-contamination. Hand hygiene is the most effective method of infection control as it removes transient organisms from the hands of the nurse (see **Skill 1.1**).

Give a clear explanation of the procedure and establish therapeutic communication
Introduce yourself, and check you have the correct patient. Discuss the procedure and gain the patient's consent. Giving a clear explanation is required to gain legal consent and to address policy requirements. It will also assist the patient to cooperate with the procedure, allay anxiety and assist in establishing a therapeutic relationship.

Patient anxiety about the procedure may result in vasoconstriction. Giving a clear explanation of the procedure and working in a confident manner helps allay fears, anxiety and other potential complications such as haematoma (Dougherty & Lister, 2015). Many people have deep-seated fears of needles. Emphasising the necessity and the benefits of the procedure helps people accept the unpleasant procedure. Do not be dishonest about the discomfort; give reassurance and emphasise it will be completed quickly.

Prepare the area and equipment
Provide privacy for the patient by closing the bedside curtains or the door to the patient's room. Adjust the lighting to provide good illumination for the procedure. If the patient is in bed, raise or lower the bed to a comfortable working position to reduce strain on back muscles and improve access to the venepuncture site.

Place the equipment in a convenient position. Assemble the vacuum collection system.

Assess the arm and site, and prepare the patient
Visually inspect the veins on both arms. Veins adjacent to an infection, bruising or phlebitis are not suitable because of the risk of causing more local tissue damage or systemic infection. Areas of previous venepuncture are avoided, reducing the

build-up of scar tissue, which makes accessing the vein difficult and painful (Dougherty & Lister, 2015). When choosing the arm to be used for venous access, be aware of such conditions as lymphoedema, a mastectomy or axillary node dissection on that side, an established intravenous access in that arm, an arteriovenous shunt or a haematoma at the potential site that preclude use of that arm for venous access.

The vein chosen for access is usually in the antecubital fossa – the median cubital vein is the usual choice. Be aware that others may be more suitable, such as the basilic and cephalic veins. The median cubital, basilic and cephalic veins are straight and strong, and suitable for large-gauge venepuncture. The basilic and cephalic veins require stabilisation as they tend to roll. Ideally, preference is given to an unused vein, easily detected by inspection and palpation, patent and healthy. These veins feel soft and bouncy and will refill when depressed (Dougherty & Lister, 2015).

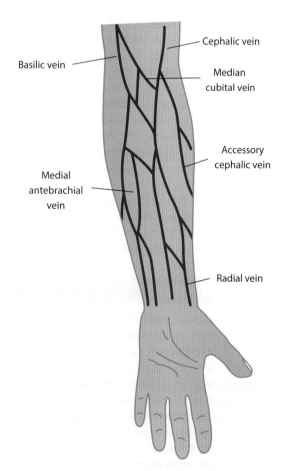

FIGURE 6.1.1 Location of veins in the antecubital fossa

To engorge veins, ask the patient to clench their fist after application of the tourniquet. This increases blood volume in the venous system and makes access of these veins easier.

Position the chosen arm extended to form a straight line from the shoulder to the wrist and well below the heart. A small pillow or towel covered with the 'bluey' under the upper arm stabilises it. The patient may be sitting or lying. Some patients feel very faint when blood is being taken, and require the lying position to accommodate that.

Apply the tourniquet

Apply the tourniquet about 12 to 15 cm above the intended puncture site. Lay the tourniquet flat against the skin, clip ends together and tighten. The nurse also places two fingers under the tourniquet while tightening to ensure it is not too tight. Check the distal pulse to make sure you have not occluded an artery. If you are unable to locate a pulse, release the tourniquet and reapply. Leave the tourniquet in place for 2 minutes only, as prolonged tourniquet application may cause stasis, localised acidaemia and haemoconcentration. If you are unable to find and access the vein in two minutes, release the tourniquet, wait a few minutes and reapply it.

Locate the vein

Locate the vein visually and, using the index and middle fingers of your non-dominant hand, palpate to determine the location and condition of the vein, distinguish veins from arteries and tendons and detect deeper veins. Palpating with the non-dominant hand increases the sensitivity and accuracy of locating the vein and also allows repalpation if the vein is missed and to realign the needle (Dougherty & Lister, 2015).

Ask the patient to open and close their fist slowly to increase the dilation and engorgement of the vein. Pumping or doing this too quickly may affect the blood test results (Dougherty & Lister, 2015). Stroke the arm towards the tourniquet to dilate the vein. The vein should feel round and firm and spring back when compressed.

Perform hand hygiene

Maintain the 5 Moments for Hand Hygiene and perform hand hygiene after touching the patient and the patient's surrounds.

Don non-sterile gloves

Put on well-fitting non-sterile gloves as part of standard precautions.

Cleanse the area with an alcohol wipe

Cleanse the area with the alcohol wipe and allow drying. Using circular strokes outward from the intended puncture point avoids bringing microorganisms into the clean area. Drying prevents stinging and discomfort when inserting the needle.

Access the vein and draw blood

With the access device in your dominant hand, anchor the vein firmly with a finger from your non-dominant hand below the intended puncture site. This will prevent the vein rolling away from the needle and the taut skin enables the needle to slide through the skin easily. The needle should be parallel to the vein and above it. The angle of insertion is less than 30 degrees elevation for a Vacutainer® and 15 degrees for a butterfly needle, to avoid going through the other side of the vein. Keeping the bevel of the needle upward also assists to avoid going through the opposite wall of the vein. Advance the needle through the skin and subcutaneous tissue and, gently but firmly, through the vein wall. You will feel the difference in pressure as the needle advances from the tissue through the vein wall (most commonly felt in adults, less often in children or in the frail elderly). A flash of blood appears in the hub of the needle or out of the tubing of the butterfly needle but not all Vacutainer® needle devices. Reduce the angle of descent when this flashback is seen or when puncture of the vein wall is felt. Advancing the needle slightly into the vein stabilises the needle within the vein and prevents dislodgement during withdrawal of blood (Dougherty & Lister, 2015). If there is no flashback, withdraw the needle slightly as it may be in contact with a valve. If the attempt was unsuccessful, release the tourniquet, wait a few minutes and try again. Most facilities have a policy of only allowing two unsuccessful attempts, to protect the patient.

Firmly hold the access device in place with the non-dominant hand and push a test tube onto the back part of the access device needle using your dominant hand. The needle must be firmly anchored by the non-dominant hand to avoid dislodging the needle. The vacuum in the test tube will pull the required amount of blood into it. If no blood appears in the container (i.e. the vein was missed), do not use that container again as the vacuum will have been broken.

Release the tourniquet

Release the tourniquet to increase comfort once a good blood flow in the tube has been established.

Withdraw the needle from the vein

Once all required blood has been collected, withdraw the needle at the same angle it was inserted to avoid tearing the vein. Using a gauze swab, apply pressure to the puncture site after the needle is fully removed. Do not apply pressure before removing the needle to reduce the risk of a needlestick injury. It will also decrease pain on removal and prevent damage to the intima of the vein (Dougherty & Lister, 2015). Activate the safety device on the needle, and place in a kidney dish or sharps container.

Pressure is applied with the gauze for 2 to 5 minutes to assist clotting, as well as to prevent bleeding and ecchymosis. Place a circular pressure dressing or tape (ask the patient if they have any allergies to tape) over the insertion site to continue the pressure to minimise bleeding. If the patient has fragile skin, do not use a tape; rather, apply pressure to the puncture site until bleeding has ceased. The patient is advised to minimise activity with the involved arm and to maintain pressure on the site for 5 minutes. Observe the site for haematoma formation.

If needed, gently rock the inverted test tube eight times to prevent haemolysis of the blood cells and to thoroughly mix the blood with any additives.

Remove and discard the gloves.

Label the test tube with the patient's information. Place the specimen in the press seal section of the biohazard bag for transporting to the laboratory. The request form is placed in the separated outside sleeve that is part of the biohazard bag, to prevent contamination of the form by the specimen or specimen container. Send the specimen and the request form to the laboratory as soon as possible.

Perform hand hygiene

Maintain the 5 Moments for Hand Hygiene and perform hand hygiene after touching the patient and the patient's surrounds.

CLEAN, REPLACE OR DISPOSE OF EQUIPMENT

Needles are placed in the sharps container for safety. Other items will be disposed of in the normal rubbish or contaminated waste bin. For efficiency, restock any equipment and specimen containers used.

DOCUMENT AND REPORT RELEVANT INFORMATION

Documentation of blood taken usually consists of a brief notation in the progress notes, including time, date, type of tests and patient response, the nursing care plan or patient observation and response chart. Results of the blood tests will be sent from the laboratory to the ward area and will be filed into the patient's notes.

CASE STUDY

Alfredo Martinez, aged 68, has been ordered blood tests for a fasting blood glucose level. He is required to have this blood taken before eating breakfast. His current medications are an oral antihypertensive and an anticoagulant injection twice daily. You are the enrolled nurse caring for Alfredo, and the facility requires the nursing staff to collect the early morning blood specimens for the laboratory.

1. Describe how you will explain this blood test to Alfredo.
2. What veins are preferable for the collection of the blood, and where are they located?
3. Considering his current medications, why is it important to apply pressure over the venepuncture site post collection of blood?

Note: These notes are summaries of the most important points in the assessments/procedures, and are not exhaustive on the subject. The naming of documents or charts may differ from state to state, and facility to facility. In all possible situations the guidelines of the ACSQHC are used when describing national charts or documents (e.g. the ACSQHC Observation and Response Chart is named the Adult Observation and Response Chart in WA, and the Rapid Detection and Response Observation Chart in SA). References of the materials used to compile the information have been supplied. The student is expected to have learned the material surrounding each skill as presented in the references. No single reference is complete on the subject.

REFERENCES

Dougherty, L. & Lister, S. (eds). (2015). *The Royal Marsden Hospital Manual of Clinical Nursing Procedures* (9th ed.). Oxford: Wiley-Blackwell.

Makhumula-Nkhoma, N., Whittaker, Vicki, B. & McSherry, R. (2015). Level of confidence in venepuncture and knowledge in determining causes of blood sample haemolysis among clinical staff and phlebotomists. *Journal of Clinical Nursing*, 24(3–4), p. 370.

Martel, A. (2017). Using a quality management system to implement best practice standards for phlebotomy processes. *MLO: Medical Laboratory Observer*, 49(10), p. 20.

Muegge, S. (2017). Stick to procedure when performing phlebotomy. *AAACN Viewpoint*, 39(3), pp. 1–11.

RECOMMENDED READINGS

Meiri, N., Ankri, A., Hamad-Saied, M., Konopnicki, M. & Pillar, G. (2016). The effect of medical clowning on reducing pain, crying, and anxiety in children aged 2–10 years old undergoing venous blood drawing—a randomized controlled study. *European Journal of Pediatrics*, 175(3), pp. 373–9

ESSENTIAL SKILLS COMPETENCY

Venepuncture
Demonstrates the ability to effectively and safely obtain a blood sample from a vein

CRITERIA FOR SKILL PERFORMANCE	Y	D
(Numbers indicate *Enrolled Nurse Standards for Practice*, 2016)	(Satisfactory)	(Requires development)
1. Identifies indication (8.3, 8.4)		
2. Outlines safety considerations (1.2)		
3. Gathers equipment (1.2, 1.6, 4.4, 6.4, 8.4, 9.4): ■ 'bluey', sharps container ■ non-sterile gloves, tourniquet ■ access device and vacuum collection system ■ appropriate vacuumed test tubes ■ alcohol wipes, gauze, tape or bandaid		
4. Performs hand hygiene (1.2, 1.4, 1.8, 3.9, 6.4, 9.4)		
5. Evidence of effective communication with the patient; e.g. gives patient a clear explanation of procedure, gains patient consent (2.1, 2.3, 2.4, 2,5, 6.3)		
6. Displays problem-solving abilities; e.g. positions patient, provides privacy (4.1, 4.2, 8.3, 8.4, 9.4)		
7. Assesses arm and selects site (1.2, 4.1, 8.4, 9.4)		
8. Assembles equipment conveniently (1.2, 1.6, 4.4, 6.4, 8.4, 9.4)		
9. Applies tourniquet (1.2)		
10. Locates vein and cleanses area (1.2, 1.4, 3.2, 3.9, 8.4, 9.4)		
11. Performs hand hygiene and dons non-sterile gloves (1.2, 1.4, 1.8, 3.2, 3.9, 6.4, 9.4)		
12. Accesses vein (1.2, 1.4, 1.8, 3.9, 4.4, 6.4, 8.4, 9.4)		
13. Draws blood (1.2, 1.4, 1.8, 3.1, 3.2, 3.9, 4.4, 6.4, 8.4, 9.4)		
14. Releases tourniquet (1.2)		
15. Withdraws needle, activates needle safety device, applies pressure to site (1.2, 1.4, 1.8, 3.2, 3.9, 4.4, 6.4, 8.4, 9.4)		
16. Doffs gloves and performs hand hygiene (1.2, 1.4, 1.8, 3.9, 6.4, 9.4)		
17. Cleans, replaces or disposes of equipment appropriately (1.2, 1.4, 3.9, 6.5, 9.4)		
18. Documents relevant information (1.2, 1.3, 1.8, 3.2, 5.3, 6.6, 7.1, 7.2, 7.3, 7.4, 7.5)		
19. Demonstrates ability to link theory to practice (8.3, 8.4, 8.5, 9.4)		

Student:

Clinical facilitator: Date:

CHAPTER **6.2**

PERIPHERAL INTRAVENOUS CANNULA (PIVC) – ASSISTING WITH ESTABLISHMENT

IDENTIFY INDICATIONS

Peripheral intravenous cannulas (PIVC) are the most commonly used intravenous devices in hospitalised patients and are often inserted for therapeutic purposes such as administration of medications, fluids and/or blood products (Bolton, 2015). Current guidelines from the ACSQHC (2019) recommend that a PIVC should only be inserted for

the administration of fluid or medication when all other routes are not suitable. The insertion of the PIVC is the responsibility of the medical staff or registered nurses who have undergone specialist education and maintained their competency in cannulation.

DEMONSTRATE PROBLEM-SOLVING ABILITIES

Peripheral intravenous cannulae (PIVC) provide direct access to the patient's bloodstream and therefore pose a serious risk for infection from microorganisms introduced either at the time of insertion or while the cannula is in situ.

(WA Health, 2017).

Use of an aseptic technique is essential to reduce the risk of introducing infection to the patient. Standard precautions are also essential when managing a PIVC to reduce the risk of exposure to blood. Closed intravenous access systems and needleless ports are recommended as they are associated with fewer infections (Queensland Health, 2019; WA Health, 2017). They also reduce the nurse's risk of exposure to the patient's body fluids.

The doctor or registered nurse inserting the PIVC will assess the patient's overall health status and

possible IV sites. Usually, initial IV access is at the most peripheral suitable site to leave the more proximal sites for subsequent access. It is also preferable for the PIVC to be inserted into the patient's non-dominant hand. Avoid areas of flexion (antecubital fossa, wrist), the site of a previous mastectomy, the affected side of a stroke patient or arteriovenous shunt, or the affected side if surgery is proposed for the arm/hand/shoulder. Children should have their IV access sited away from joints.

Assess the patient's baseline vital signs, allergies (to medications, iodine, latex, adhesive), planned interventions and general condition prior to PIVC establishment. PIVCs can remain in place for 72 to 96 hours before they are re-sited (Queensland Health, 2019; SA Health, 2020; WA Health, 2017). PIVCs should be removed when no longer required or immediately if complications develop (phlebitis, infection or malfunction) (ACSQHC, 2019; Queensland Health, 2019). Review facility and state health department policy on the re-siting and maintenance of PIVCs.

GATHER EQUIPMENT

Gather equipment prior to starting the procedure. Organisation increases your own confidence and permits a rehearsal of the procedure. It also increases the patient's confidence in the nursing care and minimises the time needed to accomplish the procedure.

- *IV trolley* is generally used to transport equipment to and from the bedside. Trolleys are usually stocked with all required items.

- *Required IV cannula (catheter), infusion port/connector and extension tubing.* These items should already be stocked in the IV trolley. Cannulae come in a variety of gauges, lengths and types. The doctor or registered nurse will determine which one to use. Generally, the chosen cannula is the smallest size that can deliver the volume of fluid or medication needed. The cannula, port and extension tubing will have a closed, needleless system to reduce infection risks for the patient and to reduce the

risk of exposure to body fluids for healthcare workers. *Other items* such as IV line sticker may be required.
- *Chlorhexidine gluconate 2% or alcohol (70%) solution* should always be used for skin preparation prior to insertion of intravascular devices (IVDs) and allowed to air dry (Queensland Health, 2019).
- *Sterile gloves* are required to maintain an aseptic technique and for protection of the person inserting the PIVC or connecting the PIVC port and extension tubing.
- *The tourniquet* is applied above the intended IV site to reduce the flow of venous blood back to the heart. This

distends the venous vessels, making insertion of an IV cannula more easily accomplished.
- *Transparent IV site dressing.* Transparent dressings enable continuous observation of the IV insertion site.
- *Tape* for securing the extension tubing.
- *The sharps container* is taken to the bedside so that the used inner cannula from the insertion set can be immediately disposed of, thus reducing the chance of needlestick injuries.
- *Clippers (if required)* to remove excess hair from the skin around the insertion site to allow for adherence of the dressing to the skin (Queensland Health, 2019).

ASSISTING WITH PIVC ESTABLISHMENT

Perform hand hygiene
Perform hand hygiene before touching the patient or the patient's surrounds and prior to any procedure involving patient contact to reduce the possibility of cross-contamination. Hand hygiene is the most effective method of infection control as it removes transient organisms from the hands of the nurse (see **Skill 1.1**).

Give a clear explanation of the procedure and establish therapeutic communication
Introduce yourself, and check you have the correct patient. Discuss the procedure and gain the patient's consent. Giving a clear explanation is required to gain legal consent and to address policy requirements. It will also assist the patient to cooperate with the procedure, allay anxiety and assist in establishing a therapeutic relationship.

Many people have a fear of needles. Explaining the necessity and the benefits of the procedure can help the patient be more settled during an unpleasant procedure. Warn the patient that they may experience some discomfort during insertion of the PIVC, or vein irritation during infusion of fluids or medication administration. Some policies promote the use of a topical or local anaesthetic to minimise the pain during insertion and reduce the associated anxiety (ACSQHC, 2019; Queensland Health, 2018; WA Health, 2017). Discuss adverse effects that are common with the PIVC therapy and ask the patient to alert the nurses to any changes that they note following insertion of the PIVC, or during any ongoing treatment.

Assist the doctor or cannulating nurse to establish an IV access
Ensure patient privacy by drawing the curtains or closing the door. Adjust the bed height to promote principles of workplace health and safety. Remove any jewellery from the arm where the PIVC is being inserted. Assist the doctor or cannulating nurse to establish an IV access by assembling and preparing

the equipment, supporting the patient and applying the dressing after any blood has been cleaned from the site. The person inserting the PIVC will be required to wear sterile gloves to maintain an aseptic technique.

Apply the dressing
An aseptic technique is required for PIVC insertion and application of the site dressing. As key parts (IV cannula and port) or key sites (IV insertion point) are being touched, sterile gloves are recommended to maintain an aseptic technique and to comply with standard precautions. Refer to **Skill 4.9** for how to don sterile gloves using an open gloving technique.

Stabilise the cannula with your non-dominant hand and apply the transparent dressing using an aseptic technique. Carefully remove the adherent backing from one edge of the dressing. Apply the dressing from that edge, smoothing it onto the skin as you remove the backing. It should cover the insertion site and most of the hub of the cannula but not the adapter, also leaving the junction clear of dressing material. Ensure the insertion site and surrounding tissues are not obscured with any tapes. Write the date and time of insertion on the dressing (WA Health, 2017). Securing the PIVC in place is essential to limit the increased risk of infection or phlebitis (ACSQHC, 2019; Queensland Health, 2018).

Attach extension tubing
Hold the IV cannula hub, and then gently insert the extension tubing. Extension sets help reduce movement of the cannula, trauma to the vein and potential complications (WA Health, 2017). The extension tubing should be secured using tape. Ensure no tape is placed over the PIVC insertion site or site dressing.

Refer to subsequent skills for any further procedures related to a PIVC and general care of a PIVC.

Doff gloves and perform hand hygiene
Remove sterile gloves and then perform hand hygiene. Maintain the 5 Moments for Hand Hygiene and perform hand hygiene after touching the patient and the patient's surrounds.

CLEAN, REPLACE OR DISPOSE OF EQUIPMENT

Clean, replace and dispose of equipment appropriately. The person inserting the cannula is responsible for the correct disposal of sharps. The trolley is cleaned using disinfecting wipes, restocked and returned to its storage area.

DOCUMENT AND REPORT RELEVANT INFORMATION

The insertion of an IV cannula is noted in the IV monitoring chart, patient progress notes and nursing care plan, and should include the date and the site of insertion.

Insertion site observations are noted every shift as a minimum in the IV monitoring chart and during clinical handover. (see **Skill 7.3**).

CASE STUDY

You are an enrolled nurse working in an acute medical ward. The doctor has requested your patient to commence IV fluids, for hydration and administration of medication. A new PIVC will need to be inserted by the doctor.

1. Use dot points to list your responsibilities as an enrolled nurse to assist with the establishment of IV therapy and insertion of the PIVC for your patient.

Note: These notes are summaries of the most important points in the assessments/procedures, and are not exhaustive on the subject. The naming of documents or charts may differ from state to state, and facility to facility. In all possible situations the guidelines of the ACSQHC are used when describing national charts or documents (e.g. the ACSQHC Observation and Response Chart is named the Adult Observation and Response Chart in WA, and the Rapid Detection and Response Obervation Chart in SA). References of the materials used to compile the information have been supplied. The student is expected to have learned the material surrounding each skill as presented in the references. No single reference is complete on the subject.

REFERENCES

Australian Commission on Safety and Quality in Health Care (ACSQHC). (2019). *Peripheral Intravenous Catheters.* https://www.safetyandquality.gov.au/standards/clinical-care-standards/peripheral-venous-access-clinical-care-standard

Bolton, D. (2015). Clinically indicated replacement of peripheral cannulas. *British Journal of Nursing*, 24, S4–12.

Queensland Health. (2018). *Peripheral Intravenous Catheter (PIVC) Guidelines.* Queensland Government. https://www.health.qld.gov.au/__data/assets/pdf_file/0025/444490/icare-pivc-guideline.pdf

Queensland Health. (2019). *Recommendations for the Prevention of Infection in Intra-vascular Devices.* Queensland Government. https://www.health.qld.gov.au/clinical-practice/guidelines-procedures/diseases-infection/infection-prevention/intravascular-device-management

SA Health. (2020). *Peripheral Intravenous Catheter (PIVC) Infection Prevention Clinical Directive Version No.: 1.1* Approval date: 9 June 2020. Government of South Australia. https://www.sahealth.sa.gov.au/wps/wcm/connect/b8b0b71d-899e-42aa-ac3b-ca37d905f9a8/Clinical_Directive_PIVC_Infection_Prevention_v1.0_22.11.2019.pdf?MOD=AJPERES&CACHEID=ROOTWORKSPACE-b8b0b71d-899e-42aa-ac3b-ca37d905f9a8-mWhfA4q

WA Health. (2017). *Insertion and Management of Peripheral Intravenous Cannulae in Western Australian Healthcare Facilities Policy.* © Department of Health, Government of Western Australia. https://ww2.health.wa.gov.au/-/media/Files/Corporate/Policy-Frameworks/Public-Health/Policy/Insertion-and-Management-of-Peripheral-Intravenous-Cannulae/MP38-Insertion-and-Management-of-Peripheral-Intravenous-Cannulae.pdf

RECOMMENDED READINGS

Brooks, N. (2016). Intravenous cannula site management. *Nursing Standard*, 30(52), p. 53.

Shaw, S.J. (2016). How to insert a peripheral cannula. *Nursing Standard*, 31(12), p. 42.

ESSENTIAL SKILLS COMPETENCY

Intravenous Therapy (IVT) – Assisting with Establishment

Demonstrates the ability to effectively and safely assist in the establishment of intravenous therapy

Criteria for skill performance	Y	D
(Numbers indicate *Enrolled Nurse Standards for Practice*, 2016)	(Satisfactory)	(Requires development)
1. Identifies indication (8.3, 8.4)		
2. Demonstrates problem-solving abilities; e.g. recognises need for PIVC (or replacement cannula), maintains standard precautions (4.1, 4.2, 8.3, 8.4, 9.4)		
3. Gathers equipment (1.2, 1.6, 4.4, 6.4, 8.4, 9.4): ■ IV trolley ■ cannula, IV connectors and IV extension tubing ■ chlorhexidine gluconate 2% or alcohol 70% solution ■ sterile gloves ■ tourniquet ■ transparent IV site dressing ■ tape for securing extension tubing ■ sharps container ■ hair clippers if required		
4. Performs hand hygiene (1.2, 1.4, 1.8, 3.9, 6.4, 9.4)		
5. Evidence of effective communication with the patient; gives explanation of procedure, gains patient consent; allays patient's anxiety by adequately explaining the procedure (2.1, 2.3, 2.4, 2.5, 6.3)		
6. Assists the doctor/registered nurse to establish an IV access by preparing the patient and then assisting where required (1.2)		
7. Applies and dates the transparent dressing (1.2, 1.4, 6.4, 8.4, 9.4)		
8. Connects and secures extension tubing (1.2, 1.4, 6.4, 8.4, 9.4)		
9. Doffs gloves and performs hand hygiene (1.2, 1.4, 1.8, 3.9, 6.4, 9.4)		
10. Cleans, replaces or disposes of equipment appropriately (1.2, 1.4, 3.9, 6.5, 9.4)		
11. Documents and reports relevant information (1.2, 1.3, 1.8, 3.2, 5.3, 6.6, 7.1, 7.2, 7.3, 7.4, 7.5)		
12. Demonstrates ability to link theory to practice (8.3, 8.4, 8.5, 9.4)		

Student:

Clinical facilitator: Date:

CHAPTER 6.3

PERIPHERAL INTRAVENOUS CANNULA (PIVC) AND THERAPY (PIVT) MANAGEMENT

IDENTIFY INDICATIONS

Intravenous (IV) infusion into a peripheral vein is a common therapeutic intervention in an acute care setting. A peripheral intravenous cannula (PIVC) is inserted for the purpose of providing a portal for therapeutic purposes such as administration of medications, fluids and/or blood products. PIVC create a high risk for infection and other complications from IV therapy; therefore, the site should be assessed regularly, any fluid or medication administration monitored closely and non-essential IV devices removed promptly (ACSQHC, 2019; Queensland Health, 2019; WA Health, 2017). Other nursing care actions also need to ensure they reduce movement or knocking the site and avoid pulling on any attached IV lines to prevent the dislodging of an IV line and the infection or irritation of a PIVC site.

Indications for IV administration of fluids are to restore fluid or maintain fluid and electrolyte balance and administer medications. They are also inserted when a patient has a procedure (e.g. surgery) or urgent medical interventions that will require IV access. The acronym DRIP can be used to identify criteria for IV insertion: D – deterioration, R – rehydration, I – IV medication, P – procedures such as surgery. IV infusions introduce sterile fluids into the patient's circulation when the use of oral or enteral fluids is not possible, sufficient or appropriate. Examples are pre- or postoperatively, during trauma recovery or for IV medication administration.

DEMONSTRATE PROBLEM-SOLVING ABILITIES

Closed IV access systems and needleless ports are recommended for all IV access devices, connector ports, tubing and medication administration as they are associated with fewer infections (Queensland Health, 2019; WA Health, 2017). They also reduce the nurse's risk of exposure to the patient's body fluids. Use of an aseptic technique is essential when touching or accessing an IV port to reduce the risk of introducing infection to the patient. Standard precautions are also essential when managing a PIVC to reduce the risk of exposure to the patient's blood. Care of the PIVC is the responsibility of all nurses caring for the patient, unless the enrolled nurse (EN)

has a notation for medication administration against their name on the Nursing and Midwifery Board of Australia register (NMBA, 2020). However, the ability to monitor and administer IV fluid will be based on the EN's current scope of practice and IV competency (NMBA, 2020).

To manage an IV infusion, the nurse must be aware of the solution ordered, the rate of flow ordered and if there are further solution/s to be used after the current one is absorbed. This will be recorded on the IV fluid order chart. Administration sets (including extension tubing) are single-use devices and should be discarded after each use (i.e. between intermittent medication doses). For a continuous infusion, they must be changed after 72 to 96 hours (Queensland Health, 2018; SA Health, 2020; WA Health, 2017).

GATHER EQUIPMENT

Gather equipment prior to starting the procedure. Organisation increases your own confidence and permits a rehearsal of the procedure. It also increases the patient's confidence in the nursing care and minimises the time needed to accomplish the procedure.

- *IV risk assessment or phlebitis assessment chart* and all other documentation to record information for

monitoring the PIVC such as insertion date, site review and removal of PIVC.
- *A fluid balance chart* to record all fluid administered plus fluid output, and also to monitor the patient's fluid status.
- *The intravenous fluid order chart* with the written order is used to identify the IV fluid and administration rate. The fluid order chart has the patient's name, ID

number, date of birth and doctor on it and is used during identification of the patient to ensure that the correct fluid and amount are being given to the correct patient.

- *The prescribed fluid* (one bag) is obtained from stock. Check the bag for an intact outer bag, date of expiry, type and strength of fluid and remove the outer bag/packaging. The inner bag may be damp from condensation. Check the sterile contents of the inner bag for colour and clarity of the fluid by holding it up against both a dark and a light background. Gently squeeze the bag to check for leaks. Determine if additives are required. Two nurses (one is a registered nurse [RN]) are required to check the fluid against the fluid order and sign the order sheet.

- *IV administration set* depends on the fluid being infused (e.g. 0.9% sodium chloride versus blood) and the patient and infusion pump being used. Each pump will require a specific giving set. For infusions not using a pump, adults usually have a macrodrip giving set with a chamber providing 20 drops per mL. Frail elderly people,

children and infants generally require a giving set with a microdrip (60 drops per mL) chamber to make the regulation of the fluid more precise.

- *The IV stand/pole* is an extendable support for the fluid bag. It is inserted into a specific space located at the top of the bed head or has wheels attached to assist the patient with mobilisation.

- *Infusion pump*, if one is to be used. Most IV infusions in general ward areas are administered using a pump. Children, infants and frail elderly generally require a pump.

- *IV line sticker* for noting the date of when the IV line was changed. A watch with a second hand is used to time the flow of IV fluids, if an infusion pump is not used.

- *Sterile gloves* are required to maintain an aseptic technique when connecting the IV administration line. Kidney dish is used for collecting fluid when priming the IV administration set.

- *Alcohol wipes* are used for cleaning the administration port before connecting other tubing or after removing the IV administration set.

IMPLEMENT CARE OF A PIVC

Perform hand hygiene
Perform hand hygiene before touching the patient or the patient's surrounds and prior to any procedure involving patient contact to reduce the possibility of cross-contamination. Hand hygiene is the most effective method of infection control as it removes transient organisms from the hands of the nurse (see **Skill 1.1**). When managing the PIVC, the ACSQHC recommends performing hand hygiene visually in front of the patient (ACSQHC, 2019).

Give a clear explanation of the procedure and establish therapeutic communication
Introduce yourself, and check you have the correct patient. Discuss the procedure and gain the patient's consent. Giving a clear explanation is required to gain legal consent and to address policy requirements. It will also assist the patient to cooperate with the procedure, allay anxiety and assist in establishing a therapeutic relationship.

Effective communication with the patient who has a PIVC in situ and IV therapy includes discussing the comfort of the site with the patient; reassurance that the frequent checks done on the peripheral PIVC and the infusion flow rate (or pump) are a normal routine; and requesting the patient to disclose any pain or other abnormal sensation at the insertion site.

Assess the patient with a PIVC and/or IV therapy
Both the PIVC insertion site and the infusion require ongoing assessment for a patient with a PIVC. If the patient only has a cannula inserted, and not infusion, the site still requires regular routine assessment, as a minimum every 8 hours. Continuous infusions require monitoring of the IV flow rate, as well as assessment

of the patient. During clinical handover, the PIVC site, pre-existing rating score and IV fluids being administered should be checked by both the current nurse and nurse for the next shift.

PIVC insertion site
The PIVC insertion site should be visually assessed at least once each shift, every time the site is accessed or the patient expresses any concern about the PIVC (ACSQHC, 2019). A PIVC site should also continue to be assessed for 48 hours post completion of IV medication administration or removal of PIVC.

The IV insertion site is assessed using the facility risk assessment and/or phlebitis and infection risk assessment tool. Assessment includes looking at the PIVC, listening to any input from the patient and gently palpating the site. Different tools (e.g. peripheral intravenous assessment score [PIVAS] or visual infusion phlebitis [VIP] score) are used for assessing the infusion site and are determined by facility policy (ACSQHC, 2019; WA Health, 2017). A rating score is given according to symptoms of phlebitis (inflammation of the vein) or thrombophlebitis, such as pain, redness (erythema), swelling and palpable vein. The score will determine the ongoing response and management of the IV site (Moola, 2020). Other observations of the site include assessment for fluid leakage at the insertion site, occlusion or infiltration, indicated by discomfort, blanching, coolness of skin and a slow IV rate, and that the site dressing has remained intact. The results of this assessment should be recorded on the nursing care plan or other IV documentation. Check the date of the PIVC insertion and if the catheter needs to be reinserted. PIVCs can remain in place for 72 to 96 hours (Queensland Health, 2018; SA Health, 2020; WA Health, 2017) before they are re-sited. All PIVCs are removed immediately at the first sign of phlebitis.

IV infusion

The IV infusion is checked for several factors.

- *Systemic assessment.* This includes monitoring for signs of circulatory overload, fluid volume deficit, septicaemia, hypersensitivity and pulmonary or air embolism.
- *Fluid and equipment assessment.* The established IV infusion is assessed and recorded hourly to determine that it is being administered at the correct rate; the solution is the prescribed one; the amount absorbed is calculated; and the amount remaining to be infused is noted. When the administration rate is checked, it should be adjusted if it is not the correct rate. Also check required labels for the IV administration set and any IV medications are correct and intact (ACSQHC, 2015). Change the administration set every 72 to 96 hours (Queensland Health, 2018; SA Health, 2020; WA Health, 2017).

Establishing and connecting an IV infusion

Use general concepts and the 'rights of medication administration'

Use the 'rights of medication administration' to check, prepare and administer the fluid to the patient. IV fluids are therapeutic prescriptions and are thus treated as medications. The prescribed fluid (i.e. medication order), volume and flow rate will be stated on the IV fluid order chart.

Prepare the giving set and check the IV pump

Before priming and connecting the IV administration set, check the IV pump for currency of maintenance and any manufacturer's instructions for programming the pump. Ensure alarms are working, batteries are charged and connect the pump to the mains supply.

Prepare the administration set by removing it from its packaging and moving the clamp to just below (about 5 cm) the drip chamber. Tighten the clamp to prevent fluid flow until you are ready to prime the line and adjust the flow.

Perform hand hygiene

After completing a care action required to manage the care of an IV infusion or PIVC, maintain the 5 Moments for Hand Hygiene and perform hand hygiene after touching the patient and the patient's surrounds.

Spike the fluid bag

Remove the protective sheath over the spike on the top end of the drip chamber. Take care to maintain the sterility of the spike. Spike the fluid bag after exposing the port on the fluid bag by pulling off the protective sheath. Rest the fluid bag on a table, to ensure that the port is straight and the spike does not go through the sides of the port. Hold the side of the port with the fingers of your non-dominant hand. Take care not to touch the outer edges of the port with the spike while firmly pushing the spike all of its length into the port.

Prime and label the line

Follow the manufacturer's instructions for specific guidelines on priming lines for an IV pump. Generally, the line is primed with fluid by hanging the bag of fluid on the IV pole. For gravity flow administration sets with a drip chamber, gently squeeze and release the drip chamber until it is half-full (ensuring the roller clamp is still closed). Open the roller clamp and allow fluid to fill the IV line. You may need to remove the protective cap at the distal end of the IV line (some caps permit priming while still in place). Hold the distal end of the line over the kidney dish and higher than its dependent loops so that air is expelled and fluid is not spilled. When the line is full and there are no air bubbles, close the roller clamp, reapply the protective cap and hang the line on the IV pole until it is needed (note: if a smaller volume of IV fluids is prescribed, a smaller 50 mL bag of sodium chloride 0.9% may be used to prime the line and prevent wastage of fluid and/or medication). Remember that this is an aseptic technique and the key parts of the connection should not be touched or contaminated.

Place the required blue IV line label on the IV tubing, noting the date of tubing commencement (ACSQHC, 2015). Make sure the dependent loop of the line is clear of the floor and the end is easily reached. If there are air bubbles, gently tap the line at the point where the air bubbles are, keeping the line between the bubbles and the drip chamber straight. The bubbles will dislodge from the line and ascend into the drip chamber. Raise the IV pole to a height not more than 1 metre above the patient.

Establish the ordered flow using the infusion pump

Infusion pumps differ from one manufacturer to another. Familiarise yourself with the infusion pump in use at the facility and ensure that the giving set is the one required for use with the pump. Close any safety clamps on the IV line. Open the door on the face of the pump. Thread the IV tubing through the pump according to the manufacturer's instructions, usually in the direction of the flow. Close the door. Turn the power on. As per the doctor's orders, set the pump to volume per hour as appropriate to the pump. Determine the flow rate by calculating an hourly rate. Open the clamp so it does not impede the flow of fluid. Press the start button on the infusion pump. Check the flow to ensure that the pump is working effectively.

The formula for calculating flow rate: divide the volume (in mL) to be infused by the number of hours over which the volume is to infuse.

$$\frac{\text{volume}}{\text{time}} = \text{mL per hour}$$

For example, 1 litre of fluid in an 8-hour period is calculated by dividing 1000 mL by 8 = 125 mL/hr.

Establish the ordered flow rate for gravity flow IV giving sets

Calculate the flow rate to a 'drops per minute' rate by using one of the following formulae:

$$\text{macrodrip giving set:} \quad \frac{\text{volume}}{\text{time}} \times \frac{20 \text{ drops per mL}}{60 \text{ minutes}} = \frac{\text{drops per}}{\text{minute}}$$

$$\text{microdrip giving set:} \quad \frac{\text{volume}}{\text{time}} \times \frac{60 \text{ drops per mL}}{60 \text{ minutes}} = \frac{\text{drops per}}{\text{minute}}$$

Time the flow by counting the drops as they fall into the drip chamber for 1 minute. Adjust the rate of flow by tightening or loosening the roller clamp. Again, time the flow, until the rate is as ordered.

Perform hand hygiene

After completing a care action required to manage the care of an IV infusion or PIVC, maintain the 5 Moments for Hand Hygiene and perform hand hygiene after touching the patient and the patient's surrounds.

Don sterile gloves

Don sterile gloves (see **Skill 4.9**). This is an aseptic technique and sterile gloves should be worn.

Connect the IV infusion

Check the infusion port on the extension tubing and replace if necessary. For non-changed ports, clean the port with an alcohol wipe for a minimum of 15 seconds and then allow to dry. Remove the cap from the administration set and avoid contamination. While avoiding touching the key parts, stabilise the connection port with the non-dominant hand and insert the open end of the administration set into the port.

To avoid a bolus dose being given to the patient using an infusion pump, the line should be connected after the pump completes its set-up procedure and the correct flow rate is programmed. Place the pump in standby mode while connecting the administration set. Other IV administration sets are connected before the flow rate is adjusted.

Doff sterile gloves and perform hand hygiene

After completing a care action required to manage the care of an IV infusion or PIVC, remove gloves and maintain the 5 Moments for Hand Hygiene and perform hand hygiene after touching the patient and the patient's surrounds.

Monitor the flow rate for an IV infusion

Monitor the flow rate and compare it to that prescribed. The flow rate is monitored hourly. IV infusion pumps ensure that fluid infusion is precise in millilitres per hour. Each pump will be different and you will need to familiarise yourself with the model used in the facility. For areas where a pump is not being used, a flow rate control device (burette; see **Skill 6.6**) should be considered for elderly, paediatric and/or critically ill patients. Some clinical areas will record the amount infused hourly on the fluid balance chart. Ensure you record the volume infused in the relevant IV column in the input part of the fluid balance chart.

Some PIVC are positional, causing the IV pump to alarm (or show an occlusion) or the flow rate to change for lines with an IV pump. The flow rate may require regular checking and adjustment. Encourage the patient to limit movement of the arm where the PIVC is inserted. Maintain the height of the infusion at 1 m or slightly more above the IV insertion site. Inspect the IV tubing for kinks or large air bubbles. Look for dependent loops and place excess tubing on the bed. Assess connections for leaks and tighten any loose connections.

Change solutions on an established IV infusion

Changing solutions on an established IV is similar to the initial establishment of IV infusion, except that the line is already fully primed. IV fluids need to be checked by two nurses as per policy (one is an RN) who both sign the infusion order. Check the IV fluid orders and bring the selected solution to the bedside and check the patient's identification ('rights of medication administration').

When the bag is nearly empty, perform hand hygiene and pause the pump, or if using a gravity flow administration set use the clamp to stop the flow of solution. Don non-sterile gloves and remove the old fluid bag from the IV stand. Remove the spike by firmly pulling it from the old bag, taking care not to contaminate it. Expose the port on the new fluid bag and spike the new bag as described above. Hang the new bag. Check the flow rate and pump programming, clear administered volumes and then recommence the IV pump. If an IV pump is not used, ensure that the drip chamber is half-full and loosen the clamp to re-establish the prescribed flow rate. Remove non-sterile gloves and perform hand hygiene.

Change a gown for a patient with a continuous IV infusion

Specific IV gowns are available in many facilities. They are designed with fasteners (buttons, ties, velcro) along the upper side of each sleeve and can be easily put on and removed. However, many patients prefer to use their own clothing. To remove a shirt or pyjama top, provide privacy and have the clean shirt prepared (unfolded and in the proper orientation). With the assistance of an RN (or advanced skills EN), put the IV pump on pause, close the safety clamp and open the pump door to temporarily remove the IV tubing. Assist the patient to remove their unaffected arm from the original shirt. Move the shirt carefully over the IV insertion site and off the hand (so it is lying on the bed with the IV line still running through it). Take the IV bag off the IV stand and, keeping it above the level of the insertion site, slide the shirt off the line and bag. Discard the soiled shirt. Thread the clean shirt or top over the IV bag and line (bag first) from the armhole to the wrist of the sleeve. Rehang the fluid bag. Carefully slip the shirt sleeve over the patient's hand and insertion site and then help them to put their unaffected arm through the other sleeve. Adjust the shirt for comfort. The IV line is then returned to the IV pump, the safety clamp released and the infusion recommenced. For a gravity flow administration set, the same principles are followed.

Assist a patient with a continuous IV infusion to ambulate

This consists of providing a wheeled IV stand and being mindful of the PIVC insertion site and lines. Many patients prefer to use the IV stand to steady themselves as they walk. Take care to assist the person from their unaffected side, to help them to manage the tubing and to keep the IV stand far enough in front or to the side to prevent the patient from tripping on the wheels.

Discontinue a continuous IV infusion

Turn off the infusion pump. Clamp the tubing of the administration set so no fluid can flow out onto the patient or their bed. Perform hand hygiene and don non-sterile gloves, steady the PIVC/administration port with the non-dominant hand, then release the connection and remove the administration set from the administration port at the end of the extension tubing. Wipe the end of the administration port with a single-use alcohol wipe for 15 seconds. Principles of an aseptic technique should be maintained while completing this procedure. The closed IV access system and needleless port will reduce any risk of exposure to body fluids, as well as maintain the integrity of the remaining PIVC. The administration set is a single-use device and should be discarded after removal. Record the removal of the IV infusion and the volume of fluid absorbed in the appropriate patient progress notes and charts, as per facility policy. Remove non-sterile gloves and discard in the waste bin.

Perform hand hygiene

After completing a care action required to manage the care of an IV infusion or PIVC, maintain the 5 Moments for Hand Hygiene and perform hand hygiene after touching the patient and the patient's surrounds

CLEAN, REPLACE OR DISPOSE OF EQUIPMENT

Clean, replace or dispose of equipment appropriately. Packaging, used gloves and other rubbish is disposed of in the regular waste. Excess solution in the discontinued IV fluid bag is emptied down the sink and the emptied bag placed into the general rubbish. The kidney dish is washed and returned to storage or disposed of, if disposable. Clean any re-useable equipment with the disinfecting solution or wipes recommended by your facility.

DOCUMENT AND REPORT RELEVANT INFORMATION

The documentation for IV interventions is completed on the IV monitoring chart, fluid balance chart and nursing care plan. The minimum documentation for a PIVC should include information about insertion, reviewing the insertion site and removing the PIVC (ACSQHC, 2019). The time of an IV fluid bag change (or commencement), type of solution infused and the volume infused is recorded on the fluid balance chart. All fluids administered are signed on the IV orders chart. Verbally report the amount of IV fluid remaining to be infused and the rate it is infusing during clinical handover. IV site assessment is recorded on the relevant phlebitis assessment scale or IV risk assessment tool and reported during clinical handover. Accurate documentation of PIVC should be maintained to ensure patient safety (ACSQHC, 2019; Queensland Health, 2019).

CASE STUDY

Esme Bennet, a 58-year-old woman was admitted to your ward following surgery for a hip replacement. Postoperatively (at 1000 hours) Esme has decreased blood pressure. She has a PIVC in situ for IV fluids and antibiotics.

1. The doctor has ordered 1 L of sodium chloride 0.9% to be administered over 5 hours, via the infusion pump. What is the correct flow rate for this infusion?
2. You are asked to attach a label to Esme's IV line.
   a. What labels should be attached to the IV line?
   b. What information will it contain?
   c. Explain the purpose of the label.

3. What assessments would you implement to monitor Esme's PIVC site?
4. The alarm sounds on Esme's IV pump and she is complaining of discomfort at the IV insertion site. When you check the site, the area is red and swollen.
   a. What is your assessment of these signs?
   b. Access an IV site risk assessment tool (PIVAS or VIP score), identify the correct score and chart these observations.
   c. After charting your observations, what are your next actions for these results?

Note: These notes are summaries of the most important points in the assessments/procedures, and are not exhaustive on the subject. The naming of documents or charts may differ from state to state, and facility to facility. In all possible situations the guidelines of the ACSQHC are used when describing national charts or documents (e.g. the ACSQHC Observation and Response Chart is named the Adult Observation and Response Chart in WA, and the Rapid Detection and Response Observation Chart in SA). References of the materials used to compile the information have been supplied. The student is expected to have learned the material surrounding each skill as presented in the references. No single reference is complete on the subject.

REFERENCES

Australian Commission on Safety and Quality in Health Care (ACSQHC). (2015). *National Standard for User-applied Labelling of Injectable Medicines, Fluids and Lines*. https://www.safetyandquality.gov.au/sites/default/files/migrated/National-Standard-for-User-Applied-Labelling-Aug-2015.pdf

Australian Commission on Safety and Quality in Health Care (ACSQHC). (2019). *Consultation Draft – Peripheral Venous Access Clinical Care Standard*. https://www.safetyandquality.gov.au/sites/default/files/2019-08/pva_ccs_-_consultation_draft_-_2019.pdf

Moola, S. (2020). *Evidence Summary. Phlebitis: Risk Assessment*. The Joanna Briggs Institute EBP Database.

Nursing and Midwifery Board of Australia (NMBA). (2020). *Fact Sheet: Enrolled Nurses and Medicine Administration*. https://www.nursingmidwiferyboard.gov.au/Codes-Guidelines-Statements/FAQ/Enrolled-nurses-and-medicine-administration.aspx

Queensland Health. (2018). Peripheral intravenous catheter (PIVC) guidelines. *Intravascular Device Management (I-Care)*. https://www.health.qld.gov.au/__data/assets/pdf_file/0025/444490/icare-pivc-guideline.pdf

Queensland Health. (2019). *Intravascular Device Management (I-Care)*. Queensland Government. https://www.health.qld.gov.au/clinical-practice/guidelines-procedures/diseases-infection/infection-prevention/intravascular-device-management

SA Health. (2020). *Peripheral Intravenous Catheter (PIVC) Infection Prevention Clinical Directive Version No.: 1.1* Approval date: 9 June 2020. Government of South Australia. https://www.sahealth.sa.gov.au/wps/wcm/connect/b8b0b71d-899e-42aa-ac3b-ca37d905f9a8/Clinical_Directive_PIVC_Infection_Prevention_v1.0_22.11.2019.pdf?MOD=AJPERES&CACHEID=ROOTWORKSPACE-b8b0b71d-899e-42aa-ac3b-ca37d905f9a8-mWhfA4q

WA Health. (2017). *Insertion and Management of Peripheral Intravenous Cannulae in Western Australian Healthcare Facilities Policy*. © Department of Health, Government of Western Australia. https://ww2.health.wa.gov.au/-/media/Files/Corporate/Policy-Frameworks/Public-Health/Policy/Insertion-and-Management-of-Peripheral-Intravenous-Cannulae/MP38-Insertion-and-Management-of-Peripheral-Intravenous-Cannulae.pdf

RECOMMENDED READINGS

Brooks, N. (2016). Intravenous cannula site management. *Nursing Standard*, 30(52), p. 53.

Ray-Barruel, G. (2017). Infection prevention: peripheral intravenous catheter assessment and care. *Australian Nursing & Midwifery Journal*, 24(8), p. 34.

Spencer, S. & Gilliam, P. (2017). The KISSSS method of peripheral I.V. catheter care. *Nursing*, 47(6), p. 64.

ESSENTIAL SKILLS COMPETENCY

Peripheral Intravenous Therapy (PIVT) Management
Demonstrates the ability to effectively and safely manage intravenous therapy

Criteria for skill performance	Y	D
(Numbers indicate *Enrolled Nurse Standards for Practice*, 2016)	(Satisfactory)	(Requires development)
1. Identifies indication (8.3, 8.4)		
2. Demonstrates problem-solving abilities (4.1, 4.2, 8.3, 8.4, 9.4)		

3. Gathers equipment (1.2, 1.6, 4.4, 6.4, 8.4, 9.4):
  ■ IV fluid order chart
  ■ correct IV fluid
  ■ IV giving set
  ■ IV line sticker
  ■ IV stand
  ■ infusion pump
  ■ sterile gloves
  ■ alcohol wipes
  ■ fluid balance chart
  ■ IV site assessment chart
  ■ watch with a second hand		

4. Performs hand hygiene (1.2, 1.4, 1.8, 3.9, 6.4, 9.4)		
5. Evidence of effective communication with the patient; gives explanation of procedure, gains patient consent; allays patient's anxiety by adequately explaining the procedure (2.1, 2.3, 2.4, 2.5, 6.3)		
6. Assesses the patient and the IV site (1.2, 4.1, 8.4, 9.4)		
7. Performs hand hygiene and dons sterile gloves (1.2, 1.4, 1.8, 3.9, 6.4, 9.4)		
8. Connects IV fluid line (wearing sterile gloves) and IV bag/changes IV fluid bag (1.2, 1.4, 6.4, 8.4, 9.4)		
9. Monitors and calculates correct flow rate (1.2, 1.4, 6.4, 8.4, 9.4)		
10. Changes a gown for the client with an IV prn (1.2, 1.4, 3.2, 3.9, 4.4, 6.4, 8.4, 9.4)		
11. Assists the client with an IV to ambulate prn (1.2, 1.4, 1.8, 3.2, 3.9, 4.4, 6.4, 8.4, 9.4)		
12. Discontinues IV therapy when ordered (1.2, 1.4, 3.2)		
13. Doffs gloves and performs hand hygiene (1.2, 1.4, 1.8, 3.9, 6.4, 9.4)		
14. Cleans, replaces or disposes of equipment appropriately (1.2, 1.4, 3.9, 6.5, 9.4)		
15. Documents and reports relevant information (1.2, 1.3, 1.8, 3.2, 5.3, 6.6, 7.1, 7.2, 7.3, 7.4, 7.5)		
16. Demonstrates ability to link theory to practice (8.3, 8.4, 8.5, 9.4)		

Student:

Clinical facilitator: Date:

CHAPTER 6.4

REMOVAL OF A PERIPHERAL INTRAVENOUS CANNULA (PIVC)

IDENTIFY INDICATIONS

A peripheral intravenous cannula (PIVC) should be re-sited every 72 to 96 hours or when clinically indicated.
It is removed when no longer required for administration of medication or IV fluid (ACSQHC, 2019; Queensland Health, 2019; SA Health, 2020; WA Health, 2017). If a PIVC is accidentally dislodged or partially withdrawn, it will also require removal and re-siting.

DEMONSTRATE PROBLEM-SOLVING ABILITIES

A doctor's or nurse practitioner's order is required to confirm the removal of a PIVC. The nurse may identify that the PIVC is due to be changed or removed; however, they will need to contact the doctor to gain written orders for its removal. As the PIVC is sited in the patient's vein, there is a risk of exposure to the patient's body fluids, as well as a bleeding risk for the patient post removal. Check the patient's medication chart to determine if the patient is on any anticoagulants, as this may affect the bleeding risk after removal.

GATHER EQUIPMENT

Gather equipment to increase efficient use of time and increase the confidence of the patient in the nurse's ability.
- *Non-sterile gloves and goggles* (personal protective equipment) to be worn while completing removal of the device and to protect the nurse from exposure to body fluids.
- *Sterile gauze swab.*
- *Sterile, small, circular adhesive dressing.*
- *Paper bag and/or kidney dish* for collecting the removed cannula.

REMOVING THE PIVC

Give a clear explanation of the procedure and establish therapeutic communication

Introduce yourself, and check you have the correct patient. Discuss the procedure and gain the patient's consent. Giving a clear explanation is required to gain legal consent and to address policy requirements. It will also assist the patient to cooperate with the procedure, allay anxiety and assist in establishing a therapeutic relationship.

Some patients may be apprehensive when removing a PIVC as they anticipate pain or movement of a needle in the vein. It is important to reinforce that only a polyurethane cannula remains in the vein and removal does not cause discomfort. While PIVC are usually not uncomfortable while in situ, removal may reduce discomfort experienced while the PIVC was in situ.

Position the patient and prepare the area

Provide privacy for the patient by closing the bedside curtains or the door to the patient's room. Adjust the lighting to provide good illumination for the procedure. If the patient is in bed, raise or lower the bed to a comfortable working position to reduce strain on the nurse's back muscles and improve access to the PIVC. Place the small dressing in an easily accessible position.

Perform hand hygiene and don personal protective equipment (PPE)

Perform hand hygiene before touching the patient or the patient's surrounds and prior to any procedure involving patient contact to reduce the possibility of cross-contamination. Hand hygiene is the most effective method of infection control as it removes transient organisms from the hands of the nurse (see **Skill 1.1**). After performing hand hygiene, don protective eye wear and non-sterile gloves.

Remove the cannula

If not already ceased, turn off the IV infusion and clamp the administration set. Remove the IV infusion, as described in **Skill 6.3**.

Carefully remove the transparent dressing securing the PIVC, while holding the cannula firmly in place to prevent trauma to the patient's vein. Also take care not to damage the patient's skin, especially that of elderly patients. Discard the dressing into the kidney dish. Place the sterile gauze over the insertion site without application of any pressure. Gently pull the cannula out following the line of the vein to avoid injury to the vein. Place the cannula into the kidney dish.

Keeping the gauze in place, apply firm digital pressure to the insertion site for approximately 2 to 3 minutes, until haemostasis is achieved (Queensland Health, 2018). While removing the gauze, immediately place the circular dressing over the site and maintain pressure for a further couple of minutes. Remove PPE and perform hand hygiene.

Monitor PIVC site after cannula removal

The PIVC site should be rechecked 15 minutes post removal for any bleeding and the dressing should remain intact for 24 hours. Peripheral intravenous assessment score [PIVAS] observations should continue for 48 hours if the patient remains in hospital to detect any post-infusion phlebitis (ACSQHC, 2019; Queensland Health, 2018). Advise the patient to call the nurse immediately if bleeding occurs. If this happens, apply pressure and a new dressing.

Doff PPE and perform hand hygiene

Remove non-sterile gloves and discard appropriately and then perform hand hygiene. Then remove protective eye wear, discard and perform further hand hygiene. Maintain the 5 Moments for Hand Hygiene and perform hand hygiene after touching the patient and the patient's surrounds.

CLEAN, REPLACE OR DISPOSE OF EQUIPMENT

Clean, replace and dispose of equipment appropriately. The cannula is disposed of in the regular waste along with the gloves, kidney dish and dressing material.

DOCUMENT AND REPORT RELEVANT INFORMATION

Removal of the PIVC should be recorded in the patient's notes, PIVC monitoring chart and nursing care plan. Any removed IV fluids and the volume infused should be recorded on the fluid balance chart. IV site assessment is recorded on the relevant phlebitis assessment scale or IV risk assessment tool and reported during clinical handover.

CASE STUDY

Cyril Kickett's IV therapy has been discontinued and the PIVC is required to be removed. He seems concerned about the removal.

1. Outline your explanation to Cyril.
2. Describe how you will remove the cannula.
3. Why is it necessary to place pressure over the removal site after removal?
4. How long will you continue observations of the site once the PIVC is removed?

Note: These notes are summaries of the most important points in the assessments/procedures, and are not exhaustive on the subject. The naming of documents or charts may differ from state to state, and facility to facility. In all possible situations the guidelines of the ACSQHC are used when describing national charts or documents (e.g. the ACSQHC Observation and Response Chart is named the Adult Observation and Response Chart in WA, and the Rapid Detection and Response Observation Chart in SA). References of the materials used to compile the information have been supplied. The student is expected to have learned the material surrounding each skill as presented in the references. No single reference is complete on the subject.

REFERENCES

Australian Commission on Safety and Quality in Health Care (ACSQHC). (2019). *Peripheral Venous Access Clinical Care Standard.* https://www.safetyandquality.gov.au/standards/clinical-care-standards/peripheral-venous-access-clinical-care-standard

Queensland Health. (2018). Peripheral intravenous catheter (PIVC) guidelines. *Intravascular Device Management (I-Care).* https://www.health.qld.gov.au/__data/assets/pdf_file/0025/444490/icare-pivc-guideline.pdf

Queensland Health. (2019). *Intravascular Device Management (I-Care).* Queensland Government. https://www.health.qld.gov.au/clinical-practice/guidelines-procedures/diseases-infection/infection-prevention/intravascular-device-management

SA Health. (2020). *Peripheral Intravenous Catheter (PIVC) Infection Prevention Clinical Directive Version No.: 1.1* Approval date: 9 June 2020. Government of South Australia. https://www.sahealth.sa.gov.au/wps/wcm/connect/b8b0b71d-899e-42aa-ac3b-ca37d905f9a8/Clinical_Directive_PIVC_Infection_Prevention_v1.0_22.11.2019.pd

f?MOD=AJPERES&CACHEID=ROOTWORKSPACE-b8b0b71d-899e-
42aa-ac3b-ca37d905f9a8-mWhfA4q

WA Health. (2017). *Insertion and Management of Peripheral
Intravenous Cannulae in Western Australian Healthcare Facilities
Policy.* Department of Health, Government of Western Australia.

https://ww2.health.wa.gov.au/-/media/Files/Corporate/Policy-
Frameworks/Public-Health/Policy/Insertion-and-Management-
of-Peripheral-Intravenous-Cannulae/MP38-Insertion-and-
Management-of-Peripheral-Intravenous-Cannulae.pdf

RECOMMENDED READINGS

Brooks, N. (2016). Intravenous cannula site management. *Nursing
Standard* (2014+), 30(52), p. 53.

NSW Health. (2019). *Policy Directive – Intravascular Access
Devices (IVAD) – Infection Prevention & Control.* https://www1.
health.nsw.gov.au/pds/ActivePDSDocuments/PD2019_040.pdf

Nursing and Midwifery Board of Australia (NMBA). (2020).
Fact Sheet: Enrolled Nurses and Medicine Administration.

https://www.nursingmidwiferyboard.gov.au/Codes-Guidelines-
Statements/FAQ/Enrolled-nurses-and-medicine-administration.
aspx

Ray-Barruel, G. (2017). Infection prevention: peripheral intravenous
catheter assessment and care. *Australian Nursing & Midwifery
Journal*, 24(8), p. 34.

ESSENTIAL SKILLS COMPETENCY

Removal of Peripheral Intravenous Cannula (PIVC)

Demonstrates the ability to effectively and safely manage intravenous therapy

Criteria for skill performance	Y	D
(Numbers indicate *Enrolled Nurse Standards for Practice*, 2016)	(Satisfactory)	(Requires development)
1. Identifies indication (8.3, 8.4)		
2. Demonstrates problem-solving abilities (4.1, 4.2, 8.3, 8.4, 9.4)		
3. Gathers equipment (1.2, 1.6, 4.4, 6.4, 8.4, 9.4): ■ non-sterile gloves (and goggles) ■ sterile gauze swabs ■ rubbish bag/kidney dish ■ small circular adhesive dressing (or equivalent)		
4. Performs hand hygiene (1.2, 1.4, 1.8, 3.9, 6.4, 9.4)		
5. Evidence of effective communication with the patient; gives explanation of procedure, gains patient consent; allays patient's anxiety by adequately explaining the procedure (2.1, 2.3, 2.4, 2.5, 6.3)		
6. Assesses the patient and the IV site; ceases/removes existing IV therapy (1.2, 4.1, 8.4, 9.4)		
7. Loosens transparent adhesive dressing (and any other tapes) (1.2, 1.4, 3.2)		
8. Performs hand hygiene and dons PPE (protective eyewear and non-sterile gloves) (1.2, 1.4, 1.8, 3.9, 6.4, 9.4)		
9. Gently remove cannula (1.2, 1.4, 3.2)		
10. Places pressure over removal site with sterile gauze for 2–3 minutes (1.2, 4.1, 8.4, 9.4)		
11. Ensures bleeding has stopped, and applies new dressing to site (1.2, 4.1, 8.4, 9.4)		
12. Removes PPE in correct sequence and performs hand hygiene (1.2, 1.4, 1.8, 3.9, 6.4, 9.4)		
13. Checks site 15 minutes later to ensure no further bleeding (1.2, 4.1, 8.4, 9.4)		
14. Performs hand hygiene (1.2, 1.4, 1.8, 3.9, 6.4, 9.4)		
15. Cleans, replaces or disposes of equipment appropriately (1.2, 1.4, 3.9, 6.5, 9.4)		
16. Documents and reports relevant information (1.2, 1.3, 1.8, 3.2, 5.3, 6.6, 7.1, 7.2, 7.3, 7.4, 7.5)		
17. Demonstrates ability to link theory to practice (8.3, 8.4, 8.5, 9.4)		

Student:

Clinical facilitator: Date:

CHAPTER 6.5

INTRAVENOUS MEDICATION ADMINISTRATION – ADDING MEDICATION TO PIVC FLUID BAG

IDENTIFY INDICATIONS

Intravenous (IV) administration of medication is the fastest route of administration, as the medication is administered directly into the vein and then carried through the body by the bloodstream. Many medications are administered intravenously to reduce the discomfort from subcutaneous or intramuscular injections and to maintain dosage control of the medication. Indications for administration of medications via an IV fluid bag are to provide a constant level of medication in the blood and to administer irritating medications in a diluted form at a continuous rate. Some

IV fluids containing medication come from the pharmacy, prepared and labelled. However, nurses often prepare the medication on the ward. Two nurses are required to check IV medications, one of whom must be a registered nurse (RN). Enrolled nurses (ENs) who can administer IV medications do not have a notation on their registration because they have completed the required medication administration education (NMBA, 2020). Specific facility policies for medication competency should also be followed.

GATHER EQUIPMENT

Gather equipment prior to starting the procedure as a time-management strategy and to prevent distractions once preparation of the medication has commenced, so errors are reduced.

- *A medication chart* with the written order for the required drug. The medication chart will need to meet all the requirements for the national medication chart, and is used to identify the correct patient, patient allergies risk and to ensure that the correct drug, dose, time and route are being given.
- *Peripheral intravenous assessment score (PIVAS) observation chart.*
- *Required medication and ordered IV fluid.* The medication will usually be in a vial or ampoule. If the medication needs to be reconstituted, a sterile diluent that is recommended for the medication will be required. Refer to hospital policy or the *Australian Injectable Drugs Handbook (AIDH)* for the correct diluent.
- *The fluid order chart* will state which IV fluid is to be used. Check that the drug and IV fluid are compatible.

The reconstitution of medication and preparation of the IV require use of an aseptic technique.
- *A medication additive label* according to Australian labelling standards is completed with: the patient's name and number; the drug, dose, date and time of administration; and the signatures of the preparing and checking nurses.
- *A sterile Luer lock syringe* is required to draw up and inject the medication into the IV bag.
- *A needleless syringe cannula or a sterile needle* for drawing up the medication, usually an 18-gauge needle.
- *Alcohol wipes* are used to cleanse and disinfect the tops of vials and the latex seal on the medication access port.
- *Non-sterile gloves/sterile gloves* are used to protect the nurse from exposure to medication and to maintain an aseptic technique (according to facility policy).
- *The sharps container* is used for the immediate disposal of needles, glass ampoules and vials, thus reducing the chance of needlestick injuries.

PREPARE AND ADD THE MEDICATION TO PIVC FLUID BAG

Perform hand hygiene

Perform hand hygiene as an infection-control measure. The medication being prepared is going directly into a vein and care needs to be taken in the preparation to maintain an aseptic technique. Non-sterile gloves are used to protect the nurse's hands from contact with medications, comply with standard precautions and maintain an aseptic technique.

Give a clear explanation of the procedure and establish therapeutic communication

Introduce yourself, and check you have the correct patient. Discuss the procedure and gain the patient's consent. Giving a clear explanation is required to gain legal consent and to address policy requirements. It will also assist the patient to cooperate with the procedure, allay anxiety and assist in establishing a therapeutic relationship.

Many patients will be apprehensive about receiving medication via a peripheral intravenous catheter (PIVC). Discussion about the need for IV therapy and medications will enlist most patients' cooperation. Warn the patient that they may experience some discomfort. Determine the patient's understanding of the purpose of the medication and provide education about common side effects for the drug to be administered, and ask the patient to alert the nurses to any changes that they note.

Assess the patient prior to PIVC administration of a drug

Patient assessment prior to IV administration of a drug includes baseline vital signs, allergies to medications, IV line patency and IV site assessment (see **Skill 6.3**) for inflammation, infiltration, thrombus or phlebitis of the insertion site or of the vein. The drug must be assessed for: compatibility with the fluid that it is infusing; its normal dosage, action and side effects; the time recommended over which to administer the drug; and its peak action time. Mixing of medications is not recommended as it increases the risk of medication incompatibility. Administration via a secondary line is the preferred method when using a separate mini bag to infuse the medication.

Use general concepts and the 'rights of medication administration'

Follow the 'rights of medication administration' to prepare and administer the medication to the patient. IV medications are checked by two nurses (one must be an RN), according to policy.

Use an aseptic technique

The preparation and administration of IV medication requires the use of an aseptic technique, ensuring that key parts are not touched within micro-aseptic fields (see **Skill 4.1**). Follow facility policy regarding the use of sterile gloves or non-sterile gloves when accessing and touching these areas. Syringes, IV ports and connectors use needleless systems to reduce the risk of needlestick injury.

Assess the preparation area

Assess the preparation area for adequate lighting, ventilation and space. Preparing any medication requires concentration and the nurse should be free from distraction during the procedure. Clean the work surface with alcohol or soap and water wipes.

Prepare the medication label

All containers (i.e. IV fluid bag) used to administer IV medications should be labelled using the blue IV label and remain intact throughout administration of the medication (ACSQHC, 2015). Prepare the label prior to preparing the medication so it can then be easily attached to the IV fluid bag immediately after the medication has been injected into the IV bag. The label should be legible and contain the following information: patient's name and identification number; patient's date of birth; medication name and total dose; total volume in the fluid container; concentration; date and time prepared; route of administration; and signatures of the nurses preparing the medication.

Perform hand hygiene and don non-sterile gloves

Perform hand hygiene as an infection control measure. The medication being prepared is going directly into a vein and care needs to be taken in the preparation to maintain an aseptic technique. Non-sterile gloves are used to protect the nurse's hands from contact with medications, comply with standard precautions and maintain an aseptic technique.

Prepare the syringe

Collect the required IV fluid, medication, diluent, alcohol wipe, access cannula/needle and syringe. Refer to hospital policy or the *Australian Injectable Drugs Handbook* (AIDH) for the correct diluent. Draw up the required diluent into a 20 mL syringe or as per facility policy. Swab the top of the medication vial with an alcohol wipe for 15 seconds, allow it to dry and then insert the syringe into the rubber bung. Add 5 to 10 mL of the diluent to the vial to reconstitute and mix the medication. Without removing the syringe, gently roll the medication vial between your hands to mix the medication. Ensure all the dry powder is dissolved and then withdraw the dissolved medication into the syringe. The medication should now be immediately added to the IV fluid bag, and not left on the bench. Be aware that all IV medication volumes added to a fluid bag need to be recorded on the fluid balance chart and included when calculating total volume of fluid to be administered to the patient.

Inject medication into the IV fluid bag

- With the IV fluid bag sitting on the bench, identify the medication additive port. This is different from the IV tubing insertion port.
- Clean the additive port with an alcohol wipe for 15 seconds to remove microorganisms. Allow the alcohol to dry. The injection port is designed to be self-sealing.
- Remove the access cannula/drawing up needle from the syringe while the port is drying, and dispose in the sharps container.
- Insert the tip of the syringe into the centre of the IV fluid bag's injection port.
- Inject the medication, withdraw the syringe and dispose of into the sharps container.
- Attach the IV medication label to the front of the bag, ensuring the fluid name, batch number and expiry date remain visible.
- Gently rotate the IV fluid bag, turning it end over end 10 times, to mix the fluids.
- Ensure there is no crystallising or clouding of the content occurring. If this occurs it indicates a reaction between the medication and the IV fluid, and the bag should be discarded.

Doff personal protective equipment (PPE) and perform hand hygiene

Remove non-sterile gloves, maintain the 5 Moments for Hand Hygiene and perform hand hygiene after touching the patient and the patient's surrounds.

Check the patient and PIVC site

Identify the correct patient, check for allergies (see **Skill 5.1**) and complete an assessment of the PIVC insertion site prior to administering any IV medications (see **Skill 6.3**). Medications should not be given if any signs of infiltration or phlebitis exist.

Perform hand hygiene and don non-sterile gloves

Maintain the 5 Moments for Hand Hygiene and perform hand hygiene after touching the patient and the patient's surrounds. Put on non-sterile gloves according to the required process (i.e. attaching the IV bag or IV line).

Connect the IV fluid bag to the IV line

Intermitted IV medication via a mini bag

If the medication being given is an intermittent IV medication, the IV cannula should be flushed with normal saline (sodium chloride 0.9% for injection) 3 to 5 mL (see **Skill 6.7**) to ensure patency of the PIVC and to prevent mixing of any incompatible medications in the IV tubing or catheter. Prime the IV line with normal saline (see **Skill 6.2**), then attach the labelled IV fluid bag containing the required prepared medication as above. Wearing non-sterile gloves, swab the IV access port for 15 seconds with an alcohol wipe, allow it to dry and then attach the IV line using an aseptic technique, ensuring not to touch any key parts and protecting the micro-aseptic field.

Continuous IV medication

After checking the patency of the patient's PIVC attach the labelled IV fluid bag containing the prescribed medication, as per the procedure for changing an IV fluid bag as described in **Skill 6.3**.

For both methods following the attachment of the IV fluid bag containing medication, adjust the flow rate on the IV pump or the clamp below the drip chamber to establish the IV flow to the ordered rate (see **Skill 6.3**). A fresh giving set should be used for each intermittent medication. Care needs to be taken when connecting and disconnecting needleless IV devices to prevent breaks, leaks or contaminants in the system.

Return to assess the patient

Return to assess the patient regularly during and after the medication administration. Monitor the flow rate and the patient's reaction to the medication as per **Skill 6.3**. When the medication administration has been completed, don non-sterile gloves and remove the intermittent line and IV medication bag. Then flush the PIVC with 10 to 20 mL of normal saline 0.9% (see **Skill 6.7**) and discard the line, IV medication bag and gloves.

Doff gloves and perform hand hygiene

Doff gloves and perform hand hygiene. Maintain the 5 Moments for Hand Hygiene and perform hand hygiene after touching the patient and the patient's surrounds.

CLEAN, REPLACE OR DISPOSE OF EQUIPMENT

The needles, syringes and vials/ampoules are placed into the sharps container to prevent needlestick injuries to either the nursing or domestic staff. Used gloves and alcohol wipes are disposed of in the general rubbish. The IV line is disposed of with the IV bag intact according to facility policy.

DOCUMENT AND REPORT RELEVANT INFORMATION

Documentation of IV medications is the same as for any other medication. The nurse signs or initials the time slot on the medication chart to indicate that the ordered dose of the medication was given to the patient by the IV route at the designated time. Any IV fluid volumes are recorded on the fluid balance chart. The checking nurse countersigns the medication chart. PIVAS observations should be recorded on the PIVAS monitoring chart.

CASE STUDY

You are caring for Esme Bennett, a 58-year-old woman who was admitted to your ward following surgery for a hip replacement. Postoperatively Esme has decreased blood pressure. She has an IV in situ for IV fluids and antibiotics.

Esme is ordered amoxicillin 500 mg, reconstituted vial with 10 mL water for injection and then diluted in 100 mL NaCl 0.9%, and administered over 50 minutes.

1. What patient assessments should you complete prior to administering the IV amoxicillin?
2. Why is it important to maintain an aseptic technique and not touch key parts when preparing and administering this medication?
3. How many millilitres per hour will you set the infusion pump at if administering the amoxicillin over 50 minutes?

Note: These notes are summaries of the most important points in the assessments/procedures, and are not exhaustive on the subject. The naming of documents or charts may differ from state to state, and facility to facility. In all possible situations the guidelines of the ACSQHC are used when describing national charts or documents (e.g. the ACSQHC Observation and Response Chart is named the Adult Observation and Response Chart in WA, and the Rapid Detection and Response Observation Chart in SA). References of the materials used to compile the information have been supplied. The student is expected to have learned the material surrounding each skill as presented in the references. No single reference is complete on the subject.

REFERENCES

Australian Commission on Safety and Quality in Health Care (ACSQHC). (2015). *National Standard for User-applied Labelling of Injectable Medicines, Fluids and Lines.* https://www.safetyandquality.gov.au/sites/default/files/migrated/National-Standard-for-User-Applied-Labelling-Aug-2015.pdf

Nursing and Midwifery Board of Australia (NMBA). (2020). *Fact Sheet: Enrolled Nurses and Medicine Administration.* https://www.nursingmidwiferyboard.gov.au/Codes-Guidelines-Statements/FAQ/Enrolled-nurses-and-medicine-administration.aspx

RECOMMENDED READINGS

Abbott, B. & DeVries, S. (2016). *Monitoring and Administration of IV Medications for the Enrolled Nurse.* Melbourne: Cengage.

Australian Commission on Safety and Quality in Health Care (ACSQHC). (2019). *Peripheral Venous Catheters.* https://www.safetyandquality.gov.au/standards/clinical-care-standards/peripheral-venous-access-clinical-care-standard

NSW Health. (2019). *Policy Directive: Intravascular Access Devices (IVAD) – Infection Prevention & Control.* NSW Government. https://www1.health.nsw.gov.au/pds/ActivePDSDocuments/PD2019_040.pdf

Queensland Health. (2019). *Intra-vascular Device Management.* Queensland Government. https://www.health.qld.gov.au/clinical-practice/guidelines-procedures/diseases-infection/infection-prevention/intravascular-device-managements

Ray-Barruel, G. (2017). Infection prevention: peripheral intravenous catheter assessment and care. *Australian Nursing & Midwifery Journal,* 24(8), p. 34.

WA Department of Health. (2016). *National Standard for User-applied Labelling of Injectable Medicines, Fluids and Lines.* Government of Western Australia, http://ww2.health.wa.gov.au/Articles/N_R/National-standard-for-user-applied-labelling-of-injectable-medicines-fluids-and-lines

WA Health. (2017). *Insertion and Management of Peripheral Intravenous Cannulae in Western Australian Healthcare Facilities Policy.* Department of Health, Government of Western Australia. https://ww2.health.wa.gov.au/-/media/Files/Corporate/Policy-Frameworks/Public-Health/Policy/Insertion-and-Management-of-Peripheral-Intravenous-Cannulae/MP38-Insertion-and-Management-of-Peripheral-Intravenous-Cannulae.pdf

ESSENTIAL SKILLS COMPETENCY

Intravenous Medication Administration – Adding Medication to PIVC Fluid Bag

Demonstrates the ability to effectively and safely administer intravenous medication by adding medication to an IV fluid, and then administering to the patient

Criteria for skill performance	Y	D
(Numbers indicate *Enrolled Nurse Standards for Practice*, 2016)	(Satisfactory)	(Requires development)
1. Identifies indication (8.3, 8.4)		
2. Gathers equipment (1.2, 1.6, 4.4, 6.4, 8.4, 9.4): ■ medication chart and peripheral intravenous assessment score (PIVAS) chart, fluid order chart required medication, diluent and IV fluid, *Australian Injectable Drugs Handbook* (AIDH) ■ syringe and needles ■ alcohol wipes ■ medication additive label ■ sharps container ■ non-sterile gloves or sterile gloves according to facility policy		
3. Performs hand hygiene (1.2, 1.4, 1.8, 3.9, 6.4, 9.4)		
4. Evidence of effective communication with the patient; e.g. gives patient a clear explanation of procedure, gains patient consent (2.1, 2.3, 2.4, 2.5, 6.3)		
5. Assesses the patient, IV site and drug (1.2, 1.4, 3.2, 4.1, 4.4, 6.4, 8.4, 9.4)		
6. Uses general concepts of medication administration plus 'rights' (1.1, 1.2, 1.3, 1.4, 2.2, 2.3, 3.1, 3.2, 3.9, 5.5, 8.4, 9.3, 9.4)		
7. Performs hand hygiene and dons gloves (1.2, 1.4, 3.9, 8.4, 9.4)		
8. Maintains aseptic technique and wears gloves (1.2, 1.4, 3.9, 8.4, 9.4)		
9. Prepares the syringe with medication (1.1, 1.2, 1.3, 1.4, 1.8, 2.2, 3.1, 3.2, 3.9, 8.4, 9.4)		
10. Injects medication into IV container (1.1, 1.2, 1.3, 1.4, 1.8, 2.2, 3.1, 3.2, 3.9, 8.4, 9.4)		
11. Attaches medication label (1.2, 1.4)		
12. Checks correct patient, and assesses IV insertion site; flushes IV cannula; hangs medicated IV bag (1.2, 1.4, 1.8, 2.2, 3.2, 3.9, 4.1, 6.4, 8.4, 9.4)		
13. Monitors the patient, removes the intermittent line and flushes the PIVC (1.2, 1.4, 3.2, 4.1, 6.4, 8.4, 9.4)		
14. Doffs gloves and performs hand hygiene (1.2, 1.4, 1.8, 3.9, 6.4, 9.4)		
15. Cleans, replaces or disposes of equipment appropriately (1.2, 1.4, 3.9, 6.5, 9.4)		
16. Documents and reports relevant information (1.2, 1.3, 1.8, 3.2, 5.3, 6.6, 7.1, 7.2, 7.3, 7.4, 7.5)		
17. Demonstrates ability to link theory to practice (8.3, 8.4, 8.5, 9.4)		

Student:

Clinical facilitator: Date:

CHAPTER 6.6

INTRAVENOUS MEDICATION ADMINISTRATION – ADDING MEDICATION TO A BURETTE

IDENTIFY INDICATIONS

Intravenous (IV) administration of medication is the fastest route of administration, as the medication is administered directly into the vein and then carried through the body by the bloodstream. Many medications are administered intravenously to reduce the discomfort from subcutaneous or intramuscular injections and to maintain dosage control of the medication. Indications for IV administration of medications via a burette are: 1. a medication that does not remain stable for the length of time it takes an IV prepared bag to infuse; 2. to administer multiple (but separate) medications intermittently; 3. to avoid mixing incompatible medications; 4. to further dilute a drug which is very irritating to the veins; and 5. to deliver medications in precise amounts of liquid (e.g. when the volume administered is critical).

The burette is a volume-control device that is attached to the IV fluid bag as a secondary part of the primary IV tubing. Many facilities and general ward areas opt to use an IV mini-bag (50 or 100 mL IV fluid bag) or a syringe (50 mL) attached to an infusion pump rather than a burette. Please refer to **Skill 6.5** for preparing a mini-bag and **Skill 6.7** for preparing a syringe that can then be attached to an infusion pump.

Two nurses are required to check IV medications, one of whom must be a registered nurse (RN). Enrolled nurses (ENs) who can administer IV medications do not have a notation on their registration because they have completed the required medication administration education (NMBA, 2020). Specific facility policies for medication competency should also be followed.

GATHER EQUIPMENT

Gather equipment prior to starting the procedure as a time-management strategy, and to prevent distractions once preparation of the medication has commenced, to reduce errors.

- *The medication chart* with the written order for the required drug and dose. The medication chart will need to meet all the requirements for the national medication chart, and is used to identify the correct patient and patient allergies risk, and to ensure that the correct drug, dose, time and route are being given.
- *Peripheral intravenous assessment score (PIVAS) observation chart.*
- *The required medication* is obtained from stock, usually as a vial or ampoule. If the medication needs to be reconstituted, the recommended sterile diluting solution will be required. Refer to hospital policy or the *Australian Injectable Drugs Handbook* (AIDH) for the correct diluent.
- *Burette*, which is a separate infusion set with a calibrated chamber for infusion of small volumes or controlled amounts. It is attached as a secondary line to the primary IV tubing.

- *A medication additive label* according to Australian labelling standards is completed with the patient's name, ID number, the drug, the dose, the date and time of preparation and commencement of administration and the signature of the preparing and checking nurses.
- *A sterile Luer lock 20 mL syringe* is required to draw up the medication.
- *A needleless syringe cannula or sterile needle* for drawing up the medication, usually an 18-gauge needle.
- *Alcohol wipes* are used to cleanse and disinfect the tops of vials and the medication access port of the burette.
- *A kidney dish* is used for transporting the medications, syringes and alcohol wipes to the bedside.
- *The sharps container* is taken to the bedside so that needles (if used), glass ampoules and vials can be immediately disposed of, thus reducing the chance of needlestick injuries.
- *Non-sterile gloves or sterile gloves* may be used to comply with standard precautions and assist with maintaining an aseptic technique.

PREPARE AND ADD THE MEDICATION TO THE BURETTE

Perform hand hygiene

Perform hand hygiene as an infection-control measure (see **Skill 1.1**). The medication being prepared is going directly into a vein and care needs to be taken in the preparation to maintain an aseptic technique. Non-sterile gloves are used to protect the nurse's hands from contact with medications, comply with standard precautions and maintain an aseptic technique.

Give a clear explanation of the procedure and establish therapeutic communication

Introduce yourself to the patient, check you have the correct patient and gain the patient's consent. Give a clear explanation to the patient of the purpose of the procedure and the sensations that will be felt. Checking the patient and gaining their consent will also ensure that you meet legal and policy requirements before implementing any procedures.

Many patients will be apprehensive about receiving medication via a peripheral intravenous catheter (PIVC). Warn the patient that they may experience some discomfort when the medication is administered but this should be temporary. Determine the patient's understanding of the purpose of the medication, provide education about common side effects for the drug to be administered and ask the patient to alert the nurses to any changes that they note.

Assess the patient prior to PIVC administration of a drug

Patient assessment prior to IV administration of a drug includes baseline vital signs, allergies to medications and IV site assessment (see **Skill 6.3**) for inflammation, infiltration, thrombus or phlebitis of the insertion site or of the vein. The drug must be assessed for: compatibility with the fluid that it is infusing; its normal dosage, action and side effects; the time recommended over which to administer the drug; and its peak action time. Mixing of medications is not recommended as it increases the risk of medication incompatibility.

Use general concepts and the 'rights of medication administration'

Follow the 'rights of medication administration' to prepare and administer the medication to the patient. IV medications are checked by two nurses (one must be an RN), according to policy.

Use an aseptic technique

The preparation and administration of IV medication requires the use of an aseptic technique, and ensuring that key parts are not touched within micro-aseptic fields (see **Skill 4.1**). Follow facility policy regarding the use of sterile gloves or non-sterile gloves when accessing and touching these areas. Syringes, IV ports and connectors use needleless systems to reduce the risk of needlestick injury.

Assess the preparation area

Assess the preparation area for adequate lighting, ventilation and space. Preparing any medication requires concentration and the nurse should be free from distraction during the procedure. Clean the work surface with an alcohol or soap and water wipe.

Prepare the medication additive label

Pre-prepare an IV additive label for both the syringe and the burette. All containers (i.e. IV fluid bag) and syringes used to administer IV medications should be labelled using the blue IV label and remain intact throughout administration of the medication (ACSQHC, 2015). Prepare the labels prior to preparing the medication so they can then be easily attached to the syringe immediately after the medication has been prepared and to the burette when the medication has been added. The label should be legible and contain the following information: patient's name and identification number; patient's date of birth; medication name and total amount; total volume in the fluid container; concentration; date and time prepared; route of administration; and signatures of nurses preparing the medication.

Perform hand hygiene and don non-sterile gloves

Perform hand hygiene as an infection-control measure. The medication being prepared is going directly into a vein and care needs to be taken in the preparation to maintain an aseptic technique. Non-sterile gloves are used to protect the nurse's hands from contact with medications, comply with standard precautions and maintain an aseptic technique.

Prepare the syringe

Collect the required IV fluid, medication, diluent, alcohol wipe, access cannula/needle and syringe. Refer to hospital policy or the *Australian Injectable Drugs Handbook* (AIDH) for the correct diluent. Draw up the required diluent into a 20 mL syringe. Swab the top of the medication vial with an alcohol wipe for 15 seconds, allow it to dry and then insert the syringe into the bung. Add 5–10 mL of the diluent to the vial to reconstitute and mix the medication. Without removing the syringe, gently roll the medication vial between your hands to mix the medication. Ensure all the dry powder is dissolved and then withdraw the dissolved medication into the syringe. Place the medication label on the syringe parallel to the long axis of the syringe barrel. The top end is flush with, but not covering, the graduation (ACSQHC, 2015). Place the syringe along with a second label and a new alcohol wipe into the kidney dish. Be aware that all IV medication volumes added to a burette need to be recorded on the fluid balance chart and included when calculating total volume of fluid to be administered to the patient. Remove non-sterile gloves and perform hand hygiene.

Check the correct patient

Identify the correct patient, check for allergies (see **Skill 5.1**) and complete a peripheral intravenous assessment score (PIVAS) assessment of the IV insertion site prior to administering any IV medications (see **Skill 6.3**). Medications should not be given if any signs of infiltration or phlebitis exist.

Perform hand hygiene and don non-sterile gloves

Maintain the 5 Moments for Hand Hygiene and perform hand hygiene after touching the patient and the patient's surrounds. Non-sterile gloves are used to protect the nurse's hands from contact with medications, comply with standard precautions and maintain an aseptic technique.

Attach a burette

Attach a burette (if this is the initial dose using a burette) to the IV line by inserting the spike of the burette (see **Skill 6.3**) into a new IV fluid bag (50 mL 0.9% sodium chloride for priming the burette). Hang the IV bag on the IV stand. Open the air vent clamp on the burette to allow air to escape as fluid flows in. Undo and then slide the clamp on the burette line to just below the drip chamber and clamp it so the burette chamber can fill before priming the line. Open the upper clamp (between the IV bag and the burette) and allow 30 mL of fluid into the burette chamber. Close the upper clamp. Gently squeeze the drip chamber. Release the drip chamber and gently reshape it. It should be half-full of fluid. Open the lower clamp. Prime the burette line, then close the clamp and leave this secondary line hanging on the IV pole. Ensure the end does not become contaminated.

The burette now becomes a secondary line and is attached to the primary IV line. Pause the pump or close the roller clamp on the primary IV line. Don non-sterile gloves according to facility policy (see **Skill 4.9**). Wipe the lumen (for attaching a secondary line on the primary IV line) with an alcohol wipe for 15 seconds and allow to dry while continuing to hold the line. Remove the protective cap from the end of the burette tubing and, using a non-touch technique so that key parts are not contaminated, slide the end of the burette line into the access lumen.

Inject medication into the burette

- Fill the burette with the required/ordered amount of IV fluid – usually 50 mL or 100 mL – so the medication is sufficiently diluted and dispersed throughout the fluid in the burette.
- Close the roller clamp to stop the inflow line from the IV fluid bag.
- Clean the additive port on the burette with an alcohol wipe for 15 seconds to remove microorganisms and allow to dry. The injection port is designed for multiple access.

- Insert the syringe into the additive port of the burette and carefully inject the medication. Gently rotate (agitate) the fluid chamber to mix the fluids.
- Attach the medication label to the burette. This will clearly indicate the addition of a medication to the burette. Peeling back one side or corner only and attaching that to the burette will reduce the amount of paper tape that sticks to the burette, an important consideration over time. Adjust the flow rate for the medication administration (see **Skill 6.3**) by either:
  - adjusting the infusion pump (for a piggyback administration when infusing the burette volume via the pump), or
  - keeping the clamp on the main IV line closed, and then adjusting the flow rate using the roller clamp below the burette drip chamber.

If other medication is being given continuously via the main IV line the tubing should be flushed with normal saline (sodium chloride 0.9% for injection) prior to attaching the burette and adding the medication to prevent mixing of any incompatible medications in the IV tubing. A flush would also be required following administration of the medication.

Doff gloves and perform hand hygiene

Remove non-sterile gloves and discard appropriately, then perform hand hygiene. Maintain the 5 Moments for Hand Hygiene by removing gloves and performing hand hygiene after touching the patient and the patient's surrounds.

Return to assess the patient

Return to assess the patient during administration of the medication. When the medication has been administered, flush as ordered. Don non-sterile gloves, clamp the burette line, disconnect this secondary line and then dispose of as per facility policy. Reset the flow rate and open the flow from the primary IV line.

Perform hand hygiene

Maintain the 5 Moments for Hand Hygiene and perform hand hygiene after touching the patient and the patient's surrounds.

CLEAN, REPLACE OR DISPOSE OF EQUIPMENT

The needles, syringes and vials/ampoules are placed into the sharps container to prevent needlestick injuries to either the nursing or domestic staff. Used gloves and alcohol wipes are disposed of in the general rubbish. The burette is disposed of with the line intact according to facility policy.

DOCUMENT AND REPORT RELEVANT INFORMATION

Documentation of IV medications is the same as for any other medication. The nurse signs or initials the time slot on the medication chart to indicate that the ordered dose of the medication was given to the patient by the IV route at the designated time. The checking nurse countersigns the medication chart.

Any IV fluid volumes are recorded on the fluid balance chart. The observation of the PIVC insertion site prior to medication administration should also be recorded in the IV monitoring chart.

CASE STUDY

Max Winter is a 23-year-old patient who has been admitted for management of osteomyelitis in his left tibia. He is receiving two IV antibiotics, and sometimes requires an IV antiemetic to manage the side effects of his medication. The IV antibiotics are being administered intermittently via a burette attached to the IV line. An IV pump is being used to control the IV flow rate.

1. Why would a burette be used to assist with administering the patient's IV medication?

2. A flush with sodium chloride 0.9% is ordered prior to and following the administration of each medication. What is the reason for this?

3. How would you identify the correct diluents to prepare the medication, prior to adding it to the burette?

4. What resource would you use to check the compatibility of the medication and the IV fluid used in the burette?

Note: These notes are summaries of the most important points in the assessments/procedures, and are not exhaustive on the subject. The naming of documents or charts may differ from state to state, and facility to facility. In all possible situations the guidelines of the ACSQHC are used when describing national charts or documents (e.g. the ACSQHC Observation and Response Chart is named the Adult Observation and Response Chart in WA, and the Rapid Detection and Response Observation Chart in SA). References of the materials used to compile the information have been supplied. The student is expected to have learned the material surrounding each skill as presented in the references. No single reference is complete on the subject.

REFERENCES

Australian Commission on Safety and Quality in Health Care (ACSQHC). (2015). *National Standard for User-applied Labelling of Injectable Medicines, Fluids and Lines*. https://www. safetyandquality.gov.au/sites/default/files/migrated/National-Standard-for-User-Applied-Labelling-Aug-2015.pdf

Nursing and Midwifery Board of Australia (NMBA). (2020). *Fact Sheet: Enrolled Nurses and Medicine Administration*. http://www. nursingmidwiferyboard.gov.au/Codes-Guidelines-Statements/ FAQ/Enrolled-nurses-and-medicine-administration.aspx

RECOMMENDED READINGS

Abbott, B. and DeVries, S. (2016). *Monitoring and Administration of IV Medications for the Enrolled Nurse*. Melbourne: Cengage.

Australian Commission on Safety and Quality in Health Care (ACSQHC). (2019). *Peripheral Venous Access Clinical Care Standard*. https://www.safetyandquality.gov.au/standards/ clinical-care-standards/peripheral-venous-access-clinical-care-standard

Queensland Health. (2019). *Intra-vascular Device Management*. Queensland Government. https://www.health.qld.gov.au/clinical-practice/guidelines-procedures/diseases-infection/infection-prevention/intravascular-device-management

Ray-Barruel, G. (2017). Infection prevention: peripheral intravenous catheter assessment and care. *Australian Nursing & Midwifery Journal*, 24(8), p. 34.

SA Health. (2020). *Peripheral Intravenous Catheter (PIVC) Infection Prevention Clinical Directive. Version No.: 1.1* Approval date: 9 June 2020. Government of South Australia. https://www.sahealth. sa.gov.au/wps/wcm/connect/b8b0b71d-899e-42aa-ac3b-ca37d905f9a8/Clinical_Directive_PIVC_Infection_Prevention_ v1.0_22.11.2019.pdf?MOD=AJPERES&CACHEID=ROOTWORKSPA CE-b8b0b71d-899e-42aa-ac3b-ca37d905f9a8-mWhfA4q

WA Department of Health. (2017). *Insertion and Management of Peripheral Intravenous Cannulae in Western Australian Healthcare Facilities Policy*. Government of Western Australia. https://ww2.health.wa.gov.au/-/media/Files/Corporate/Policy-Frameworks/Public-Health/Policy/Insertion-and-Management-of-Peripheral-Intravenous-Cannulae/MP38-Insertion-and-Management-of-Peripheral-Intravenous-Cannulae.pdf

ESSENTIAL SKILLS COMPETENCY

Intravenous Medication Administration – Adding Medication to a Burette

Demonstrates the ability to effectively and safely administer intravenous medication via a burette

Criteria for skill performance	Y	D
(Numbers indicate *Enrolled Nurse Standards for Practice*, 2016)	(Satisfactory)	(Requires development)
1. Identifies indication (8.3, 8.4)		
2. Gathers equipment (1.2, 1.6, 4.4, 6.4, 8.4, 9.4): ■ medication chart/PIVAS chart ■ required medication, diluent, *Australian Injectable Drugs Handbook* (AIDH) ■ burette ■ syringes and needles or needleless devices ■ alcohol wipes ■ injection tray/kidney dish ■ sharps container ■ IV additive medication labels ■ non-sterile or sterile gloves		
3. Performs hand hygiene and dons non-sterile gloves (1.2, 1.4, 1.8, 3.9, 6.4, 9.4)		
4. Evidence of effective communication with the patient; e.g. gives patient a clear explanation of procedure, gains patient consent (2.1, 2.3, 2.4, 2.5, 6.3)		
5. Assesses the patient PIVC site (1.2, 1.4, 3.2, 4.1, 4.4, 6.4, 8.4, 9.4)		
6. Uses general concepts of medication administration plus 'rights' (1.1, 1.2, 1.3, 1.4, 2.2, 3.1, 3.2, 3.9, 5.5, 8.4, 9.3, 9.4)		
7. Maintains an aseptic technique (1.2, 1.4, 3.9, 8.4, 9.4)		
8. Prepares the syringe with medication and attaches medication label to syringe (1.1, 1.2, 1.3, 1.4, 1.8, 2.2, 3.1, 3.2, 3.9, 8.4, 9.4)		
9. Doffs gloves and performs hand hygiene (1.2, 1.4, 1.8, 3.9, 6.4, 9.4)		
10. Checks correct patient and assesses IV insertion site; flushes IV cannula (if required) (1.2, 1.4, 1.8, 2.2, 3.2, 3.9, 4.4, 8.4, 9.4)		
11. Performs hand hygiene and dons non-sterile gloves (1.2, 1.4, 1.8, 3.9, 6.4, 9.4)		
12. Inserts the burette into a new IV fluid bag (1.2, 1.4)		
13. Wipes port with alcohol wipe for 15 seconds, and allows to dry; injects medication into burette (1.2, 1.4, 1.8, 2.2, 3.2, 3.9, 4.4, 8.4, 9.4)		
14. Attaches the additive medication label (1.2, 1.4)		
15. Sets the rate of IV (1.2, 1.4, 6.4, 8.4, 9.4)		
16. Returns when medication is administered; dons non-sterile gloves, disconnects burette and resets IV rate (1.2, 1.4, 5.4, 6.4, 8.4, 9.4)		
17. Removes gloves and performs hand hygiene (1.2, 1.4, 1.8, 3.9, 6.4, 9.4)		
18. Cleans, replaces or disposes of equipment appropriately (1.2, 1.4, 3.9, 6.5, 9.4)		
19. Documents and reports relevant information (1.2, 1.3, 1.8, 3.2, 5.3, 6.6, 7.1, 7.2, 7.3, 7.4, 7.5)		
20. Demonstrates ability to link theory to practice (8.3, 8.4, 8.5, 9.4)		

Student:

Clinical facilitator: Date:

CHAPTER 6.7

INTRAVENOUS MEDICATION ADMINISTRATION – INJECTION (BOLUS)

IDENTIFY INDICATIONS

Intravenous (IV) administration of medication is the fastest route of administration, as the medication is administered directly into the vein and then carried through the body by the bloodstream. Medications are administered intravenously to reduce the discomfort from subcutaneous or intramuscular injections and to maintain dosage control of the medication.

Injection of IV medication by syringe directly into an access port (lumen) is often referred to as an IV bolus or push. Direct IV injection or IV bolus is administered directly into the vein via an access lumen on an existing IV line, or into the access port of the extension tubing attached to a peripheral IV cannula (PIVC). The PIVC is kept patent using a prescribed saline solution to prevent clotting at the end of the catheter. Administration of a bolus IV medication is the most hazardous of all types of medication administration because the entire dose is administered in a short time, the effects are immediate and the drug is irretrievable. Some medications cannot be given via the IV bolus – check the manufacturer's recommendations, the *Australian Injectable*

Drugs Handbook (AIDH) or with the hospital pharmacist if unsure. Many facilities also prefer using a rapid infusion rate on an IV volumetric pump, then adding the medication to a small IV fluid bag (see **Skill 6.5**) or attaching the syringe to the IV pump (according to manufacturer's instructions) rather than the traditional 'push' method.

Indications for IV administration of medications by the bolus method are: 1. the medication does not require dilution or is diluted to a small volume; 2. the medication cannot be diluted; 3. it is an emergency situation requiring quick administration; and 4. to achieve maximum benefit from the medication.

Two nurses are required to check IV medications, one of whom must be a registered nurse (RN). Enrolled nurses (ENs) who can administer IV medications do not have a notation on their registration because they have completed the required medication administration education (NMBA, 2020). Specific facility policies for medication competency should also be followed.

GATHER EQUIPMENT

Gathering equipment is a time-management strategy and prevents distractions once commencing preparation of the medication. This reduces errors.

- *The medication chart* is the written order for the required drug and dose. The medication chart will need to meet all the requirements for the national medication chart, and is used to identify the correct patient and patient allergies risk, and to ensure the correct drug, dose, time and route are given.
- *The required medication* is obtained from stock. It will be in a vial or an ampoule. If reconstitution is needed, a sterile diluting solution as recommended for the medication is required. Refer to hospital policy or the AIDH for the correct diluents, if the medication is compatible with the infusing IV fluid and is suitable for bolus injection.

- *Medication additive labels* according to Australian labelling standards is completed with the patient's name, ID number, the drug, the dose, the date and time of preparation, commencement of administration and the signature of the preparing and checking nurses.
- *A sterile Luer lock syringe* of a size depending on the diluted volume (5 to 20 mL) is used to draw up and prepare the medication.
- *A needleless syringe cannula or a sterile needle* for drawing up the medication; usually an 18-gauge needle.
- *Alcohol wipes* to cleanse and disinfect the tops of vials and the seal on the medication access port of the IV line.
- *A kidney dish* is used to transport medications, syringes and alcohol wipes to the bedside.
- *The sharps container* so needles, glass ampoules and vials can be immediately disposed of at the bedside, thus reducing the chance of needlestick injuries or cuts from broken glass.

- *Normal saline (NS)* (saline 0.9%) in a sterile syringe is used to flush the IV line before and after administration of the medication. This prevents any medication incompatibilities and ensures patency of the PIVC. NS has been found to be effective in preventing occlusion of the cannula. Check the facility's policy for correct regimen.
- *Non-sterile or sterile gloves* are used to comply with standard precautions, maintain an aseptic technique when touching key parts and key sites, and reduce contact with the medication. Check the facility policy.

- *A watch with a second hand* is required to time the rate of the IV injection. Infusion rates vary with the medication – follow the manufacturer's recommendation. Too-rapid injection of many medications precipitates either a local reaction or more serious, systemic reactions. The rate needs to be determined prior to administration. An IV infusion pump can be programmed to deliver a bolus dose within a short timeframe (e.g. 10 to 20 minutes), and will deliver the medication more consistently.

PREPARE AND ADMINISTER THE MEDICATION

Perform hand hygiene

Perform hand hygiene before touching the patient or the patient's surrounds and prior to any procedure involving patient contact to reduce the possibility of cross-contamination. Hand hygiene is the most effective method of infection control as it removes transient organisms from the hands of the nurse (see **Skill 1.1**).

Give a clear explanation of the procedure and establish therapeutic communication

Introduce yourself, and check you have the correct patient. Discuss the procedure and gain the patient's consent. Giving a clear explanation is required to gain legal consent and to address policy requirements. It will also assist the patient to cooperate with the procedure, allay anxiety and assist in establishing a therapeutic relationship.

Many patients will be apprehensive about receiving medication via a PIVC. Advising the patient that the 'needle' is introduced into an existing IV line, not injected into their body, reassures most people. Warn the patient that they may experience some discomfort when the medication is administered but this should be temporary. Determine the patient's understanding of the purpose of the medication, provide education about common side effects for the drug to be administered and ask the patient to alert the nurses to any changes that they note.

Assess the patient and PIVC prior to IV bolus

Assessment prior to IV administration of a medication involves several areas. The patient is assessed for allergies to medications and their general condition. The PIVC site is assessed for patency, infection, inflammation, infiltration, thrombus or phlebitis of the insertion site or the vein (see **Skill 6.3**) (SA Health, 2020). The drug must be assessed for: compatibility with the fluid infusing; its normal dosage, action and side effects; the recommended infusion time of the drug; and its peak action time.

Use general concepts and 'rights of medication administration'

Follow the 'rights of medication administration' to prepare and administer the medication to the patient. IV medications are checked by two nurses (one must be an RN), according to the facility's protocol.

Perform hand hygiene

Perform hand hygiene before touching the patient or the patient's surrounds and prior to any procedure involving patient contact to reduce the possibility of cross-contamination. The medication being prepared is administered directly into a vein and an aseptic non-touch technique should be used.

Use an aseptic technique

The preparation and administration of IV medication requires the use of an aseptic technique, ensuring that key parts are not touched within micro-aseptic fields (see **Skill 4.1**). Follow facility policy regarding the use of sterile gloves or non-sterile gloves when accessing and touching these areas. Syringes, IV ports and connectors use needleless systems to reduce the risk of needlestick injury.

Assess the preparation area

Assess the preparation area for adequate lighting, ventilation and space. Preparing any medication requires concentration and the nurse should be free from distraction during the procedure. Clean the work surface with alcohol or soap and water wipes.

Prepare the medication additive label

All syringes used to administer IV medications should be labelled using the blue IV label and remain intact throughout the administration of the medication (ACSQHC, 2015). Prepare the label prior to preparing the medication so it can be easily attached to the syringe immediately after the medication has been prepared. The label should be legible and contain the following information: patient's name and identification number; patient's date of birth; medication name and total dose; total volume in fluid container; concentration; date and time prepared; route of administration; and signatures of nurses preparing the medication.

Perform hand hygiene and don non-sterile gloves

Perform hand hygiene as an infection-control measure. The medication being prepared is administered directly into a vein and an aseptic non-touch technique should be used. Non-sterile gloves are used to protect the nurse's hands from contact with medications, comply with standard precautions.

Prepare the syringes

Collect the required medication, diluent, flush, alcohol wipe, access cannula/needle and syringe. Refer to hospital policy or the *Australian Injectable Drugs Handbook* (AIDH) for the correct diluent. Draw up the required diluent into a 20 mL syringe. Swab the top of the medication vial with an alcohol wipe for 15 seconds, allow it to dry and then insert the syringe into the bung and add 5 to 10 mL of the diluent to the vial to reconstitute and mix the medication. Without removing the syringe, gently roll the medication vial between your hands to mix the medication. Ensure all the dry powder is dissolved and then withdraw the dissolved medication into the syringe. Alternatively, draw the medication from the ampoule and then dilute by drawing up the correct diluents into the same syringe. Place the medication label on the syringe parallel to the long axis of the syringe barrel. The top end is flush with, but not covering, the graduation (ACSQHC, 2015).

Place all the labelled medication syringes in the kidney dish with a new alcohol wipe, ready to carry to the patient's area. Remove and dispose of gloves.

Perform hand hygiene

Maintain the 5 Moments for Hand Hygiene and perform hand hygiene after touching the patient and the patient's surrounds.

Check the correct patient

Identify the correct patient, check for allergies (see **Skill 5.1**) and complete an assessment of the PIVC insertion site prior to administering any IV medications (see **Skill 6.3**). Medications should not be given if any signs of infiltration or phlebitis exist.

Perform hand hygiene and don gloves

Perform hand hygiene and don gloves. Maintain the 5 Moments for Hand Hygiene and perform hand hygiene after touching the patient and the patient's surrounds. Non-sterile gloves are used to protect the nurse's hands from contact with medications and comply with standard precautions.

Inject medication into an existing line or PIVC

- Pause any continuous IV administration by pausing the pump or closing the roller clamp.
- Don non-sterile gloves to maintain an aseptic technique, reduce risk from exposure from any body fluids and to protect the nurse's hands from contact with medications.
- Clean the injection port of the IV line or the extension tubing with an alcohol wipe for 15 seconds to remove microorganisms. Allow the alcohol to dry.

For a PIVC without an existing fluid administration

- Don non-sterile gloves to maintain an aseptic technique, reduce risk from exposure from any body fluids and to protect the nurse's hands from contact with medications.
- Clean the injection port of the IV line or the extension tubing with an alcohol wipe for 15 seconds to remove micro-organisms. Allow the alcohol to dry.
- Attach the Luer lock syringe with the saline flush to the access port and test that the IV cannula is in the vein by gently attempting to inject the saline while feeling for resistance. Do not use excess force. If any resistance is felt, it is possible that the cannula is occluded and needs to be replaced. If there is no resistance, flush with 5 to 10 mL of the prescribed saline 0.9%. Detach the syringe and place it in the kidney dish.

For both procedures

- Attach the Luer lock syringe with the medication to the access port and inject the medication at the recommended rate. Use a watch to maintain the preferred rate to prevent irritation or damage to vein walls by too high a concentration of the medication. Alternatively, a 20 mL syringe can be attached to the infusion pump as a secondary line (follow the manufacturer's instructions) and the pump set at the required bolus dose flow rate. This will create a more consistent and safer delivery of the medication. Please note that some pump manufacturers recommend the use of the larger 20 mL syringe, even when administering a small volume, to ensure the accuracy of the pump. Disconnect the syringe when all the medication has been administered.
- Attach fresh syringe containing the post-flush, and flush the line with 10 to 20 mL of saline to remove any irritant caused by the medication to the vein. Disconnect the syringe and place in the kidney dish.
- Re-establish the flow of the IV by unclamping the line and resetting the IV rate.
- If multiple medications are being given, the line should be flushed between each medication to prevent mixing of medication in the IV tubing. Remove and dispose of gloves.
- Check if there is also a required time to wait between medications being administered.

Assess the patient

Assess the patient during administration of the medication and also after the medication has been administered. Desired outcomes and adverse effects from the medication can occur during administration or in the time briefly after the medication has been administered.

Doff gloves and perform hand hygiene

Remove gloves and perform hand hygiene. Maintain the 5 Moments for Hand Hygiene after touching the patient and the patient's surrounds.

CLEAN, REPLACE OR DISPOSE OF EQUIPMENT

The needles, syringes and vials/ampoules are placed into the sharps container to prevent needlestick injuries by either the nursing or domestic staff. Dispose of alcohol wipes, kidney dish and used gloves in the general rubbish.

DOCUMENT AND REPORT RELEVANT INFORMATION

Documentation of IV medications is similar to any other medication. The nurse signs or initials the medication chart, indicating the ordered dose was given to the patient by the IV route at the designated time. The nurse who checked the drug usually countersigns the medication (as per the facility's policies). Any untoward reactions are immediately reported to the shift coordinator and the medical officer. PIVC observations should be recorded on the PIVC monitoring chart.

CASE STUDY

Irene Jones, aged 62, was admitted to your ward 3 hours ago following surgery to her right wrist, after a fall while gardening at home. She is reasonably fit and healthy. She has osteoarthritis in her hands, feet and right knee. She has no known allergies.

On arrival to the ward post-op, she is alert and orientated. Her observations have been stable, and she has taken a small amount of fluids and diet, but is hesitant to continue her oral intake due to nausea and possible

vomiting. The doctor has ordered a stat dose of ondansetron 4 mg IV to help manage this.

As the medication-competent EN looking after her, you will administer this medication under the supervision of the RN.

1. Where will you be able to access all the required information that you need to know to ensure safe administration of this medication?
2. Research possible side effects of ondansetron and explain how you will monitor the patient post injection.

Note: These notes are summaries of the most important points in the assessments/procedures, and are not exhaustive on the subject. The naming of documents or charts may differ from state to state, and facility to facility. In all possible situations the guidelines of the ACSQHC are used when describing national charts or documents (e.g. the ACSQHC Observation and Response Chart is named the Adult Observation and Response Chart in WA, and the Rapid Detection and Response Observation Chart in SA). References of the materials used to compile the information have been supplied. The student is expected to have learned the material surrounding each skill as presented in the references. No single reference is complete on the subject.

REFERENCES

Australian Commission on Safety and Quality in Health Care (ACSQHC). (2015). *National Standard for User-applied Labelling of Injectable Medicines, Fluids and Lines.* https://www.safetyandquality.gov.au/sites/default/files/migrated/National-Standard-for-User-Applied-Labelling-Aug-2015.pdf

Nursing and Midwifery Board of Australia (NMBA). (2020). *Fact sheet: Enrolled Nurses and Medicine Administration.* http://www.nursingmidwiferyboard.gov.au/Codes-Guidelines-Statements/FAQ/Enrolled-nurses-and-medicine-administration.aspx

SA Health. (2020). *Peripheral intravenous catheter (PIVC) infection prevention clinical directive. Version No.: 1.1* Approval date: 9 June 2020. Government of South Australia. https://www.sahealth.sa.gov.au/wps/wcm/connect/b8b0b71d-899e-42aa-ac3b-ca37d905f9a8/Clinical_Directive_PIVC_Infection_Prevention_v1.0_22.11.2019.pdf?MOD=AJPERES&CACHEID=ROOTWORKSPACE-b8b0b71d-899e-42aa-ac3b-ca37d905f9a8-mWhfA4q

---

RECOMMENDED READINGS

Abbott, B. & DeVries, S. (2016). *Monitoring and Administration of IV Medications for the Enrolled Nurse.* Cengage Australia.

Australian Commission on Safety and Quality in Health Care (ACSQHC). (2019). *Peripheral Venous Access Clinical Care Standard.* https://www.safetyandquality.gov.au/standards/clinical-care-standards/peripheral-venous-access-clinical-care-standard

Queensland Health. (2019). *Intra-vascular Device Management.* Queensland Government. https://www.health.qld.gov.au/clinical-practice/guidelines-procedures/diseases-infection/infection-prevention/intravascular-device-management

Ray-Barruel, G. (2017). Infection prevention: peripheral intravenous catheter assessment and care. *Australian Nursing & Midwifery Journal,* 24(8), p. 34.

ESSENTIAL SKILLS COMPETENCY

Intravenous Medication Administration – Injection (Bolus)

Demonstrates the ability to effectively and safely administer intravenous medication by injecting medication via an IV lumen

Criteria for skill performance	Y	D
(Numbers indicate *Enrolled Nurse Standards for Practice*, 2016)	(Satisfactory)	(Requires development)
1. Identifies indication (8.3, 8.4)		
2. Gathers equipment (1.2, 1.6, 4.4, 6.4, 8.4, 9.4): ■ medication chart ■ required medication ■ syringes and needles ■ alcohol wipes ■ NS flush ■ medication additive labels ■ injection tray/kidney dish ■ sharps container ■ non-sterile/sterile gloves ■ watch with a second hand		
3. Performs hand hygiene (1.2, 1.4, 1.8, 3.9, 6.4, 9.4)		
4. Evidence of effective communication with the patient; e.g. gives patient a clear explanation of procedure, gains patient consent (2.1, 2.3, 2.4, 2.5, 6.3)		
5. Assesses patient PIVC site (1.2, 1.4, 3.2, 4.1, 4.4, 6.4, 8.4, 9.4)		
6. Performs hand hygiene (1.2, 1.4, 1.8, 3.9, 6.4, 9.4)		
7. Uses general concepts of medication administration plus 'rights' (1.1, 1.2, 1.3, 1.4, 2.2, 3.1, 3.2, 3.9, 5.5, 8.4, 9.3, 9.4)		
8. Maintains an aseptic technique and dons non-sterile gloves (1.2, 1.4, 3.9, 8.4, 9.4)		
9. Prepares the medication and attaches the additive medication label; removes non-sterile gloves and takes medication to patient's bedside (1.1, 1.2, 1.3, 1.4, 1.8, 2.2, 3.1, 3.2, 3.9, 8.4, 9.4)		
10. Performs hand hygiene and dons non-sterile gloves (1.2, 1.4, 1.8, 3.9, 6.4, 9.4)		
11. Swabs port, flushes PIVC and then injects medication into an existing line at correct rate; flushes line after injection administered (1.1, 1.2, 1.3, 1.4, 1.8, 2.2, 3.1, 3.9, 8.4, 9.4)		
12. Assesses patient, PIVC site and drug after administering medication (1.2, 1.4, 3.2, 4.1, 6.4, 8.4, 9.4)		
13. Removes gloves and performs hand hygiene (1.2, 1.4, 1.8, 3.9, 6.4, 9.4)		
14. Cleans, replaces or disposes of equipment appropriately (1.2, 1.4, 3.9, 6.5, 9.4)		
15. Documents and reports relevant information (1.2, 1.3, 1.8, 3.2, 5.3, 6.6, 7.1, 7.2, 7.3, 7.4, 7.5)		
16. Demonstrates ability to link theory to practice (8.3, 8.4, 8.5, 9.4)		

Student:

Clinical facilitator: Date:

CHAPTER 6.8

CENTRAL VENOUS ACCESS DEVICE (CVAD) DRESSING

IDENTIFY INDICATIONS

Central venous catheters (CVCs) and peripherally inserted central catheters (PICCs) are a type of central venous access device (CAVD) that terminate at or close to the heart or in one of the great vessels (Australian Nursing Federation, 2020). They may be used when the patient requires medications, blood transfusions, intravenous fluids or nutrients, and are usually for a period of weeks or months.

There are a variety of CVC lines in use:

- *tunnelled cuffed CVCs*, usually used for long-term treatment
- *un-cuffed CVCs*, usually in place for a shorter duration

- *non-tunnelled CVCs*, usually short-term and for an emergency, usually less than 3 weeks.

The patient with a CVC or PICC line is at greater risk of infection. Dressings will be carried out on a regular basis, usually weekly, or sooner if the dressing becomes soiled, wet or loose (SA Health, 2017). Always check the policy of your organisation regarding the frequency for dressing change. The dressing acts as a protection to the insertion site. Always follow the facility's policy for this procedure and possible learning module requirements.

GATHER AND PREPARE EQUIPMENT

Gathering equipment for use during the procedure is a time-management strategy. It allows the nurse to mentally rehearse the steps in the procedure. Having all necessary items available prevents having to seek assistance – leaving a sterile set-up to obtain forgotten items would risk contamination. Being organised creates self-confidence in the nurse and promotes patient confidence. The following items may be required.

- *Dressing trolley*, used to transport materials to and from the bedside; the trolley must be cleaned both before and after the dressing.
- *Dressing packs* are usually commercially supplied and contain a waterproof wrapper that serves as the sterile field when the pack is unwrapped. There is a receptacle containing gauze swabs that is used as a solution bowl. These are usually sufficient but additional supplies of gauze swabs for cleaning and drying the insertion site of the CVC or PICC line may be added.

- *A sterile solution* (usually alcohol-based skin cleaning preparation, 2% chlorhexidine in 70% alcohol) is used to cleanse the insertion site.
- *Normal saline 0.9%* may be required if exit site is visibly soiled.
- *Dressings*, used to protect the site. A sterile transparent semipermeable dressing is used to cover the site. Check the policy and protocol of your facility.
- *Non-sterile gloves* (clean) used to remove the old dressing so that contamination is minimised. An aseptic technique is used for the dressing procedure.
- *Sterile gloves* for dressing procedure.
- *A waste disposable waterproof bag* is necessary for the disposal of all used and contaminated material to prevent transmission of microorganisms.
- *Extra sterile gauze squares* may be required.

All unopened items should be placed on the bottom shelf of the trolley, leaving the top surface as clean as possible for use during the procedure. This includes dressing packs and other sterile items. Take the trolley to the patient's bedside.

PERFORM THE DRESSING

Perform hand hygiene

Perform hand hygiene before touching the patient or the patient's surrounds and prior to any procedure involving patient contact to reduce the possibility of cross-contamination. Hand hygiene is the most effective method of infection control as it removes transient organisms from the hands of the nurse (see **Skill 1.1**).

Demonstrate problem-solving abilities

Positioning the patient comfortably will eliminate movement during the procedure, which can contaminate sterile items. The patient's position should be considered in relation to the time that it is expected they will need to stay still for treatment. The site should be comfortably accessible to the nurse to eliminate contamination or self-injury from using an awkward position for the treatment. Offering the bedpan or urinal or assisting the patient to the toilet prior to the procedure will reduce unnecessary interruptions and increase patient comfort. Time the dressing change in consultation with the patient, so that visiting hours or mealtimes are not disrupted.

Give a clear explanation of the procedure and establish therapeutic communication

Introduce yourself, and check you have the correct patient. Discuss the procedure and gain the patient's consent. Giving a clear explanation is required to gain legal consent and to address policy requirements. It will also assist the patient to cooperate with the procedure, allay anxiety and assist in establishing a therapeutic relationship.

Explanation of the positioning and the expectations of the patient will ensure their cooperation, reducing the risk that they will touch and contaminate something sterile.

Prepare the room and environment

Privacy is provided for the patient, to minimise embarrassment, by pulling the curtains around the patient in a shared room or closing the door in a private room. Airflow is restricted by closing the door, reducing vacuuming or bed making by other staff so that airborne microorganisms are less likely to contaminate the insertion site. The site must be well-lit to assist with assessment and treatment. A waterproof waste disposal bag is placed near the patient to receive contaminated articles so that transmission of microorganisms is prevented.

Remove the soiled dressing

Some practitioners advocate leaving the dressing on until the sterile field is established, then removing it. This reduces the chance of contamination (either by patient or from the environment) while the nurse is performing hand hygiene and setting up the aseptic field. Tape is removed carefully by supporting the skin around the tape and pulling towards the insertion site. Use short gentle pulls parallel to the skin to minimise pain. Take care not to dislodge the line while removing the dressing. Non-sterile gloves are used when removing the dressing. If the dressing is soiled, remove the dressing with the soiled surface away from the patient. Assess for any drainage, noting amount, colour, consistency and odour. The dressing and the gloves are carefully placed in the disposable bag without contaminating the outside of the bag.

Perform hand hygiene

Perform hand hygiene to remove microorganisms and prevent cross-contamination.

Establish a critical aseptic field

See **Skill 4.2** for establishing an aseptic field and setting up the dressing. Key parts will be touched during this procedure so sterile gloves are also required.

Cleanse and assess the insertion site

Use forceps to transfer the sterile drape to your fingertips, holding at the top edge and place the sterile drape as close as possible to the insertion site. This extends the critical aseptic field and helps prevent contamination of equipment. Keep the setting-up forceps for cleansing.

Don sterile gloves using an open-gloving technique, as described in **Skill 4.9**.

A non-touch technique is implemented by picking up a swab with the clean forceps in the aseptic field, then using the forceps to pass the swab to the swabbing forceps. One gauze swab is used for each stroke, to cleanse the insertion site. Place each used swab in the waste disposal bag. Maintain the following principles utilising a non-touch aseptic technique.

- Clean around the insertion site in a circular motion, moving outwards from exit site and ensuring the whole area to be covered with a dressing is cleaned (Royal Children's Hospital Melbourne, 2017; SA Health, 2020).
- Repeat with a second swab.
- Clean along the lumen, starting from the exit site and moving outwards.
- Allow to air dry for 1 to 2 minutes (SA Health, 2020); do not dry with gauze swabs.
- Apply sterile transparent semipermeable dressing.
- For tunnelled CVC lines, loop the catheter under the dressing, carefully avoiding coverage of the exit site. This prevents the lumen being accidentally pulled out.
- Note and record external length of catheter if applicable.

Always follow the policy of your organisation and ensure that this procedure is within your scope of practice.

During and after the cleansing of the insertion site, assess to determine status of the insertion site. Inspect for:

- infection (are there signs of exudate?)
- inflammation/swelling at site
- dislodgement of the lumen – some lumens will be measured on a daily basis
- splitting or cracking of the lumen
- leaking and discharge
- patency of CVC or PICC
- external length of catheter, if applicable.

Apply a dressing

Sterile, transparent, semipermeable polyurethane dressings (unless there is known sensitivity) are applied over the lumen and insertion site. Use the two remaining forceps and a non-touch technique to pick up the dressing and pass to your gloved hand, and then apply the dressing.

Secure the dressing

Once the outer dressing has been put in place, secure the dressing with the selected tape, if required. Ensure that the entry site is not occluded. The patient is assisted to a position of comfort. The date is documented on the appropriate dressing tag/label.

Doff gloves and perform hand hygiene

Remove gloves and discard appropriately and then perform hand hygiene. Maintain the 5 Moments for Hand Hygiene and perform hand hygiene after touching the patient and the patient's surrounds.

CLEAN, REPLACE OR DISPOSE OF EQUIPMENT

Clean, replace and dispose of equipment appropriately. After securing the wound dressing, contaminated materials are wrapped in the (disposable) wrapper that has formed the aseptic field and placed in the waste disposal bag, which is then placed in the contaminated waste. The trolley is wiped down with the recommended disinfecting solution or wipes. The trolley is returned to its position in the clean service area of the unit. Disposable metal forceps (if used) are placed in the sharps container.

DOCUMENT AND REPORT RELEVANT INFORMATION

Document relevant information in the wound management plan, care plan and patient notes and CVAD management record, including:

- infection (are there signs of exudate?)
- inflammation/swelling at site
- dislodgement of the lumen – some lumens will be measured on a daily basis
- splitting or cracking of the lumen
- leaking and discharge
- external length of catheter, if applicable
- type of dressing applied
- patient's response to the procedure.

Note any alteration in comfort levels or changes noted at the insertion site and report these to the registered nurse.

CASE STUDY

You are caring for Abdul Habid, a 48 year-old male patient who has a PICC line inserted for treatment with intravenous antibiotics over a period of 4 to 6 weeks. Abdul requires his PICC line dressing to be changed. As an enrolled nurse, you have completed the required learning package and are authorised to perform this dressing.

1. Explain the difference between a CVC and PICC line.

2. Identify additional precautions that you need to take when performing this PICC line dressing.
3. What should be documented at the completion of the PICC line dressing?
4. Identify three possible complications for a patient with a PICC line in situ.

Note: These notes are summaries of the most important points in the assessments/procedures, and are not exhaustive on the subject. The naming of documents or charts may differ from state to state, and facility to facility. In all possible situations the guidelines of the ACSQHC are used when describing national charts or documents (e.g. the ACSQHC Observation and Response Chart is named the Adult Observation and Response Chart in WA, and the Rapid Detection and Response Observation Chart in SA). References of the materials used to compile the information have been supplied. The student is expected to have learned the material surrounding each skill as presented in the references. No single reference is complete on the subject.

REFERENCES

Australian Nursing Federation. (2020). Nursing management of peripherally inserted central catheters. *Western Nurse Magazine*, January–February.

Royal Children's Hospital Melbourne. (2018). *Central Venous Access Device Management.* https://www.rch.org.au/policy/public/Central_Venous_Access_Device_Management/

SA Health. (2020). *Peripherally Inserted Central Catheter (PICC) Dressing Management Clinical Guideline.* Government of South Australian. https://www.sahealth.sa.gov.au/wps/wcm/connect/ba19850042c387a78165f78cd21c605e/PICC+Dressing+procedure+guideline+v1.0_27092017.pdf?MOD=AJPERES&CACHEID=ROOTWORKSPACE-ba19850042c387a78165f78cd21c605e-mMHfDQN

RECOMMENDED READINGS

National Health and Medical Research Council (NHMRC). (2020). *Australian Guidelines for the Prevention and Control of Infection in Healthcare (2019).* https://www.nhmrc.gov.au/about-us/publications/australian-guidelines-prevention-and-control-infection-healthcare-2019#block-views-block-file-attachments-content-block-1

WA Country Health Service. (2019). *Central Venous Access Devices (CVAD) and Long Peripheral Venous Catheter (Long PVC) Management Clinical Practice Standard.* http://www.wacountry.health.wa.gov.au:443/index.php?id=1200

ESSENTIAL SKILLS COMPETENCY

Performs Central Venous Access Device (CVAD) Dressings
Demonstrates the ability to effectively and safely change the dressing for a central venous access device

Criteria for skill performance	Y	D
(Numbers indicate *Enrolled Nurse Standards for Practice*, 2016)	(Satisfactory)	(Requires development)
1. Identifies indication (8.3, 8.4)		
2. Gathers and prepares equipment (1.2, 1.6, 4.4, 6.4, 8.4, 9.4): ■ dressing trolley ■ dressing pack ■ sterile solution for cleansing (as per facility policy) ■ extra sterile gauze swabs if needed ■ sterile transparent dressing (as per facility policy) ■ non-sterile gloves for removing dressing ■ sterile gloves for dressing procedure ■ a waste disposable waterproof bag for rubbish		
3. Performs hand hygiene and dons non-sterile gloves (1.2, 1.4, 1.8, 3.9, 6.4, 9.4)		
4. Demonstrates problem-solving abilities; e.g. assesses the patient, positions the patient (4.1, 4.2, 8.3, 8.4, 8.5, 9.4)		
5. Evidence of effective communication with the patient; e.g. gives patient a clear explanation of procedure, gains patient consent (2.1, 2.3, 2.4, 2.5, 6.3)		
6. Removes soiled dressing (1.2, 1.4, 1.8, 2.7, 3.2, 3.9, 8.4, 9.4)		
7. Performs hand hygiene (1.2, 1.4, 1.8, 3.9, 6.4, 9.4)		
8. Dons sterile gloves (1.2, 1.4, 1.8, 2.2, 3.2, 3.9, 8.4, 9.4)		
9. Performs dressing to site (1.2, 1.4, 2.2, 2.7, 2.10, 3.2, 3.4, 4.4, 6.4, 8.4, 9.4)		
10. Doffs sterile gloves and performs hand hygiene (1.2, 1.4, 1.8, 3.9, 6.4, 9.4)		
11. Cleans, replaces or disposes of equipment appropriately (1.2, 1.4, 3.9, 6.5, 9.4)		
12. Documents and reports relevant information (1.2, 1.3, 1.8, 3.2, 5.3, 6.6, 7.1, 7.2, 7.3, 7.4, 7.5)		
13. Demonstrates ability to link theory to practice (8.3, 8.4, 8.5, 9.4)		

Student:

Clinical facilitator: Date:

CHAPTER 6.9

BLOOD TRANSFUSION MANAGEMENT

IDENTIFY INDICATIONS

The administration of blood and its constituents is important not only to replace body fluids but also to restore other body functions when used appropriately. Blood is made up of several components, including albumin, platelets, plasma and globulins, and has complex functions. Significant blood loss or loss of one or more of the components has far-reaching consequences, such as clotting abnormalities, immunological deficits and tissue oxygenation problems. Indications for a blood or blood product transfusion include blood loss (trauma, surgery, haemorrhage), severe anaemia, replacement of fluid and protein, restoration of oncotic pressure and replacement of essential clotting factors.

There are specific national guidelines to minimise the administration of blood or blood products, and reduce the potential of harm to the patient. All other therapies and the patient's overall clinical condition will also be considered before a blood transfusion is ordered. The doctor will order the blood product and the number of units to be infused. This is a legal prescription. Patient education and consent are required prior to the transfusion. Written consent must be verified prior to initiating the transfusion, and must be documented in the patient's notes.

GATHER AND PREPARE EQUIPMENT

Gathering equipment for use during the procedure is a time-management strategy. It allows the nurse to mentally rehearse the steps in the procedure. Having all necessary items available prevents having to seek assistance. Being organised creates self-confidence in the nurse and promotes patient confidence. The following items may be required:

- *blood product administration order and blood management chart*
- *dressing trolley*
- *blood transfusion set* used for administration of blood – an approved type with a filter to remove clots and aggregate

- *personal protective equipment (PPE) – non-sterile gloves, goggles and plastic apron* to protect the nurse from exposure to the blood and reduce infection risk
- *required blood product* as ordered by the doctor
- *sodium chloride 0.9%* as ordered for flushing the line (if required)
- *vital signs monitoring equipment including sphygmomanometer, stethoscope and BP cuff of appropriate size, pulse oximeter, thermometer and a watch with a second hand.*

DISPLAY KNOWLEDGE OF BLOOD GROUPING AND BLOOD CROSS-MATCHING

Blood grouping and blood cross-matching must be carried out prior to initiating the transfusion. Blood is obtained from volunteers in Australia. The possibility of a transfusion reaction exists, which can vary from a mild fever to organ failure or anaphylaxis. The recipient's blood type must be matched for all blood or blood products. A rigorous procedure for identification of the patient and of the blood product must be carried out to prevent potential reactions.

Human blood is grouped into four classifications based on immune reactivity and is tested for grouping, Rh factor and other antigens. The groups are A, B, O and AB. The blood of any one group is incompatible with the blood of another group, and donor blood must be matched to the patient's blood. Mismatched blood in grouping, Rh factor or other antigens will cause transfusion reactions. In emergency situations, type O-negative blood may be used for patients with other blood groups because it reacts minimally with the other blood types and Rh-positive antibodies.

As well as compatibility testing, blood in Australia is tested for various viral infections including hepatitis and HIV. COVID-19 has been classified as a low risk, and is not currently known to be transmitted by transfusion (Australian Red Cross Lifeblood, 2020a).

DISPLAY KNOWLEDGE OF BLOOD PRODUCTS

- National *Patient Blood Management Guidelines* are managed by the National Blood Authority Australia (NBA, n.d.) and provide guidelines for decision-making about the use of blood and blood products according to a patient's clinical need. These guidelines support the criteria of administering blood products when the benefits outweigh the potential hazards, recommended in the *Blood Management Standard* (ACSQHC, 2019).
- Whole blood is no longer supplied by the 'Australian Red Cross Lifeblood' and is used only for preparing other blood components.
- Red cells result from removing the plasma from whole blood. They are also filtered to remove most leucocytes (Australian Red Cross Lifeblood, 2020b). They are used for patients who require increased oxygen-carrying capacity without excess fluid. They may also be used in combination with other blood products or treatments in situations of severe blood loss.
- Plasma is used to treat coagulation disorders where there is a high risk of bleeding (Australian Red Cross Lifeblood, 2020b). Plasma is usually frozen to preserve the clotting factors. However, rewarming can degrade the clotting factors, so frozen plasma must be used within 6 hours of thawing.
- Platelets are used to assist patients with severe bleeding due to low levels of platelets or clotting abnormalities. Platelets are separated out of the plasma. Platelets should be gently rocked during administration to prevent clumping in the bag.
- Cryoprecipitate is a solution containing factor VIII, fibrinogen, factor XIII, von Willebrand factor and fibronectin from fresh frozen plasma. Cryoprecipitate is indicated for the treatment of fibrinogen deficiency. It should not be used to treat haemophilia, von Willebrand's disease or deficiencies of factor XIII unless other therapies are not available. Small amounts (30 to 40 mL/10 kg) are usually administered (Australian Red Cross Lifeblood, 2021).
- Prior to the commencement of a transfusion, the IV line should be primed with either saline 0.9% or the blood component (Australian Red Cross Lifeblood, 2020b). Blood should not be mixed with any other IV fluids or medications.

PREPARE THE PATIENT AND ADMINISTER THE BLOOD

Perform hand hygiene
Perform hand hygiene before touching the patient or the patient's surrounds and prior to any procedure involving patient contact to reduce the possibility of cross-contamination. Hand hygiene is the most effective method of infection control as it removes transient organisms from the hands of the nurse (see **Skill 1.1**).

Give a clear explanation of the procedure and establish therapeutic communication
Introduce yourself, and check you have the correct patient. Discuss the procedure and gain the patient's consent. Giving a clear explanation is required to gain legal consent and to address policy requirements. It will also assist the patient to cooperate with the procedure, allay anxiety and assist in establishing a therapeutic relationship. According to facility policy, written consent may also be required for administration of blood and blood products.

Explaining the entire procedure and its benefits to the patient will gain their cooperation. The patient should be aware of the signs and symptoms that may indicate a problem. Alert the patient to back pain, fever and chills, itching or alterations in respiratory status. Also ask them to report any alterations (sensations, feelings) that may occur during the transfusion. Resources to assist with explaining the transfusion of blood and blood products are easily available from the Australian Red Cross.

Record vital signs
A baseline is established prior to commencing the transfusion so that changes in the patient's condition during the transfusion can be monitored. Blood pressure, temperature, pulse and respiratory rate are recorded on the observation and response chart (ORC) (see **Skills 2.3**, **2.4** and **2.5**) An elevated temperature and any other abnormalities must be reported. Ask the patient about known allergies or any reactions to previous products. Other baseline data relating to the patient's pathology is noted (e.g. haemoglobin, haematocrit), and the patient is observed for pre-existing rashes.

Don PPE and follow standard precautions
Blood and blood products are a body fluid, and non-sterile gloves should be worn whenever you are handling the blood bag and IV line. This includes attaching or changing the blood bag from the IV line and while discarding the blood bag and the IV tubing. Some facilities may also recommend wearing goggles and a plastic apron when changing the bag or IV administration set to reduce the risk of blood exposure.

Identify patient and blood product according to policy

The patient's blood order will include the written order for blood as well as an identification of the patient. When the patient has given consent and the peripheral intravenous catheter (PIVC) has been inserted, the chart is taken to the blood bank to cross-check with the blood product being retrieved. The blood transfusion must then commence within 30 minutes of being removed from the approved blood storage. If this is not possible, it must be returned to the blood bank immediately to minimise the risk of bacterial contamination.

The nurse brings the blood product to the patient and, with a registered nurse (RN), completes a three-point check for patient identification. Ask the patient to state their name and date of birth, and check the armband for the same information and the patient identification number. The blood order chart and the information on the blood product should also be checked to ensure they are all the same. The type of blood product (and type ordered), the expiration date of the blood product and the blood's ID number should also be checked. If there are any discrepancies, the blood should not be administered and advice should be sought immediately. The patient's consent to the transfusion is rechecked.

The blood bag is then checked for any clots, discolouration or abnormalities. Ensure the pack is intact. Turn the blood bag upside down to thoroughly mix the contents (Australian Red Cross Lifeblood, 2020b). Once the transfusion has commenced it should be completed within 4 hours. Different types of blood products have different recommended infusion rates, with red cells being transfused over 1 to 3 hours.

Perform hand hygiene

Maintain the 5 Moments for Hand Hygiene and perform hand hygiene after touching the patient and the patient's surrounds.

Don PPE as required

PPE requirements will vary according to the care being delivered and the patient's health status, and may include plastic apron/gown, mask, protective eyewear and gloves to reduce the risk of exposure to body fluids.

Prepare the IV line prior to commencing the transfusion

The IV line should be prepared using sodium chloride 0.9% or the blood product and connected to the PIVC as per **Skill 6.3**. If the patient requires insertion of a PIVC, assist the doctor or RN as per **Skill 6.2**. Check the IV administration chart and the blood order chart for the blood orders. The IV administration set must be an approved type with a filter to remove clots and aggregate.

Commence the transfusion and monitor the patient

Complete a set of baseline vital signs (see **Skills 2.3**, **2.4** and **2.5**) before connecting and administering the blood. Wearing PPE, the blood bag is then connected to the IV line and the required flow rate set (as per **Skill 6.3**).

Patient monitoring should include temperature, pulse, respiration, oxygen saturations and blood pressure plus other potential transfusion reactions:
- prior to commencing the transfusion
- 15 minutes after commencing
- 1 hour after commencing
- each hour after that
- at completion of transfusion (Australian Red Cross Lifeblood, 2020b).

Stay with the patient and closely observe them during the first 15 minutes of a transfusion, as this is when most life-threatening reactions occur. Assessment should include observation for any symptoms of a possible transfusion reaction or fluid overload (especially in the elderly or when large volumes are being infused). Facility policies may vary in their guidelines for monitoring the patient during the process of the transfusion. More frequent observations may be required, depending on the patient's health status.

The transfusion should be completed within 4 hours.

The following assessment findings indicate the need for immediate nursing interventions:
- The signs and symptoms of an allergic reaction include flushing, urticaria (hives) and an itchy rash. A more severe allergic reaction, and possible anaphylaxis, has the symptoms of dyspnoea, airway obstruction and hypotension. This more severe reaction is a medical emergency.
- The signs and symptoms of a febrile non-haemolytic reaction are fever (38°C to 39°C), chills and malaise.
- The signs and symptoms of haemolytic reaction are restlessness, anxiety, flushing, chest/lumbar pain, tachypnoea, tachycardia, hypotension, fever above 39°C and chills.
- The signs and symptoms of circulatory overload are dyspnoea, chest pain, rales and rhonchi, anxiety, tachycardia, diaphoresis and blood-tinged sputum.

If any of these signs and symptoms occur, stop the transfusion immediately and contact the RN and the doctor. The transfusion should not be recommenced until a medical review has been completed. Medical emergencies would require a medical emergency team (MET) call. Different actions can be implemented, depending on the reaction and the doctor's orders. All transfusion reactions should also be well documented, including a transfusion reaction form sent to the transfusion laboratory. The blood product should also be returned to the lab for assessment.

Flush and disconnect the IV line

Once the transfusion has been completed, the IV line should be changed. PPE will be required for this procedure. Flushing of the line with normal saline 0.9% is only required to ensure that all blood has been administered. Flushing of the line between units of blood may not be necessary but may be used to maintain IV access for the next unit of blood (Australian Red Cross Lifeblood, 2020b). Care should be taken to ensure the patient does not experience fluid overload.

A new IV line should be used if IV therapy is to be recommended. The blood bag is disposed of in the medical biological waste according to facility policy.

Doff PPE

Remove PPE in the following sequence: non-sterile gloves, hand hygiene, eyewear/face shield, plastic apron/gown and mask and then perform hand hygiene (ACSQHC, 2020). Dispose of in the rubbish bag.

Perform hand hygiene

Maintain the 5 Moments for Hand Hygiene and perform hand hygiene after touching the patient and the patient's surrounds.

Continue to monitor the patient

Continue to monitor the patient for alterations in vital signs or the appearance of symptoms of a reaction, according to policy. If symptoms do occur, notify the doctor. Monitor the patient's fluid balance closely, and ensure they are passing urine. Fluid overload can occur with a blood transfusion.

Perform hand hygiene

Maintain the 5 Moments for Hand Hygiene and perform hand hygiene after touching the patient and the patient's surrounds.

CLEAN, REPLACE OR DISPOSE OF EQUIPMENT

Clean, replace and dispose of equipment appropriately. The blood products and IV line should be disposed of in the medical biological waste as per facility policy.

DOCUMENT AND REPORT RELEVANT INFORMATION

Specific documentation is used for recording blood transfusions. This will include a chart for the blood pack peel-off identification tab that is identical to the blood unit ID number, grouping and Rh factor. This tab should be removed from the blood pack and placed on the chart, noting when the transfusion started. A note is also made of the sequence number of the blood pack, if more than one pack is given, and the time of completion of each pack. The patient ORC should be used for recording all vital signs before and during the transfusion. A fluid balance chart may also be maintained during the transfusion.

CASE STUDY

You are caring for Anne-Marie Reynolds who is aged 65 and has been admitted for an upper gastric bleed. The medical team have ordered 2 units of red blood cells to be administered. Each unit is to be administered over 3 hours.

1. Locate and read the policies and procedures for blood and blood product administration at your local major hospital. Why is it important for the patient to provide written consent for a blood transfusion?

2. Explain why two nurses (one an RN) are required to check the patient's identity, their consent, the blood order and the blood product before administration.

3. What vital signs are you required to complete prior to administering the blood?

4. What observations will you complete during the first 15 minutes of the transfusion?

5. How frequently should you monitor the patient over the next 3 hours while the transfusion is being administered?

During the first 15 minutes of the transfusion Anne-Marie complains of feeling sweaty and itchy.

6. What action/s will you implement?

7. What specific documentation would you include in the patient's notes when Anne-Marie's blood transfusion has been completed?

Note: These notes are summaries of the most important points in the assessments/procedures, and are not exhaustive on the subject. The naming of documents or charts may differ from state to state, and facility to facility. In all possible situations the guidelines of the ACSQHC are used when describing national charts or documents (e.g. the ACSQHC Observation and Response Chart is named the Adult Observation and Response Chart in WA, and the Rapid Detection and Response Observation Chart in SA). References of the materials used to compile the information have been supplied. The student is expected to have learned the material surrounding each skill as presented in the references. No single reference is complete on the subject.

PART 6

CRITICAL THINKING

Consider the previous clinical skills while answering the questions below.

1. According to the NMBA 'Enrolled Nurses and Medicine Administration – Fact Sheet' when is an enrolled nurse (EN) permitted to administer IV medications?
2. You are an EN working in a community setting. Identify how you would maintain an aseptic technique while preparing and administering IV medication or IV fluids in this environment.
3. How will you maintain your EN scope of practice when administering IV medications in a community setting?

REFERENCES

Australian Commission on Safety and Quality Health Care (ACSQHC). (2019). *Blood Management Standard.* https://www.safetyandquality.gov.au/standards/nsqhs-standards/blood-management-standard

Australian Commission on Safety and Quality in Health Care (ACSQHC). (2020). *Sequence for Putting on and Removing PPE.* https://www.safetyandquality.gov.au/sites/default/files/2020-03/putting_on_and_removing_ppe_diagram_-_march_2020.pdf

Australian Red Cross Lifeblood. (2020a). *Health Professionals: Coronavirus Disease (COVID-19) and the Impact on the Blood Supply.* https://transfusion.com.au/coronavirus

Australian Red Cross Lifeblood. (2020b). *Health Professionals: Preparing to Administer a Blood Component Including Equipment.* https://transfusion.com.au/transfusion_practice/administration

Australian Red Cross Lifeblood. (2021). *Blood Products and Transfusion Practice for Health Professionals.* http://www.transfusion.com.au

National Blood Authority Australia. (n.d.). *Patient Blood Management Guidelines.* https://www.blood.gov.au/pbm-guidelines

RECOMMENDED READINGS

Australian Commission on Safety and Quality Health Care (ACSQHC). (2018). *What is Patient Blood Management?* https://www.safetyandquality.gov.au/national-priorities/pbm-collaborative/what-is-patient-blood-management/

ESSENTIAL SKILLS COMPETENCY

Blood Transfusion Management

Demonstrates the ability to effectively and safely manage a blood transfusion

Criteria for skill performance (Numbers indicate *Enrolled Nurse Standards for Practice*, 2016)	**Y** (Satisfactory)	**D** (Requires development)
1. Identifies indication (8.3, 8.4)		
2. Displays knowledge of blood groups and cross-matching (1.2, 8.3, 8.4, 10.5)		
3. Displays knowledge of blood products (1.2, 8.3, 8.4, 10.5)		
4. Gathers equipment (1.2, 1.6, 4.4, 6.4, 8.4, 9.4): ■ blood product administration order and blood management chart ■ blood transfusion set used for administration of blood – an approved type with a filter to remove clots and aggregate ■ PPE – non-sterile gloves, goggles and plastic apron ■ required blood product as ordered by the doctor ■ sodium chloride 0.9% as ordered for flushing the line (if required) ■ trolley if required ■ vital signs monitoring equipment		
5. Performs hand hygiene (1.2, 1.4, 1.8, 3.9, 6.4, 9.4)		
6. Evidence of effective communication with the patient; e.g. gives patient a clear explanation of procedure, gains patient consent (2.1, 2.3, 2.4, 2.5, 6.3)		
7. Records vital signs (1.2, 1.4, 3.2, 4.1, 4.2, 4.4, 6.3, 6.4, 6.6, 7.1, 8.4, 9.4)		
8. Performs hand hygiene, dons gloves and maintains standard precautions (1.2, 1.4, 1.8, 3.9, 6.4, 9.4)		
9. Identifies patient and blood product according to policy (1.2, 1.3, 1.8, 2.1, 2.3, 2.4, 2.5, 6.3)		
10. Prepares IV line and commences transfusion (1.2, 1.4, 6.4, 8.4, 9.4)		
11. Monitors the patient during transfusion (1.2, 1.4, 1.8, 3.2, 3.9, 4.1, 4.2, 4.3, 4.4, 6.4, 6.6, 7.1, 7.2, 8.4, 9.4)		
12. Continues to monitor the patient after the transfusion (1.2, 1.4, 1.8, 3.2, 3.9, 4.1, 4.2, 4.3, 4.4, 6.4, 6.6, 7.1, 7.2, 8.4, 9.4)		
13. Flushes the IV line and disconnects IV line wearing PPE (1.2, 1.4, 6.4, 8.4, 9.4)		
14. Doffs PPE and performs hand hygiene (1.2, 1.4, 1.8, 3.9, 6.4, 9.4)		
15. Cleans, replaces or disposes of equipment appropriately (1.2, 1.4, 3.9, 6.5, 9.4)		
16. Documents and reports relevant information (1.2, 1.3, 1.8, 3.2, 5.3, 6.6, 7.1, 7.2, 7.3, 7.4, 7.5)		
17. Demonstrates ability to link theory to practice (8.3, 8.4, 8.5, 9.4)		

Student:

Clinical facilitator: Date:

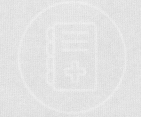

DOCUMENTATION

Note: These notes are summaries of the most important points in the assessments/procedures and are not exhaustive on the subject. References of the materials used to compile the information have been supplied. The student is expected to have learnt the material surrounding each skill as presented in the references. No single reference is complete on each subject.

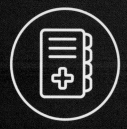

CHAPTER

CHAPTER 7.1

DOCUMENTATION

IDENTIFY INDICATIONS

Indications for documentation include admission or baseline notation of assessments and any changes in the patient's condition. The recording of accurate, complete and timely information is important, and helps to ensure correct treatment is given by nurses and health professionals. Patients are in hospital because their health condition is relatively unstable. Therefore, changes in their condition need to be reported and documented. In the acute setting, hospital policy usually requires an entry per shift; some may permit a minimum of a written entry once every 24 hours if there are no patient problems that require comment. In these situations, ensure all care plans and other documents accurately record care given per shift and other relevant patient data. Different requirements apply for residential care settings.

REVIEW TYPES OF CLINICAL DOCUMENTATION

Professional documentation of a patient's status is both a legal requirement and a professional responsibility. It ensures continuity of care by providing written and permanent communication of patient information. Hospital accreditation is dependent on sound basic documentation and nurses are legally protected if their charting demonstrates that a professional standard of care has been delivered. In a court of law, if it is not charted, it was not done. Documentation also has educational and research applications, as students and researchers can use the information for scientific purposes. Additionally, funding or staff levels may be reduced or fines imposed if documentation is incorrect.

There are many different types of documentation and charting, depending on the facility and the circumstances. These include various flow sheets, assessment tools, incident forms, risk assessment tools, transfer and discharge planning forms and nursing care planning forms. All staff need to become familiar with the protocols for completing documents used at the facility where you are attending clinical practice. Although principles of documentation apply to all patient documentation, this section will focus more on the 'integrated progress notes' or 'nursing notes', usually recorded at the end of each shift.

Patient progress notes, depending on the facility's choice, can be narrative, problem-oriented or focused, but all must be objective and accurate. Many facilities have access to electronic medical records (EMR) documentation.

- *Problem-oriented documentation* is a holistic approach that makes the patient needs or problems the focus of care. Nursing reports may be organised using *Data*, *Action* and *Response* (DAR). *Data* includes observation of patient status and behaviours. *Action* refers to nursing interventions, and *Response* is evaluating how the patient responds to the interventions. Problems are named (e.g. pain, nausea, diarrhoea). Current practice in some areas uses a body systems approach (e.g. central nervous system [CNS], respiratory [resp], cardiovascular [CVS]) or follows the section headings in the nursing care plan to help structure the content and report relevant information. This type of documentation tends to be more nursing-focused and flexible, with specific information easier to find. Duplication of routine care recorded in care plans or other charts should be avoided.

- *Documentation by exception* is used by some facilities. This mode of documentation focuses on exceptions to the normal or deviations from the usual standards. These events are documented and documentation continues until there is a return to the previous status or establishment of a new level of wellbeing for the individual. Documentation by exception reduces the amount of time and documentation required. Documentation by exception relies on nurses using the established flow sheets, charting/graphic records, standard protocols and care plans or pathways so that continuous appropriate care is provided and recorded as being delivered.

■ *Narrative documentation* is simply recording what has happened as it happens, with the observations, interventions and the patient's response to the interventions noted. This type of documentation is being used less frequently and can be contrary to facility policy.

RECORD CONTENT

Content of the documentation depends on the patient and their condition. For instance, the documentation for a patient who is in hospital for a myocardial infarct would include charts for pain levels, their circulation and perfusion, and levels of anxiety. A person who has had a surgical procedure such as a knee replacement would have different assessment parameters reported; for example, neurovascular observations (NVO) on the affected leg, pain assessment of the site, drainage from the wound, and circulatory and respiratory status following anaesthetic. Both patients would have notations about nursing interventions attended (e.g. repositioning, oxygen administration, supporting the leg on a pillow, analgesic administration) and the patient's response to these.

On admission to the unit, a thorough physical assessment and nursing history is documented as a baseline. As each nurse takes over the care of the patient, their assessment of the patient at that time should be noted. After that, alterations in the physical or psychosocial findings are noted. Use the patient's own words when reporting subjective data.

Generally, changes in medical, physical, emotional or psychological conditions are documented to alert other healthcare professionals of potential complications (e.g. unrelieved leg or foot pain in the patient with orthopaedic surgery to the leg).

RECORD RESPONSE TO TREATMENT

Response to treatment, including analgesia or other prescribed medication, is important to note so that ineffective treatment can be stopped or effective interventions continued. This might take the following form.

Nursing documentation 0230 hours: Patient complained of feeling nauseated (nausea score 2/10) post administration of IV antibiotic at 2400 hours. Patient commenced vomiting at 0130 hours, vomited bile-stained fluid × 2, nausea score 6/10, antiemetic given as per medication chart at 0150 hours. No further vomiting as at 0230 hours and patient reported nausea score 0/10.

You do not always need to report the information that is charted on charts such as the observation and response chart unless that information is relevant to other pertinent information you are recording; for example, '0730 – patient found on the floor, pale, diaphoretic, states "felt dizzy", BP 100/68, P. 58, BGL 2.3'. This uses both observed information

and measured information to give a more complete picture.

Interventions and their effect that are not on other charts or assessment tools should be documented. An example might be for a patient with fatigue: 'Initial strategy for managing fatigue discussed. Able to explain need to plan activities early in the day. Stated that "this makes sense" and will adopt this idea.'

ADHERE TO LEGAL REQUIREMENTS FOR DOCUMENTATION

Because all patient documentation is a legal document, there are minimum standards that must be met. Your entry must be:

■ in the correct patient's notes
■ legible
■ written in black ink
■ dated using the dd/mm/yy system and timed using the 24-hour clock
■ error-free or errors acknowledged with a single line through them and 'error' plus your initials written above
■ free of blank areas (draw a line through an unused portion of a line)
■ written using plain language using the acceptable facility abbreviations and without jargon; non-accepted abbreviations should not be used as they can lead to errors and potential patient harm
■ signed (this means that it was you who acted or observed – not someone else), with a printed name and designation after the signature for identification purposes
■ contemporaneous (i.e. made as close to the time of the observation or intervention as is reasonable)
■ in chronological order.

A late entry must follow the last entry (do not try to squeeze additional information into the notes) and be noted as such (i.e. use either 'addit' or 'late entry' beside the time you actually wrote the notation). Include the time of the occurrence within the notation.

Only document care once it is given, and never pre-empt care. Correct spelling and grammar are important because they make the entry readable. The entry should be factual, with specific information (time of the occurrence; exact findings; the patient's, doctor's or your response) and objective, not subjective. Do not interpret the facts or use vague or tentative wording (e.g. appears, seems), and do not use the words 'mistake' or 'accident'. Write what happened. Any change in the patient's condition (physical, medical, emotional, psychological) requires documenting in the relevant chart/s and progress notes.

Regularly update the patient's progress notes and care plan. Failure to document care or record patient observations/data is interpreted as care not being completed. Therefore, good documentation is critical for every patient, not only for their safety and comfort, but also for the nurse's security.

BECOME FAMILIAR WITH ELECTRONIC DOCUMENTATION

As technological advances become more affordable, EMR in hospitals and healthcare facilities have become more common. Much of the material presented so far in this skill will be applicable to EMR. There are additional precautions; for example, since you cannot 'sign' your note, indicating that it was you who saw or did something, you will need to use a password and PIN that will be unique to you and you will need to guard it carefully. Errors in data entry will still have to be acknowledged and left in the record.

Transmitting documentation from one facility to another or from the doctor's office to a facility, laboratory or other external provider requires the nurse to be aware of ensuring security of information, confidentiality and transmissibility of materials. The facility where you are working will have protocols and policies for moving and photocopying material from a patient's chart to another setting.

CASE STUDY

Utilising the Internet, obtain and read the article 'Stay out of court with proper documentation', which you can find at http://journals.lww.com/nursing/Fulltext/2011/04000/Stay_out_of_court_with_proper_documentation.11.aspx

1. Using the information/guidelines in this article and the documentation guidelines of this skill, practise writing/ documenting progress notes that follow the principles of 'focus documentation' and 'documentation by exception' to complete an end-of-shift report for the a.m./morning shift for a patient that you had cared for while on clinical practicum.

Note: These notes are summaries of the most important points in the assessments/procedures, and are not exhaustive on the subject. The naming of documents or charts may differ from state to state, and facility to facility. In all possible situations the guidelines of the ACSQHC are used when describing national charts or documents (e.g. the ACSQHC Observation and Response Chart is named the Adult Observation and Response Chart in WA, and the Rapid Detection and Response Observation Chart in SA). References of the materials used to compile the information have been supplied. The student is expected to have learned the material surrounding each skill as presented in the references. No single reference is complete on the subject.

RECOMMENDED READINGS

Arnold, P. (2015). Rising with accurate documentation to shine in the justice system: a nurse's experience. *ACORN: The Journal of Perioperative Nursing in Australia*, 28(2), pp. 16–19.

Austin, S. (2011). Stay out of court with proper documentation. *Nursing*. 41(4), pp. 24–9. doi: 10.1097/01.NURSE.0000395202.86451.d4

Gray, S., Ferris, L., White, L.E., Duncan, G. & Baumle, W. (2018). *Foundations of Nursing: Enrolled Nurses* (2nd ANZ ed.). Melbourne: Cengage.

Griffith, R. (2015). Understanding the Code: keeping accurate records. *British Journal of Community Nursing*, 20(10), pp. 511–14.

Joustra, C. & Moloney, A. (2019). *Clinical Placement Manual* (1st ed.). Melbourne: Cengage.

Royal Children's Hospital Melbourne. (2019). *Nursing Documentation Principles*. March. https://www.rch.org.au/rchcpg/hospital_clinical_guideline_index/nursing-documentation-principles/

ESSENTIAL SKILLS COMPETENCY

Documentation
Demonstrates the ability to accurately record information about a patient in a timely manner

Criteria for skill performance	Y	D
(Numbers indicate *Enrolled Nurse Standards for Practice*, 2016)	(Satisfactory)	(Requires development)
1. Identifies indications for documentation in the patient's chart/record (7.1, 7.2, 8.3, 8.4)		
2. Uses appropriate medical terminology and approved abbreviations (1.2, 1.3, 1.4, 2.2, 7.3, 7.4, 7.5, 9.4)		
3. Content is relevant and accurate (1.1, 1.2, 1.3, 2.2, 4.2, 7.1, 7.2, 7.3, 7.4, 7.5, 9.4)		
4. Adheres to legal requirements (1.1, 1.2, 1.3, 2.2, 7.1, 9.4)		
5. Demonstrates ability to effectively use facilities' standard forms (1.3, 4.2, 4.4, 7.1, 7.2, 7.3, 7.4, 7.5, 9.4)		
6. Performs hand hygiene (1.2, 1.4, 1.8, 3.9, 6.4, 9.4)		

Student:

Clinical facilitator: Date:

CHAPTER **7.2**

NURSING CARE PLANS

IDENTIFY INDICATIONS

Nurses provide nursing care 24 hours per day, every day. They are described by Duffield and colleagues (2007 in Levett-Jones, 2017) as the caregivers most directly involved with patients, being responsible for monitoring and assessing clinical changes in the patient and ensuring appropriate intervention and coordination of patient care. The depth and scope of their work makes nurses different to other allied health professionals. Nursing care plans are the core documents that help nurses to implement and maintain consistent 24-hour care for their patients across different shifts. When maintained correctly, care plans are an essential tool that communicates the care required for the patient each shift, along with a record of the previous nursing care implemented. Consistency of care is created because all nurses caring for a specific patient will follow the same plan, and not create a new plan for the patient each shift. Additionally as a legal document, they provide a record of all the nursing care a patient has received during their admission. The nursing care plan commences on patient admission and continues to be updated until the patient is discharged.

There are different types of nursing care plans, and they will vary in format between facilities or care environments (e.g. residential care, community-based care, acute care, surgical, rehabilitation). However, their underlying use as a tool to plan the patient's required care and maintain consistency of care remains unchanged. In residential care settings, the nursing care plan is a comprehensive document that is also linked to funding.

TYPES OF NURSING CARE PLANS

Nursing care plans come in different formats and types. Care plans can be in an electronic format or paper-based documents placed at the end of the patient's bed. Use of electronic care plans is increasing within the acute care sector, and is a well-established format in the community and residential care settings.

There are different types of care plans. The type of patient and care area will influence the type of care plan being used and the layout for recording the nursing care actions. Nurses within specialty areas (e.g. theatre or emergency department) may also use a nursing care plan that will appear quite different in layout and content to those used in a general ward area. Care plans can be standardised (preprinted with expected care actions, timeframes and expected patient outcomes) or individualised (created by the nurse). Standardised care plans do include the ability to edit and personalise the care needs for a patient. Individualised care plans are completed by the nurse for each patient. The final layout of a care plan is based on the type (i.e. standardised or individualised) and the work area. Examples of these include the following.

- Flow charts. These care plans look like a grid, with the care listed on the side of the page. The nursing care is written in by the nurse and is specific to each patient, although some routine care (e.g. daily checking of oxygen and suction) may be prefilled on the form. The nurse signs each care action for each shift.
- Clinical pathway/care pathways. A page or column is usually allocated to each day in the care pathway, with the standardised care listed for each day. These care plans also include care actions being implemented by other allied health team members. Often used in surgical areas where the expected pathway of care usually follows a routine pattern for the patients, they are preprinted with anticipated routine care changes and are used in specific environments.

While the nursing care plan can vary between facilities and care services in their preferences for layout, they all include required nursing interventions for patient care. Some will be more complex, including nursing diagnosis and expected outcomes for the patient care. Most care plans group care actions within common headings, such as observation, hygiene and grooming, elimination, mobility, nutrition and fluids, respiratory needs (or oxygenation) and comfort.

DEMONSTRATE PROBLEM-SOLVING ABILITIES

Problem solving and critical thinking are a core part of planning and implementing nursing care. The nurse is required to assess patient information (patient data) and decide on the relevant care for the patient, thus creating the nursing care plan. The care plan is also reviewed and updated when required as the nurse reviews the nursing care implemented and determines its effectiveness, or identifies changes in the patient's health status that then requires changes to any nursing care. The nurse uses underlying knowledge and nursing experience within this process to determine and plan the correct care for the patient. These critical thinking and problem-solving skills that are part of care planning are essential for nurses to not only assess a patient and identify their care needs within a stable care situation, but also within the more dynamic or unpredictable situations where changes occur within a patient's condition. Patients have complex health needs and come from diverse backgrounds. The nursing care they receive needs to be specific to their needs.

THE CARE PLANNING PROCESS

Nursing care planning is part of the nursing process, a simple problem-solving and decision-making process. The same type of decision-making and problem-solving cycle is used in many other industries and within daily life. The five steps of this process are as follows.

1. Collect patient information (data). This can be new admission information, or changes (deterioration or improvement) in the patient's condition.
2. Review this patient data and identify the patient problems and nursing needs.
3. Plan the patient nursing care requirements to resolve the identified patient problems, including patient risks and needs.
4. Implement the required care.
5. Review (evaluate) the effectiveness of the care given.

The process becomes a cycle because data are collected based on a patient's response to care implemented. The nursing care plan is then edited and updated for the patient's current health status and nursing problems or needs. Caution needs to be taken when identifying a patient problem (also described as a nursing diagnosis) to ensure you are not stating a medical diagnosis.

As described by Gray and colleagues (2018), the nursing process also requires critical thinking because each patient situation will be different, and each patient will respond differently to the implemented nursing care. Nurses also need to be aware that this problem-solving process often happens in action, during actual care implementation. The nurse may need to adjust how or what they are doing based on the patient's response or health status. They will need to later edit the nursing care plan, based on the decision making they used.

CONSULTATION WITHIN THE ALLIED HEALTH TEAM

Documentation within healthcare guides the caregiver and records the patient's status or response. This information is seen and acted upon by different health team members as part of their responsibilities for patient treatment and management. It will include treatment decisions that influence the nursing care implemented for the patient (e.g. a doctor has requested interventions or treatments that are implemented by the nurse).

USING THE NURSING CARE PLAN DURING THE SHIFT

Nursing care plans are written by nurses, stating all the nursing care required for a patient. The care plan is specific to the patient's cultural and social background as well as their specific health problems. It states the nursing interventions required and is the blueprint that directs the nurse's work for the shift. As described in Skill 3.1, the nurse commences a shift by reading the care plans for the allocated patients and identifies all the care required for each patient during that shift. The nurse then collates this information to create a work plan for that shift. Understanding and prioritising the nursing care stated in each patient's nursing care plan helps the nurse to manage and allocate time for the required patient care actions within that shift, and ensure all patients receive the correct nursing care. The care plan is then referred to during the shift as the nurse clarifies the care to be implemented, and the specific directions for how to implement care for that patient (e.g. the level of assistance required for the patient for hygiene and grooming).

Individual nursing care actions are signed by the nurse implementing that care after it has been completed. This is a legal record of the care being implemented and should never be pre-signed. The area and process for signing the care plan will depend on the type of care plan being used. If care actions are being initialled, then a specimen signature area is also usually required. Electronic signing of care completed will be linked to the user's personal ID and access.

The nursing care plan is used as a reference point for care provided when the nurse is completing the shift handover report and shift written report. It may not be necessary to state all of the care listed on the nursing care plan, but any changes to care or specific care actions should be stated within the report. At the completion of the shift, review each patient's nursing care plan to double-check all the required care has been implemented, and that the nursing care plan is up to date. Ensure all required areas have been initialled or signed. If required, edit the patient's stated nursing interventions.

EDITING AND REVISING A NURSING CARE PLAN

A nursing care plan should be revised each shift and updated as the patient's condition changes. Within some settings (e.g. residential care), the nursing care plan will remain unchanged for extended periods of time, while patients in acute care settings may experience changes each shift to the planned nursing interventions. Maintain the nursing process, and collect data about each patient based on:

- evaluating the nursing care implemented
- observations and assessments.

In consultation with the registered nurse (RN), this data is then reviewed, and required nursing interventions changed. The previous interventions are dated and ceased, with the new intervention dated for commencement. Changes may be recorded during the shift or while reviewing the care plan, and interventions implemented at the end of the shift.

Care plans in the residential care setting are linked to funding processes and have a more comprehensive process for editing the described care. The RN is usually responsible for this, and facility guidelines should be followed.

CASE STUDY

Maria Evangelista is a 47-year-old woman who has been admitted for a cholecystectomy. She has recently moved to Australia from Italy to live with her daughter, who married an Australian. She speaks limited English. Her nursing admission has been completed, but her nursing care plan has been handed over from the nurse on the a.m. shift. Maria is planned for surgery this afternoon at 5 p.m.

1. The RN has advised you to use a clinical pathway for Maria. What type of nursing care plan is this?

2. Are there any adjustments (i.e. variances) that need to be made to this care plan for Maria?

3. How will you use Maria's nursing care plan to organise your work during the shift?

4. When will you sign the care plan for the nursing care you have implemented?

Note: These notes are summaries of the most important points in the assessments/procedures, and are not exhaustive on the subject. The naming of documents or charts may differ from state to state, and facility to facility. In all possible situations the guidelines of the ACSQHC are used when describing national charts or documents (e.g. the ACSQHC Observation and Response Chart is named the Adult Observation and Response Chart in WA, and the Rapid Detection and Response Observation Chart in SA). References of the materials used to compile the information have been supplied. The student is expected to have learned the material surrounding each skill as presented in the references. No single reference is complete on the subject.

REFERENCES

Gray, S., Ferris, L., White, L.E., Duncan, G. & Baumle, W. (2018). *Foundations of Nursing: Enrolled Nurses* (2nd ANZ ed.). Melbourne: Cengage.

Levett-Jones, T. (2017). *Clinical Reasoning: Learning to Think Like a Nurse* (2nd ed.). Melbourne: Pearson.

RECOMMENDED READINGS

Ballantyne, H. (2016). Developing nursing care plans. *Nursing Standard*, 30(26), p. 51.

Berman, A., Frandsen, G., Snyder, S., Levett-Jones, T., Burston, A., Dwyer, T., Hales, M., Harvey, N., Moxham, L., Langtree, T., Reid-Searl, K., Rolf, F. & Stanley, D. (2020). *Kozier &*

Erb's Fundamentals of Nursing, Volumes 1–3. (5th ed.) Melbourne: Pearson.

Joustra, C. & Moloney, A. (2019). *Clinical Placement Manual* (1st ed.). Melbourne: Cengage.

ESSENTIAL SKILLS COMPETENCY

Nursing Care Plan
Demonstrates the ability to use a nursing care plan to deliver patient care

Criteria for skill performance	Y	D
(Numbers indicate *Enrolled Nurse Standards for Practice*, 2016)	(Satisfactory)	(Requires development)
1. Identifies indication (8.3, 8.4)		
2. Identifies different types of nursing care plans (4.2, 4.3)		
3. Demonstrates problem-solving abilities (4.1, 4.2, 8.3, 8.4, 9.4)		
4. Displays understanding of the care planning process and the nursing process (1.4, 4.2, 4.3)		
5. Uses the nursing care plan/s to plan workload for the shift, and prioritise patient care (1.2, 1.4, 1.5, 2.10, 3.2, 4.2, 4.3, 5.4, 6.5, 8.4)		
6. Refers to nursing care plan to determine specific care actions and the patient's specific care needs when implementing patient care (1.2, 4.2, 4.3, 5.4)		
7. Edits and revises the nursing care plan at the end of the shift (1.2, 4.2, 4.3, 5.4)		
8. Completes the required signing/documentation requirements for the nursing care plan, after care is implemented. (1.2, 1.3, 3.2, 5.3, 6.6, 7.1, 7.2, 7.3, 7.4, 7.5)		
9. Documents and reports relevant information (1.2, 1.3, 1.8, 3.2, 5.3, 6.6, 7.1, 7.2, 7.3, 7.4, 7.5)		
10. Demonstrates ability to link theory to practice (8.3, 8.4, 8.5, 9.4)		

Student:

Clinical facilitator:　　　　　　　　　　　　　　　　　Date:

CHAPTER **7.3**

CLINICAL HANDOVER – CHANGE OF SHIFT

IDENTIFY INDICATIONS

Clinical handover is the transfer of professional responsibility and accountability for the care of a patient, or patients, to another person or professional group (ACSQHC, 2019a). National standards for clinical handover have created standardised processes to increase patient safety and enable continuity of care. Handover includes a verbal report on the condition of the patient, and occurs at different times, such as change of shift within the care team, patient transfer to a specialty area for a test or procedure, transfer to a new ward or facility and transfer to or from community-based care. A handover communication also occurs when reporting the escalation of a deteriorating patient to another healthcare professional. Clinical handovers help to update knowledge about patients, enable teamwork, permit debriefing and create an opportunity to clarify patient information or point out the need for further action.

Clinical handover for the change of shift often occurs in two stages. The first stage will involve a team handover or huddle and the second a bedside handover.

IDENTIFY SAFETY CONSIDERATIONS

Knowledge of the patient you are handing over is imperative. You need to be aware of what information is important and what is superfluous. Missing or incorrect information can impact on a patient's safety. Patients can die as a result of healthcare personnel not passing on information relevant to their care or condition. Their recuperation can be impaired and their comfort compromised if the healthcare personnel who will be looking after them are unaware of important aspects of their condition, progress or deterioration. Information should also be communicated in a concise and timely manner.

As part of patient safety, clinical handover also requires a check of three approved patient identifiers (patient full name, date of birth and patient ID number/medical record number [MRN]) to ensure the correct patient is being discussed (ACSQHC, 2019a). To protect patient confidentiality, any handover notes should be shredded and disposed of on the ward at the end of your shift.

USE A TEMPLATE TO PREPARE OR LISTEN TO HANDOVER

When preparing to give a handover, it is important to take a few minutes to plan what you are going to say.

Using a template provides consistency, and using it every time a handover is given will assist those who are receiving the report to listen and understand the material more easily. Prior to listening to the handover at the start of your shift, prepare handover notes based on the area template and a time management grid with all of your patients for the day listed, and cells for the important information. This will assist you to organise the work for the day and give a guide to preparing your handover at the end of the shift. Many areas provide printed handover notes or use an electronic patient journey board that can also create printed notes.

A template guides the communication process. It also helps to ensure quality content and prioritising of information. State/territory health departments have policies about clinical handover procedures and include tools such as iSoBAR, ISBAR, SBAR and SHARED. Facilities may develop or adjust these tools to suit their work area (ACSQHC, 2019b), and facility handover policies should be followed. If the facility does not have a preferred procedure, resources can be accessed from the OSSIE Guide to Clinical Handover Improvement (ACSQHC, 2010) (search for it at http://www.safetyandquality.gov.au) or state/territory health department websites. TABLE 7.3.1 shows some of the different tools that can assist with a shift change handover.

TABLE 7.3.1 Examples of handover templates

ISOBAR (WA HEALTH)	ISBAR (NSW HEALTH)	SHARED	SBAR
Identify	Introduction	Situation	Situation
Situation	Situation	History	Background
Observations	Background	Assessment	Assessment
Background	Assessment	Risk	Recommendations
Agree to a plan	Recommendations	Expectations	
Read back		Documentation	

CONDUCT HANDOVER

An initial team meeting (huddle) will be held. Private information about the patient is being transmitted and this requires the handover to be conducted in surroundings that are conducive to confidentiality and free from distractions. This is a brief meeting that includes an overview of the patients and key issues including patients of concern and new admissions. Current risks within the ward or unit should also be identified. Sensitive issues are also communicated at this time, and not at the patient's bedside.

Bedside handover occurs at the patient's bedside. Although there may be concerns about information being presented during the handover, current clinical standards recommend greeting the patient and introducing oncoming staff, plus inclusion of the patient in the handover process (e.g. questions, clarifications, care requirements). Patient participation in the handover has shown an increase in patient satisfaction, trust in the staff and understanding of their health status. Patients who are confused, have decreased consciousness or expressed a preference not to participate may not be involved with the bedside handover. A 'three-point check' should also occur at this point to identify the correct patient (ACSQHC, 2019a). The verbal report should follow the facility's required template, with the most important patient information being delivered first. Information should be objective and concise and refrain from any personal comments. The patient, their charts and any drainage or infusion lines are also checked as part of the handover process. Information recommended for inclusion in bedside handover is:

- date and reason for admission
- relevant medical history
- investigations
- treatments and patient's response

- nursing care and patient's response
- safety concerns including alerts and allergies
- discharge planning
- recommendations for future care/awaiting follow-up response from other health team member.

USE CORRECT MEDICAL TERMINOLOGY

Appropriate use of medical terminology is an important consideration as it results in a report that is complete and concise. Using medical terminology when giving a handover demonstrates knowledge and acknowledges the professional status of the person/s to whom you are handing over. Remember, different facilities and wards may have medical terminology and abbreviations that are specific to that area. The receivers of the information must be allowed to question the deliverer of the handover for clarification and extension of information.

DOCUMENT AND REPORT RELEVANT INFORMATION

No formal documentation is currently maintained for clinical handover, but some facilities have handover notepads accessible for use in making notes for the delivery of handover. Facilities do maintain specific policies about patient confidentiality and the safe disposal of preprinted and individual nurses' handover notes. They must not leave the hospital, and are shredded at the end of the shift or placed in a specific waste location or bin for secure disposal. These notes should also be kept in your pocket during the shift and not left in unsecure locations in the ward.

CASE STUDY

Ron Blackwell is a 55-year-old man who has been admitted to the emergency department at 1820 hours via ambulance that evening. He had been cleaning out his house gutters that afternoon. While climbing down the ladder, his foot slipped off a rung (which was situated about halfway down) and he fell onto the lawn area below.

He is complaining of severe pain to his right shoulder area and right arm, with soreness to both knees, and appears to be in distress. He has a past medical history of mild hypertension, treated with an anti-hypertensive medication daily.

Currently Ron is on hourly full neurological observations (FNO), with the Observation Response Chart (ORC) last completed at 2000 hours. The medical officer has ordered X-rays and scans which have been organised.

His Glasgow Coma Scale (GCS) is 14/15, with limb deficits as he is unable/hesitant to move due to the pain/ soreness in his arms and legs. His temperature is 37.6°C, pulse is 108 bpm, blood pressure is 150/94 mmHG and his respiratory rate is 20.

His pain assessment score (at rest) is 6/10, and he is awaiting review from both the resident medical officer and the surgeon this evening for a decision regarding pain relief and possible theatre. He has a peripheral intravenous catheter (PIVC) in situ.

His wife has just arrived in the emergency department, and is understandably very upset and concerned.

1. You are the enrolled nurse [EN] caring for Ron. Using the information above, write the content for the end-of-shift handover by accessing and completing a handover format template relevant to your state/territory health department or facility.

Note: These notes are summaries of the most important points in the assessments/procedures, and are not exhaustive on the subject. The naming of documents or charts may differ from state to state, and facility to facility. In all possible situations the guidelines of the ACSQHC are used when describing national charts or documents (e.g. the ACSQHC Observation and Response Chart is named the Adult Observation and Response Chart in WA, and the Rapid Detection and Response Observation Chart in SA). References of the materials used to compile the information have been supplied. The student is expected to have learned the material surrounding each skill as presented in the references. No single reference is complete on the subject.

REFERENCES

Australian Commission on Safety and Quality in Health Care (ACSQHC). (2010). *OSSIE Guide to Clinical Handover Improvement*. https://www.safetyandquality.gov.au/our-work/communicating-safety/clinical-handover/ossie-guide-clinical-handover-improvement

Australian Commission on Safety and Quality in Health Care (ACSQHC). (2019a). *Communication at Clinical Handover.*

https://www.safetyandquality.gov.au/standards/nsqhs-standards/communicating-safety-standard/communication-clinical-handover

Australian Commission on Safety and Quality in Health Care (ACSQHC). (2019b). *Communicating for Safety*. https://www.safetyandquality.gov.au/our-work/communicating-safety

RECOMMENDED READINGS

Queensland Health. (2019). *Clinical Handover*. Queensland Government. https://www.health.qld.gov.au/cq/patients-and-visitors/your-rights-and-responsibilities/clinical-handover

SA Health. (2020). *Clinical Handover and Teamwork*. Government of South Australia. https://www.sahealth.sa.gov.au/wps/wcm/connect/public+content/sa+health+internet/clinical+resources/clinical+programs+and+practice+guidelines/

safety+and+wellbeing/communicating+for+safety/clinical+handover+and+teamwork

Victorian State Government. (2020). *Handing Over Care*. https://www2.health.vic.gov.au/hospitals-and-health-services/patient-care/older-people/resources/clinical-handover/handover

WA Health. (2020). *Clinical Handover*. Government of Western Australia. https://ww2.health.wa.gov.au/Articles/A_E/Clinical-handover

ESSENTIAL SKILLS COMPETENCY

Clinical Handover – Change of Shift

Demonstrates the ability to clearly and concisely report the condition of a patient or group of patients to another healthcare professional

Criteria for skill performance	Y	D
(Numbers indicate *Enrolled Nurse Standards for Practice*, 2016)	(Satisfactory)	(Requires development)
1. Identifies indications (1.2, 8.3, 8.4)		
2. Identifies safety considerations (1.3, 1.5, 1.8, 1.10, 3.2, 3.9, 4.2, 7.4, 8.4, 9.4)		
3. Uses a template (1.4, 7.1, 7.4, 8.3, 8.4, 9.4)		
4. Information is accurate, concise and complete (1.2, 4.2, 7.1, 7.2, 7.3, 7.4, 7.5, 9.4)		
5. Conducts verbal handover at initial team meeting (e.g. nursing huddle) and then at bedside (1.2, 1.4, 2.3, 2.4, 3.2, 4.2, 4.3, 7.1, 7.2, 7.3, 7.4, 7.5, 8.4, 9.4)		
6. Medical terminology is used appropriately (1.2, 1.3, 2.2, 7.3, 7.4, 7.5, 9.4)		
7. Delivery of information is timely (6.5, 6.6, 7.1, 7.2, 7.3, 7.4, 7.5)		
8. Demonstrates ability to link theory to practice (8.3, 8.4, 8.5, 9.4)		

Student:

Clinical facilitator: Date:

CHAPTER 7.4

ADMISSION, DISCHARGE AND PATIENT TRANSFER

IDENTIFY INDICATIONS

All patients admitted or transferred into a ward, care facility or community care service require the collection of patient information to establish nursing care to be implemented, and to contribute to overall patient assessment by the healthcare team. It involves the initial stages of the nursing process – patient assessment, analysing and interpreting the data and creation of a nursing care plan. The process and requirements for admission will vary according to the area or institution policy. The admission interview is an important time to establish a positive nurse–patient relationship with the use of effective communication skills. It also creates the opportunity to begin any necessary health teaching processes and commence discharge planning.

Patients will be admitted from a variety of situations, including the following.

- Emergency admissions, where preparation for admission to hospital has not occurred. The patient and their family will require support and education to help overcome a potentially higher level of anxiety or fear about hospitalisation.
- Elective (planned/booked) admissions where there has been time to prepare for and understand what will happen during hospitalisation. Admission processes for these patients may begin prior to admission in the preadmission or preoperative clinic.
- Transfer from another ward or hospital/institution – most admission data and care planning processes will

already be completed. Patients are also accustomed to the hospital experience, although they may be unsure about the new ward. This would also include patients transferring from being an inpatient to 'hospital in the home' or community-based care services.

All patients will usually have completed paperwork covering some basic personal data with hospital admission staff. They are then transferred to the ward where the nurse collects specific patient health history and a physical assessment, assesses the collected data and then compiles a nursing care plan. The doctor will also complete an admission assessment of the patient.

Discharge planning is a process of anticipating and planning ongoing patient care for when the patient leaves the ward or facility. The aim is to meet patient needs by creating a continuity of care. Ongoing care providers include family, community services, outpatient clinics and patient self-care actions. Discharge planning is a crucial part of all patients' ongoing health care and is an essential part of each patient's care plan. It commences on admission. The importance of good discharge planning is reinforced by the length of stay for patients in acute hospital settings becoming shorter. Patients are frequently discharged with the goal of continuing care in the community (e.g. wound management), a long-term care facility or Home and Community Care (HACC) service providers or disability service providers.

GATHER EQUIPMENT

Gather equipment needed prior to the admission interview. This will include thermometer, sphygmomanometer, stethoscope, pulse oximeter, hospital admission forms and nursing charts, patient ID band/s, patient information brochures, hospital contact names (e.g. social worker, patient advocates, pastoral care) and a valuables record book (if required). Patient scales and height measurement tools may be in a common area.

COMMUNICATE EFFECTIVELY WITH THE PATIENT

Effective communication during the admission process helps to allay a patient's fears and establish a positive nurse–patient relationship. It is vital that the admission interview is organised and not rushed. Establish a conversation or discussion with the patient to obtain relevant data, rather than just 'interrogating' them with a list of questions. Initiate an open and trusting communication process, and avoid looking as though you are just going through the motions when asking the patient questions. A quiet, calm, private environment is provided when admitting the patient.

Effective communication is also needed with discharge planning, as the patient can be anxious about going home and there is a need to understand their concerns and the environment into which they are being discharged. Trust is also needed for health teaching, and the nurse must recognise that patients may not always retain information because of their illness or personal stress levels.

DEMONSTRATE PROBLEM-SOLVING ABILITIES

Patients being admitted to acute care areas may require implementation of some immediate interventions or care actions (e.g. oxygen therapy or pain management). Review the medical notes for any required interventions, and complete a quick assessment of the patient prior to commencing the full admission interview and assessment.

While the admission form asks routine questions, and requires the collection of all data, adjust your questioning style and length of interview to the patient's immediate needs, health status (e.g. critically ill or fatigued patients) or mental state/cognitive ability. It may sometimes be necessary to complete the interview in two sessions, so prioritise the information collected first. Use time-management skills to plan and ensure enough time is available to complete the admission process.

Some patients may not be able to answer questions due to confusion/dementia or they may be unconscious. Use family input to assist you with the necessary information. Patients with speech problems may be assisted by using cue cards. If the patient speaks minimal English or English as a second language, an official interpreter will be needed to complete the full patient admission. For a planned admission, an interpreter can be booked through the telephone interpreter service, and all healthcare team members will need to use this service in the time allocated.

Discharge processes begin with the admission procedure. Establishing correct information about a patient's family, social background and home situation and environment are vital to discharge planning. If family is providing care in the home, their physical ability and emotional state should be noted to help determine their personal ability to continue the patient's care after discharge. Identify community services that may already be used by the patient and the patient's normal levels of mobility or independence. The telephone interpreter service may be required when explaining the discharge process for patients who speak minimal English or English as a second language.

Perform hand hygiene

Perform hand hygiene before touching the patient or the patient's surrounds and prior to any procedure involving patient contact to reduce the possibility of cross-contamination. Hand hygiene is the most effective method of infection control as it removes transient organisms from the hands of the nurse (see **Skill 1.1**).

CONDUCT ADMISSION PROCESS

Begin the admission process by introducing yourself and other staff to the patient, and welcoming them to the ward, facility or service. For inpatients, inform the patient about mealtimes, visiting hours, ward/hospital facilities (e.g. patient lounge, visitors' waiting area, hospital shop), smoking rules and use of mobile phones. Familiarise the patient with the patient call bell, bathroom, space for their belongings, TV, radio and adjusting the electronic bed, and introduce them to other patients in the ward (if a shared room). Also check if the patient has brought in any valuables, as generally they will have been informed not to bring any valuables into hospital. As per area policy, complete a minimum 'three-point identification check' to ensure you have the correct notes, identification band and patient. National standards for patient identification procedures require this to be completed as part of the admission process. Attach patient identification bands to wrist and ankle if not already completed.

The admission process includes a 'head-to-toe' assessment (see **Skill 2.1**). Complete a set of vital signs, height, weight and urinalysis that will act as baseline patient data, plus give input to their current physiological status. Assess the status of the patient's skin, noting any bruises, tattoos, piercings or impaired skin integrity. A skin assessment and pressure injury risk, using the organisation's preferred tools, should be completed within 6 to 8 hours of admission (see **Skill 3.13**). Note the patient's general physical appearance and their ability to communicate or understand English. A 'falls risk assessment' (see **Skill 2.2**) should be completed for all patients. Depending on the patient's age, health status and reason for admission, further assessments such as mini mental state assessment or Barthel Index for activities of daily living (ADL) may also need to be completed. Identify any allergies (including food, medication and general allergies), and attach an allergy alert band if required. Complete a nursing history that records data about the patient's social and cultural background, brief surgical and medical history and history of the current illness or reason for admission. Identify next of kin contact details and who to contact when the patient is ready for discharge.

List all the medications currently being taken by the patient – this should include prescription and non-prescription medication, plus any herbal remedies. Any medications brought in by the patient should be locked in their medication drawer or in the ward cupboard, and can be returned to them on discharge (some private hospitals may also use this medication during the patient's period of hospitalisation).

Patient health teaching occurs throughout the admission process, where relevant. Before leaving the patient, settle them and ensure they have a jug of water (if not fasting) and the call bell to hand; and answer any further questions they or their family may have. Provide any relevant information and brochures about the patient's illness or planned procedures.

All collected information is recorded on the patient admission forms and other specific assessment tools during the admission interview. At completion of the admission, check all data has been recorded and charted. It will then be necessary to create a nursing care plan and implement any relevant patient treatments or interventions that have been ordered by the doctor. Report any abnormalities or concerns identified during the admission. If the patient is booked for a procedure on the same day as admission, complete any required preprocedure/preoperative checklists, then assist the patient to change into a hospital gown.

CONDUCT DISCHARGE PLANNING

Discharge planning can occur at different points during the hospital admission, but should always begin during the primary admission process, or within preadmission clinics. Facility discharge planning checklists ensure all requirements are met and ensure that the patient has received all necessary appointments and equipment. Good discharge planning is based on patient needs and assessment, and should include input from the patient to determine their preferences in long-term care decisions. It will also include formal and informal health teaching sessions. Some facilities employ nurses dedicated to discharge planning and care who will accept primary responsibility for implementing all discharge care. Yet it still remains the primary responsibility of all nurses caring for the patient.

Discharge planning is an ongoing procedure that will be discussed in team meetings. It will include evaluating the need for outpatient procedures and other community support services. The patient's self-care ability and need for rehabilitation will also be evaluated. Nursing care plans will have a section for ongoing discharge documentation and records of health teaching sessions.

Assess the patient and family needs for health teaching – self-care actions, use of equipment, changes to lifestyle from illness (e.g. dietary changes or exercise regimens), understanding illness or changing personal behaviours that influence health and use of medications. If wound care is required, identify and teach the person who will be providing that care (unless it is a community nurse). Review all discharge advice at actual discharge time and answer any final questions. Ensure the patient and family understand potential complications following discharge and what to do if these occur. Give printouts of routine guidelines (e.g. postoperative advice, cast care).

Identify the discharge location (e.g. family home, other facility) and who will pick up the patient/how they will travel to their discharge location. Check the time the patient will be picked up and if there is a need to use a hospital 'transit lounge' while waiting to go home. It may be necessary to telephone relevant family members or others who are collecting the patient on discharge to confirm a discharge time. Check all referrals to community agencies, such as HACC, 'hospital in the home', physiotherapy and 'meals on wheels', have been completed and the patient has all follow-up outpatient or specialist appointment cards. Ensure they have all discharge medications (with instructions on when to take these), personal X-rays, laboratory request forms (if needed) and hospital-supplied equipment or appliances (shower chair, crutches, etc.). Give advice about where they can obtain any long-term supplies or equipment if they need to hire or purchase these. These details may be listed on a discharge summary; the patient is given a copy of this. The patient should also be given phone numbers for the ward and emergency contact numbers and instructions.

Help the patient collect and pack all their personal belongings. Assist the patient from the area with a wheelchair, if needed, and assist them to transfer into the vehicle.

CONDUCT PATIENT TRANSFER

Patient transfer may occur between hospital wards or facilities. If the patient is going to another ward in the same institution, an internal 'patient transfer' form is usually completed to communicate vital information to the nursing staff. Patient charts and care plans will also be transferred and used in the new ward area. Standards for continuity of patient care and clinical handover require a 'face-to-face' verbal handover in the patient's presence/bedside as part of the patient transfer (see **Skill 7.3**). Use any supplied hospital templates and procedure guidelines as part of this process, and introduce the patient to the new nursing staff.

Transfers between facilities will require the completion of transfer letters and other relevant documentation that communicate patient information and nursing care information. Use facility forms, envelopes and guidelines. Because charts will not be transferred between hospitals, it is important to include as much information as possible about care being implemented and nursing care goals. Also list medications the patient is prescribed and when these were last administered. This will help to avoid the patient missing doses or being given an extra dose of medication. Ensure other doctors' and health team transfer letters are with the patient. You should include all relevant names and contact details if the new facility requires further information. Check that all belongings, medications and personal X-rays go with the patient. Standards for continuity of patient care recommend a face-to-face verbal handover in the patient's presence when transferring patients between facilities, and to the community setting (ACSQHC, 2019). Refer to facility policies for completing this. The face-to-face handover may involve other health professionals (e.g. paramedics) responsible for the patient during the transfer to the new facility.

Patients may be anxious about being transferred, so ensure they receive an explanation about the transfer and answer any of their queries. Also notify family when the transfer occurs. Completing a verbal handover in the presence of the patient and their family can help to increase their understanding and involvement in their care (ACSQHC, 2019).

Perform hand hygiene

Maintain the 5 Moments for Hand Hygiene and perform hand hygiene after touching the patient and the patient's surrounds.

CLEAN, REPLACE OR DISPOSE OF EQUIPMENT

Clean, decontaminate, replace and dispose of equipment appropriately, as per facility policy.

DOCUMENT AND REPORT RELEVANT INFORMATION

All documentation, including admission forms and risk assessment tools, are usually completed during the admission process. Patient vital signs and other baseline data should be recorded on the observation and response chart. After the admission interview is completed, review and check all the data collected to assist in the care planning process. Assess the data collected and complete the patient's care plan in collaboration with the registered nurse (RN). Report any discrepancies in patient data and patient observations outside of normal range to the RN and other relevant healthcare personnel.

On patient discharge, ensure all required documents are completed (according to hospital policy) and signed, and that the patient has a copy of the discharge summary.

Similarly, when a patient is being transferred to either another ward area or facility, ensure that all required information and documentation are fully completed.

CASE STUDY

Admission

1. Access a nursing admission form from your facility. Using a family member or friend, complete an admission using this form.

Discharge

You are caring for Phillip Owens, aged 65. Phillip is to be discharged tomorrow, following a right hip replacement 7 days previously.

Phillip lives alone and has no family. He is retired and lives in state housing. He does not like to socialise and states he has 'no friends'. He lives in a unit on the third floor of a large complex (with a lift) and states he will manage fine at home. Prior to admission, Phillip did not require any services and was managing independently.

2. Outline the potential problems that Phillip may face on return to his unit.

3. What community services could be utilised to support Phillip?

Note: These notes are summaries of the most important points in the assessments/procedures, and are not exhaustive on the subject. The naming of documents or charts may differ from state to state, and facility to facility. In all possible situations the guidelines of the ACSQHC are used when describing national charts or documents (e.g. the ACSQHC Observation and Response Chart is named the Adult Observation and Response Chart in WA, and the Rapid Detection and Response Observation Chart in SA). References of the materials used to compile the information have been supplied. The student is expected to have learned the material surrounding each skill as presented in the references. No single reference is complete on the subject.

REFERENCES

Australian Commission on Safety and Quality in Health Care (ACSQHC). (2019). *Communicating for Safety Standard.* https://www.safetyandquality.gov.au/standards/nsqhs-standards/communicating-safety-standard

RECOMMENDED READINGS

Australian Nursing and Midwifery Federation (ANMF) (Victorian Branch). (2016). *ANMF (Vic Branch) policy: Admission and Discharge.* Melbourne: ANMF (Victorian Branch).

Gabriel, S., Gaddis, J., Mariga, N.N., Obanor, F., Okafor, O.T., Thornton, A. & Molasky, W. (2017). Use of a daily discharge goals checklist for timely discharge and patient satisfaction. *MEDSURG Nursing*, 26(4), pp. 236–41.

Joustra, C. & Moloney, A. (2019). *Clinical Placement Manual* (1st ed.). Melbourne: Cengage.

Tytler, B. (2016). Improving patient flow: Role of the orthopaedic discharge sister. *Emergency Nurse*, 23(10), p. 20.

ESSENTIAL SKILLS COMPETENCY

Admission, Discharge and Patient Transfer

Demonstrates the ability to effectively carry out admission, discharge and transfer procedures as per facility policy

Criteria for skill performance	Y	D
(Numbers indicate *Enrolled Nurse Standards for Practice*, 2016)	(Satisfactory)	(Requires development)
1. Identifies indication (8.3, 8.4)		
2. Gathers equipment and prepares environment (1.2, 6.4, 8.4, 9.4)		
3. Evidence of effective communication with the patient; establishes therapeutic relationship and gives patient a clear explanation of what to expect during and after hospitalisation; gives explanation of procedure; gains patient consent (2.1, 2.3, 2.4, 2.5, 6.3)		
4. Demonstrates problem-solving abilities (4.1, 4.2, 8.3, 8.4, 9.4)		
5. Performs hand hygiene (1.2, 1.4, 1.8, 3.9, 6.4, 9.4)		
Admission		
6. Orientates patient to ward area and routines (1.2, 1.4, 2.1, 2.2, 2.3, 2.4, 2.5, 2.6. 2.7, 3.2, 4.1, 4.2, 4.3, 4.4, 5.3, 6.4, 7.1, 7.2, 7.3, 7.5, 8.4, 9.4)		
7. Obtains a thorough nursing history (1.2, 1.4, 2.1, 2.2, 2.3, 2.4, 2.5, 2.6. 2.7, 3.2, 4.1, 4.2, 4.3, 4.4, 5.3, 6.4, 7.1, 7.2, 7.3, 7.5, 8.4, 9.4)		
8. Conducts assessment of the patient (including head-to-toe assessment) (1.2, 2.3, 2.4, 2.7, 3.2, 4.1, 4.2, 4.3, 4.4, 7.1, 7.2, 7.3, 8.4, 9.4)		
9. Completes patient nursing care plan and all other relevant admission forms. (1.2, 1.3, 1.8, 3.2, 5.3, 6.6, 7.1, 7.2, 7.3, 7.4, 7.5)		
10. Cleans, replaces and disposes of equipment appropriately (1.2, 1.4, 3.9, 6.5, 9.4)		
11. Performs hand hygiene (1.2, 1.4, 1.8, 3.9, 6.4, 9.4)		
12. Documents and reports relevant information (1.2, 1.3, 1.8, 3.2, 5.3, 6.6, 7.1, 7.2, 7.3, 7.4, 7.5)		
13. Demonstrates ability to link theory to practice (8.3, 8.4, 8.5, 9.4)		
Discharge		
14. Identifies discharge destination, makes contact with relevant person and ensures safe transport organised (1.2, 1.4, 2.1, 2.3, 2.4, 2.7, 3.2, 4.1, 4.2, 4.3, 4.4, 5.3, 6.4, 7.1, 7.2, 7.3, 7.5, 8.4, 9.4)		
15. Explains discharge process to patient and ensures patient has all required details on discharge (1.2, 1.4, 2.1, 2.3, 2.4, 2.7, 3.2, 4.1, 4.2, 4.3, 4.4, 5.3, 6.4, 7.1, 7.2, 7.3, 7.5, 8.4, 9.4)		
16. Liaises with relevant community services and support for post discharge care (1.2, 1.4, 2.1, 2.3, 2.4, 2.7, 3.2, 4.1, 4.2, 4.3, 4.4, 5.3, 6.4, 7.1, 7.2, 7.3, 7.5, 8.4, 9.4)		
17. Cleans, replaces and disposes of equipment appropriately (1.2, 1.4, 3.9, 6.5, 9.4)		
Patient transfer		
18. Identifies transfer destination, makes contact with relevant person and ensures safe transport organised (1.2, 1.4, 2.1, 2.3, 2.4, 2.7, 3.2, 4.1, 4.2, 4.3, 4.4, 5.3, 6.4, 7.1, 7.2, 7.3, 7.5, 8.4, 9.4)		
19. Informs patient and patient's family of transfer arrangements organised (1.2, 1.4, 2.1, 2.3, 2.4, 2.7, 3.2, 4.1, 4.2, 4.3, 4.4, 5.3, 6.4, 7.1, 7.2, 7.3, 7.5, 8.4, 9.4)		
20. Completes all required documentation for transfer (1.2, 1.3, 1.8, 3.2, 5.3, 6.6, 7.1, 7.2, 7.3, 7.4, 7.5)		
21. Completes verbal handover with paramedical staff or staff of new facility/ward (1.2, 1.4, 2.1, 2.3, 2.4, 2.7, 3.2, 4.1, 4.2, 4.3, 4.4, 5.3, 6.4, 7.1, 7.2, 7.3, 7.5, 8.4, 9.4)		
22. Performs hand hygiene (1.2, 1.4, 1.8, 3.9, 6.4, 9.4)		
23. Documents and reports relevant information (1.2, 1.3, 1.8, 3.2, 5.3, 6.6, 7.1, 7.2, 7.3, 7.4, 7.5)		
24. Demonstrates ability to link theory to practice (8.3, 8.4, 8.5, 9.4)		

Student:

Clinical facilitator: Date:

CHAPTER 7.5

HEALTH TEACHING

IDENTIFY INDICATIONS

Patient education is an integral part of the role of a nurse, with nurses teaching patients and their families in a variety of clinical and community settings. Within the Standards for Practice: Enrolled Nurses 2016, health teaching comes under the 'Provision of Care' domain which:

> encompasses all aspects of care from assessment to engaging in care, and includes health education and evaluation of outcomes.
>
> (NMBA, 2016, p. 3)

Early discharge from hospital, increasing complexity of healthcare options, financial constraints and increased home healthcare services have combined to make the teaching of skills and knowledge required to enhance health, independence and quality of life to patients imperative in quality health care. Patient education empowers patients to gain better control of their health. It is a nursing action that aids patients in becoming aware, making choices and moving towards a higher level of wellness. Informal teaching can be part of the daily routine and support other formal teaching sessions.

Patients have a right to receive understandable information about their health care so they can make informed decisions about treatment options and their lifestyle. Offering information relevant to the patient's health supports their efforts to assume responsibility for their own health and wellbeing. Health teaching can cover concepts of promoting health, preventing illness or injury, restoring health and adapting to current health status and altered function. Patients and caregivers need to understand the issues that can impact on a patient's health status: how to deal with their feelings, attitudes, interests and values that influence how they behave; make choices that influence health; and learning skills, such as giving oneself an injection or changing a dressing. Most patient teaching should include the patient's support person as well, so that there is reinforcement of the information/attitude/skill. Including family members in the teaching sessions may assist them to help the patient in their recovery and understand changes the patient is experiencing.

ASSESS THE PATIENT

A patient's willingness to learn, ability to learn and attitude towards learning are influenced by age, gender, level of maturity, level of fear and anxiety relating to their illness, intelligence, education, cultural and socioeconomic background, lifestyle, language and support. When assessing a patient and their educational needs, include an assessment of the patient's personal motivation, developmental and physical capabilities, culture, English skills, literacy skills, ability to take responsibility for their own learning, the learning environment and the applicability of the information to their situation. The nurse also needs to know the patient's level of existing knowledge and skills, so that previous knowledge can be used to build on. Do not assume a level of prior knowledge. During an assessment (e.g. basic physical assessment) explore the patient's knowledge of the issues in question (e.g. medications, pathophysiology).

Assessment of these factors allows the teaching to be tailored to the individual and helps to prioritise learning needs.

IDENTIFY BARRIERS TO LEARNING AND PLAN SESSION/S

Barriers to learning reduce the effectiveness of any teaching. Understanding these barriers is the first step in assisting the nurse to identify their role in helping the patient overcome barriers. It enables the nurse and the patient to clarify and develop strategies to individualise treatment guidelines, implement continuing education and improve communication skills, assisting the patient to achieve the desired behavioural change. Careful planning of the timing of the teaching session can reduce physiological barriers such as fatigue and pain. Other physiological problems such as hearing loss, poor vision, aphasia, organic brain syndrome, loss of muscle strength and coordination will require the nurse to use other strategies (e.g. enlarged visual aids, short sessions, simple concrete explanations, multiple repetitions, primary teaching of the significant other).

Psychological barriers to learning, such as fear, anxiety and perceived loss of control, can be addressed by first identifying the problem/s and then discussing important concerns of the patient and reducing these feelings so that learning can occur. Personalised, accurate, consistent and structured information that is paced to the individual will reduce the perceived threat of the new learning. Health promotion programs can be especially challenging because lifestyle behaviour change is difficult. Individuals may be gaining many positive outcomes and feelings from their current behaviour and feel very negative about making changes. A patient's motivation to learn and create change is greatest when they believe their need will be met through what they are learning.

Cultural factors may become barriers to learning because there are varying perceptions of illness, pain and health care in different cultures. The patient's locus of control, beliefs about religion, gender, ageing and ethnicity will affect beliefs about health maintenance and preventing and treating disease. The nurse must be aware that learning is often culturally based and take this into account when teaching. Because of the negative consequences of inadequate understanding, information must be transferred in a way the patient can comprehend. Providing healthcare information in the patient's language and the use of medical interpreting services assists in overcoming communication problems and improves the quality of care for patients who do not have English as their primary language.

Knowledge of the content is important. The nurse must be perceived by the patient as being competent, trustworthy and supportive. This results from thorough knowledge of self, the procedural, sensory and factual aspects of the subject, the ability to be considerate of the learner's fears and anxieties, and the flexibility to adapt the delivery of the material accordingly.

COMMUNICATE EFFECTIVELY WITH THE PATIENT

Good verbal and non-verbal communication skills are imperative. Establish a positive rapport with the patient, and communicate clearly and concisely. Introduce yourself, use the patient's preferred name, and explain what you will do and the timeframe. The level of knowledge to impart is also part of the content and is determined by the patient's ability and interest, and the amount of time available for the teaching. Correct teaching strategies and organisation of the teaching session is crucial to its success. Understanding the principles of adult learning is helpful when teaching adult patients.

- Adults learn best when there is a perceived need. The nurse must ensure the patient understands the underlying health issue (to be prevented) or illness (to be resolved), prior to teaching.
- The teaching of adults should build on their existing knowledge, after first having clarified what they already understand.
- Teaching should progress from simple to more complex topics.
- Adults learn best using active participation. Asking the patient to restate material discussed will encourage learning and permit clarification.
- Adults require opportunities to practise new skills (e.g. drawing up insulin).
- Adults need the behaviour reinforced (e.g. allow the patient to draw up and give their insulin each time it is due).

Similar principles can be followed when teaching children or adolescents, with specific attention given to the age or growth and development stage of the patient. Adjust teaching sessions to meet these abilities and their levels of understanding. Teaching aids for children can include games, toys, simple books, puppets, role play, 'apps' or electronic games, and visits to hospital areas. Parents also need to be involved with structured education sessions. (Further information regarding life span considerations in teaching are outlined by Gray and colleagues (2018, pp. 257–65).

GATHER EQUIPMENT

- *Audiovisual materials* must take into consideration the patient's learning ability, vocabulary, reading ability and concentration span. Audiovisual and online resources usually range from written instructions to online resources presenting information. The nurse should stay with the patient when they initially go over the audiovisual material to answer questions, direct attention and individualise standardised material. Use of valid online resources, such as apps or a health organisation website, are helpful because the patient can also access these later or when they are at home.

- *All equipment for teaching a skill* needs to be gathered and checked for completeness and working order before the teaching begins. Good organisation demonstrates accuracy and reliability. A well-lit room that is private, maintains confidentiality and is free of distractions makes learning easier.
- *Any teaching aid used* must be assessed for suitability for the learner. Determine the readability of the written material; for example, print size, complexity of words used, number of concepts/facts presented and if it is suitable for the patient.

Perform hand hygiene

Perform hand hygiene before touching the patient or the patient's surrounds and prior to any procedure involving patient contact to reduce the possibility of cross-contamination. Hand hygiene is the most effective method of infection control as it removes transient organisms from the hands of the nurse (see **Skill 1.1**).

EXPLAIN THE PURPOSE OF THE TEACHING SESSION

Explain the purpose of each teaching session. Link the new knowledge to previous knowledge. Explain the purpose of the new skill to increase the patient's interest and motivation. With the patient, set learning outcomes for each session since learning is more effective if it is directed towards specified and achievable outcomes. Individualisation of standardised material promotes consistency and accuracy.

DEMONSTRATE THE SKILL

Demonstrate the skill to be learned from beginning to end, with no interruptions. This allows the patient to see the skill in its entirety and performed in a seamless and flowing fashion. Demonstrate the skill again, breaking it into simple steps that are easily understood and can be explained. Giving small steps to the skill makes the skill easier to learn as it can be assimilated a small amount at a time. Explaining the rationale for each step increases the ease with which it can be recalled. Repeat the demonstration, with the patient directing your actions and giving explanations for each of the steps. This process helps the patient consolidate the progression of the skill without needing to use the motor movements of actually manipulating the equipment. The patient then handles each piece of equipment and is urged to ask questions, try parts of the procedure and practise the steps.

REQUEST A RETURN DEMONSTRATION

A return demonstration is done by the patient with the nurse coaching them through the steps. This gives the patient a chance to master the fine motor movements of the skill. A second return demonstration with the patient coaching themselves through the steps helps them to consolidate and integrate the skill and the rationale. These steps may require many repetitions before the patient masters the skill. Short practice sessions are more effective than one sustained practice period. Finally, the patient demonstrates how to deal with errors and unexpected situational variations (with the nurse coaching as needed). Written instructions, checklists, posters, pictures and audiovisual presentations are used in conjunction with these practical demonstrations.

ONGOING HEALTH TEACHING ACTIONS

These further health teaching actions are implemented over several teaching sessions and in collaboration with other health professionals. They may occur within the ward area or other specialty clinics.

Facilitate affective change

Affective change involves a patient's emotions and feelings, and is usually facilitated by group discussion and role-playing, with the patient as an active participant. One-to-one discussions offer support during change. Changing values and beliefs is not easy and requires time and effort, and a well-motivated patient.

Provide feedback

Feedback should be given throughout the teaching of the patient. Feedback needs to be positive and constructive to increase self-esteem and therefore the self-confidence of the patient. Any corrections should only follow positive feedback, so that self-confidence is preserved. Constructive feedback is more valuable if it clearly specifies what the error is, why the response was wrong and the actions for correcting it. Feedback needs to be timely; that is, occur at the time of the error to prevent the establishment of inaccurate mind-sets and (bad habits). Feedback must also be honest to preserve the therapeutic relationship and is essential in learning new skills. Patients should be encouraged to reflect on their progress as their skills develop and they achieve their goals.

Encourage the patient to perform the new skill

Encouragement to perform the new skill or display the new knowledge assists the patient to reinforce new learning and increases the likelihood of the knowledge being incorporated into their repertoire of skills.

Perform hand hygiene

Maintain the 5 Moments for Hand Hygiene and perform hand hygiene after touching the patient and the patient's surrounds

DOCUMENT AND REPORT RELEVANT INFORMATION

Documentation of the teaching provides for continuity of care and provides evidence that time was spent teaching the patient. What was taught, when it was taught, the resources used and whether the learning goals were met or not is documented in the patient's notes and the discharge planning record. Record any written material, apps or links provided to the patient. Referral to other healthcare personnel and recommendations for further teaching should be noted, both in writing and verbally, during clinical handover or team meetings to ensure that there is appropriate follow-up by staff.

CASE STUDY

Brett Jones is a 14-year-old school student on your medical ward in a large public hospital who has just been diagnosed with type 1 diabetes.

You are required to commence education sessions today to teach him how to perform blood glucose monitoring twice daily.

1. List the steps you would take to demonstrate performing a blood glucose assessment.

2. Identify a possible barrier you might anticipate Brett may have to this procedure. Brett has already said that he doesn't like needles.

The diabetes educator has organised for Brett to come to the diabetic clinic tomorrow afternoon.

3. What information will you document in relation to your health education session today with Brett?

4. Where will you document this information?

Note: These notes are summaries of the most important points in the assessments/procedures, and are not exhaustive on the subject. The naming of documents or charts may differ from state to state, and facility to facility. In all possible situations the guidelines of the ACSQHC are used when describing national charts or documents (e.g. the ACSQHC Observation and Response Chart is named the Adult Observation and Response Chart in WA, and the Rapid Detection and Response Observation Chart in SA). References of the materials used to compile the information have been supplied. The student is expected to have learned the material surrounding each skill as presented in the references. No single reference is complete on the subject.

REFERENCES

Gray, S., Ferris, L., White, L.E., Duncan, G. & Baumle, W. (2018). *Foundations of Nursing: Enrolled Nurses* (2nd ANZ ed.). Melbourne: Cengage.

Nursing and Midwifery Board of Australia (NMBA). (2016). *Standards for Practice: Enrolled Nurses*. Australia

Health Practitioner Regulation Agency, p. 3. http://www.nursingmidwiferyboard.gov.au/Codes-Guidelines-Statements/Professional-standards/enrolled-nurse-standards-for-practice.aspx

RECOMMENDED READINGS

Alberti, T.L. & Morris, N.J. (2017). Health literacy in the urgent care setting: What factors impact consumer comprehension of health information? *Journal of the American Association of Nurse Practitioners*, 29(5), pp. 242–7.

Joustra, C. & Moloney, A. (2019). *Clinical Placement Manual* (1st ed.). Melbourne: Cengage.

Kennard, D.K. (2016). Health literacy concepts in nursing education. *Nursing Education Perspectives*, 37(2), pp. 118–19.

ESSENTIAL SKILLS COMPETENCY

Health Teaching

Demonstrates the ability to effectively teach a skill to a patient

Criteria for skill performance	Y	D
(Numbers indicate *Enrolled Nurse Standards for Practice*, 2016)	(Satisfactory)	(Requires development)
1. Identifies indication (8.3, 8.4)		
2. Identifies potential patient barriers to learning and plans session/s (1.2, 4.4, 6.4, 8.4, 9.4)		
3. Performs hand hygiene (1.2, 1.4, 1.8, 3.9, 6.4, 9.4)		
4. Evidence of effective communication with the patient; gives explanation of procedure, gains patient consent (2.1, 2.3, 2.4, 2.5, 6.3)		
5. Assesses the patient (1.2, 2.1, 2.3, 2.4, 2.10, 4.1, 4.2, 7.1)		
6. Individualises standard material (2.1, 2.3, 2.4, 2.5, 2.6, 2.10, 6.3)		
7. Provides information at the patient's level (cognitive) (2.1, 2.3, 2.4, 2.6, 2.10, 6.3)		
8. Demonstrates the skill; has patient repeat the demonstration (if relevant) (2.1, 2.10, 6.3)		

9. For ongoing teaching sessions:
    a. facilitates affective learning (2.1, 2.5, 2.10, 6.3)
    b. gives feedback (6.3, 7.3, 7.5)
    c. encourages the patient to use the new skill/information (6.3, 7.3, 7.5)		

10. Performs hand hygiene (1.2, 1.4, 1.8, 3.9, 6.4, 9.4)		
11. Documents and reports relevant information (1.2, 1.3, 1.8, 3.2, 5.3, 6.6, 7.1, 7.2, 7.3, 7.4, 7.5)		
12. Demonstrates ability to link theory to practice (8.3, 8.4, 8.5, 9.4)		

Student:

Clinical facilitator: Date:

CHAPTER 7.6

NURSING INFORMATICS

IDENTIFY INDICATIONS

Nursing Informatics is the science and practice [that] integrates nursing, its information and knowledge, with information and communication technologies to promote the health of people, families and communities worldwide.

(American Medical Informatics Association [AMIA], 2018)

Information and communication technology is an increasing presence in health care and is part of routine daily practice in facilities or community organisations. Although there have been long-term concerns about managing issues such as patient confidentiality and legal requirements for reporting, the development of new technology is enabling safe documentation and reporting practices. Health informatics includes health information systems, e-health services, electronic health records, clinical decision support systems and telehealth. Telehealth and e-health services have become established providers of care.

Telehealth is an established system within the Australian healthcare system. Telehealth services deliver health services and transmit health information over long and short distances. Voice, images and information is transmitted among healthcare professionals and the care recipient. It is used to deliver care services to aged care facilities, medical services to Aboriginal and Torres Strait Islander peoples across Australia and staff training across the rural health services area. Patients are also using videoconferencing for a health assessment with the GP, specialist or area health services, rather than travelling large distances to a city area, or to minimise infection risks between patients

and healthcare providers. The Australian Government has also established digital and e-health records for patients that maintain a summary of their health information online. With the patient's permission, this information can then be accessed by healthcare providers. A nurse working within a GP practice or the emergency department will need to understand how to access and use this information as part of their daily work routine.

Within a healthcare facility, many departments will use clinical information systems so staff can gain quick access to information (e.g. pharmacy and laboratory results) about their patients. Nurses may also use these systems to order specific equipment, linen and other urgent supplies from a central source, as well as barcode systems linked to a database when administering medications as part of reducing patient identification errors. Patients may also use online systems to complete their daily meal preferences.

Software is available to assist with care planning, shift reporting and patient charting processes. Networked mobile devices are able to record patient data at the bedside that can then be immediately accessed from other data access points. Similarly, nurses working within community settings are able to access and record patient information using mobile data access and portable devices. As the largest area of the healthcare workforce, nurses are potentially one of the largest users of health information technology. Acceptance, computer literacy and ability are essential in being able to embrace and use the emerging and already existing technologies.

USING INFORMATION AND COMMUNICATION TECHNOLOGY IN THE WORKPLACE

Computer and information technology skills

Nurses should have established basic computer skills and an understanding of common information technology such as internet, intranet, instant messaging and email. When using workplace technology, ensure privacy of personal login ID, access codes and remote access links. Breach of facility privacy policies can potentially allow non-employees to access the information stored within the care provider's systems. Ensure you log off after accessing or inputting data to the network, and do not share passwords or access links with others. All employees should use their own access ID.

Positive attitude and acceptance of technology

Nurses need to develop a positive belief about the value of informatics and its increasing use in health care. Their acceptance will also enable them to give input to their facility to ensure the systems they are using are effective in helping improve their work and enhance patient care. If information or communication systems being used in a workplace are new or unfamiliar, then the nurse needs to ensure their personal participation in staff training.

Use of care planning and digital patient records

Care planning and digital patient records follow the same principles as any paper-based documentation. Follow facility guidelines for login and completing any documentation. Some nursing information systems use a menu to collect required data and develop individualised care plans, work lists, documenting of patient data, including vital signs, and documenting nursing care in the patient's progress notes.

My Health Record is a national database containing an online summary of an individual's health information that is accessible by authorised providers. Patients need to activate and provide consent for their data to be stored, and may require the nurse to explain this service.

Use of telehealth

When participating in care delivery using telehealth or e-health, the nurse will need to become comfortable communicating with doctors, patients and other allied health workers using videoconferencing or other online communication. Data may be transmitted separately using email and other online services. Equipment such as ECG machines, wearable biometric devices or other home-based medical equipment include software to transmit data to medical specialists and GPs. Alternatively, they can store data for retrieval at an appointment.

The actions of patient assessment and care, plus communication with the healthcare team still exist but are applied in a different format. These patient interactions may become virtual visits, where a sense of presence and caring still needs to be shared with the patient.

CASE STUDY

You are a new employee of a large tertiary hospital that uses computer-based care planning and patient digital records. As part of your orientation you are given a personal staff ID code in order to access patient and hospital information.

1. Why is it essential that you do not share your staff ID access and that you log out after entering relevant patient information?

2. What is the potential outcome of not following workplace procedures for keeping your login details and workplace systems secure?

3. What is your responsibility if you are unsure about how to use the facility software?

4. On an afternoon shift you are required to access a patient file (Cedric Jacobs) online, and update information online related to the following changes.
   - Diet/fluids: patient can commence clear fluids this evening
   - Mobility: To sit out of bed twice daily; commence ambulation after assessment by physiotherapist.

5. When on placement in a tertiary hospital, review the electronic patient record system available and identify how changes such as these could be successfully updated.

Note: These notes are summaries of the most important points in the assessments/procedures, and are not exhaustive on the subject. The naming of documents or charts may differ from state to state, and facility to facility. In all possible situations the guidelines of the ACSQHC are used when describing national charts or documents (e.g. the ACSQHC Observation and Response Chart is named the Adult Observation and Response Chart in WA, and the Rapid Detection and Response Observation Chart in SA). References of the materials used to compile the information have been supplied. The student is expected to have learned the material surrounding each skill as presented in the references. No single reference is complete on the subject.

CRITICAL THINKING

Growth and Development

1. Access the intranet at your work placement and review the relevant documents relating to Skills 7.2 to 7.4.
   How do you think these forms/paperwork may vary within the following types of facilities:
   - public hospital
   - private hospital
   - aged care facility
   - community nursing?

2. Consider how you would adapt a patient teaching session for a child aged 5 compared to an adult aged 30.

3. Explain why nursing care plans should be individualised to each patient's personal needs and their stage of growth and development.

REFERENCES

American Medical Informatics Association (AMIA). (2018). *Nursing Informatics*. https://www.amia.org/programs/working-groups/nursing-informatics

RECOMMENDED READINGS

ACN, HISA and NIA. (2017). *Nursing Informatics Position Statement*. https://www.acn.edu.au/wp-content/uploads/joint-position-statement-nursing-informatics-hisa-nia.pdf

DeLaune, S., Ladner, P.K., McTier, L., Tollefson, J. & Lawrence, J. (2016) *Fundamentals of Nursing* (Australian and New Zealand rev. ed.). Melbourne: Cengage.

Department of Health. (2015). *Telehealth*. Australian Government. http://www.health.gov.au/internet/main/publishing.nsf/content/e-health-telehealth

Lee, A. (2014). The role of informatics in nursing. *Nursing Made Incredibly Easy*. 12(4), p. 55.

WA Country Health Service. (2019). *WA Country Health Service Digital Innovation Strategy 2019–2022*. Government of Western Australia. http://www.wacountry.health.wa.gov.au/fileadmin/sections/publications/Publications_by_topic_type/Service_Strategies/ED-CO-18-84303__eDoc_-_CO_-_2019-05-13_Digital_Innovation_Strategy_Final_Version_13_May_2019.pdf

ESSENTIAL SKILLS COMPETENCY

Nursing Informatics
Demonstrates the ability to use workplace information technology

Criteria for skill performance	Y	D
(Numbers indicate *Enrolled Nurse Standards for Practice*, 2016)	(Satisfactory)	(Requires development)
1. Identifies indication (8.3, 8.4)		
2. Able to demonstrate basic computer and information technology skills, as per facility online program (1.1, 1.2, 2.2, 4.2, 4.4, 6.4, 10.3)		
3. Displays positive attitude and acceptance of technology (4.4, 6.4, 10.3)		
4. Uses care planning and digital patient records (1.2, 1.4, 1.5, 4.4, 6.4, 7.1, 7.2, 7.3, 8.4)		
5. Uses telehealth or biometric equipment (1.2, 4.1, 4.2, 4.3, 4.4, 6.4, 7.3, 7.4)		
6. Demonstrates ability to link theory to practice (8.3, 8.4, 8.5, 9.4)		

Student:

Clinical facilitator: Date:

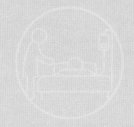

PART 8

SPECIFIC NURSING CARE

Note: These notes are summaries of the most important points in the assessments/procedures and are not exhaustive on the subject. References of the materials used to compile the information have been supplied. The student is expected to have learnt the material surrounding each skill as presented in the references. No single reference is complete on each subject.

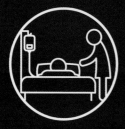

CHAPTER 8.1

OXYGEN THERAPY (INCLUDES PEAK FLOW METER)

IDENTIFY INDICATIONS

Oxygen therapy is the provision of supplemental oxygen to patients. It is an administered substance and principles for ordering oxygen are the same as medication administration guidelines. The doctor orders oxygen therapy: the amount, the concentration, delivery method and the desired oxygen saturation levels. As per the Thoracic Society of Australia and New Zealand Clinical Practice Guidelines 'An oxygen prescription should be documented in the patient records and medication chart' (Thoracic Society of Australia and New Zealand [TSANZ], 2015, pp. 3, 6). Oxygen can be given on a nurse's initiative in emergency situations, but a doctor's order must then be obtained. The eight 'rights' of medication administration apply to oxygen administration.

TSANZ (2015) identifies many concepts, concerns and recommendations regarding the use of oxygen therapy in patients. Oxygen should be considered and administered for specific indications, with a documented target oxygen saturation range, and with regular monitoring of the patient's response to the treatment. This monitoring involves the use of pulse oximetry (SpO_2), or if more accurate results/estimates are required, arterial blood gas (ABG) measurement.

Prior to any oxygen administration, the patient should have had a respiratory assessment. This includes observation/determination of:

- respiratory rate, abnormal breath rhythm and depth
- oxygen saturation levels
- patient's perception of respiratory effort, their ability to complete activities of daily living and their ability to speak in sentences
- abnormal vital signs (e.g. tachycardia, fever)
- breathing patterns and chest movements, such as cough, accessory muscle use, nasal flaring or mouth breathing

- chest wall configuration; for example, kyphosis, barrel chest
- air entry, adventitious lung sounds or sputum production
- diagnosis of chronic obstructive pulmonary disease (COPD) (see below)
- clinical signs of hypoxaemia – the early signs are tachycardia and tachypnoea, anxiety, agitation and restlessness, dyspnoea, pallor or cyanosis (especially buccal mucosa and lips); a later and more severe sign of hypoxaemia is confusion
- clinical signs of hypercapnia (restlessness, headache, hypertension, lethargy and tremor) or oxygen toxicity (tracheal irritation and cough, dyspnoea, decreased pulmonary ventilation)
- diagnostic and laboratory studies (haemoglobin, haematocrit, complete blood count, arterial blood gases, pulmonary function studies).

COPD is a group of pulmonary diseases (e.g. emphysema or chronic bronchitis) that cause the patient to have chronic hypoxaemia and hypercapnia. In patients without COPD, the usual stimulus to breathe is hypercapnia (a PCO_2 level of 40 to 45 mmHg). People with COPD may become desensitised to high CO_2 over time and do not respond to the hypercapnia stimulus, but only to hypoxaemia (low oxygen levels). Therefore, the patient with COPD needs to remain slightly hypoxaemic in order to have a stimulus to continue breathing.

According to the oxygen guidelines, in COPD and other conditions associated with chronic respiratory failure, oxygen should be administered if the SpO_2 is less than 88%, and titrated to a target SpO_2 range of 88% to 92% (TSANZ, 2015). In other acute medical conditions, oxygen should be administered if the SpO_2 is less than 92%, and titrated to a target SpO_2 range of 92% to 96% (TSANZ, 2015).

GATHER AND PREPARE EQUIPMENT

This is a time-management strategy as well as a confidence-increasing strategy. The nurse will be able to mentally rehearse the procedure as equipment is gathered.

The patient will feel more confidence in the nurse (thereby decreasing anxiety and reducing distress) if there are no interruptions in the procedure to return to the storage room for forgotten equipment.

- *Oxygen order or treatment chart.*
- *Oxygen sources* are wall outlets in hospitals, and various sizes of cylinders are available for portable oxygen therapy. Wall outlets are supplied from large central tanks and the oxygen is delivered under low pressure. The flow meter is set to 'off' to prevent loss of oxygen.

    Cylinders come in a variety of sizes for hospital and home use. The oxygen is under high pressure in the tanks and requires a pressure regulator to be used when administering oxygen therapy for a safe and desirable rate. The flow meter will be attached to the pressure regulator. Cylinders must be checked for the remaining level of oxygen before, during and after use.
- *The flow meter* measures and regulates the oxygen output from either the wall outlet or the cylinder in L/min. There are two types of flow meters: the cylindrical tube and a round gauge. Both are calibrated in L/min. The flow meter should be adjusted to the ordered concentration of L/min by turning the knob before the delivery device is placed on the patient.
- A *humidifier* may be used in certain circumstances/medical conditions (e.g. a tracheostomy), or oxygen delivered at above 6 L/per min via a face mask for more than 24 hours (WA Country Health Service, 2019) and in certain areas of the hospital, such as the emergency department, high dependency units or intensive care units (ICU). Generally, they are not utilised in ward areas.
- A *pulse oximeter* is used to monitor the effect of oxygen administration in order to maximise the benefit to the patient, and should always be available in all clinical situations where oxygen is used (TSANZ, 2015). Oxygen saturation levels should be performed at the same frequency as all other observations.
- *Oxygen tubing* is specifically designed for use with oxygen equipment. Each end is reinforced with a thicker 'nipple', which is pushed onto the adaptors on the flow meter or the delivery device. Oxygen tubing is disposable.
- *Oxygen delivery systems.* Oxygen is delivered via small-bore tubing and the inhalation of the oxygen percentage is dependent on the patient's respiratory rate, oxygen saturation, tidal volume and the flow rate of the oxygen. This is considered a low-flow system.

Standard nasal cannula (prongs)

The standard nasal cannula (prongs) is generally considered a low-flow delivery system consisting of a plastic tube that extends across the face, with short (0.6 to 1.5 cm) projections curving into the nostrils (see FIGURE 8.1.1). For most patients, it is the preferred method of oxygen delivery, with the flow rate varied to achieve the target oxygen saturation (TSANZ, 2015). It delivers oxygen at 1–4 L/min depending on the patient's breathing patterns (Dougherty & Lister, 2015; TSANZ, 2015). It is inexpensive, comfortable, well tolerated and allows the patient to eat, drink and talk. Also, there is no risk of rebreathing of carbon dioxide (TSANZ, 2015). It is secured by either an elastic strap or an extension of the plastic face tube that fits around the patient's head or around the patient's ears and under their chin.

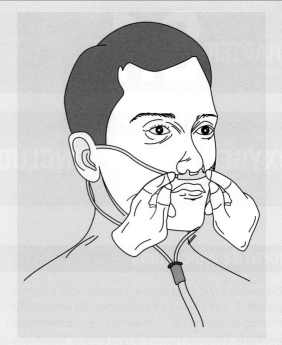

FIGURE 8.1.1 Nasal cannula

Face masks

Face masks are essentially similar to each other. They are clear or green plastic with a nose clip to mould them for a snug fit and an elastic band that is adjustable to fit the patient's head for a secure fit. Face masks come in a variety of sizes, so one of a suitable size must be chosen for each individual patient.

- A *simple face mask* covers the patient's nose and mouth (see FIGURE 8.1.2). These are low-flow masks and deliver oxygen at flow rates of 5 to 15 L/min, which creates concentrations between 40% and 60% (Dougherty & Lister, 2015). According to TSANZ (2015, p. 9), a flow rate of < 5 L/min should be avoided due to the potential risk of carbon dioxide rebreathing.

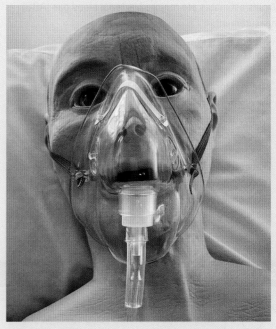

FIGURE 8.1.2 Simple face mask

- *A Venturi mask* can deliver specified percentage concentrations of oxygen at flow rates of 4 to 12 L/min, depending on the prescribed percentage of oxygen (see FIGURE 8.1.3). Adaptors are attached to regulate the intake of room air with various flow rates of oxygen. This is suitable for patients with known concentration requirements; for example, COPD.

Face masks have similar disadvantages: they may irritate the patient's skin; are hot and confining; require a tight seal which is both uncomfortable and claustrophobic; and cannot be used while eating or drinking, during personal hygiene or while talking. For these reasons, face masks are not suitable for long-term use.

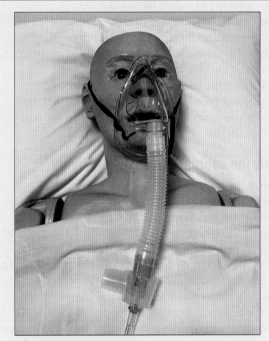

FIGURE 8.1.3 Venturi mask

Note: A Venturi-type mask permits the administration of an exact amount of O_2.

IMPLEMENT OXYGEN THERAPY

Perform hand hygiene
Perform hand hygiene before touching the patient or the patient's surrounds and prior to any procedure involving patient contact to reduce the possibility of cross-contamination. Hand hygiene is the most effective method of infection control as it removes transient organisms from the hands of the nurse (see **Skill 1.1**).

Give a clear explanation of the procedure and establish therapeutic communication
Introduce yourself, and check you have the correct patient. Discuss the procedure and gain the patient's consent. Giving a clear explanation is required to gain legal consent and to address policy requirements. It will also assist the patient to cooperate with the procedure, allay anxiety and assist in establishing a therapeutic relationship. Explanation also fosters trust, and enables the building of a working therapeutic relationship.

Patients who are hypoxaemic are often restless and agitated, lack judgement and motor coordination, and are highly anxious. Their nares may flare, they may use accessory muscles for breathing, their pulse and respiratory rates rise and they may become cyanotic. Patients often associate difficulty breathing with the possibility of death, which exacerbates the anxiety. Assisting the patient to assume an upright, position will help reduce breathlessness and, thus, anxiety. Gentle, confident

and relaxed movements, calm tone of voice while talking to the patient and use of closed questions requiring a brief yes/no answer will assist the patient to relax and become more cooperative. Breathing with the patient and slowing your own rate down is sometimes effective, as is teaching breathing exercises such as pursed-lip breathing and relaxation techniques.

Demonstrate problem-solving abilities
Positioning can assist the patient to breathe more easily. Positioning depends on the patient's condition and level of consciousness. An upright position will assist the patient to breathe more easily by moving the abdominal contents away from the diaphragm. Patients must be conscious and alert to maintain this position. Support is often needed. The orthopnoeic position (sitting upright with arms bent and elbows supported on an over-bed table, or arms braced against the knees when sitting out of bed) is also effective if the patient is able to maintain it. This position lifts the shoulder girdle, allowing for greater lung expansion. Some patients are more comfortable sitting out in a chair. The recovery position is necessary if the patient is unconscious to prevent the tongue from obstructing the airway.

Attend to safety precautions
Safety precautions are necessary because oxygen facilitates explosive combustion. The recommended safety precautions include:
- teaching the patient and visitors about the hazards of oxygen

- no smoking or naked flames/candles
- using only appropriately earthed, hospital-inspected and tagged electrical equipment (e.g. shavers, hairdryers) to prevent the occurrence of short circuits/sparks
- avoiding the use of volatile or inflammable materials such as oils, grease, alcohol, ether, nail polish remover, and so on near oxygen use (Gray et al., 2019).

Apply the appropriate oxygen delivery device

Refer to the oxygen therapy order to determine the correct mask and flow rate. Attach the mask and oxygen tubing together, and then attach the free end of the oxygen tubing to the wall outlet. Adjust the flow meter for the correct rate by reading the floating ball against the marked level on the flow meter, according to the manufacturer's guidelines. Ensure that the system is working correctly.

- *Nasal cannula (prongs)*. These are positioned so they curve towards the nares and oxygen is directed upward into the nose. The plastic tubing is fitted over the patient's ears and under the chin, and the toggle is tightened until the tubing is comfortably snug. Gauze squares may be used as padding over the ears if the tubing is irritating. On some prongs, an elastic strap is fitted over the head and tightened to keep the prongs snug but not tight on the face. The patient needs to be reassured that normal breathing patterns are effective even for mouth breathers, since oxygen is heavier than air. It tends to flow down the trachea along with air breathed in through the mouth. Provide nasal care for the nares using water-based products every 4 hours.
- *Simple face mask*. With the mask placed over the nose and mouth, the oxygen output is set to the required flow rate and the nose clip and elastic band are adjusted to ensure a snug fit, so oxygen does not escape from beneath the mask.
- *Venturi mask*. Select the adaptor (on some models set the dial) to give the ordered concentration of oxygen. Connect the adaptor to the wide corrugated tubing of the mask, and attach the oxygen tubing to the narrow end of the adaptor. Apply the mask as above.

All patients should be instructed to leave the delivery device in place at all times so the flow of oxygen is unimpeded. They should be instructed to ask for assistance if they feel dyspnoeic and to not adjust the flow rate since it has been set at the concentration ordered by their doctor. The oxygen tubing for patients who are ambulatory needs to be long enough so that they can move about the room without disconnecting their oxygen. For trips beyond the reach of the tubing, a portable cylinder must be attached.

Monitor the patient during therapy

Ensure the patient is comfortable with the oxygen delivery device since some find initial use of a mask or cannula uncomfortable. Monitor the patient's oxygenation status – oxygen saturation, pulse, respiration, colour, anxiety levels – during this initial time at least every 15 to 30 minutes, extending the timeframe depending on the patient's condition. With nasal prongs, the prongs and nares should be inspected for mucus encrustations. These should be cleaned off with water-dampened cotton applicators and a water-soluble lubricant applied. Check the placement of the prongs frequently because they are easily displaced. With all face masks, the facial skin and ears require attention to prevent pressure injury and deterioration because of the constant irritation and pressure from the plastic. The mask may also require cleaning with a disposable wipe to remove perspiration or other nasal secretions. The skin should be cleaned, dried and inspected at least every 4 hours. Provide regular mouth care and oral fluids to prevent drying of the mouth and lips.

Once the patient is stable, their ability to tolerate reduction and cessation of O_2 therapy must be assessed regularly. The oxygen dose is gradually reduced, as per medical orders, and the patient is 'trialled' on room air. Remain with the patient during this trial and assess their respiratory status. A pulse oximeter will be used to monitor the saturation levels.

Inspect equipment regularly

Inspect equipment regularly to ensure the integrity of the system and compliance with the ordered concentration of oxygen. The flow meter is checked to see if adjustments are needed, tubing is checked to ensure it is completely connected and not kinked and masks/prongs are checked to ensure proper working position or order. With some Venturi masks, the large-bore tubing needs to be checked for water accumulation and emptied frequently to prevent bacterial colonisation. Mask and tubing are changed as per the facility's protocol.

Peak flow meters

Assess the patient's respiratory status using a peak flow meter. *Peak flow meters* are a simple device used to measure the highest forced expiratory volume and are an indicator of respiratory status. Peak flow readings are often taken before and after nebulisation and preferably recorded on a standardised peak flow chart. When peak flow is monitored regularly, the standardised peak flow chart allows the doctor and the patient to measure how much and when the airways are changing. It is recommended to use the same peak flow meter every time (National Asthma Council of Australia, 2017). Ensure the indicator is at the zero mark. The patient takes a deep breath and then places their mouth over the mouthpiece. Ask the patient to blow out through the meter as hard as possible. Observe the reading achieved and re-set the indicator to zero. This process is repeated three times and the highest reading is taken.

Perform hand hygiene

Maintain the 5 Moments for Hand Hygiene and perform hand hygiene after touching the patient and the patient's surrounds.

CLEAN, REPLACE OR DISPOSE OF EQUIPMENT

Oxygen masks are single-use equipment and are disposed of in the general waste after use. If the mask is being used for an extended time (i.e. more than 2 to 3 days), it should be replaced with a new one, although many patients in the community may regularly clean and recycle their mask.

DOCUMENT AND REPORT RELEVANT INFORMATION

On initiation of oxygen therapy, the time, date, assessment data, oxygen concentration and/or flow rate, delivery method, patient's response and any adverse effects need to be recorded. Ongoing documentation (as per organisation policy or doctor's orders) is required. Oxygen therapy should be recorded on an oxygen therapy chart or medication chart, as well as the nursing care plan. It is also recorded on the observation and response chart and included as part of the calculation of the Adult Deterioration Detection System (ADD) score.

CASE STUDY

You are an enrolled nurse caring for the following patients in an acute medical ward. For each patient scenario listed below state:
- the correct type of oxygen delivery device
- the correct oxygen flow rate
- the required documentation to be completed.
1. Paul Evans is a 34-year-old man admitted with acute asthma. The doctor has ordered oxygen at 6 L/min.
2. Matilda Jeeves is aged 63 and has COPD. She is continuing her long-term oxygen at 2 L/min.

3. Jim Bowen is aged 72 and has been admitted with severe respiratory distress and hypoxia. He has a medical history of COPD.
   a. He initially requires oxygen at 28%.
   b. Based on improved blood gas results the doctor adjusts the oxygen order to 24% oxygen.
4. Identify special precautions/safety precautions that must be considered when oxygen is in use in the hospital ward area.

Note: These notes are summaries of the most important points in the assessments/procedures, and are not exhaustive on the subject. The naming of documents or charts may differ from state to state, and facility to facility. In all possible situations the guidelines of the ACSQHC are used when describing national charts or documents (e.g. the ACSQHC Observation and Response Chart is named the Adult Observation and Response Chart in WA, and the Rapid Detection and Response Observation Chart in SA). References of the materials used to compile the information have been supplied. The student is expected to have learned the material surrounding each skill as presented in the references. No single reference is complete on the subject.

CRITICAL THINKING/LIFESPAN

Thinking of the clinical skills discussed in this skill, and the stages of growth and development, what are some of the key components you would need to consider in the following scenarios?
1. Jade is 2 years old and requires continuous oxygen therapy via a mask. She continually tries to remove the mask. How will you manage this situation?
2. You are required to shower Simon, aged 68 years, who will 'de-saturate' unless he is on continuous oxygen as charted. How will you manage this situation and ensure he is showered safely?

REFERENCES

Dougherty, L. & Lister, S. (eds). (2015). *The Royal Marsden Hospital Manual of Clinical Nursing Procedures* (9th ed.). Oxford: Wiley-Blackwell.

Gray, S., Ferris, L., White, L.E., Duncan, G. & Baumle, W. (2018). *Foundations of Nursing: Enrolled Nurses* (2nd ANZ ed.). Melbourne: Cengage.

National Asthma Council of Australia. (2017). *Peak Flow Chart*. https://www.nationalasthma.org.au/living-with-asthma/resources/health-professionals/charts/peak-flow-chart

Thoracic Society of Australia and New Zealand (TSANZ). (2015). *Oxygen Guidelines for Acute Oxygen use in Adults*. pp. 3, 6.

https://www.thoracic.org.au/journal-publishing/command/download_file/id/34/filename/TSANZ-AcuteOxygen-Guidelines-2016-web.pdf

WA Country Health Service. (2019). *Oxygen Therapy and Respiratory Devices – Adults Clinical Practice Standard*. Government of Western Australia. http://www.wacountry.health.wa.gov.au/fileadmin/sections/policies/Managed/Oxygen_Therapy_and_Respiratory_Devices_Adults_Clinical_Practice_Standard_TS4KSNFPVEZQ_210_6735.pdf

RECOMMENDED READINGS

Australian Commission on Safety and Quality in Health Care (ACSQHC). (2017). *Observation and Response Charts*. https://www.safetyandquality.gov.au/our-work/recognising-and-responding-to-clinical-deterioration/observation-and-response-charts/

Australian Commission on Safety and Quality in Health Care (ACSQHC). (2019). *Communicating for Safety Standard*. https://www.safetyandquality.gov.au/standards/nsqhs-standards/communicating-safety-standard

ESSENTIAL SKILLS COMPETENCY

Oxygen Therapy (Including Use of Peak Flow Meter)
Demonstrates the ability to effectively and safely provide oxygen and related therapy

Criteria for skill performance	Y	D
(Numbers indicate *Enrolled Nurse Standards for Practice*, 2016)	(Satisfactory)	(Requires development)
1. Identifies indication (8.3, 8.4)		
2. Gathers and prepares equipment (1.2, 1.6, 4.4, 6.4, 8.4, 9.4): ■ oxygen source (wall outlet, cylinder) ■ flow meter ■ oxygen delivery device (nasal cannula, specified mask) ■ oxygen order/medication chart ■ tubing appropriate to device to be used ■ pulse oximeter ■ humidifier if required		
3. Performs hand hygiene (1.2, 1.4, 1.8, 3.9, 6.4, 9.4)		
4. Evidence of effective communication with the patient; e.g. gives patient a clear explanation of procedure, gains patient consent (2.1, 2.3, 2.4, 2.5, 6.3)		
5. Demonstrates problem-solving abilities; e.g. positions patient in upright/semi-upright position (4.1, 4.2, 8.3, 8.4, 9.4)		
6. Attends to safety precautions (1.2, 1.4, 3.2)		
7. Applies the appropriate oxygen delivery device and adjusts the oxygen flow rate correctly (1.2, 1.4, 1.8, 3.2, 3.9, 4.4, 6.4, 8.4, 9.4)		
8. Monitors the patient at regular intervals (1.2, 1.4, 1.8, 3.2, 3.9, 4.1, 4.2, 4.3, 4.4, 6.4, 6.6, 7.1, 7.2, 8.4, 9.4)		
9. Regularly inspects equipment (1.2, 1.4)		
10. Performs peak flow reading (1.2, 1.4, 3.2, 4.1, 4.4, 6.4, 8.4, 9.4) as required		
11. Performs hand hygiene (1.2, 1.4, 1.8, 3.9, 6.4, 9.4)		
12. Cleans, replaces and disposes of equipment appropriately (1.2, 1.4, 3.9, 6.5, 9.4)		
13. Documents and reports relevant information (1.2, 1.3, 1.8, 3.2, 5.3, 6.6, 7.1, 7.2, 7.3, 7.4, 7.5)		
14. Demonstrates ability to link theory to practice (8.3, 8.4, 8.5, 9.4)		

Student:

Clinical facilitator: Date:

CHAPTER 8.2

PREOPERATIVE CARE

IDENTIFY INDICATIONS

Preoperative preparation of the patient has been proven to be effective. Patients who are well prepared:
- understand more about their planned surgery
- feel more in control of the actions and consequences affecting their care

- often experience less postoperative pain and anxiety
- are better motivated for self-care
- often require less time in the hospital
- have a shortened recuperative period.

IDENTIFY TYPE OF SURGERY

The type of surgery that the patient is to have will affect the preoperative care given, the amount of time in which to do it and, at times, the actual care. For instance, a patient booked for an elective gall bladder removal will have had time to have a full medical assessment, and any underlying disease or symptoms would have been explored and either eradicated or controlled. That patient would have had sufficient time to ask their surgeon questions, to have had pre-op exercises and teaching done, to be properly physically prepared (e.g. fasting, skin preparation) and to have at least some of their anxiety allayed before the day of surgery. In contrast, a patient with emergency surgery (e.g. a ruptured appendix) will not

have had the opportunity to have much, if any, of the preoperative care carried out, with the exception of the basic safety requirements. If surgery is to be day surgery, the admission and preparation of the patient are done on the same day and this will also affect the amount and timing of the preoperative care.

Similarly, the preparation of the patient for surgery also depends on the surgical procedure that will be done. The preparation of two patients, one for a tonsillectomy and the other for an abdominal perineal resection, will have elements of similarity, but there will be different information given, different emphasis placed on postoperative exercises and different physical preparation for these two patients. This skill provides only a basic outline that will need to be adapted to each individual circumstance.

GATHER EQUIPMENT

Gathering equipment before initiating the procedure is part of effective time management for implementing the procedure and provides an opportunity for the nurse to rehearse the procedure mentally.

Pre-op checklist
- *Patient ID bands* (if not already in situ)
- *Equipment as needed to measure vital signs*

- *Patient's theatre clothing*
- *Denture cup* if required
- *Anti-embolic stockings/pneumatic boots*
- *Pre-op checklist and other relevant charts*
- *Patient's notes, including signed consent form*
- *Fasting sign*

IMPLEMENT PREOPERATIVE CARE

Perform hand hygiene
Perform hand hygiene before touching the patient or the patient's surrounds and prior to any procedure involving patient contact to reduce the possibility of cross-contamination. Hand hygiene is the most effective

method of infection control as it removes transient organisms from the hands of the nurse (see **Skill 1.1**).

Give a clear explanation of the procedure and establish therapeutic communication
Introduce yourself, and check you have the correct patient. Discuss the procedure and gain

the patient's consent. Giving a clear explanation is required to gain legal consent and to address policy requirements. It will also assist the patient to cooperate with the procedure, allay anxiety and assist in establishing a therapeutic relationship. Explanation also fosters trust, and enables the building of a working therapeutic relationship.

Patients regard the following areas as most important to receive teaching about:

- information regarding pain management postoperatively
- psychosocial support (e.g. reassurance, honest information)
- roles and expectations (e.g. desired behaviours such as early ambulation)
- skills training (e.g. splinting the incision, deep breathing exercises).

The provision of preoperative information and skills training is more effective if the patient receives it in the pre-admission clinic and the information is reviewed with the patient (either individually or in a group) following admission. This information is available in the form of pamphlets, online tutorials, brochures and staff teaching.

Provide psychological support

Surgery is an experience that evokes anxiety in most patients. Facilitating communication, so that concerns and fears can be expressed, is an effective strategy to reduce the stressors of impending surgery. Being available to provide the patient with the opportunity to discuss fears and feelings is an essential step. The fears and concerns that are felt by patients are individual, but are influenced by factors such as: diagnosis; proposed surgical procedure; age; educational, cultural and social background; occupation; social support; and family responsibilities. Information and education on the procedure and the expectations regarding common concerns will reduce psychological stress. Common concerns include such questions as:

- What is the surgical procedure and what will it do to my body?
- What happens when I get to the theatre?
- What will happen to me when I am unconscious – will I feel anything, lose control of bowels or bladder, say things I would be embarrassed about?
- What will the incision look like?
- What will I have to deal with after surgery? Tubes and drips? Blood transfusions?
- Will I have pain when I wake up?
- When will I be able to eat and drink? Will I be sick?
- When will I be able to go home/return to work/ return to school?
- Will I be able to lead a normal life? Will I be disfigured?

Information given in answer to these questions will need to be tailored to the individual patient, but will need to be honest, factual and complete to the patient's level of need. A registered nurse should assist the student when answering these questions. Spiritual needs must also be taken into account. A visit by the patient's minister, priest, rabbi or other spiritual adviser may be arranged on request.

Provide pain management information

Pain is a major fear of most people facing surgery. Reassurance that the pain will be managed effectively will assist some patients to relax, and where relevant, patients are taught how to use a patient-controlled analgesia (PCA) system. Some people require more detailed information about medications usually used, and routes, times and effects of the analgesia. Reassurance that drug addiction is virtually non-existent when a drug is given for pain relief will assist some patients to utilise the pain management program more comfortably. Teaching the patient how to use the pain assessment tool before surgery is effective in increasing the accuracy of pain assessment postoperatively.

Teach techniques for preventing respiratory complications

The risk of respiratory complications occurring in patients who are essentially healthy is increased by factors such as: enforced inactivity, which reduces ventilation; lack of fluid intake prior to surgery tends to thicken respiratory secretions; anaesthetic/ oxygen inhalation dries mucous membranes; and postoperative pain reduces respiratory excursion. Deep breathing exercises, incentive spirometry and pursed-lip breathing assist the patient to maintain open airways and inflate the lungs fully, and to move secretions up out of the respiratory tract. Deep breathing exercises (see **Skill 3.15**) should be done frequently for the first 2 to 3 days following surgery. Coughing exercises for patients (not done routinely for patients with hernia repairs, eye surgery or brain surgery) help to loosen secretions so they can be expectorated. These are done as frequently as needed to keep the air passages free of secretions.

Teach techniques for avoiding venous thromboemboli (VTE)

Inactivity/immobility and gravity cause blood to pool in the lower body, blood tends to become more viscous from fluid restrictions, and positioning during and after surgery may trap blood in the legs. These factors contribute to the formation of thrombi and emboli. Reminders about positioning (no prolonged sitting, crossing legs or pillows under the knees) will assist the patient to prevent clot formation. Leg exercises promote circulation and prevent clot formation. Anti-embolic stockings (e.g. TEDs) (as per **Skill 2.2**) prevent thrombi formation by applying pressure to support the walls and valves of the leg veins, and as blood is pumped towards the heart, the TEDs prevent blood from pooling in the leg veins. Intermittent pneumatic compression (IPC) is a device that intermittently compresses the veins in the calf and/or thigh, commonly used on surgical patients (ACSQHC, 2020). Pneumatic boots may be worn by the patient and connected to the device.

Promote activity and exercise

Pain and fear of problems with the incision keep most postoperative patients relatively inactive. As mentioned earlier, inactivity can contribute to complications such as thrombi and emboli, respiratory complications, slow return of bowel peristalsis and reduced gastric emptying, all of which increase the postsurgical convalescent time. Patients need to know that they will be active following surgery. They will be expected to assist the nurse when they are turned and moved in bed, and in most cases will be expected to get out of bed and walk a short distance within the first 12 to 24 hours post operation. The time out of bed and walking will increase daily. To do this, they may need to be given adequate analgesia. They will need reassurance regarding the operative site. They may need to be taught how to splint the incision. Expectations regarding walking upright will be made clear prior to the operation and reinforced when the patient is sitting and walking. Take into consideration the patient's cultural background, as this may affect their response to postoperative care.

Prepare the surgical site

The surgical site is specially prepared preoperatively to reduce the chances of contaminating the incision with the microorganisms harboured in hair or skin. Different types of surgery have different preparations. Skin preparation will require the patient to have a preoperative shower with an antimicrobial or normal soap. Shaving of the surgical area is completed less frequently in the ward, as it may increase the risk of microabrasions of the skin and infection. For some procedures, hair in the vicinity of the incision may be clipped, but most facilities complete any shaving or clipping in theatre.

Carry out the preoperative routine

This routine involves identification, fasting, elimination, consent signature and valuables. Most facilities have a checklist of priority actions that must be completed before surgery. The checklist eliminates wasted time as various healthcare personnel search through the chart to verify that specific actions have been carried out (often in the pre-op clinic), and ensures that all priority actions have received attention. The patient is identified by checking the details on the two ID bands (on the arm and/or leg) and the chart with the patient. This eliminates misidentification and serious physical and legal repercussions.

Fasting for a specified time (generally 6 to 8 hours) produces an empty and non-active gastrointestinal tract. This prevents aspiration of undigested food if vomiting occurs, and reduces the incidence of postoperative nausea and abdominal distension. Elimination of bowel contents (on the surgeon's order or protocol) reduces postoperative distension and constipation. This can be accomplished by measures such as bowel preparations and modified diet in the days prior to surgery, or enemas. The patient is asked to void prior to surgery to reduce discomfort and to avoid interference with the surgical procedure.

The patient's consent to surgery is checked by asking the patient to discuss their understanding of the procedure and asking them to confirm it is their signature on the form. This is to comply with legal requirements that the patient has understood the surgical procedure.

Physical status for routine surgery is assessed. This could include physical assessment, medical/surgical history, laboratory tests, special examinations or X-rays to reduce surgical risks, avoid complications and prevent unexpected difficulties during and after surgery (often these are done in the pre-op clinic). Allergies are identified so that patients are protected from inadvertent administration of a drug or contact with a substance to which they are allergic. Any allergies, and the patient's reaction, are written in the patient's notes and medication chart. A red patient identification band is also attached to the patient (ACSQHC, 2019). The allergies and reaction are also highlighted on the preoperative check list. This communicates the information to all members of the multidisciplinary team in the various departments.

Valuables are removed (or taped in the case of some wedding rings that may be difficult to remove) and handled according to the policies of the facility to prevent their loss or damage and subsequent legal problems for the facility. Metal jewellery and piercings also constitute a hazard when diathermy is being used. Oral and lip piercing (and potentially nasal piercings) create an anaesthetic risk and should be removed. Hygiene (shower/bath) and mouth care are attended to for hygiene purposes. A hospital gown, theatre pants and cap are worn to prevent damage to the patient's clothing and to reduce the transfer of microorganisms from the patient's hair. Hair clips should not be used to secure long hair as they might damage the scalp when the patient is unconscious and are also a hazard when diathermy is used.

Prostheses and dentures may be removed to protect them from loss or damage. Loose teeth and crowns are noted to alert the anaesthetist to them, as extra care will be taken not to dislodge them when intubating. Some facilities allow patients to wear dentures and hearing aids to theatre and the circulating nurse becomes responsible for their care during surgery. Glasses and contact lenses are removed to prevent their loss or damage. Lenses can also damage the eye if left in during surgery. Cosmetics are removed to enable healthcare personnel to assess circulation.

Anti-embolic stockings (compression stockings; e.g. TEDs) and IPC (ACSQHC, 2020) are usually applied and worn throughout surgery to promote venous return. These have proven effective in preventing deep venous thromboses in moderate-risk surgical patients. They need to be fitted to the individual patient, applied to dry feet and legs prior to surgery and then worn throughout the postsurgical period. Check that any other special preoperative procedures ordered by the surgeon have been done. Complete a preoperative checklist, and document and report relevant information. This pre-op checklist ensures important information has been collected, and that all preoperative preparations and care have been completed. It is signed by the nurse preparing the patient for theatre, then by theatre nurses. The amount of further information required to complete this form will depend on the facility policy or the type of procedure.

Personnel in the theatre and recovery area will require the information to be completed in all other patient charts and checklists (e.g. Observation Response Chart [ORC], fluid balance chart) so that appropriate decisions can be made. All documentation must be completed prior to administering premedication (if prescribed), as the patient is considered legally unable to provide information after the premedication has been given.

Administer preoperative medication if ordered

Premedications are rarely prescribed. However, if one is ordered, it can be ordered at a specific time or 'on call', so the patient will need to be completely ready for surgery prior to that time. The patient needs to know that the medication will help them feel relaxed and possibly drowsy. They will need to be cautioned to stay in bed. Have the side-rails raised to remind them to stay in bed and the call bell within reach to obtain assistance.

DOCUMENT AND REPORT RELEVANT INFORMATION

Personnel in the theatre and recovery area will require the information to be complete in the charts and checklists so that appropriate decisions can be made. All documentation must be completed prior to administering premedication, as the patient is considered legally unable to provide information if premedication has been given.

Accompany the patient to theatre

The ward nurse who is responsible for the preparation of the patient for surgery accompanies the patient to the theatre. The patient will usually go to theatre on their own bed. Privacy and dignity are maintained. The patient's notes, the preoperative checklist and any X-rays accompany the patient to theatre. Labelled containers for dentures, spectacles and/or hearing aids as necessary are taken with the patient to theatre. The patient is handed over to the theatre nurse following the facility clinical handover template (see **Skill 7.3**), with both nurses identifying the patient and verifying the preoperative checklist (ACSQHC, 2019). These are safety precautions.

Perform hand hygiene

Maintain the 5 Moments for Hand Hygiene and perform hand hygiene after touching the patient and the patient's surrounds.

CLEAN, REPLACE OR DISPOSE OF EQUIPMENT

All hospital equipment is returned to the relevant areas.

The bed area is tidied in preparation for the return of the patient. Depending on the surgery, equipment is brought to this area for use by staff on the patient's return. The oxygen and suction apparatus should be checked to ensure that it is working correctly, and that there is sufficient stock present.

CASE STUDY

1. Access a copy of a preoperative checklist from your healthcare facility. Use this document to complete a preoperative checklist for a total hip replacement, using either a family member or nursing colleague to interview.
2. As part of completing the preoperative checklist, also complete a patient education session for a 22-year-old footballer who has had a repair of a torn anterior cruciate ligament (ACL) of his right knee. He is to be discharged the next morning to his home. This patient lives with his parents who both are at work during the day Monday to Friday.

Note: These notes are summaries of the most important points in the assessments/procedures, and are not exhaustive on the subject. The naming of documents or charts may differ from state to state, and facility to facility. In all possible situations the guidelines of the ACSQHC are used when describing national charts or documents (e.g. the ACSQHC Observation and Response Chart is named the Adult Observation and Response Chart in WA, and the Rapid Detection and Response Observation Chart in SA). References of the materials used to compile the information have been supplied. The student is expected to have learned the material surrounding each skill as presented in the references. No single reference is complete on the subject.

CRITICAL THINKING/LIFESPAN

Thinking of the clinical skills discussed in this skill, and the stages of growth and development, what are some of the key components you would need to consider in the following scenarios?

1. Oscar, a 5-year-old child, is booked for insertion of grommets to treat recurrent otitis media. Why is pre-op education important to both Oscar and his parents?
2. Jaden, aged 15 years, has a fracture of his humerus that requires surgical treatment (ORIF – open reduction internal fixation). He remains very quiet while lying in bed, is hesitant and his mother keeps interrupting and answers questions on his behalf. How will you manage his pre-op education?
3. Mai is a 38-year-old woman, with English as her second language. She is being admitted for a lumpectomy to her right breast that morning. She tells you that up to now, she has been drinking water, but has fasted from food. How will you manage this situation?

REFERENCES

Australian Commission on Safety and Quality in Health Care (ACSQHC). (2019). *Communicating for Safety Standard.* https://www.safetyandquality.gov.au/standards/nsqhs-standards/communicating-safety-standard

Australian Commission on Safety and Quality in Health Care (ACSQHC). (2020). *Venous Thromboembolism Prevention Clinical Care Standard.* https://www.safetyandquality.gov.au/publications-and-resources/resource-library/venous-thromboembolism-prevention-clinical-care-standard

RECOMMENDED READINGS

Joustra, C. & Moloney, A. (2019). *Clinical Placement Manual* (1st ed.). Melbourne: Cengage.

Koutoukidis, G. & Stainton, K. (2020). *Tabbner's Nursing Care: Theory and Practice* (8th ed.). Sydney: Elsevier.

ESSENTIAL SKILLS COMPETENCY

Preoperative Care
Demonstrates the ability to effectively prepare a patient for theatre

Criteria for skill performance	Y	D
(Numbers indicate *Enrolled Nurse Standards for Practice*, 2016)	(Satisfactory)	(Requires development)
1. Identifies indication (8.3, 8.4)		
2. Gathers equipment (1.2, 1.6, 4.4, 6.4, 8.4, 9.4): ■ patient ID bands (if not already in situ) ■ equipment as needed to measure vital signs ■ patient's theatre clothing ■ denture cup ■ anti-embolic stockings/pneumatic boots ■ pre-op checklist and other relevant charts ■ patient's notes, including signed consent form ■ fasting sign		
3. Performs hand hygiene (1.2, 1.4, 1.8, 3.9, 6.4, 9.4)		
4. Evidence of effective communication with the patient; e.g. gives patient a clear explanation of procedure, gains patient consent (2.1, 2.3, 2.4, 2.5, 6.3)		
5. Provides psychological support (1.2, 1.4, 2.1, 2.2, 2.5, 2.10, 3.2, 6.1, 8.4, 9.4)		
6. Provides pain management information (1.2, 1.4, 2.1, 3.2, 3.3, 6.4, 8.4, 9.4)		
7. Carries out preoperative teaching appropriate to patient and procedure (1.8, 3.9, 4.2, 6.3, 8.4, 9.4)		
8. Prepares the surgical site as ordered (1.2, 1.4, 2.7, 3.2, 6.4, 8.4, 9.4)		
9. Performs hand hygiene (1.2, 1.4, 1.8, 3.9, 6.4, 9.4)		
10. Carries out the preoperative routine; e.g. patient identification, fasting, elimination, procedure consent signature, valuables, clothing (1.2, 1.4, 3.2, 4.1, 4.2, 4.4, 7.1, 7.3, 7.5, 8.4, 9.4)		
11. Administers preoperative medication (if ordered) (1.1, 1.2, 1.4, 1.8, 2.2, 3.2, 3.9, 6.1, 8.4, 9.4)		
12. Documents and reports relevant information (1.2, 1.3, 1.8, 3.2, 5.3, 6.6, 7.1, 7.2, 7.3, 7.4, 7.5)		
13. Accompanies patient to theatre (1.2, 1.4, 2.7, 3.2, 3.9, 4.4, 6.4, 8.4, 9.4)		
14. Performs hand hygiene (1.2, 1.4, 1.8, 3.9, 6.4, 9.4)		
15. Cleans, replaces and disposes of equipment appropriately (1.2, 1.4, 3.9, 6.5, 9.4)		
16. Demonstrates ability to link theory to practice (8.3, 8.4, 8.5, 9.4)		

Student:

Clinical facilitator: Date:

CHAPTER 8.3

RECOVERY ROOM CARE AND HANDOVER

IDENTIFY INDICATIONS

Following surgery, the surgical patient is at great risk in the immediate post-anaesthetic period. The effects of surgery, anaesthesia, alterations in thermoregulation, fluid shifts, airway patency, cardiovascular complications and neurological dysfunction are all factors that contribute to this risk. The goals of nursing care in the post-anaesthetic care unit (PACU) are to support respiratory and haemodynamic stabilisation following anaesthesia and surgery, promote recovery from anaesthesia, promote physical comfort and healing, prevent injury and prevent postoperative complications. The patient remains in the PACU until their physiological signs have stabilised. During this time, the patient is carefully and thoroughly monitored to identify possible complications. This usually entails one-to-one nursing.

FAMILIARISE YOURSELF WITH ANTICIPATED COMPLICATIONS OF THE PATIENT'S SURGICAL PROCEDURE

Since each of the various surgical procedures entails specific risks, the nurse must be familiar with the anticipated complications that could arise from the surgical procedure. The patient's age should be known since patients who are very elderly or very young are at a greater risk of some complications than a younger adult patient. Furthermore, since each patient is unique and has a unique medical history, any of their specific problems should be conveyed to the PACU staff before or during surgery so that problems can be anticipated. Many patients have a complex medical history with multiple conditions such as diabetes mellitus, obesity, impaired vision or hearing, peripheral vascular disease, a previous cerebrovascular accident or cigarette and alcohol intake, which can all have an impact on the patient's immediate recovery from anaesthesia and surgery. Knowledge of the anticipated problems and complications that might arise allows the nurse to prepare for reasonable eventualities and to have sufficient specific equipment available.

GATHER AND PREPARE EQUIPMENT

All equipment used must be functioning and at the bedside before the patient arrives. The PACU is generally set out with all of the basic equipment (airway maintenance, pulse oximetry, non-invasive blood pressure and cardiac monitoring, plus oxygen and suctioning) needed at each individual recovery bay, arranged for ease of access and always in clean and full working order. Nurses must familiarise themselves with the essential equipment for respiratory and cardiac support, which is generally located centrally. The resuscitation trolley has additional equipment to that of a general ward. Specific equipment will have to be supplied and tested prior to use. When the patient arrives following a general anaesthetic, they will be unconscious and will require one-to-one nursing, which obligates the nurse to remain at the bedside and prevents them from obtaining forgotten equipment. Patients who have a local or spinal anaesthetic also require a period of postoperative observation, although the priorities of care will focus on different considerations, such as hypotension, dizziness and headaches (Dougherty & Lister, 2015).

Equipment that may be needed includes the following.

- *A stethoscope, sphygmomanometer, tympanic thermometer, probe covers, pulse oximeter and a watch* are all required to monitor vital signs. Generally, an automatic blood pressure machine is used, although some situations require a manual sphygmomanometer (e.g. for shivering or profoundly bradycardic patients) (Dougherty & Lister, 2015).
- *An intravenous fluid stand* is required to hang an intravenous bag. Patients who have undergone surgery almost always have an intravenous infusion to balance and maintain their fluid levels as well as provide access routes for intravenous medications.

- *Oxygen equipment.* A flow meter to connect the patient's oxygen tubing that will be in situ post-op will be required, plus extra tubing, face masks and full range of oropharyngeal and nasopharyngeal airways. The patient has been anaesthetised and their respiratory system needs assistance to maintain oxygenation to the tissues.
- *Suctioning equipment* is required since the patient's gag reflex and swallowing reflex have been temporarily eliminated or reduced by the depressive effects of anaesthetic and the paralytic drugs used during surgery.

- *Dressing supplies* are needed in case the surgical site requires reinforcement because of excess bleeding/drainage.
- *A warm blanket* is used to provide comfort. Altered thermoregulation as well as a colder ambient temperature of the operating theatre contribute to the discomfort felt by the patient.
- *Other equipment* may be needed as indicated by the patient's surgical procedure.

IMPLEMENT CARE IN THE POSTOPERATIVE PERIOD

Most of the following activities occur simultaneously or at least in very rapid succession and will depend on the patient's condition. For instance, often during the handover, the circulating nurse and the PACU nurse are assessing the patient together.

Perform hand hygiene

Perform hand hygiene before touching the patient or the patient's surrounds and prior to any procedure involving patient contact to reduce the possibility of cross-contamination. Hand hygiene is the most effective method of infection control as it removes transient organisms from the hands of the nurse (see **Skill 1.1**). Immediately postoperatively, the patient is extremely at risk of invasion by micro-organisms, making it imperative that all measures are taken to prevent cross-infection.

Receive a verbal handover from the operating theatre staff

The handover includes the name, age, language spoken, allergies, pre-existing medical condition (e.g. diabetes mellitus), type and extent of the surgical procedure, preoperative and intraoperative vital signs, positioning during surgery, type of anaesthetic used, estimated blood loss, medications and intravenous solutions administered, complications, location and type of catheters, the presence, position and nature of any arterial devices, drains or packs, altered sensory or motor functions and intraoperative events that might affect the postoperative course. PACU staff need to know what has occurred during surgery. Such things as fluid loss and replacement, haemorrhage, medications given, time under anaesthetic, the medications used to reverse anaesthesia and any difficulties encountered, such as prolonged bleeding time, must be reported to the PACU staff as they will affect the patient during the recovery from anaesthetic. The actual surgery performed, any deviations from that surgery, specific orders left by the surgeon and postoperative standing orders should also be discussed. The anaesthetist also gives specific instructions for postoperative care. Though all information is provided in the patient's file notes, a verbal handover is given to ensure no delay in providing immediate care. The Australian Commission on Safety and Quality in Health Care (ACSQHC, 2019) requires that the facility policy for a clinical handover (e.g. iSoBAR or ISBAR) be followed when handing over patient's care, along with the use of facility guidelines or a specific mnemonic (e.g. ABCDE format – Airway, Breathing, Circulation, Drips, Drains, Drugs (medications) and Extras) to complete a primary and secondary survey of the patient to guide the assessment structure.

- **Identify.** Nurse introduces themself to the patient, important information is gathered.
- **Situation.** What operation has been performed, type of anaesthetic used.
- **Observations.** Vital signs.
- **Background.** Any known allergies, relevant history.
- **Agree to a plan.** Based on patient's current status and progress made, identify the care actions to be implemented.
- **Read back.** Review and read the documentation together, repeat back orders and information given. Review the recommendations for handover and use of templates described in **Skill 7.3**.

Give a clear explanation of the procedure and establish therapeutic communication

Patients will display varying degrees of responsiveness, and physical and emotional states, so establishing a rapport with them will gain their confidence and cooperation and will aid assessment. Following the final stage of anaesthesia, some patients behave in an emotional and disinhibited manner, at odds with their usual behaviour. This is transient and usually forgotten (Dougherty & Lister, 2015). Give the patient a clear explanation of procedure, even if they are unconscious. Hearing is the last sense to leave and the first to return, and even if patients cannot respond, they may hear your explanations and gain some reassurance from them.

Families should not be forgotten, especially parents of children, and should be informed that the surgery is completed and their loved one/child is in the recovery room.

Assess and maintain patency of the airway

Assess for airway patency by feeling for movement of expired air. Listen for inspiration, observe for any accessory respiratory use and check for tracheal tug. General anaesthesia causes depression of many of the patient's reflexes, including pharyngeal, cough, swallowing and gag reflexes. Nausea and vomiting are also common effects of general anaesthesia. Patients usually return to the PACU with a Guedel's airway in situ. This type of airway keeps the tongue forced forward so it does not block the patient's airway, and should be left in place until the patient attempts to cough or spit it out. If the Guedel's is causing distress and gagging, it may be removed by the nurse even if the patient is not awake enough to remove it themselves. If this occurs, care must be taken to ensure that the patient's airway remains patent. The patient will return from theatre in a side-lying position (recovery position) to protect the airway from secretions and regurgitation, unless there is a specific reason for them to be placed in a different position. If necessary, support the chin with the neck extended (unless contraindicated). The patient should remain in this position until they are fully conscious and able to maintain their own airway. Keep the bed flat if not contraindicated. Monitor breath sounds to detect airway obstruction. Suction the oral cavity if breath sounds such as noisy respirations, snoring, wheezes and gurgling (which indicate partial airway obstruction) are heard. The registered nurse (RN) may need to do nasopharyngeal suction. Oxygen is administered continuously during the patient's stay in the PACU to facilitate gas exchange and to assist with the removal of the anaesthetic from the patient's lungs. A pulse oximeter is used to monitor oxygen saturation levels, which should be maintained at 95% to 100% (unless the patient has a known respiratory condition, in which case the doctor/anaesthetist will give more specific instructions). The patient may require verbal stimulation to maintain their respiratory rate above 10 since the anaesthetic acts as a general depressant. Encourage the patient to cough and breathe deeply when awake (as appropriate).

Obtain readings of vital signs and assess circulatory status

Connect the patient to the monitoring system. Blood pressure (BP), pulse, temperature and respiratory assessments are done immediately on arrival at the unit and every 5 to 15 minutes thereafter until the patient is stable and returned to the ward. Monitor the patient's skin for warmth, moisture and colour (check the colour of the lips and conjunctiva, then peripheral colour and perfusion). Central cyanosis indicates impaired gaseous exchange between the alveoli and pulmonary capillaries. Peripheral cyanosis indicates low cardiac output (Dougherty & Lister, 2015). Haemodynamic instability and altered tissue perfusion occur because of pooling of the blood during surgery, peripheral vasodilation, hypothermia and hypovolaemia. Cardiac monitors that assess the heart rate and rhythm may be used. Hypoxia can manifest as irritability, restlessness, confusion and/or aggression. Temperature is monitored initially and then as needed. Hypothermia can occur due to the anaesthesia, ambient temperature in the theatre and length/extent of the procedure. Shivering may result from either a compensatory response or the effects of anaesthetic agents. Though it is not as common as hypothermia, hyperthermia is a serious complication of surgery caused by accidental over-warming during surgery, sepsis or transfusion reactions. An elevated temperature increases oxygen demands and ventilatory and cardiac workloads. The possibility of malignant hyperthermia (MH) (a genetically determined condition) must always be considered, because successful management of MH depends on early assessment and prompt intervention (Dougherty & Lister, 2015).

Assess the level of consciousness

Assessment of the level of consciousness is carried out by rousing the patient, using both touch and verbal stimulation. At first the patient will be unable to respond appropriately, but by the time they are ready to be returned to the ward, they should be drowsy but easily roused and able to answer questions appropriately. Frequent stimulation, such as every 5 minutes or even more often, may be required. Premedications and anaesthesia can induce a degree of amnesia and disorientation. The nurse orients the patient to time and place frequently to assist in alleviating anxiety and to reassure. Observe for return of movement and sensation, especially if the patient has received a regional, spinal or epidural anaesthetic.

Assess fluid balance

Assessment of fluid balance is ongoing throughout the recovery period. Initially, the PACU nurse will note the intravenous infusion solution, amount remaining to be infused, rate of flow, the fact that it is infusing at the correct rate and that further orders are available. The infusion site will be assessed for inflammation and infiltration.

A note will be made of the urinary output – whether the patient is catheterised or not. If catheterised, the amount of urine in the collection bag is recorded hourly, along with odour, consistency, colour and concentration. Review the facility policy for the minimum amount of urine output to be expected hourly.

Inspect drainage tubes and dressings

All drainage tubes, including nasogastric tubes, are initially inspected for patency and connection to the appropriate receptacle. Their patency is checked when completing other postoperative observations along with the amount, colour, odour and consistency of the drainage documented on the postoperative chart. All surgical dressings are inspected initially for intactness, soakage or drainage, or frank haemorrhage. If necessary, the surgical dressing can be reinforced with additional dressing material. However, do not remove the dressing without the surgeon's order.

Monitor specific parameters

These assessments will vary depending on the surgery and the patient. Some surgical procedures require specific assessments. For instance, musculoskeletal surgery carries a high risk of compartment syndrome. Therefore, any patient who has had musculoskeletal surgery should have frequent neurovascular observations to determine any neurovascular deterioration or compromise. Similarly, patients who have had neurological surgery will require assessment of their neurological functioning. A patient who is a diabetic would have their blood glucose level monitored frequently (see **Skill 2.6**).

Check the medication chart

Medications may need to be administered during the immediate postoperative period (e.g. commencement of patient-controlled analgesia, antiemetics). Follow the eight rights of medication administration.

Continue to monitor vital signs, circulatory status and fluid balance

The patient's status is monitored and documented on arrival, every 5 to 10 minutes for the first half-hour or until stable, and every 15 minutes until discharged from the PACU. This is a general guideline and may vary in different facilities; however, all recovery room monitoring and documentation is very frequent.

Provide comfort measures

Pain assessment and relief is an important consideration during the postoperative recovery time. Because of all the drugs they have been given, patients are monitored carefully for respiratory depression. Talking to the patient can help them wake up and overcome their slow respiratory rate, plus reduce any anxiety. Reassurance is essential for the psychological comfort of the patient. Repeating that the surgery is finished and that the patient is safe provides reassurance during the early stages of recovery from anaesthetic.

Warmth is essential for comfort and to prevent vasoconstriction from shivering. This can be accomplished by supplying warm blankets. Monitor the patient's temperature to avoid over-warming. Frequent repositioning helps to prevent pressure injuries as well as to provide comfort. The nurse can assess body prominences and areas of potential pressure injuries. The risk of development of pressure injuries is very high until the patient's vascular and motor functions return. The patient may have been lying on the theatre table in one position for several hours and compromised the vascular circulation to specific areas.

Determine stability of physiological signs prior to transfer to unit

The criteria for discharge from the PACU to the general ward include the following.

- The patient is sufficiently conscious (e.g. easily aroused, able to answer simple questions), can maintain own airway and exhibits protective airway reflexes (e.g. gag reflex, cough).
- Respiratory function and good oxygenation are being maintained (e.g. SpO_2 greater than 92% on room air or supplemental oxygen to maintain saturations above 95%). Again be aware of requirements for patients with chronic respiratory conditions).
- The cardiovascular system is stable; no unexpected cardiac irregularities. The specific values of pulse and BP are within the patient's preoperative limits on consecutive observations.
- No persistent or excessive bleeding from wound or drainage sites.
- Those with urinary catheters have an output greater than 0.5 mL/kg/hr (i.e. approximately half their body weight in mL/hr).
- Pain and vomiting are controlled; suitable analgesia/antiemetic regimens have been prescribed by the anaesthetist.
- Body temperature is at least 36°C.
- The patient is able to move limbs; peripheral pulses distal to the surgical site are present.
- Postoperative complications are resolved or controlled (Dougherty & Lister, 2015; Royal Children's Hospital Melbourne, 2019; Smith et al., 2016).

Some facilities use a scoring system to assist in determining whether the patient is stable enough to return to the unit. Various types of scoring systems are in use. Follow the facility's policy.

The nurse must recognise and report any abnormalities in all of the above assessments to the RN promptly.

Provide a thorough handover for ward staff

The ward staff are notified when a patient is ready to return to the ward. The ward nurse goes to the PACU to assess the patient and transfer them back to the ward, accompanied by a patient care assistant or the PACU staff. The report given at this handover includes the same items addressed on entry to the PACU plus a summary of the patient's stay in the PACU and should again follow the facility policy for a clinical handover (e.g. iSoBAR or ISBAR), along with the use of a mnemonic (e.g. ABCDE format – Airway, Breathing, Circulation, Drips, Drains, Drugs [medications] and Extras) to complete a primary and secondary survey of the patient (ACSQHC, 2019). Also complete a check of the patient's identity during this handover. Special instructions and postoperative orders are reviewed with the ward staff. The ward nurse needs to assess the patient's level of consciousness, pain and ability to maintain their airway, check that there are appropriate analgesia, antiemetic and IV fluid orders and that the postoperative instructions are clearly documented, as the surgeon and anaesthetist may not be available later due to their operating list. Safety of the patient during transfer to the ward is of great concern, as most patients remain drowsy. Ensure that safety rails are used, beds have locked wheels and that the patient transfer is accomplished with sufficient staff to prevent injury to the patient or staff.

DOCUMENT AND REPORT RELEVANT INFORMATION

Maintain accurate documentation on the appropriate sheets. PACU documentation is made on specific sheets that are individual to each facility. All observations should be recorded on the observation and response chart.

CLEAN, REPLACE OR DISPOSE OF EQUIPMENT

Requirements for cleaning, replacement and disposal of equipment and disposable materials will vary, depending on what equipment is used for each patient. It is imperative that all necessary materials are immediately available at each bedside for use in a possible emergency. Nursing in a one-to-one situation does not permit leaving a patient to find frequently used material and equipment. It is the responsibility of each nurse to see that the stethoscope earpieces are cleaned (if it is a ward stethoscope); that the sphygmomanometer is cleaned or the cuff replaced if there is visible soiling; that there is a thermometer and sufficient covers, an intravenous fluid pole and commonly used fluids; that all the airway, oxygen and suctioning equipment are present, clean and functioning; and that there are sufficient dressing supplies and linen available.

CASE STUDY

You are an enrolled nurse working in an acute surgical ward. You have received a phone call from PACU stating that your patient, Josh Baker, is ready to return to the ward post-op. Josh is 26 years old and was a booked admission for a shoulder reconstruction following an injury while playing football. Josh is very concerned as to how long he will need to recuperate after this surgery and rehabilitation. He is very keen to return to football training.

1. List the type of information you would expect to receive from the PACU nurse during handover. Review relevant texts to gain information about this procedure, including any post-op drains, IV lines, wound dressing, and so on.
2. Identify any issues that you, as his nurse, could anticipate in his post-op recovery.

Note: These notes are summaries of the most important points in the assessments/procedures, and are not exhaustive on the subject. The naming of documents or charts may differ from state to state, and facility to facility. In all possible situations the guidelines of the ACSQHC are used when describing national charts or documents (e.g. the ACSQHC Observation and Response Chart is named the Adult Observation and Response Chart in WA, and the Rapid Detection and Response Observation Chart in SA). References of the materials used to compile the information have been supplied. The student is expected to have learned the material surrounding each skill as presented in the references. No single reference is complete on the subject.

REFERENCES

Australian Commission on Safety and Quality in Health Care (ACSQHC). (2019). *Communicating for Safety Standard.* https://www.safetyandquality.gov.au/standards/nsqhs-standards/communicating-safety-standard

Dougherty, L. & Lister, S. (eds). (2015). *The Royal Marsden Hospital Manual of Clinical Nursing Procedures* (9th ed.). Oxford: Wiley-Blackwell.

Royal Children's Hospital Melbourne. (2019). *Routine Post Anaesthetic Observation.* https://www.rch.org.au/rchcpg/hospital_clinical_guideline_index/Routine_post_anaesthetic_observation/

Smith, S., Duell, D., Martin, B., Gonzalez, L. & Aebersold, M. (2016). *Clinical Nursing Skills: Basic to Advanced Skills* (9th ed.). Pearson.

RECOMMENDED READINGS

Australian Commission on Safety and Quality in Health Care (ACSQHC). (2019). *Comprehensive Care Standard.* https://www.safetyandquality.gov.au/standards/nsqhs-standards/comprehensive-care-standard

Brindley, P.G., Beed, M., Law, J.A., Hung, O., Levitan, R., Murphy, M.F. & Duggan, L.V. (2017). Airway management outside the operating room: How to better prepare. *Canadian Journal of Anesthesia*, 64(5), pp. 530–9.

Plowman, E. (2017). A2K: A comprehensive and systematic approach to the physical assessment of postoperative patient. *Australian Nursing and Midwifery Journal*, 24(10), p. 43.

Royal Children's Hospital Melbourne. (2019). *Neurovascular Observations.* https://www.rch.org.au/rchcpg/hospital_clinical_guideline_index/Neurovascular_observations/#:~:text=Assessment%20of%20neurovascular%20status%20is,trauma%2C%20surgery%20or%20cast%20application

ESSENTIAL SKILLS COMPETENCY

Recovery Room Care and Handover

Demonstrates the ability to effectively and safely complete a verbal handover to or from the PACU and safely care for a patient in the PACU

Criteria for skill performance	Y	D
(Numbers indicate *Enrolled Nurse Standards for Practice*, 2016)	(Satisfactory)	(Requires development)
1. Identifies indication (8.3, 8.4)		
2. Familiarises self with anticipated complications of the patient's surgical procedure (1.2, 1.6, 3.1, 3.2, 3.3, 10.1, 10.3, 10.5, 10.6)		
3. Gathers equipment (1.2, 1.6, 4.4, 6.4, 8.4, 9.4): ■ stethoscope, sphygmomanometer, tympanic thermometer, pulse oximeter, probe covers ■ intravenous fluid pole ■ oxygen equipment ■ suctioning equipment ■ dressing supplies ■ warm blanket ■ other equipment as indicated by the patient's surgical procedure		
4. Performs hand hygiene (1.2, 1.4, 1.8, 3.9, 6.4, 9.4)		
5. Receives PACU verbal handover (1.2, 1.4, 1.8, 3.2, 4.2, 7.1, 7.2, 7.3, 7.4, 7.5, 8.4, 9.4)		
6. Evidence of effective communication with the patient; e.g. gives a clear explanation of procedure (2.1, 2.3, 2.4, 2.5, 6.3)		
7. Assesses/maintains patency of the airway, level of consciousness, fluid balance (1.2, 1.4, 1.8, 3.2, 3.9, 4.1, 4.2, 4.3, 4.4, 6.1, 6.4, 6.6, 7.1, 7.2, 7.3, 8.4, 9.4)		
8. Monitors vital signs and circulatory status (1.2, 1.4, 1.8, 3.2, 3.9, 4.1, 4.2, 4.3, 4.4, 6.1, 6.4, 6.6, 7.1, 7.2, 7.3, 8.4, 9.4)		
9. Inspects drainage tubes, intravenous infusion and oxygen equipment; inspects dressing/cast (1.2, 1.4, 1.8, 3.2, 3.9, 4.1, 4.2, 4.3, 4.4, 6.1, 6.4, 6.6, 7.1, 7.2, 7.3, 8.4, 9.4)		
10. Monitors specific parameters (1.2, 1.4, 1.8, 3.2, 3.9, 4.1, 4.2, 4.3, 4.4, 6.1, 6.4, 7.1, 7.2, 7.3, 8.4, 9.4)		
11. Continues to monitor vital signs, circulatory status and fluid balance, and reports any abnormalities (1.2, 1.4, 1.8, 3.2, 3.9, 4.1, 4.2, 4.3, 4.4, 6.1, 6.4, 6.6, 7.1, 7.2, 7.3, 8.4, 9.4)		
12 Provides for comfort measures (1.2, 1.4, 3.2, 8.4, 9.4)		
13. Determines stability prior to transfer (1.2, 1.4, 3.2, 3.9, 6.6, 7.3, 8.4, 9.4)		
14. Maintains documentation appropriately (1.1, 1.2, 1.3, 1.4, 2.2, 3.2, 4.2, 6.6, 7.1, 7.2, 7.3, 7.4, 7.5, 9.4)		
15. Provides a thorough handover for ward staff (1.2, 1.4, 3.2, 7.1, 7.2, 7.3, 7.4, 7.5, 8.4, 9.4)		
16. Cleans, replaces and disposes of equipment appropriately (1.2, 1.4, 3.9, 6.5, 9.4)		
17. Demonstrates ability to link theory to practice (8.3, 8.4, 8.5, 9.4)		

Student:

Clinical facilitator: Date:

POSTOPERATIVE CARE

IDENTIFY INDICATIONS

Postoperative care is given to patients following surgery and stabilisation in the recovery room or post-anaesthetic care unit (PACU). Postoperative care consists of prevention or recognition of common postoperative complications and supporting the patient until they have regained normal physiological functioning. The effects of anaesthesia and physiological stressors can place the patient at risk for a variety of physiological alterations.

Postoperative care is divided into two phases. Initial care occurs in the postoperative recovery room (sometimes the intensive or coronary care units as well) and extends until the patient has regained consciousness

and is physiologically stable. The second phase is the postoperative convalescent phase, which extends from transfer of the patient to the ward until the patient is discharged from hospital. This skill will deal with the second phase only. The information in this section is very general and should be taken as such.

The nurse must always be aware of the hospital policy and procedure for postoperative care. Also, many surgeons have very specific postoperative protocols for their patients. Take care to make yourself familiar with both, preferably before the patient goes to surgery, but at least before they return to the ward.

GATHER AND PREPARE EQUIPMENT

Postoperative care begins preoperatively with adequate teaching and continues when the patient has left the ward for the operating theatre. The bed area and room are prepared to receive the patient postoperatively. The bedside locker is cleared of any personal material in anticipation of its possible use during an emergency situation, or for placing equipment on. *A sphygmomanometer, stethoscope, thermometer* and *pulse oximeter* should be easily accessible for monitoring vital signs. *An intravenous (IV) stand* and pumps required are both brought to the bedside area in anticipation for use when the patient returns.

Extra pillows are available so the patient can be supported in appropriate positions. The room is cleared of clutter so the bed can be more easily manoeuvred. *Oxygen and suction equipment* would be checked before the patient returns to the ward. Other specific equipment would be added for different surgical procedures. Time of return is estimated and the nurse plans for the care of other patients so that extra time can be devoted to the acute postoperative patient. Required relevant charts (e.g. fluid balance chart [FBC], neurovascular observations [NVO], and so on) will be included in the patient's notes on their return from theatre.

IMPLEMENT IMMEDIATE POST-OP CARE

Perform hand hygiene

Perform hand hygiene before touching the patient or the patient's surrounds and prior to any procedure involving patient contact to reduce the possibility of cross-contamination. Hand hygiene is the most effective method of infection control as it removes transient organisms from the hands of the nurse (see **Skill 1.1**).

The post-surgical patient is particularly vulnerable to infection because of breaks in their skin integrity and diminished protective mechanisms in the respiratory system from the effects of anaesthetic.

Transfer the patient to their room

Transfer of the patient to their room is done maintaining patient safety and minimising muscle strain on the staff. The patient's oxygen tubing is immediately attached to the wall unit to maintain the required flow. IV fluid is hung and tubing attached to the appropriate IV pump and the flow rate checked.

Assess the postoperative patient

Assessment of the postoperative patient is performed immediately on return to the unit. A verbal handover from the recovery room nurse, using the hospital clinical handover template, is gained prior to accepting the patient from the PACU or into the ward so that appropriate assessment and nursing care measures can be planned (ACSQHC, 2019). The theatre notes and charts are consulted for baseline information, previous medical conditions, nature of surgery and any complications that occurred during surgery, so that the more likely complications are anticipated. Assessment – head-to-toe and/or use of a mnemonic such as ABCDE format (Airway, Breathing, Circulation, Drips, Drains, Drugs [medications] and Extras) to complete a primary and secondary survey of the patient – is in accordance with organisational policy, and may include the following:

- level of consciousness
- vital signs
- oxygen saturation level with pulse oximeter
- pain levels
- position of the patient during surgery
- condition and colour of the skin
- circulation – peripheral pulses and sensation of extremities as applicable
- condition and location of dressings
- condition of the suture line if no dressing
- type and patency of drains and catheters as applicable
- amount and type of drainage
- muscle strength and response
- pupillary response as indicated
- fluid therapy, location of lines, type and amount of solution infusing
- level of physical and emotional comfort
- blood glucose level (BGL) monitoring if patient is diabetic.

Postoperative orders are consulted to assist in planning care.

Position the patient

Positioning of the patient on the side with head extended minimises chances of aspiration while the patient remains semiconscious. This is not always practicable, depending on the surgery and the underlying condition of the patient. As they regain awareness, and taking into account the type of surgery done, position for comfort, maintaining correct body alignment to avoid stressing the incision and to increase comfort and relaxation.

Carry out nursing actions indicated during assessment

Check the drains and wound sites for the quantity, quality and nature of drainage. For example, the dressing may have fresh bleeding. If there is a small amount mark the edges with a pen and monitor. If there is a larger amount, reinforce the dressing, report it to the registered nurse and monitor closely.

The surgeon may need to be notified. Haemorrhage is a serious complication. Monitor fluid intake and output to maintain fluid balance. If the patient does not have an indwelling catheter (IDC), ask about the need to void. Anaesthetics and analgesia depress the sensation of bladder fullness. Other drugs used in the theatre may affect the bladder tone temporarily. Palpation of the bladder or assessing bladder volume with a bladder scanner may be required to determine urinary retention. Assess for pain using a 10-point pain scale, and use careful questioning to determine the location and type of the pain. Do not assume that the pain is due to surgical intervention – it may be due to positioning during surgery or to the endotracheal tube or to a previous medical condition (e.g. arthritis). Prescribed analgesia may be administered after determining the status of the vital signs and consulting recovery room notes to determine if analgesia is due. Reassess the patient after the administration of pain-relieving interventions. Failure to reassess results in less than optimal management, and higher levels of pain and discomfort.

Communicate effectively with the patient

Discuss with the patient that you will be checking on them frequently until their condition is stable. This reduces anxiety over frequent checks and increases their sense of wellbeing. Leave the bedrails up and the call bell within reach until all effects of anaesthesia have worn off. Give information to the patient's family since they will also be anxious. Discuss with them the reason for frequent monitoring and the purpose of equipment being used, since unfamiliar sights provoke anxiety. They also need to be aware that the patient will be drowsy for several hours. The family can participate in the patient's care where appropriate.

Monitor the patient

Monitoring of the patient occurs according to facility policy. This can vary between half-hourly observations for 1 hour, followed by hourly observations for 4 hours; or hourly for 4 hours, followed by 4-hourly observations for 24 hours as long as the patient's condition remains stable. Changes in baseline measures can reveal the early onset of complications. Observations include the vital signs, pain levels, dressing/drain assessment, oxygen saturation and fluid status. Other observations are determined by the patient's procedure and condition (e.g. a diabetic patient will require regular/routine BGL measurement).

General postoperative complications can occur immediately or days after surgery, and may include the following:

- *respiratory system* – pneumonia, hypoxia, pulmonary embolism
- *cardiovascular system* – haemorrhage, hypovolaemic shock, thrombophlebitis, embolism

- *gastrointestinal system* – nausea and vomiting, constipation, abdominal distension from paralytic ileus
- *genitourinary system* – urinary retention, urinary tract infection
- *integumentary system* – wound infection, dehiscence, pressure injury
- *nervous system* – pain and postoperative cognitive decline in the elderly
- *endocrine system* – unstable BGLs if the patient is a diabetic.

Complications can occur quickly in the early postoperative period. Monitoring of each of the above assessment criteria is determined by the patient's condition and the surgery performed.

Provide personal hygiene

Providing personal hygiene following surgery is an important comfort measure. Within the first 6 hours postoperatively, change the patient out of theatre clothes and offer a wash. This removes the antiseptic solution and blood, and assists the patient to relax. Pain medication may be required prior to a sponge bath.

Mouth care is essential since anaesthetics and oxygen tend to dry mucous membranes, the patient has been nil by mouth for several hours and various medications used during surgery leave an unpleasant taste in the mouth.

Assist with fluids and nutrition

Fluids and nutrition are necessary to healing and to help the body return to normal functioning. Patients usually return from theatre with an IV cannula in situ for administering fluids until they can tolerate sufficient oral fluids to maintain fluid balance. Postoperative nausea and vomiting may be a problem for a number of patients due to various factors: anaesthetic agents, opiates, hypotension, abdominal surgery, pain and high-risk patients who have a history of postoperative nausea and vomiting. Administer antiemetics as ordered and monitor effectiveness. There may be fluid and dietary restrictions according to the type of surgery performed. Fluids are introduced cautiously, starting with sips of water. Patients then progress to full fluids and onto a normal diet as they tolerate each step. A fluid balance chart is used until the patient is taking oral fluids freely and the voiding pattern has returned to normal. If the patient's condition is unstable or of concern, urinary output is measured hourly. An output of less than 0.5 mL/kg/hr must be reported (Dougherty & Lister, 2015). Fluid balance includes measurement and recording of all fluid intake (IV, blood products, volume expanders, oral, enteral) and output (drainage, vomitus and nasogastric tube [NGT] output as well as urine). A suitable diet is required to promote postoperative recovery.

Assist with elimination of urine and faeces

It is important to monitor the patient for the elimination of urine following surgery. Epidural or spinal anaesthetics contribute to urinary retention. Usually, patients are able to resume voiding in a normal pattern within 6 to 8 hours, if a catheter is not in situ. Depending on the postoperative orders, offer the patient use of a bedpan/bottle, or assist to the toilet if it is 4 to 6 (or more) hours post operation and the patient is stable. If the patient is unable to void, assess the bladder volume using a bladder scanner or palpate the bladder for fullness. Depending on facility policy for volume in the bladder, it may be necessary to catheterise the patient (see **Skill 8.6**). There are many surgical procedures that require the patient to have an IDC, in which case the surgeon will insert it in theatre and order the removal when they feel it is appropriate. With any IDC, care is required during insertion and ongoing care is necessary to minimise the possibility of a bladder infection.

The postoperative patient is at risk of constipation following major surgery due to the combination of fasting, anaesthesia, dehydration and pain relief medication. Patients can also be reluctant to 'bear down/strain' to pass faeces because of the increased incisional pain, and will require assistance to support the incisional site. Oral medications, suppositories or enemas may be ordered. Some surgical procedures (e.g. gastrointestinal tract surgery) have specific protocols for bowel management.

Maintain patient comfort

Comfort is one of the most important aspects of nursing care of the post-surgical patient because pain delays healing. Pain management is paramount. The presence or absence of pain should be assessed each time the vital signs are obtained, whenever the patient reports pain or after interventions to manage the pain. Analgesia is often self-administered by patient-controlled analgesia (PCA), resulting in greater patient comfort. Analgesia may be given IV and, after nausea has diminished, orally. The effect of the analgesia and its administration (e.g. nausea, vomiting, pruritis, sedation and urinary retention) requires assessment and attention. Administration of analgesia is an important aspect of providing comfort but it is not the only intervention that is of assistance. Maintaining comfort may be fostered by splinting of the incision, position changes, massage of cramped muscles, attention to personal hygiene, attention to tubing, meditation or sometimes just by the presence of the nurse. Warmth is a comfort measure immediately following surgery because of the decreased metabolic rate, the low environmental temperature in the theatre, an open body cavity during surgery and the length of the surgical procedure. Warm blankets are usually sufficient to restore normal body temperature.

FURTHER POST-OP CARE

Encourage postoperative activity and exercise

Encouraging postoperative activity and exercise includes turning the patient frequently with their active assistance, reminding and supervising them with their deep breathing/coughing (as indicated) and leg exercises hourly, and assisting the patient to sit out of bed at the earliest opportunity, taking into account the individual's surgery. If the patient is wearing graduated compression stockings or pneumatic boots, monitor the placement of these and the neurovascular status of the patient's legs. Remove the stockings at least daily to clean and inspect the skin. If allowed, ambulation should be encouraged as soon as possible, with the patient increasing the distance walked each time they are up. These nursing actions help to prevent postoperative complications such as thrombosis, embolism and constipation. They also help the patient to become more independent, which raises self-esteem. (All postoperative activity is individual and depends on the patient's condition and the surgery performed.) Knowledge of the surgical site and incision helps the nurse to answer questions, reinforce the surgeon's instructions, assist the patient to splint the incision and perform the most effective exercises.

Provide wound care

Wound healing takes 10 to 14 days after most surgeries. A dressing is usually required to protect the tissue from further injury or contamination. It is the nurse's responsibility to keep the wound clean, assess it for improvement or deterioration and report on its condition to other relevant staff. Dressings are changed as ordered, with many remaining intact for 2 to 3 days. The surgeon will usually wish to inspect the incision when visiting the patient. If the wound dressing is not waterproof, it should be covered with plastic when the patient is showering.

Implement discharge teaching

Discharge teaching commences when the patient enters hospital and is inclusive of the patient's family or significant other. It is dependent on the patient and the surgery performed, as well as the surgeon's protocol and instructions. Instructions about self-care and emergency medical care should be given verbally and reinforced with written material. Discharge teaching should include but not be restricted to:

- guidelines concerning self-care for the specific surgery
- activity and increases in activity
- medication and treatment reviews
- dressing and wound care
- signs of complications and who to contact if they arise
- an appointment for follow-up, with the relevant telephone numbers.

DOCUMENT AND REPORT RELEVANT INFORMATION

Documentation of each nursing assessment and intervention is expected when it occurs. Documentation will be specific for each type of surgery and for each facility – or even each unit within a facility. The documentation will include nursing care plans (or clinical pathways), wound management plan, patient notes, patient observation and response chart, neurovascular observations and a fluid balance chart. Short-stay surgical areas may have more compact forms of documentation.

CASE STUDY

As an enrolled nurse you are working on an acute surgical ward. Your patients include Juan Eduardo, a 67-year-old man who has just returned to the ward following a right total hip replacement. Identify the immediate care (first 6 to 8 hours) you would deliver to Juan when he returns to your ward from the theatre recovery area.

Research this type of surgery and identify the postoperative limitations (e.g. mobility and self-care deficits) this patient will experience during his surgical recovery. Create a nursing care plan for the next 2 days following surgery.

Note: These notes are summaries of the most important points in the assessments/procedures, and are not exhaustive on the subject. The naming of documents or charts may differ from state to state, and facility to facility. In all possible situations the guidelines of the ACSQHC are used when describing national charts or documents (e.g. the ACSQHC Observation and Response Chart is named the Adult Observation and Response Chart in WA, and the Rapid Detection and Response Observation Chart in SA). References of the materials used to compile the information have been supplied. The student is expected to have learned the material surrounding each skill as presented in the references. No single reference is complete on the subject.

CRITICAL THINKING/LIFESPAN

Thinking of the clinical skills discussed in this skill, and the stages of growth and development, what are some of the key components you would need to consider in the following scenarios?

1. James is a 6-year-old boy who had a tonsillectomy that morning, and has been back from theatre for 5 hours. He is crying, and afraid to drink and eat because his throat hurts. He is due for discharge tomorrow morning, provided he can drink fluids and eat food. His mother is concerned.
   a. How will you manage James's need to eat and drink?
   b. Consider his age and how you will assess his pain.
2. Winifred is a 72-year-old woman who is recovering from a general anaesthetic (GA) post major abdominal surgery. She is 1 day postoperative. Her family are concerned because she is confused, disorientated and very different to her normal self. Consider the effects of a GA on the older adult and how you will support this patient and her family.

REFERENCES

Australian Commission on Safety and Quality in Health Care (ACSQHC). (2019). *Communicating for Safety Standard.* https://www.safetyandquality.gov.au/standards/nsqhs-standards/communicating-safety-standard

Dougherty, L. & Lister, S. (eds). (2015). *The Royal Marsden Hospital Manual of Clinical Nursing Procedures* (9th ed.). Oxford: Wiley Blackwell.

RECOMMENDED READINGS

Australian Commission on Safety and Quality in Health Care (ACSQHC). (2020). *Sequence for Putting on and Removing PPE.* https://www.safetyandquality.gov.au/sites/default/files/2020-03/putting_on_and_removing_ppe_diagram_-_march_2020.pdf

Canberra Hospital Health Services. (2018). *Canberra Hospital and Health Services Clinical Procedure Post Operative Handover and Observations – Adult Patients (First 24 hours).* http://www.health.act.gov.au/sites/default/files/2020-02/Post%20Operative%20Handover%20and%20Observations%20-%20Adult%20Patients%20%28First%2024%20hours%29.docx

Joustra, C. & Moloney, A. (2019). *Clinical Placement Manual* (1st ed.). Melbourne: Cengage.

Plowman, E. (2017). A2K: A comprehensive and systematic approach to the physical assessment of postoperative patient. *Australian Nursing and Midwifery Journal*, 24(10), p. 43.

Royal Children's Hospital Melbourne. (2019). *Routine Post Anaesthetic Observation.* https://www.rch.org.au/rchcpg/hospital_clinical_guideline_index/Routine_post_anaesthetic_observation/

WA Country Health Service. (2017). *Pre and Post Procedural Management Clinical Practice Standard.* Government of Western Australia. http://www.wacountry.health.wa.gov.au:443/fileadmin/sections/policies/Managed/Pre_and_Post_Procedural_Management_Clinical_Practice_Standard_TS4KSNFPVEZQ_210_6758.pdf

ESSENTIAL SKILLS COMPETENCY

Postoperative Care

Demonstrates the ability to effectively and safely care for a patient following a theatre experience

Criteria for skill performance	Y	D
(Numbers indicate *Enrolled Nurse Standards for Practice*, 2016)	(Satisfactory)	(Requires development)
1. Identifies indication (8.3, 8.4)		
2. Gathers equipment (1.2, 1.6, 4.4, 6.4, 8.4, 9.4) ■ vital signs equipment ■ other equipment as required		
3. Performs hand hygiene (1.2, 1.4, 1.8, 3.9, 6.4, 9.4)		
4. Assists with transfer to bed area and attaches in situ equipment (1.2, 1.4, 2.7, 3.2, 3.9, 4.4, 6.4, 8.4, 9.4)		
5. Assesses the patient (1.2, 1.4, 3.2, 4.1, 4.2, 4.3, 4.4, 6.4, 7.1, 7.2, 7.3, 8.4, 9.4)		
6. Positions the patient for safety and comfort (1.2, 1.4, 3.2, 3.9, 4.4, 6.1, 6.4, 8.4, 9.4)		
7. Completes required nursing interventions (1.2, 1.4, 3.2, 4.4, 6.1, 6.4, 8.4, 9.4)		
8. Evidence of effective communication; e.g. gives a clear explanation of procedure, gains patient consent (2.1, 2.3, 2.4, 2.5, 6.3)		
9. Monitors the patient according to hospital protocol (1.2, 1.4, 1.8, 3.2, 3.9, 4.1, 4.2, 4.3, 4.4, 6.4, 6.6, 7.1, 7.2, 8.4, 9.4)		
10. Provides personal hygiene (1.2, 1.4, 1.8, 2.3, 2.4, 2.7, 3.2, 3.9, 6.1, 6.3, 8.4, 9.4)		
11. Assists with fluids and nutrition as ordered (1.2, 1.4, 2.1, 3.2, 3.9, 6.1, 6.3, 6.4, 8.4, 9.4)		
12. Assists the patient to resume normal elimination patterns (1.2, 1.4, 2.1, 2.7, 3.2, 3.9, 6.1, 8.4, 9.4)		
13. Maintains comfort including pain relief (1.2, 1.4, 3.2, 6.1, 8.4, 9.4)		
14. Encourages postoperative activity and exercise (1.2, 1.4, 2.1, 3.2, 3.9, 6.1, 6.3, 6.4, 8.4, 9.4)		
15. Provides wound care (1.2, 1.4, 2.3, 2.4, 2.7, 3.2, 3.9, 4.1, 4.2, 7.1, 8.4, 9.4)		
16. Implements discharge teaching (1.2, 1.4, 3.2, 6.3, 7.3, 7.5, 8.4, 9.4)		
17. Documents and reports relevant information (1.2, 1.3, 1.8, 3.2, 5.3, 6.6, 7.1, 7.2, 7.3, 7.4, 7.5)		
18. Demonstrates ability to link theory to practice (8.3, 8.4, 8.5, 9.4)		

Student:

Clinical facilitator: Date:

CHAPTER 8.5

NASOGASTRIC TUBE – GASTRIC DRAINAGE

IDENTIFY INDICATIONS

A nasogastric tube (NGT) is a flexible plastic tube that is inserted through the nostrils, down the nasopharynx and into the patient's stomach or the upper portion of the small intestine. It is used for:

- feeding a patient (PLEASE NOTE: not discussed here; see **Skill 8.12**)
- removing the gastric contents.

  When used to remove gastric contents, it can have a drainage bag or suction apparatus added to decompress or empty the stomach of accumulated gas and fluid. In this situation, it is classified as a gravity drain. It can be inserted after abdominal surgery to decompress the stomach; as part of the non-surgical treatment of a small bowel obstruction; to prevent excess nausea, vomiting or gastric distension; or as part of a gastric lavage to remove substances (e.g. ingested poisons) from a patient's stomach. In these situations the type of tube used is different to a feeding tube, as this type of nasogastric tube (e.g. Ryles tube or Salem Sump tube) has a wider bore to allow easy drainage of fluid from the stomach.

DEMONSTRATE CRITICAL THINKING AND IDENTIFY SAFETY CONSIDERATIONS

It is essential that nurses do not confuse nasogastric tubes used for drainage with nasogastric tubes used to maintain a patient's nutrition and hydration (i.e. nasogastric feeding; see **Skill 8.12**). Aside from visually reviewing the type of tube inserted and any attached drainage bags, check the care plan, patient charts, the doctor's orders and the reason for the tube to be inserted. Review the patient's theatre notes or admission diagnosis, as this will also help to clarify the purpose of the nasogastric tube. Research has demonstrated that all inserted NGT create a risk of aspiration and potential pneumonia, including NGT used for drainage (Fonseca et al., 2013). Review the patient's vital signs or other indicators of respiratory change that may indicate a respiratory infection.

Each skill described as part of the care for gastric drainage via a nasogastric tube is a separate care action. Review the nursing care plan and patient notes to determine which actions are required.

GATHER EQUIPMENT

Gathering equipment before initiating the procedure is part of effective time management for implementing the procedure and provides an opportunity for the nurse to rehearse the procedure mentally.

- *A straight drainage bag* to drain fluid from the stomach. This system works using gravity for drainage.
- *Drainage bag holder.*
- *Personal protective equipment (PPE)* that may be required for this procedure include *gown, mask, eyewear/face shield and plastic apron* and are worn to comply with standard precautions and reduce the infection control risks.
- *Non-sterile, clean measuring jug (500 mL to 1 L).*
- *Alcohol wipe.*
- *The low suction apparatus*, if required, is used to apply suction to decompress the stomach and remove excess fluids and gas without damaging the intestinal mucosa.
- *20 mL syringe and paper cup* for aspirating the tube, if required.
- *An adaptor* may be required to connect the NGT to the drainage bag or other equipment.
- *Tape* is used to secure the NGT in position.
- *Mouth care* – soft toothbrush, toothpaste, water, disposable foam mouth swabs, lip balm.
- *A 'bluey'* keeps the patient and bedclothes clean and dry.

Note: For safety reasons, equipment and disposable items used for giving nasogastric feeds are identified with coloured flanges (e.g. purple or yellow), plungers, tips, and so on. If the tube is inserted as a drain, the tube and other equipment should not have purple colouring.

IMPLEMENT CARE OF GASTRIC DRAINAGE VIA AN NGT

Perform hand hygiene

Perform hand hygiene before touching the patient or the patient's surrounds and prior to any procedure involving patient contact to reduce the possibility of cross-contamination. Hand hygiene is the most effective method of infection control as it removes transient organisms from the hands of the nurse (see **Skill 1.1**).

Give a clear explanation of the procedure and establish therapeutic communication

Introduce yourself, and check you have the correct patient. Discuss the procedure and gain the patient's consent. Giving a clear explanation is required to gain legal consent and to address policy requirements. It will also assist the patient to cooperate with the procedure, allay anxiety and assist in establishing a therapeutic relationship.

Don PPE

PPE requirements will vary according to the care being delivered. Don plastic apron, goggles and non-sterile gloves to reduce the risk of exposure to body fluids.

Care of an NGT with a straight drainage bag

Straight drainage via an NGT uses gravity to drain the gastric contents into a drainage bag and can also be referred to as free drainage. The end of the NGT is connected to a straight drainage bag that is then placed below the level of the patient's stomach. A bag holder (or handles on the top of the bag) is used to hang the bag on the side of the bed (hook the holder on the bottom of the bed rails) and keep the bag off the floor. Gravity will empty the stomach contents into the bag.

Ensure there are no kinks in the tube and that the NGT is not placing tension against the patient's nose. Position the bag or ensure there is adequate tubing so that mobile patients are able to move safely in bed. Move the bag carefully when repositioning the patient to also reduce the risk of dislodging the tube.

Emptying the drainage bag

To empty the drainage bag, don PPE as required. Put a 'bluey' on the floor under the outlet of the drainage bag and place the jug under the outlet. Open the clamp and guide the flow into the jug. When all contents are emptied, close the clamp and wipe the end with an alcohol wipe to remove any residue. The type, colour and amount of drainage is charted on the fluid balance chart and any other facility drainage charts each shift (or more frequently if ordered).

Aspirating the NGT

Some patients may be ordered further aspiration of the tube every 2–4 hours. Don PPE as required. Using a 20 mL syringe, follow the procedure for aspirating the nasogastric tube described in **Skill 8.12**. Use gentle pressure when aspirating the tube, and remove all the fluid that can be removed until resistance is felt. If the syringe becomes full, disconnect from the NGT and empty the contents of the syringe into a disposable cup. Then reconnect the syringe and continue aspirating the tube. When the aspiration is complete, measure and then dispose of the secretions in the sluice. Record and describe the volume removed in the fluid balance chart. If there are any concerns about the type, colour or amount of aspirate obtained, notify the registered nurse or medical staff promptly.

Changing/attaching the drainage bag

The drainage bag should be changed at least daily. Don required PPE, disconnect the nasogastric tube from the old drainage bag. Remove the cap from the new drainage bag and attach to the end of the nasogastric tube. Use a connector if required to help the end attach. Take care not to pull on or dislodge the nasogastric tube during this procedure.

NGT attached to suction

Low-level suction may be ordered for an NGT. Constant suction can potentially damage the lining of the patient's stomach, and the pressure should not be above 20 to 30 mmHg. Alternatively, intermittent low-level suction may be used, as per the doctor's orders. Attach the low-level suction apparatus to the end of the NGT as per the manufacturer's instructions. Drainage bottles should be changed and discarded when they become three-quarters full.

Spigot the NGT

Prior to removing the NGT drain, the drainage bag may be removed and the tube spigoted while the patient commences oral fluids. The cap on the end of the NGT is left in place to close the end of the tube.

Carry out oral hygiene

Oral hygiene should be carried out every 2 to 4 hours for a patient with an NGT drain, after completing the other care. They will not be receiving any oral fluids, and their mouth will be dry. Oral hygiene using a soft toothbrush and toothpaste should be completed at least twice daily (see **Skill 3.5**). Prepackaged foam mouth swabs with water can be used at other times, and are often kept on a tray next to the patient's bed area. Use lip balm to prevent the lips becoming dry and cracked. Regular mouth care will increase patient comfort, remove plaque and reduce the risk of developing halitosis and gingivitis.

Check insertion-site skin integrity

Insertion-site skin integrity around nostrils must be checked regularly for potential pressure injuries and irritation. Replace any loose tape to ensure the NGT does not become dislodged. The nares may need cleansing with a washcloth or normal saline to remove any dried secretions.

Check the position of the NGT

Coughing, and movement in bed can dislodge an NGT. Although no NGT feeds are being administered, there is still an aspiration risk (and consequent pneumonia) with NGT used for drainage. To check that the NGT has not been dislodged, assess the length of the tube at the patient's nares if there are numbered markings on the tube. Alternatively, use a tape measure to measure the external length of the tube. Compare this to the length documented when the tube was inserted. It should remain the same.

Doff PPE

Remove PPE in the following sequence: gloves, hand hygiene, eyewear/face shield, plastic apron/gown and mask and then perform hand hygiene (ACSQHC, 2020). Dispose of in the rubbish bag.

Perform hand hygiene

Maintain the 5 Moments for Hand Hygiene and perform hand hygiene after touching the patient and the patient's surrounds.

CLEAN, REPLACE OR DISPOSE OF EQUIPMENT

Dispose of any gastric secretions in the sluice. Emptied drainage bags can be disposed of in the general waste, according to facility policy. Bags being disposed of without being emptied should be placed in the biological waste. Non-disposable equipment should be wiped over using the facility's disinfecting wipes and returned to their storage area. Tidy and replace any items on the mouth care tray, or any other equipment kept by the patient's bed area for managing the NGT drainage.

DOCUMENT AND REPORT RELEVANT INFORMATION

Drainage and aspirate are recorded on the fluid balance chart. Information about the aspirate and drainage should be included in the shift handover and patient's notes.

CASE STUDY

You are caring for Annie Logan, who has been transferred to the ward from theatre after abdominal surgery. She has an NGT inserted and connected to a drainage bag. Her post-op orders include nil orally and the NGT to be used for straight drainage

1. What does 'NGT to straight drainage' mean?
2. Why are enteral feeds not administered to Annie?
3. Describe how you would empty and then measure the gastric fluid in the drainage bag at the end of the shift.

Note: These notes are summaries of the most important points in the assessments/procedures, and are not exhaustive on the subject. The naming of documents or charts may differ from state to state, and facility to facility. In all possible situations the guidelines of the ACSQHC are used when describing national charts or documents (e.g. the ACSQHC Observation and Response Chart is named the Adult Observation and Response Chart in WA, and the Rapid Detection and Response Observation Chart in SA). References of the materials used to compile the information have been supplied. The student is expected to have learned the material surrounding each skill as presented in the references. No single reference is complete on the subject.

REFERENCES

Australian Commission on Safety and Quality in Health Care (ACSQHC). (2020). *Sequence for Putting on and Removing PPE.* https://www.safetyandquality.gov.au/sites/default/files/2020-03/putting_on_and_removing_ppe_diagram_-_march_2020.pdf

Fonseca, A.L., Schuster, K.M., Maung, A.A., Kaplan, L.J. & Davis, K.A. (2013). Routine nasogastric decompression in small bowel obstruction: Is it really necessary? *The American Surgeon,* 79(4), pp. 422–8.

RECOMMENDED READINGS

Australian Commission on Safety and Quality in Health Care (ACSQHC). (2018). *Selected Best Practices and Suggestions for Improvement for Clinicians and Health System Managers Hospital-Acquired Complication 3 Healthcare Associated Infections.* https://www.safetyandquality.gov.au/sites/default/files/migrated/SAQ7730_HAC_Factsheet_HealthcareAssociatedInfections_LongV2.pdf

Berman, A., Frandsen, G., Snyder, S., Levett-Jones, T., Burston, A., Dwyer, T., Hales, M., Harvey, N., Moxham, L., Langtree, T., Reid-Searl, K., Rolf, F. & Stanley, D. (2020). *Kozier & Erb's*

Fundamentals of Nursing, Volumes 1–3. (5th ed.) Melbourne: Pearson.

Berman, A., Snyder, S., Levett-Jones, T., Burton, T. & Harvey, N. (2021). *Skills in Clinical Nursing* (2nd ed.). Melbourne: Pearson.

Dougherty, L. & Lister, S. (eds). (2015). *The Royal Marsden Hospital Manual of Clinical Nursing Procedures* (9th ed.). Oxford: Wiley-Blackwell.

Gray, S., Ferris, L., White, L.E., Duncan, G. & Baumle, W. (2018). *Foundations of Nursing: Enrolled Nurses* (2nd ANZ ed.). Melbourne: Cengage.

ESSENTIAL SKILLS COMPETENCY

GASTRIC DRAINAGE

Demonstrates the ability to safely and efficiently manage the care of a nasogastric tube (NGT) used for gastric drainage

Criteria for skill performance	Y	D
(Numbers indicate *Enrolled Nurse Standards for Practice*, 2016)	(Satisfactory)	(Requires development)
1. Identifies indication (8.3, 8.4)		
2. Demonstrates problem-solving abilities and safety considerations (4.1, 4.2, 8.3, 8.4, 9.4)		
3. Verifies written order (1.2, 1.4, 3.2, 3.9, 5.5, 9.4)		
4. Gathers equipment (1.2, 1.6, 4.4, 6.4, 8.4, 9.4): ■ 20 mL syringe ■ drainage bag and stand ■ bluey ■ low suction apparatus, if required ■ adaptor ■ PPE as required for this procedure ■ jug and alcohol wipes ■ hypoallergenic tape cut to appropriate length ■ small disposable cup ■ oral hygiene equipment		
5. Performs hand hygiene (1.2, 1.4, 1.8, 3.2, 3.9, 6.4, 9.4)		
6. Demonstrates problem-solving abilities; e.g. provides privacy, comfort measures, pain relief; positions patient (4.1, 4.2, 8.3, 8.4, 9.4)		
7. Monitors gastric output for NGT used as a drain (1.2, 1.4, 3.2, 3.9, 4.4, 6.4, 8.4, 9.4)		
8. Dons protective PPE as required (1.2, 1.4, 1.8, 2.1, 3.2, 3.9, 8.4, 9.4)		
9. Empties or changes drainage bag and records output (1.2, 1.4, 3.2, 3.9, 4.4, 6.4, 8.4, 9.4)		
10. Aspirates the nasogastric tube (1.2, 1.4, 3.2, 3.9, 4.4, 6.4, 8.4, 9.4)		
11. Attaches nasogastric tube to suction (1.2, 1.4, 3.2, 3.9, 4.4, 6.4, 8.4, 9.4)		
12. Spigots nasogastric tube (1.2, 1.4, 3.2, 3.9, 4.4, 6.4, 8.4, 9.4)		
13. Implements oral hygiene 2–4 hourly (1.2, 1.4, 1.8, 2.1, 2.3, 2.4, 2.7, 3.2, 3.9, 6.1, 6.3, 6.6, 8.4, 9.4)		
14. Checks skin integrity of insertion site (1.2, 1.4, 3.2, 3.9, 4.4, 6.4, 8.4, 9.4)		
15. Checks position of the nasogastric tube (1.2, 1.4, 3.2, 3.9, 4.4, 6.4, 8.4, 9.4)		
16. Doffs PPE and performs hand hygiene (1.2, 1.4, 1.8, 3.9, 6.4, 9.4)		
17. Cleans, replaces and disposes of equipment appropriately (1.2, 1.4, 3.9, 6.5, 9.4)		
18. Documents and reports relevant information (1.2, 1.3, 1.8, 3.2, 5.3, 6.6, 7.1, 7.2, 7.3, 7.4, 7.5)		
19. Demonstrates ability to link theory to practice (8.3, 8.4, 8.5, 9.4)		

Student:

Clinical facilitator: Date:

CHAPTER 8.6

CATHETERISATION (URINARY)

IDENTIFY INDICATIONS

Indications for catheterisation of the urinary bladder are for diagnosis (monitoring urine output, obtaining specimen), treatment (urinary obstruction, urinary retention following childbirth or anaesthesia – although portable bladder scanners are more readily available to determine retention without the need for catheterisation) and prevention of complications of the urinary tract associated with surgery or childbirth. Intermittent urinary catheters are inserted to obtain a specimen, and then withdrawn. Indwelling catheters are left in situ so that the urine can drain freely for hours or days at a time.

Catheterisation carries risks and should only be done in the patient's best interest and when necessary. The complications of catheterisation include urinary tract infections (which are the most prevalent cause of hospital-acquired urinary tract infections [ACSQHC, 2018]), mucosal trauma and hydronephrosis. To reduce the infection control risks, and because the procedure will involve touching key parts, a surgical aseptic technique and establishing a critical aseptic field is required.

Continence control is not an indication for urinary catheterisation until all other continence measures have been explored and have failed, and there is a compelling patient reason for catheterising. Some facilities do not allow nurses to catheterise male patients, and generally all nurses are required to complete a skills package and assessment upon commencing employment. Consult the policy and procedure manual or a senior nurse. The indication for male catheterisation should prompt the nurse for possible difficulties such as prostate enlargement.

GATHER EQUIPMENT

Equipment varies in each facility. Some facilities supply a disposable catheterisation pack with all of the requirements except the catheter and sterile gloves included. Others supply a basic pack to which most necessary items need to be added. The following is a list of all the requirements for catheterising the urinary bladder.

- *A sheet* is used to cover the patient during the procedure to reduce the patient's feelings of exposure and maintain the patient's dignity.
- *Non-sterile gloves, a washcloth, warm water and a towel* may be required for the preliminary cleansing of the perineum, if soiled.
- *Personal protective equipment (PPE)* is used as required and as per facility policy.
- *A portable light source* is used to provide sufficient illumination (for female catheterisation) that is not possible in normal room light. If a free-standing light is not available, an assistant will be required to focus a torch on the patient's urethral and perineal area.
- *A waterproof pad ('bluey')* is placed under the buttocks to protect bed linen from being soiled by solutions or urine.

- *Catheterisation or dressing pack.* The inner sterile wrapper provides the sterile field when opened.
- *Forceps* (contained in the dressing pack) are used to hold the gauze swabs during cleansing of the urinary meatus.
- *A rubbish bag* is placed appropriately for disposal of used supplies.
- *Sterile gloves* help prevent the introduction of microorganisms into the urinary tract and maintenance of a surgical aseptic technique within a critical aseptic field.
- *Sterile drapes* are used to extend the critical sterile field and reduce the transfer of microorganisms.
- *A kidney dish* is used to apply solution to the gauze and to act as an initial container for the urine when the catheter is inserted.
- *Gauze swabs and solution* (e.g. normal saline 0.9%) are used to clean the urinary meatus.
- *Lubricant (the type incorporating a local anaesthetic agent)* is spread on the first 5 to 7 cm of the catheter for a female and the first 15 to 20 cm for a male catheterisation. It is also instilled into the urethral

→

meatus using the applicator provided. Dougherty and Lister (2015) highlight that if the anaesthetic lubricating gel is not instilled for at least 4 minutes, it will only have a lubricating effect. They also suggest lignocaine must be used with caution in the elderly, those with cardiac arrhythmias and those with a sensitivity to the drug. The lubricant is sterile and water-soluble.

- *The catheter* is dependent on the type of catheterisation and the size of the patient's urinary tract. The smallest catheter possible should be used (Gilbert et al., 2018; NHMRC, 2019). The most common types are straight catheters used for intermittent catheterisation and indwelling catheters (IDCs), which have an inflatable balloon near their tip so that when the catheter is inserted, the balloon is inflated and will keep the catheter in place. Both straight and indwelling catheters vary in size from French 8 to 10 (usually for children), 10 to 14 (women) and 14 to 18 (men) (Gilbert et al., 2018). It is advisable to have a spare catheter on the trolley.

- *A 10 to 30 mL syringe and sterile water* are used to inflate the IDC balloon after it has been inserted. Balloons come in a variety of sizes, from 5 to 30 mL, with 10 mL or less being preferable. Check the size of the balloon on the catheter you have chosen by checking the balloon port for the stated millilitres to be used.
- *A specimen container* is required if a catheter specimen of urine (CSU) is to be collected. *A patient ID label* is also required, as well as a laboratory requisition form.
- *A urinary collection bag and tubing* are needed if the catheter is an indwelling catheter for the continued collection of urine as it drains.
- *Tape or leg bands* are required for securing an IDC to the leg (if ordered) and to reduce potential trauma to the bladder neck and urethra (Dougherty & Lister, 2015). Nowadays most facilities use commercially produced catheter stabilisation tapes and devices in preference to regular tape.

PREPARING THE PATIENT FOR CATHETERISATION

Perform hand hygiene
Perform hand hygiene before touching the patient or the patient's surrounds and prior to any procedure involving patient contact to reduce the possibility of cross-contamination. Hand hygiene is the most effective method of infection control as it removes transient organisms from the hands of the nurse (see **Skill 1.1**).

Demonstrate problem-solving abilities
Provision of privacy includes closing the room door, putting a 'Procedure in progress' sign in a prominent place and closing the curtains. Interruptions are extremely embarrassing for the patient. Place the sheet over the patient. Determine allergies with latex, adhesive tape or the cleansing solution. Positioning the patient in the dorsal recumbent position with knees bent and abducted provides access to the urinary meatus of the female patient. The male patient should be supine. Placing a 'bluey' under the buttocks eliminates the need to change the bottom sheet if soiling occurs during the procedure. Obtaining assistance if needed indicates forward planning and good assessment skills – some patients need assistance to maintain the position, someone may be needed to hold a light source or another nurse may be required to help calm an anxious patient. Raising the bed to a workable height for the nurse reduces strain on muscles. Place the equipment within easy reach of the nurse's dominant hand, and the rubbish bag in an appropriate position.

Give a clear explanation of the procedure and establish therapeutic communication
Introduce yourself, and check you have the correct patient. Discuss the procedure and gain the patient's consent. Giving a clear explanation is required to gain legal consent and to address policy requirements. It will also assist the patient to cooperate with the procedure, allay anxiety and assist in establishing a therapeutic relationship.

Catheterisation of the urinary bladder is an embarrassing invasion of the body and most patients are psychologically affected by the procedure. They are also often anxious about the cause of the requirement for the procedure – be it diagnostic, treatment or prevention. They may also be exceedingly uncomfortable if the need for catheterisation arises out of urinary retention or obstruction. For these reasons, clear and full explanation of what will happen, why it is necessary and how the patient can help to facilitate the procedure is needed. Keep explanations simple and remember to include the sensations the patient should feel in the explanation. The catheterisation will create a sensation similar to voiding or, albeit rarely, pressure and mild burning, and the sensation will cease or diminish when the catheter is in place. If the patient knows what to expect, anxiety is diminished and trust is increased. This also gives the nurse the opportunity to assess the patient's anxiety level, ability to cooperate and level of mobility, all of which can affect the procedure.

Attend to perineal care
Don non-sterile gloves to clean the perineal area if the patient has been incontinent or if there is excessive discharge.

Adjust the light

Adjust the light for female patients so that the beam is directed at the perineum to help locate the urinary meatus.

PERFORM THE CATHETERISATION

Repeat hand hygiene

Perform hand hygiene again at this stage to reduce the risk of cross-contamination and to maintain an aseptic technique.

Don PPE

PPE requirements will vary according to the care being delivered. Don plastic apron, mask and goggles if required to reduce the risk of exposure to body fluids.

Establish a critical sterile field

Establish a critical sterile field using an aseptic technique (see **Skill 4.1**). Add any sterile supplies that are not in the catheterisation pack, such as the selected catheter. Pour solutions and add lubricant while still maintaining an aseptic technique.

Wash hands and don sterile gloves

Wash hands and don sterile gloves (see **Skill 4.9**). This is a surgical aseptic technique that involves touching key parts and key sites, and maintaining a critical aseptic field (NHMRC, 2019).

Extend the sterile field

Extend the sterile field by placing the sterile drape between the legs. If provided, the fenestrated drape will be placed over the urinary meatus area.

Prepare equipment

Lubricate the catheter to ease insertion. Soak swabs in solution and squeeze until not dripping. While some facilities may still advise the pre-inflation and testing of an indwelling catheter balloon, this process has been found to alter the shape of the catheter tip, potentially leaving a ridge that can cause friction on the urethra (McDevitt & McDevitt, 2015). (If facility policy requires testing the balloon, fill the syringe with air and attach it to the balloon port. Gently insert the air until the capacity of the balloon is reached as indicated on the catheter. Deflate the balloon.) Coil the catheter into the kidney dish with the proximal end within easy reach. Preparation of the field and equipment requires two hands, so it must be completed before the nurse begins cleansing the perineum, which will contaminate the non-dominant hand. Sterile gloved hands should only touch sterile items.

Clean the urinary meatus

Clean the urinary meatus using the chosen solution and gauze swabs held in forceps. For a female patient, spread the labia majora up and outward by placing the thumb and middle finger of your non-dominant hand about midway down the labia. Gently spread your fingers and pull the tissue upward. This promotes the cleansing of the skin folds and meatus, reducing the risk of introducing microorganisms into the urinary meatus. Using one swab for each stroke, cleanse from the labia majora inwards: that is, strokes 1 and 2 are inside the labia majora and downward, strokes 3 and 4 are inside the labia minora and downward, and stroke 5 is around the clitoris and downward over the urinary meatus. Friction and chemical action reduces the bacterial population around the meatus. Keep your hand in place after cleansing, as the labia must remain open until the catheter is inserted to minimise the chance of contamination. Move the kidney dish containing the catheter and lubricating gel to the sterile drape. Insert the nozzle of the lubricating jelly tube into the urethra and squeeze the gel into the urethra. Remove and discard the tube. Wait approximately 5 minutes to allow the anaesthetic to take effect.

For a male patient, hold the penis shaft just below the glans with the non-dominant hand. Gently retract the foreskin if necessary. Using the forceps and swabs, clean the glans in a circular motion from the meatus outwards. Use three swabs to repeat the action three times. Swabbing and chemical action reduces the bacterial population of the meatus. Gently insert the nozzle of the lubricating jelly tube into the urethra and squeeze the gel into the urethra. Remove and discard the tube. Wait approximately 5 minutes to allow the anaesthetic to take effect. The penis is held upright to prevent transfer of microorganisms until the catheter has been inserted. Keep your hand in place after cleansing. If the male patient has an erection, the procedure must be abandoned until the erection has subsided. If this occurs, respond to the situation professionally.

Insert the urinary catheter

Tell the patient that you are ready to insert the catheter, and ask them to take a deep breath and exhale to facilitate sphincter relaxation and minimise irritation. Pick up the tip of the catheter from the kidney dish using the forceps and, as the patient exhales, insert the catheter in the anatomical direction of the urethra (in females, parallel to the bed then slightly downward 5 to 8 cm; in males, towards the abdomen 25 cm). When urine begins to flow into the kidney dish, advance a further 3 to 5 cm to ensure the catheter balloon is entirely in the bladder. Do not force the catheter. In males, changing the angle of the penis may help, while strictures, prostate enlargement or other abnormalities may cause unusual resistance. If a smaller diameter catheter cannot be passed, consult the doctor. In females, if the catheter has been advanced 10 to 12 cm without urine return, it is probably in the vagina. Leave it in place to mark the vaginal opening until catheterisation is successfully completed. If no assistant is available, remove gloves, open another catheter, perform hand hygiene, replace sterile gloves and begin the catheterisation again.

Obtain a sterile specimen of urine if required by allowing several millilitres to drain, then clamping/pinching the catheter and holding the distal end over the specimen jar. If the catheterisation is an intermittent one, allow the urine to drain into the receptacle to complete emptying of the bladder. Tell the patient you are ready to withdraw the catheter, and ask them to take a breath and exhale. As they do, clamp/pinch the catheter and withdraw it in the same direction it was inserted. Place it in the collection basin.

Inflate the balloon if the catheter is indwelling

If an indwelling catheter is being inserted, inflate the balloon by attaching the syringe and inserting the required amount of fluid, as a partially filled balloon may irritate the bladder neck and an over-inflated balloon causes discomfort. Tug gently at the catheter to ensure the catheter is anchored. Remove the fenestrated drape (if used) so that it does not cause difficulties once the collecting bag is attached.

Attach the drainage collection bag and secure

Attach the drainage bag to the catheter, open the clamp and hang the drainage bag on the bed frame. Check that the outflow clamp on the drainage bag is closed. Inform the patient that lying on the tubing impedes the flow of urine, that pulling on the catheter may cause pain and injury, and that raising the level of the collection bag above the level of the bladder may cause problems.

Secure the catheter

Secure the catheter to prevent tension on it and thus the bladder neck as the patient moves. A commercially prepared catheter stabilisation tape or device may be available. Female patients may have their catheter taped to the inner thigh; male patients may have theirs taped to the anterior thigh or to the abdomen. Check hospital policy as to whether or not the catheter is taped. Many facilities supply leg bands that are secured around the thigh and to which the catheter is attached using velcro tapes. Manipulation and movement of

the catheter are a common cause of bladder trauma (Berman et al., 2021; Gilbert et al. 2018).

Clean the perineal area

Clean the perineal area of residual solution and lubricant as a comfort measure.

Doff PPE

Remove PPE in the following sequence: gloves, hand hygiene, eyewear/face shield, plastic apron/gown and mask and then perform hand hygiene (ACSQHC, 2020). Dispose of in the rubbish bag.

CLEAN, REPLACE OR DISPOSE OF EQUIPMENT

The urine specimen container is closed, labelled and sent to the laboratory with appropriate requisitions. Contaminated material is sealed in the disposable plastic bag and disposed of in the appropriate bin. The urine is measured and recorded, and the remaining urine emptied into the sluice. Soiled linen is placed in the laundry bag on the unit.

DOCUMENT AND REPORT RELEVANT INFORMATION

Relevant information including date, time, amount and characteristics of the urine, type and size of catheter used, amount of water in the balloon and the patient's response to the procedure should be recorded on the nursing care plan and progress notes. This validates the care given and provides a progress report of the patient's condition. The date is also used for forward planning if the patient will require a catheter for a long period of time. Some catheters are replaced weekly; some (silastic) need only be replaced monthly, or in some situations every 3 months. Establish a fluid balance chart if necessary and note on the care plan to monitor intake and output.

CASE STUDY

You are caring for Charles Nolan, aged 82 years, who had an indwelling catheter inserted intra-operatively due to his left hip replacement. It is a Foley 16-G catheter, with 10 mL sterile water in the balloon, and drained 180 mL urine post insertion.

Charles is commenced on hourly urine measurement following the insertion of the catheter.

1. Identify where the above information about Charles will be accurately documented.

2. Charles is quite frail and since returning to the ward post-op, appears slightly confused and has frequently 'tugged at' his urinary catheter.
   a. What would you explain to Charles to prevent this from happening?
   b. As his nurse, what other actions will you implement to manage this nursing care need?

Note: These notes are summaries of the most important points in the assessments/procedures, and are not exhaustive on the subject. The naming of documents or charts may differ from state to state, and facility to facility. In all possible situations the guidelines of the ACSQHC are used when describing national charts or documents (e.g. the ACSQHC Observation and Response Chart is named the Adult Observation and Response Chart in WA, and the Rapid Detection and Response Observation Chart in SA). References of the materials used to compile the information have been supplied. The student is expected to have learned the material surrounding each skill as presented in the references. No single reference is complete on the subject.

REFERENCES

Australian Commission on Safety and Quality in Health Care (ACSQHC). (2018). *Selected Best Practices and Suggestions for Improvement for Clinicians and Health System Managers: Hospital-Acquired Complication 3 Healthcare-associated Infections.* https://www.safetyandquality.gov.au/sites/default/files/migrated/SAQ7730_HAC_Factsheet_HealthcareAssociatedInfections_LongV2.pdf

Australian Commission on Safety and Quality in Health Care (ACSQHC). (2020). *Sequence for Putting on and Removing PPE.* https://www.safetyandquality.gov.au/sites/default/files/2020-03/putting_on_and_removing_ppe_diagram_-_march_2020.pdf

Berman, A., Snyder, S., Levett-Jones, T., Burton, T. & Harvey, N. (2021). *Skills in Clinical Nursing* (2nd ed.). Melbourne: Pearson.

Dougherty, L. & Lister, S. (eds). (2015). *The Royal Marsden Hospital Manual of Clinical Nursing Procedures* (9th ed.). Oxford: Wiley-Blackwell.

Gilbert, B., Naidoo, T. & Redwig, F. (2018). Ins and outs of urinary catheters. *Australian Journal of General Practice.* March, 47(3). https://www1.racgp.org.au/ajgp/2018/march/ins-and-outs-of-urinary-catheters

McDevitt, D. & McDevitt, M.F. (2015). 'Yes or no? Pretesting indwelling urinary catheter balloons'. *Nursing Made Incredibly Easy*, 13(6), pp. 14–15.

National Health and Medical Research Council (NHMRC). (2019). *Australian Guidelines for the Prevention and Control of Infection in Healthcare.* https://www.nhmrc.gov.au/health-advice/public-health/preventing-infection

RECOMMENDED READINGS

Berman, A., Frandsen, G., Snyder, S., Levett-Jones, T., Burston, A., Dwyer, T., Hales, M., Harvey, N., Moxham, L., Langtree, T., Reid-Searl, K., Rolf, F. & Stanley, D. (2020). *Kozier & Erb's Fundamentals of Nursing, Volumes 1–3.* (5th ed.) Melbourne: Pearson.

Booth, F. (2014). Principles underlying urinary catheterisation in the community. *Journal of Community Nursing*, 28(5), pp. 72–4, 76–7.

Ferguson, A. (2020). Implementing a CAUTI prevention program in an acute care hospital setting. *Med-Surg Matters.* 29(2), 4–12.

ESSENTIAL SKILLS COMPETENCY

Catheterisation (Urinary)

Demonstrates the ability to effectively and safely catheterise a patient's urinary bladder

Criteria for skill performance (Numbers indicate *Enrolled Nurse Standards for Practice*, 2016)	Y (Satisfactory)	D (Requires development)
1. Identifies indication (8.3, 8.4)		
2. Gathers equipment (1.2, 1.6, 4.4, 6.4, 8.4, 9.4): ■ gloves, non-sterile and sterile ■ PPE as required ■ light source ■ catheterisation or dressing pack (contains multiple items for this procedure) ■ solutions as per policy ■ lubricant ■ syringe and sterile water (if required) ■ collection bag and tubing (if required) ■ absorbent pad or waterproof sheet ('bluey') ■ sheet ■ catheter of appropriate size ■ sterile specimen jar and patient ID label (if required) ■ tape or leg bands/velcro fastener ■ a washcloth, bowl, warm water and a towel ■ rubbish bag		
3. Performs hand hygiene (1.2, 1.4, 1.8, 3.9, 6.4, 9.4)		
4. Demonstrates problem-solving abilities; e.g. provides privacy, warmth, raises bed, positions patient, obtains assistance if needed (4.1, 4.2, 8.3, 8.4, 9.4)		
5. Evidence of effective communication with the patient; e.g. gives patient a clear explanation of procedure, gains consent (2.1, 2.3, 2.4, 2.5, 6.3)		
6. Exposes and cleanses perineal area if required (1.2, 1.4, 2.3, 2.4, 2.7, 3.2, 3.9, 9.4)		
7. Adjusts light (1.2, 9.4)		
8. Performs hand hygiene (1.2, 1.4, 1.8, 3.9, 6.4, 9.4) and dons PPE		
9. Establishes critical sterile field, dons sterile gloves, prepares equipment (1.2, 1.4, 3.2, 3.9, 9.4)		
10. Cleanses urinary meatus (1.2, 1.4, 2.7, 3.2, 9.4)		
11. Inserts urinary catheter (1.2, 1.4, 3.2, 3.9, 4.2, 4.3, 4.9)		
12. Collects urine specimen if required (1.2, 1.4, 3.2, 3.9, 4.2, 4.3, 4.9)		
13. Inflates balloon if catheter is indwelling (1.2, 1.4, 3.2, 8.4, 9.4)		
14. Attaches drainage collection bag (1.2, 1.4, 3.2, 8.4, 9.4)		
15. Secures catheter (1.2, 1.4, 8.4, 9.4)		
16. Cleans perineal area (1.2, 1.4, 2.3, 2.4, 2.7, 3.2, 3.9, 9.4)		
17. Doffs PPE in correct sequence and performs hand hygiene (1.2, 1.4, 1.8, 3.9, 6.4, 9.4)		
18. Cleans, replaces and disposes of equipment appropriately (1.2, 1.4, 3.9, 6.5, 9.4)		
19. Documents and reports relevant information (1.2, 1.3, 3.2, 5.3, 6.6, 7.1, 7.2, 7.3, 7.4, 7.5)		
20. Demonstrates ability to link theory to practice (8.3, 8.4, 8.5, 9.4)		

Student:

Clinical facilitator: Date:

CHAPTER **8.7**

CATHETER CARE (INCLUDING HOURLY URINE MEASUREMENT)

IDENTIFY INDICATIONS

An indwelling urinary catheter (IDC) can be inserted to drain urine (i.e. post-op, urinary obstruction or retention) and for monitoring the urine output or renal function. Reasons for an IDC being inserted include an injury or surgery that limits movement, to manage a urinary obstruction or urinary retention, to monitor unwell patients' renal function, as part of childbirth management or to administer a bladder irrigation. The IDC is left in situ so that the urine can drain freely until the catheter is removed.

Catheterisation carries risks and an IDC should only be inserted in consultation with the doctor; it should not be used as a substitute for other nursing care actions to manage urinary elimination. The complications of catheterisation include urinary tract infection, mucosal trauma (Gilbert, 2018) and hydronephrosis. Catheters are the most prevalent cause of healthcare-acquired urinary tract infections (ACSQHC, 2018). (See **Skill 8.6** for catheter insertion.)

GATHER EQUIPMENT

Equipment required will vary according to the action being implemented.
- *Personal protective equipment (PPE)* – non-sterile gloves, goggles and plastic apron as required, to reduce exposure to body fluids.
- *A waterproof pad* ('bluey').
- *A 10 to 30 mL syringe* used to deflate the IDC balloon before removal. Check the size of the balloon on the catheter by checking the balloon port for the stated millilitres.

- *A sterile urinary collection bag and tubing* for changing the bag.
- *A sterile drainage bag with urinometer* for hourly urine measurement.
- *A drainage bag holder.*
- *Catheter stabilisation tape/dressing* for securing an IDC to the leg (if ordered) and to reduce potential trauma to the bladder neck and urethra.
- *A clean receptacle for emptying the drainage bag* – either a clean urine bottle or clean measuring jug.

CARING FOR A PATIENT WITH AN IDC

Perform hand hygiene
Perform hand hygiene before touching the patient or the patient's surrounds and prior to any procedure involving patient contact to reduce the possibility of cross-contamination. Hand hygiene is the most effective method of infection control as it removes transient organisms from the hands of the nurse (see **Skill 1.1**).

Demonstrate problem-solving abilities
Ensure patient privacy when emptying or changing a catheter bag and assisting with other IDC care. Provision of privacy includes closing the room door and closing the curtains. Interruptions are extremely embarrassing for the patient. There is always a risk of

exposure to body fluids when implementing catheter care, so appropriate PPE should be used.

Give a clear explanation of the procedure and establish therapeutic communication
Introduce yourself, and check you have the correct patient. Discuss the procedure and gain the patient's consent. Giving a clear explanation is required to gain legal consent and to address policy requirements. It will also assist the patient to cooperate with the procedure, allay anxiety and assist in establishing a therapeutic relationship. Discussing the principles of IDC care with the patient will also gain their assistance in reducing the infection risk, reduce trauma from pulling on the tube and also maintain the flow of urine.

Don PPE

PPE requirements will vary according to the care being delivered. Don plastic apron, mask, goggles and non-sterile gloves to reduce the risk of exposure to body fluids.

Reduce infection risks from the IDC

There is always an increased risk of infection and urinary tract infections from an IDC (ACSQHC, 2018, Gilbert, 2018). Ensure the IDC drainage bag is not placed directly on the floor. Use a bag holder or the attachment on the top of the bag to hang the bag on the side of the bed. Hook the holder on the bottom of the bed rails, and keep the bag off the floor (Ferguson, 2020). Ensure that the integrity of the closed sterile drainage system is not compromised. Check that the drainage valve is not open, unless the IDC bag is being drained. Do not disconnect the drainage bag unnecessarily. Also review the need for the IDC to remain in situ. In consultation with the doctor, remove the IDC as soon as clinically indicated. Also monitor the urine output, and perform a urinalysis (see **Skill 3.8**) to identify changes that may indicate a urinary tract infection. If the IDC requires changing, use a surgical aseptic technique (see **Skill 8.6**).

Enable the flow of urine from the IDC

Monitor the flow of urine from the IDC, and check the drainage tube for any loops or kinks that may be obstructing or pooling the urine flow. Position the tube in the bed so that it is below the level of the patient's bladder, but also above the drainage bag, so that gravity will empty the urine into the bag. When a patient is walking or being transported, the drainage bag should still be positioned below the level of the bladder.

Secure the catheter

Secure the IDC with a commercially prepared catheter stabilisation tape or device to prevent tension on the catheter and also the bladder neck when the patient moves. Female patients may have their catheter taped to the inner thigh; male patients may have theirs taped to the anterior thigh or to the abdomen. Some catheter bags come with commercially prepared elasticised bands that are secured around the patient's thigh, with velcro ties to which the catheter can be attached. Check hospital policy as to whether or not the catheter should be taped. Manipulation and movement of the catheter are the most common causes of bladder trauma and consequently of urinary tract infection (Berman et al., 2021; Holroyd, 2019).

Empty the drainage bag

The drainage bag should be emptied each shift, and whenever it is three-quarters full. Specific assessment of fluid volume or urinary output may require more frequent emptying of the bag. Use a clean receptacle (e.g. clean urine bottle or measuring jug) to empty the bag. Place a bluey on the floor under the bag and then don PPE to reduce the risk from the splashing hazard. Place the end of the drainage valve in the receptacle and then open it. Avoid contact between the drainage valve and the receptacle. Allow all the urine to drain and then close the valve. Wipe the end of the valve with an alcohol wipe to remove any residual urine.

The urine is then measured in the dirty utility room, and the volume recorded on the fluid balance chart. If a drainage bag without a valve is being used, then follow the instructions for changing the bag below.

Complete hourly urine measurement

Hourly urine measures are often requested by the doctor for some unwell or post-op patients to assess renal function or closely monitor their fluid balance. A drainage bag with a urinometer enables accurate monitoring of the patient's output each hour, enabling the measurement of small volumes. Urine flows from the catheter tubing and collects in a small cylinder with 1 mL markings. The primary cylinder usually has a maximum volume of 30 to 50 mL (depending on the manufacturer) and there is a backup reservoir (usually marked in 5 mL readings) for any overflow. Precise readings are made in individual mL (e.g. you can measure an output of 3 mL, 12 mL, 37 mL, etc. each hour) and then recorded hourly on the fluid balance chart. Refer to facility guidelines and each patient's specific needs for guidelines in responding to low volumes (oliguria or anuria) recorded each hour.

Ensure the patient has a drainage bag with a 'urinometer', the hourly urine measurement device. If not, change the bag as per the description given later in this skill. Ensure the valve or pinchcock of the urinometer is closed to stop urine draining into the bag. Check the IDC tubing for any kinks and pooled urine to assist the flow into the urinometer. At the same time each hour (i.e. on the hour) the nurse needs to squat down to read the urinometer at eye level. Read the volume in the main cylinder or collection area. If the patient has produced more than the main cylinder capacity, the extra volume will be in the secondary reservoir. The measurements in both areas will be linked (i.e. the volume of the secondary reservoir will start to record from the 30 or 50 mL capacity). When the reading has been obtained, open the valve and allow the urine to flow into the drainage bag. Close the valve to ensure accuracy for reading in the next hour. Record the urine volume on the fluid balance chart.

Removing an IDC

A simple aseptic technique is maintained while removing an IDC. Collect the 20 mL syringe, tissues, non-sterile gloves, goggles, plastic apron, bluey and kidney dish. Place the bluey between the patient's legs and under the IDC. Remove the tape adhering the IDC to the patient's thigh. Do not disconnect the drainage bag.

Perform hand hygiene and then don the non-sterile gloves, plastic apron and goggles to reduce risks from a splashing hazard as the IDC is removed. Attach the 20 mL syringe to the end of the inflation port on the catheter. Maintain the attachment with your fingers (as there will be resistance) and pull back on the syringe to deflate the balloon. When all fluid is removed, disconnect the syringe. Gently pull the IDC and remove it from the patient's bladder. Wipe the urethra with the tissues as there will be residue and moisture around the catheter tips as the catheter is removed. If there is difficulty deflating the balloon or removing the IDC, consult the registered nurse. Do not force the IDC removal with the balloon inflated, or burst the balloon. Both of these actions will cause trauma to the bladder and urethra.

Reposition the patient and educate them about notifying the nurse when they feel the need to pass urine (TOV – trial of void). The patient needs to be monitored for the ability to pass urine within 6 to 8 hours after an IDC is removed and a bladder scan performed immediately post voiding to ensure there is no residual urine in the bladder.

Take the IDC and drainage bag to the dirty utility room to measure the urine in the drainage bag. Dispose of the catheter and drainage bag in the waste, according to facility policy. After removal of the IDC, record in the patient's notes the date, time and volume of urine in the drainage bag. The nursing care plan should also be updated.

Depending on facility policy, the patient will be required to notify staff immediately post voiding (two to three times post removal), so that a bladder scan can be done promptly each time post void. This is to determine if any residual urine remains in their bladder. Record the volume of urine passed and the residual urine remaining post bladder scan on the fluid balance chart and the patient notes (TOV). Follow facility policy for appropriate nursing actions and reporting of residual urine results.

Changing a drainage bag

To limit the breaking of the closed sterile drainage system and prevent bacteriuria, the drainage bag for an IDC is not usually changed unless a different type of drainage bag is required (e.g. hourly urine measure), there is a leak in the tubing or bag, or the IDC is inserted as a long-term catheter. Refer to facility policy for the frequency of changing the bag of an IDC inserted for more than 7 days, as many facilities may replace the bag at the same time as changing the catheter.

Place a bluey under the catheter and between the top of the patient's legs. Remove the catheter from the tape securing it to the patient's thigh or leg. Open the new catheter bag and position the top of the tubing, with the cap intact, on the bluey and within easy access. Wearing non-sterile gloves and goggles, kink the catheter (alternatively a tubing clamp can be used) and then gently slide the tubing connector out of the catheter. Try not to place tension on the catheter to avoid causing trauma to the urethra. Remove the cap from the new drainage bag and slide the tubing connector into the end of the IDC. Re-attach the catheter to the securing tape, and hang the new catheter bag on the side of the patient's bed. Ensure the valve on the bottom of the bag is closed.

Measure and dispose of the contents of the removed bag in the dirty utility room.

Doff PPE

Remove PPE in the following sequence: gloves, hand hygiene, eyewear/face shield, plastic apron/gown and mask and then perform hand hygiene (ACSQHC, 2020). Dispose of in the rubbish bag.

Perform hand hygiene

Maintain the 5 Moments for Hand Hygiene and perform hand hygiene after touching the patient and the patient's surrounds.

CLEAN, REPLACE OR DISPOSE OF EQUIPMENT

Dispose of used items. Non-disposable equipment should be cleaned or wiped over using the facility disinfecting wipes and returned to their storage area. The urine from the drainage bag is measured and recorded, then emptied into the sluice. Removed catheters, tubing and drainage bags can be placed in the general waste. Urine bottles or measuring jugs used to measure urine and empty the catheter bag are sanitised according to the facility policy (e.g. steam sanitiser).

DOCUMENT AND REPORT RELEVANT INFORMATION

Record the volume of urine emptied from a drainage bag on the fluid balance chart. Hourly urine measures are also recorded on the fluid balance chart. Document removal of an IDC in the nursing notes and on the fluid balance chart. Update the nursing care plan for the change in the patient's urinary elimination, and also add the need for TOV following the removal. Note the time and date of removal, plus the time of and volume of the patient's first void and the bladder scan results following the void. Ensure the information about IDC removal and volumes recorded in hourly urine measurement are reported as part of shift handover.

CASE STUDY

You are caring for Krystal Delane, aged 22 years, who had an IDC inserted post-op. It is a Foley 14-G catheter, with 10 mL sterile water in the balloon, and has drained 90 mL urine post insertion. Krystal is commenced on hourly urine measurements following the insertion of the catheter.

1. What position should the IDC bag be placed in while Krystal is in bed?
2. How frequently should you empty the catheter bag?
3. What type of catheter bag will be required to complete this nursing action?

4. Where will you position the catheter bag to read the urine excreted each hour?
   Krystal's IDC has been ordered to be removed on day 2 post-op.
5. Why would the IDC have been removed so quickly?
6. How much water will you expect to withdraw from the balloon before removing the IDC?
7. Where will you record the removal of the IDC?
8. Krystal is required to do a TOV post removal. Explain what is meant by TOV.

Note: These notes are summaries of the most important points in the assessments/procedures, and are not exhaustive on the subject. The naming of documents or charts may differ from state to state, and facility to facility. In all possible situations the guidelines of the ACSQHC are used when describing national charts or documents (e.g. the ACSQHC Observation and Response Chart is named the Adult Observation and Response Chart in WA, and the Rapid Detection and Response Observation Chart in SA). References of the materials used to compile the information have been supplied. The student is expected to have learned the material surrounding each skill as presented in the references. No single reference is complete on the subject.

CRITICAL THINKING

Thinking of the clinical skills discussed, reflect on and answer the following questions.
Catheter-acquired urinary tract infections are the most prevalent of hospital-acquired urinary tract infections.
1. What is the effect of a hospital-acquired infection on the patient?
2. What impact can this have on the patient and the hospital?

REFERENCES

Australian Commission on Safety and Quality in Health Care (ACSQHC). (2018). *Selected Best Practices and Suggestions for Improvement for Clinicians and Health System Managers: Hospital-acquired Complication 3 Healthcare-associated Infections.* https://www.safetyandquality.gov.au/sites/default/files/migrated/SAQ7730_HAC_Factsheet_HealthcareAssociatedInfections_LongV2.pdf

Australian Commission on Safety and Quality in Health Care (ACSQHC). (2020). *Sequence for Putting on and Removing PPE.* https://www.safetyandquality.gov.au/sites/default/files/2020-03/putting_on_and_removing_ppe_diagram_-_march_2020.pdf

Berman, A., Snyder, S., Levett-Jones, T., Burton, T. & Harvey, N. (2021). *Skills in Clinical Nursing* (2nd ed.). Melbourne: Pearson.

Ferguson, A. (2020). Implementing a CAUTI Prevention Program in an Acute Care Hospital Setting. *Med-Surg Matters*, 29(2), pp. 4–12.

Gilbert, B., Naidoo, T. & Redwig, F. (2018). Ins and outs of urinary catheters. *Australian Journal of General Practice*, March, 47(3). https://www1.racgp.org.au/ajgp/2018/march/ins-and-outs-of-urinary-catheters

Holroyd S. (2019). The importance of indwelling urinary catheter securement. *British Journal of Nursing*, 28(15), pp. 976–7.

RECOMMENDED READINGS

Dougherty, L. & Lister, S. (eds). (2015). *The Royal Marsden Hospital Manual of Clinical Nursing Procedures* (9th ed). Oxford: Wiley-Blackwell.

CNA Training Advisor. (2018). Urinary catheter care. *Lesson Plans for Busy Staff Trainers*, 16(11), pp. 1–6.

ESSENTIAL SKILLS COMPETENCY

Care of an Indwelling Urinary Catheter

Demonstrates the ability to effectively and safely care for a patient with an IDC

Criteria for skill performance	Y	D
(Numbers indicate *Enrolled Nurse Standards for Practice*, 2016)	(Satisfactory)	(Requires development)
1. Identifies indication (8.3, 8.4)		
2. Gathers equipment (1.2, 1.6, 4.4, 6.4, 8.4, 9.4): ■ PPE – non-sterile gloves, goggles and plastic apron ■ waterproof pad ('bluey') ■ 10–30 mL syringe ■ sterile urinary collection bag and tubing or sterile drainage bag with urinometer ■ drainage bag holder ■ catheter stabilisation tape/dressing ■ urine bottle or jug with volume measurement for emptying the drainage bag		
3. Performs hand hygiene and dons PPE (1.2, 1.4, 1.8, 3.9, 6.4, 9.4)		
4. Demonstrates problem-solving abilities (4.1, 4.2, 8.3, 8.4, 9.4)		
5. Evidence of effective therapeutic communication with the patient; gives patient a clear explanation of procedure and confirms patient understanding, gains patient consent (2.1, 2.3, 2.4, 2.5, 6.3)		
6. Reduces infection risks from the IDC (i.e. ensures drainage bag is not on the floor, maintains closed drainage system) (1.2, 1.4, 1.8, 3.2, 3.9, 4.4, 6.4, 8.4, 9.4)		
7. Checks tube for kinks and ensures flow of urine to drainage bag; hangs drainage bag from bed or on bag holder. (1.2, 1.4, 3.2, 8.4, 9.4)		
8. Secures catheter to patient's thigh or as per policy (1.2, 1.4, 8.4, 9.4)		
9. Empties drainage bag ■ performs hand hygiene ■ wearing PPE ■ measures urine ■ disposes of urine correctly ■ documents volume on fluid balance chart (1.2, 1.4, 3.2, 8.4, 9.4)		
10. Completes hourly urine measurement correctly (1.2, 1.4, 3.2, 8.4, 9.4)		
11. Removes IDC ■ performs hand hygiene ■ wearing PPE ■ loosens catheter stabilisation tape ■ deflates balloon ■ gently removes catheter ■ measures urine volume in bag and records on fluid balance chart ■ notes time of removal and time of patient's next void ■ completes bladder scan (and documents) after first void (1.2, 1.4, 3.2, 8.4, 9.4)		
12. Doffs PPE in correct order and performs hand hygiene (1.2, 1.4, 1.8, 3.2, 3.9, 6.4, 9.4)		
13. Cleans, replaces and disposes of equipment appropriately (1.2, 1.4, 3.9, 6.5, 9.4)		
14. Documents and reports relevant information (1.2, 1.3, 3.2, 5.3, 6.6, 7.1, 7.2, 7.3, 7.4, 7.5)		
15. Demonstrates ability to link theory to practice (8.3, 8.4, 8.5, 9.4)		

Student:

Clinical facilitator: Date:

CHAPTER 8.8

SUCTIONING OF ORAL CAVITY

IDENTIFY INDICATIONS

Suctioning is the aspiration of fluids and secretions through a tube using negative pressure. As part of airway management, oral suctioning involves removing mucus from the oral cavity when patients are unable to effectively do so for themselves and improves the integrity of their airway (Miller et al., 2020). It is only done as needed because it can cause trauma to the airway or hypoxaemia, and distress to the patient. Risk factors that prevent the patient from protecting their own airway often indicate the need for suctioning – impaired cough ability, impaired gag reflex, decreased levels of consciousness and difficulty swallowing.

DEMONSTRATE PROBLEM-SOLVING ABILITIES

- *Assessment.* The decision to suction the patient at any time is made on analysis of a systematic and thorough respiratory assessment. Observe for signs and symptoms of upper and lower airway obstruction: gurgling noises on inspiration or expiration, excess oral or nasal secretions, sputum (amount, colour and consistency), vomitus in the mouth and coughing without clearing the airway. Knowledge of the patient's medical condition and history is important since some conditions (e.g. chronic pulmonary diseases, stroke) place the patient at risk for airway obstruction. Knowledge of the respiratory assessments over the past 24 hours can help distinguish an acute episode from a chronic deterioration of condition.

- *Positioning.* Suctioning can be accomplished in any position; however, patients are often more comfortable in semi-upright or upright position because of difficulty with breathing. Their head should be turned towards the nurse to facilitate insertion of the catheter. Sometimes, patients will benefit from other measures such as postural drainage, chest percussion, assistance with coughing or ordered medications such as bronchodilators, expectorants, narcotics or antihistamines. Consideration of other appropriate measures also displays problem-solving abilities.

GATHER AND PREPARE EQUIPMENT

Gathering equipment is a time-management strategy. Knowledge of and experience with the set-up and use of suctioning equipment prior to actual use on a patient is essential. Many types of each piece of equipment are available. Familiarise yourself with the equipment available at the facility in which you are working. Test all equipment before use for safe nursing care. The equipment needed is as follows.

- *The suctioning apparatus* is the wall unit or portable machine with regulator that produces a vacuum, which is the negative pressure used to suction (Berman et al., 2021). The regulator can be set to various amounts of negative pressure. The suction apparatus includes a disposable closed-system receptacle to contain the secretions collected. When in use, the receptacle should be changed at least every shift, or when three-quarters full, although it may need to be more frequent depending on the amount of suctioning required.

- *Suction tubing* attaches the catheter to the vacuum machine and needs to be about 2 m long to accommodate position changes and manipulation during the procedure. Attach one end to the suction apparatus and place the other end close to the patient.

- *The sterile Y suction catheter* is a soft flexible tube used to access the oral cavity. It has one or more openings in the distal end, and a thumb port on the side of the proximal end to control the application and amount of suction. Suction catheters vary in size and include French 5 to 8 (for infants), 8 to 10 (usually for children under 10 years of age and for the frail elderly) and 12 to 18 (generally recommended for adults). The use of a catheter that is too large can cause trauma and hypoxaemia, and one that is too small is ineffective.

- *Yankauer suction catheters* are rigid angled plastic suction catheters that have one large hole at the distal end for removing secretions. This type is used when secretions are copious, thick and viscous, or for vomitus. As it is a large size, the Yankauer catheter is used for the oral cavity only.
- A *small bowl/cup of water (or bottle of sterile water)* is used between suction passes to clear the tubing of tenacious secretions and therefore increase the efficiency of the suctioning. It also lubricates the tip of the catheter to ease passage.

- *Non-sterile gloves* are used to reduce the transmission of microorganisms and to protect the nurse from bodily secretions.
- A *plastic apron* is worn to protect the nurse from possible splashes of body secretions.
- *Goggles* (eye protection) are worn to protect the eyes from splashes of body fluids during excessive coughing or sneezing during the procedure. *A face shield* covering the nose and mouth of the nurse may also be required.
- A *waterproof sheet ('bluey')* may be placed on the patient's chest and pillow to protect the bed linen and clothing from soiling with secretions.
- A *large rubbish bag* is taped to the side of the bed or to the locker so that it is within easy reach for discarding the used disposable suction equipment.

IMPLEMENT ORAL SUCTIONING

Perform hand hygiene

Perform hand hygiene before touching the patient or the patient's surrounds and prior to any procedure involving patient contact to reduce the possibility of cross-contamination. Hand hygiene is the most effective method of infection control as it removes transient organisms from the hands of the nurse (see **Skill 1.1**).

Give a clear explanation of the procedure and establish therapeutic communication

Introduce yourself to the patient, check you have the correct patient and gain the patient's consent. Give a clear explanation to the patient of the purpose of the procedure and the sensations that will be felt. This reduces anxiety (which is generally high because of the difficulty in breathing) and gains the patient's cooperation. Patients need to be told that they may sneeze, gag or cough for a short while during or after the procedure. Checking the patient and gaining their consent will also ensure that you meet legal and policy requirements before implementing any procedures.

Don personal protective equipment (PPE)

PPE requirements will vary according to the care being delivered. Don plastic apron, goggles and non-sterile gloves to reduce the risk of exposure to body fluids.

Attach suction tubing and catheter

Attach suction tubing to the device. Peel back the plastic wrapper to expose the connector end of the catheter. Join the catheter to the suction tubing. Remove the outer wrap and maintain a firm hold on the suction catheter by the inner plastic sleeve. This procedure involves the touching of key parts, so a micro-aseptic field is established with the

suction catheter. Do not allow the tip to become contaminated prior to being inserted and used to suction the patient.

Turn the suction device on

Turn the suction device on and set the regulator to the appropriate setting. Dip the distal end of the catheter into the water and apply suction by occluding the proximal port with the thumb to test the equipment and lubricate the tip. Release the suction.

Remove patient's oxygen mask

Remove oxygen mask and turn off oxygen, if the patient has a mask in situ. If a nasal cannula is in situ, no need to remove.

Apply suction

Insert the catheter into the oral cavity and then apply suction by occluding the suction port. Slowly and gently move the catheter in the mouth. Apply suction for 5- to 10-second intervals. Allow the patient to rest for 30 seconds between suctioning. If there are copious or thick secretions, change the catheter and flush the tubing with water, by briefly dipping the end of the tubing in the sterile water. The entire process should last less than 2 to 3 minutes to avoid tiring the patient, increasing secretions or decreasing the oxygen supply. Reassess the patient to determine the success of intervention. Replace the oxygen mask. Disconnect the suction tubing and dispose of the catheter in the rubbish bag. Dip the end of the suction tubing in the water, apply suction and flush the tube. Turn off the suction and connect a fresh catheter (in its wrapper) to the tube.

If a Yankauer sucker is being used, follow a similar process inserting the sucker gently into the patient's mouth. When suctioning is completed, flush the sucker with the sterile water and replace. Suction bottles are disposed of intact into the contaminated rubbish while wearing PPE.

Doff PPE

Remove PPE in the following sequence: gloves, hand hygiene, eyewear/face shield, plastic apron/gown and mask and then perform hand hygiene (ACSQHC, 2020). Dispose of in the rubbish bag.

Perform hand hygiene

Maintain the 5 Moments for Hand Hygiene and perform hand hygiene after touching the patient and the patient's surrounds.

CLEAN, REPLACE OR DISPOSE OF EQUIPMENT

Replace all used equipment to ensure an adequate supply when the patient requires suctioning again.

DOCUMENT AND REPORT RELEVANT INFORMATION

Document the frequency of suctioning and any abnormalities in the patient's notes and care plan.

CASE STUDY

Review different medical conditions and patient health problems (e.g. specific respiratory conditions, unconscious patients, postoperative patients, emergency scenarios) that might cause excess respiratory secretions and create the need for oral suctioning.

List these conditions and explain how oral suctioning will relieve their symptoms and create patient comfort and/ or safety.

Note: These notes are summaries of the most important points in the assessments/procedures, and are not exhaustive on the subject. The naming of documents or charts may differ from state to state, and facility to facility. In all possible situations the guidelines of the ACSQHC are used when describing national charts or documents (e.g. the ACSQHC Observation and Response Chart is named the Adult Observation and Response Chart in WA, and the Rapid Detection and Response Observation Chart in SA). References of the materials used to compile the information have been supplied. The student is expected to have learned the material surrounding each skill as presented in the references. No single reference is complete on the subject.

CRITICAL THINKING

Thinking of the clinical skills discussed in this skill, what are some of the key components you would need to consider in the following scenario?

You are suctioning an 81-year-old patient's mouth using a Yankauer sucker. When removing the sucker, you observe fresh/ frank blood on the end of the sucker. How will you proceed after this finding?

REFERENCES

Australian Commission on Safety and Quality in Health Care (ACSQHC). (2020). *Sequence for Putting on and Removing PPE.* https://www.safetyandquality.gov.au/sites/default/files/2020-03/putting_on_and_removing_ppe_diagram_-_march_2020.pdf

Berman, A., Snyder, S., Levett-Jones, T., Burton, T. & Harvey, N. (2021). *Skills in Clinical Nursing* (2nd ed.). Melbourne: Pearson.

Miller, E., Brooks, D. & Mori, B. (2020). Using expert consensus to develop a tool to assess physical therapists' knowledge, skills, and judgement in performing airway suctioning. *Physiotherapy Canada,* 72(2), pp. 137–46.

RECOMMENDED READINGS

Berman, A., Frandsen, G., Snyder, S., Levett-Jones, T., Burston, A., Dwyer, T., Hales, M., Harvey, N., Moxham, L., Langtree, T., Reid-Searl, K., Rolf, F. & Stanley, D. (2020). *Kozier & Erb's Fundamentals of Nursing, Volumes 1–3.* (5th ed.) Melbourne: Pearson.

Dougherty, L. & Lister, S. (eds). (2015). *The Royal Marsden Hospital Manual of Clinical Nursing Procedures* (9th ed.). Oxford: Wiley-Blackwell.

Smith, S.F., Duell, D.J., Martin, B.C., Gonzalez, L., & Aebersold, M. (2017). *Clinical Nursing Skills: Basic to Advanced Skills* (9th ed.). Upper Saddle River, NJ: Pearson Prentice Hall.

Tandon, V. & Raheja, A. (2020). Modified suction apparatus to reduce the transmission risk of COVID-19 among healthcare providers. *Neurology India,* 68(5), pp. 1170–1.

ESSENTIAL SKILLS COMPETENCY

Suctioning of the Oral Cavity

Demonstrates the ability to effectively and safely suction the oral cavity of a patient

Criteria for skill performance	Y	D
(Numbers indicate *Enrolled Nurse Standards for Practice*, 2016)	(Satisfactory)	(Requires development)
1. Identifies indication (8.3, 8.4)		
2. Demonstrates problem-solving abilities; e.g. assesses the patient, positions the patient (4.1, 4.2, 8.3, 8.4, 8.5, 9.4)		
3. Gathers equipment (1.2, 1.6, 4.4, 6.4, 8.4, 9.4): ■ suction apparatus and tubing ■ suction catheters ■ small bowl/cup with water ■ non-sterile gloves, goggles/face shield, plastic apron, 'bluey', rubbish bag		
4. Performs hand hygiene (1.2, 1.4, 1.8, 3.9, 6.4, 9.4)		
5. Evidence of effective communication with the patient; e.g. gives patient a clear explanation of procedure, gains patient consent (2.1, 2.3, 2.4, 2.5, 6.3)		
6. Dons PPE in appropriate order (1.2, 1.4, 1.8, 3.2, 3.9, 6.4, 9.4)		
7. Turns suction device on and sets regulator to desired setting (1.2, 1.4, 3.2, 4.4, 6.4, 8.4, 9.4)		
8. Attaches catheter tip to suction tubing (1.2, 1.4, 1.8, 3.2, 4.4, 6.4, 8.4, 9.4)		
9. Enters oral cavity (1.2, 1.4, 1.8, 3.2, 3.9, 4.4, 6.4, 8.4, 9.4)		
10. Applies suction 5–10 seconds at a time (1.2, 1.4, 1.8, 3.2, 3.9, 4.4, 6.4, 8.4, 9.4)		
11. Doffs PPE in correct sequence and performs hand hygiene (1.2, 1.4, 1.8, 3.9, 6.4, 9.4)		
12. Cleans, replaces and disposes of equipment appropriately (1.2, 1.4, 3.9, 6.5, 9.4)		
13. Documents and reports relevant information (1.2, 1.3, 1.8, 3.2, 5.3, 6.6, 7.1, 7.2, 7.3, 7.4, 7.5)		
14. Demonstrates ability to link theory to practice (8.3, 8.4, 8.5, 9.4)		

Student:

Clinical facilitator:　　　　　　　　　　　　　　　　　　　　　　Date:

CHAPTER 8.9

TRACHEOSTOMY CARE

IDENTIFY INDICATIONS

A tracheostomy is the surgical creation of a stoma in the upper airway to facilitate airway management. Within this stoma, a tracheostomy tube is inserted. It may be carried out to bypass any upper respiratory tract obstruction or trauma, or in patients requiring long-term ventilation (Dougherty & Lister, 2015). It is generally a temporary measure. Tracheostomy care maintains airway patency by removing dried secretions. It keeps the skin around the site clean to help prevent infections of the stoma site and lower airway, and to prevent skin breakdown. Tracheostomy suctioning is an advanced skill for the enrolled nurse (EN).

Tracheostomy tubes are chosen individually for each patient and vary in their composition, number of parts, shape and size. The diameter should be smaller than the trachea so it lies comfortably in the lumen. The length and curve are important so that dislodgement during coughing or head turning is avoided. The tube may be cuffed or uncuffed. A cuff seals the space between the trachea and tube, allowing for mechanical ventilation. Long-term tracheostomy tubes have three parts: an inner cannula (smooth tube with the locking device), an outer cannula (with a flange, cuff and pilot tube) and an obturator (with a round smooth tip to facilitate non-traumatic insertion of the tube). Short-term tracheostomy tubes usually consist of a single, cuffed tube. Tracheostomy tubes come in disposable non-reactive plastics, or permanent stainless steel and sterling silver.

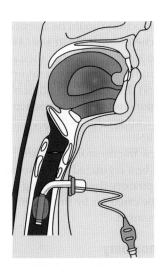

FIGURE 8.9.1 An inserted tracheostomy tube with the cuff inflated

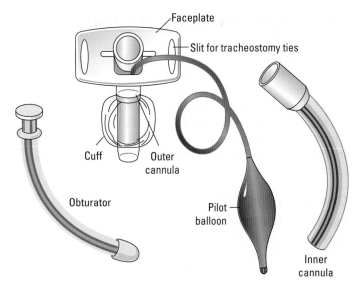

FIGURE 8.9.2 Tracheostomy tube parts

REVIEW PROBLEMS ENCOUNTERED WITH TRACHEOSTOMIES

Bleeding is a common problem immediately following insertion of the tracheostomy. Frequent assessment and dressing changes are required. Infection is also a common problem in tracheostomy stomas. A standard aseptic technique must be employed when cleansing the stoma or suctioning the trachea.

Gloves, eye protection and a plastic apron should be worn when suctioning or providing other tracheostomy care due to the high risk of contact with body secretions. A mask may also be required if there is a high risk of airborne or droplet infection. Accidental de-cannulation or dislodgement of the tracheostomy tube is possible and constitutes a medical emergency. Tracheostomy tube occlusion can occur from (usually) dried secretions. Frequent tracheostomy care, ample fluids and humidification of the air help to prevent this respiratory emergency. Communication can be a problem because the vocal cords are above the level of the tracheostomy tube. This means the patient cannot use speech. Frustration can be avoided if non-verbal strategies such as paper and pencil are used to facilitate communication. Electronic computer-type devices are also available. There are some specialised tracheostomy tubes that

make speech possible. Altered body image is also a large problem for patients who have a tracheostomy, since the stoma may be perceived as disfiguring. Fear and anxiety about the inability to speak or breathe normally will also occur. If the tracheostomy is temporary, reassurance that the ability to breathe and to speak will return post removal and that the incision will heal completely may help the patient to better accept the situation.

GATHER AND PREPARE EQUIPMENT

- *Sterile dressing pack* with gauze swabs (lint free). Most areas use a commercially prepared tracheostomy pack that includes tracheostomy ties (usually with velcro), the tracheostomy dressing and cotton tip applicators.
- *Tracheostomy dressing.* A commercial tracheostomy dressing is used because cutting gauze squares can cause frayed cotton fibres that could be aspirated into the trachea.
- *Normal saline 0.9%* is used to loosen and remove secretions from the inner cannula and around the stoma site.
- *Sterile cotton-tipped applicators* and extra gauze swabs are used to help cleanse around the stoma site.
- *Scissors* are used to cut the tracheostomy ties.
- *Personal protective equipment (PPE)* for suctioning the tracheostomy and when completing other

tracheostomy care. Non-sterile gloves are used, along with a plastic apron and goggles to reduce the risk of contamination from body fluids when the patient coughs. A mask may also be required.
- *Sterile gloves* are used to protect the patient from the nurse's microorganisms when performing a tracheostomy dressing. *Tracheostomy ties* are needed – twill tape or foam tape with velcro fasteners (prepackaged), if not in commercially prepared pack.
- *Tracheostomy suction supplies.*
- A *'Swedish nose'* is a filter/humidifier that is placed over the tracheostomy.
Note: Depending on the facility policy and requirements, the patient should have the following at the bedside: *two tracheostomy tubes* (one the size in situ and one smaller), *tracheostomy dilators, water-based lubricant and a 10 mL syringe.* This equipment should be verified at the beginning of each shift.

IMPLEMENT TRACHEOSTOMY CARE

Perform hand hygiene
Perform hand hygiene before touching the patient or the patient's surrounds and prior to any procedure involving patient contact to reduce the possibility of cross-contamination. Hand hygiene is the most effective method of infection control as it removes transient organisms from the hands of the nurse (see **Skill 1.1**).

Give a clear explanation of the procedure and establish therapeutic communication
Introduce yourself, and check you have the correct patient. Discuss the procedure and gain the patient's consent (if able). Giving a clear explanation is required to gain legal consent and to address policy requirements. It will also assist the patient to cooperate with the procedure, allay anxiety and assist in establishing a therapeutic relationship.

Don PPE
PPE requirements will vary according to the care being delivered. Don plastic apron, goggles and non-sterile gloves to reduce the risk of exposure to body fluids.

Assess the patient
The patient must be assessed for secretions around the stoma, within the trachea and on the dressing. The

respiratory status of the patient should be assessed. Factors that influence tracheal care such as hydration and the presence of infection should be assessed. Know the type of tracheostomy tube in situ. Assess the patient's ability to learn to look after their own tracheostomy. Position the patient in a semi-upright position (depending on the patient's condition) to facilitate lung expansion and make the tracheostomy area more accessible. Cuff pressure will be checked by the registered nurse (RN).

Note: Care of a new tracheostomy is a two-person procedure. One must be a registered professional (such as an RN or respiratory therapist). Long-term tracheostomies may be cared for by the patient or by suitably qualified personnel.

Suction the tracheostomy
Tracheostomy suctioning should be completed prior to a dressing change, or whenever the patient requires assistance to clear secretions from the tracheostomy tube, including audible or visible secretions (Patton, 2019). Regular suctioning is required for patients with a tracheostomy, as they produce large amounts of secretions that can easily block the tube. Tracheostomy suctioning will be completed by an RN or an advanced skills EN. To suction a tracheostomy, non-sterile gloves, a plastic apron and protective eye wear should be worn. To prevent the introduction of microorganisms to the patient an aseptic technique

should be used, and a micro-aseptic field maintained as key parts will be touched.

Turn on the suction at the wall and test by dipping the end of the suction tube in sterile water. Attach a fresh suction catheter to the suction tubing. Lubricate the end with sterile water. Holding the catheter by the small plastic sterile sleeve, insert gently into the tracheostomy tube approximately 5 to 10 cm. Cover the air hole on the catheter, and apply suction while withdrawing the suction cannula. Suction should not be applied for more than 10 seconds. Withdraw the suction catheter and discard in the waste. If further suctioning is required, a new suction catheter should be attached.

Flush the suction tubing with sterile water and then turn off the suction. Complete correct sequence for doffing PPE, and discard of PPE in the rubbish if no further patient care actions are required. Remove and dispose of gloves.

Repeat hand hygiene
Perform hand hygiene again at this stage to reduce the risk of cross-contamination and to maintain an aseptic technique.

IMPLEMENT A TRACHEOSTOMY DRESSING

Prepare the tracheostomy aseptic field
Use an aseptic technique to prepare a general aseptic field (see **Skills 4.1** and **4.2**). Add the normal saline to the basin and pre-moisten the gauze swabs. Open several (depending on the amount of secretions around the stoma) sterile cotton tip applicators. Open the tracheostomy dressing and tracheostomy ties.

Remove the old dressing
The student EN may assist the RN or advanced skills EN. Put on non-sterile gloves to remove the dressing and Swedish nose (if in place). If the patient is on oxygen, place the oxygen and humidification sources near the stoma and ask the patient to deep breathe while the dressing is removed.

Changing the inner cannula is usually done by an RN.

Repeat hand hygiene
Perform hand hygiene again at this stage to reduce the risk of cross-contamination and to maintain an aseptic technique.

Cleanse and dry the stoma
Put on sterile gloves using an open gloving technique (see **Skill 4.9**). Using cotton tip applicators dipped in normal saline and moistened gauze swabs (use forceps to hold the gauze swabs), gently but firmly remove secretions from around the stoma. Clean any dried secretions from underneath as well as the exposed outer cannula surfaces. Maintaining an aseptic technique, use the dry gauze swabs to dry the skin,

since moist surfaces promote skin excoriation and bacterial growth. Inspect the stoma site.

Redress the stoma site
Carefully slide a dry, sterile slit tracheostomy dressing under the flange and around the stoma. If necessary, use the forceps to help ease it into position. Replace the oxygen and Swedish nose/humidification source if required.

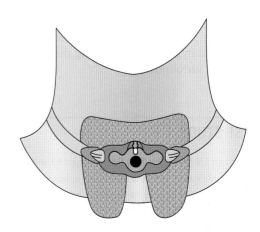

FIGURE 8.9.3 Tracheostomy with dressing and ties

Change the tracheostomy ties
Hospital policy will determine the protocol for when the ties are changed, but it is usually completed daily. Smith, Duell and Martin (2017) advocate leaving the old ties in place until the new ties are tied. The old ties should be carefully cut and removed after the new ties are securely attached. Alternatively, a second nurse can assist by holding the tracheostomy tube in place while the ties are removed and new ones attached (Credland, 2016; Russell et al., 2019).

Thread one end of the tie through one of the flange holes and pull it three-quarters through. Pass the long end behind the patient's neck and through the opposite flange hole. Again, bring the long free end back around the patient's neck. Join the velcro ends together at the side of the patient's neck. Ensure the ties are tight enough to allow one finger between the tie and the neck to prevent accidental dislodgement of the tracheostomy tube but still be comfortable and not apply pressure on the jugular veins. Cut off the old ties. Remove and discard PPE following correct doffing procedure if no further care actions are required.

Repeat hand hygiene
Perform hand hygiene again at this stage to reduce the risk of cross-contamination and to maintain an aseptic technique.

Provide oral hygiene
This is both a hygiene and a comfort measure. Since there is no air passage through the mouth on a regular basis, secretions become stale and the mouth becomes dry and foul tasting. Oral hygiene also reduces the risk of aspiration pneumonia. Due to the high risk of infection from the tracheostomy secretions, PPE

of gloves, goggles and plastic apron should be worn when implementing oral hygiene care.

Doffing of PPE

Remove PPE in the following sequence: non-sterile gloves, hand hygiene, eyewear/face shield, plastic apron/gown and mask and then perform hand hygiene (ACSQHC, 2020). Dispose of in the rubbish bag.

Perform hand hygiene

Maintain the 5 Moments for Hand Hygiene and perform hand hygiene after touching the patient and the patient's surrounds.

CLEAN, REPLACE OR DISPOSE OF EQUIPMENT

All materials contaminated with tracheal secretions, as well as PPE, gauze and cotton-tipped applicators, are discarded in the contaminated waste.

DOCUMENT AND REPORT RELEVANT INFORMATION

The time, date and procedure are documented on the progress notes and nursing care plan. Any secretions, including amount, colour, consistency and any odour noted, are documented. The patient's response to the procedure should also be documented and reported.

CASE STUDY

You are an EN caring for Troy Davies, aged 19, in the head injury rehabilitation unit of a major public hospital. He is conscious and responsive to people around him, but not mobile. He has a tracheostomy tube which has been inserted for 6 weeks. He is breathing spontaneously on room air, with the tracheostomy, that also has a Swedish nose humidifier. If Troy wants attention from the medical staff, he usually gesticulates with his hands.

When completing his routine observations, you note a large amount of secretions on the tracheostomy tube. The patient is also coughing, and you note the sound of moisture inside the tracheostomy tube indicating a collection of secretions.

1. Identify the specific nursing actions you as an EN would implement.
2. Also identify any nursing care actions that may need to be implemented by other nursing staff.

Note: These notes are summaries of the most important points in the assessments/procedures, and are not exhaustive on the subject. The naming of documents or charts may differ from state to state, and facility to facility. In all possible situations the guidelines of the ACSQHC are used when describing national charts or documents (e.g. the ACSQHC Observation and Response Chart is named the Adult Observation and Response Chart in WA, and the Rapid Detection and Response Observation Chart in SA). References of the materials used to compile the information have been supplied. The student is expected to have learned the material surrounding each skill as presented in the references. No single reference is complete on the subject.

CRITICAL THINKING

Thinking of the clinical skills discussed in this skill, what are some of the key components you would need to consider in the following scenario?

    You are caring for a patient with a tracheostomy.

1. How will you overcome the patient's inability to communicate verbally?
2. Research devices to assist a person with a permanent tracheostomy.

REFERENCES

Australian Commission on Safety and Quality in Health Care (ACSQHC). (2020). *Sequence for Putting on and Removing PPE.* https://www.safetyandquality.gov.au/sites/default/files/2020-03/putting_on_and_removing_ppe_diagram_-_march_2020.pdf

Credland, N. (2016). How to perform a tracheostomy dressing and inner cannula change. *Nursing Standard,* 23 March, 30(30), p. 34.

Dougherty, L. & Lister, S. (eds). (2015). *The Royal Marsden Hospital Manual of Clinical Nursing Procedures* (9th ed.). Oxford: Wiley-Blackwell.

Patton, J. (2019). Tracheostomy care. *British Journal of Nursing,* 28(16), pp. 1060–2.

Russell, C., MacGinley, K. & Meads, C. (2019). Tracheostomy care in community settings. *Primary Health Care.* https://journals.rcni.com/primary-health-care/cpd/tracheostomy-care-in-community-settings-phc.2019.e1548/abs

Smith, S.F., Duell, D.J., Martin, B.C., Gonzalez, L., & Aebersold, M. (2017). *Clinical Nursing Skills: Basic to Advanced Skills* (9th ed.). Upper Saddle River, NJ: Pearson Prentice Hall.

RECOMMENDED READINGS

Berman, A., Snyder, S., Levett-Jones, T., Burton, T. & Harvey, N. (2021). *Skills in Clinical Nursing* (2nd ed.). Melbourne: Pearson.

Chauhan, N., Agnihotri, M., Kaur, S. & Panda, N.K. (2020). Practices regarding the care of tracheostomy tube in the patients with

long term tracheostomy. *Nursing and Midwifery Research Journal,* 16(2), pp. 63–9.

ESSENTIAL SKILLS COMPETENCY

Tracheostomy Care
Demonstrates the ability to effectively and safely care for a patient with a tracheostomy tube

Criteria for skill performance	Y	D
(Numbers indicate *Enrolled Nurse Standards for Practice*, 2016)	(Satisfactory)	(Requires development)
1. Identifies indication (8.3, 8.4)		
2. Discusses potential problems of tracheostomies (1.2, 1.6, 3.1, 3.2, 3.3, 7.3, 10.1, 10.3, 10.5, 10.6)		

3. Gathers equipment (1.2, 1.6, 4.4, 6.4, 8.4, 9.4):
  ■ sterile tracheostomy or dressing pack, sterile cotton-tipped applicators
  ■ normal saline 0.9%
  ■ PPE – plastic apron, goggles, non-sterile gloves, mask if required, sterile scissors, sterile gloves
  ■ tracheostomy suction supplies
  ■ Swedish nose		

4. Performs hand hygiene (1.2, 1.4, 1.8, 3.9, 6.4, 9.4)		
5. Evidence of effective communication with the patient; e.g. gives patient a clear explanation of procedure, gains consent (2.1, 2.3, 2.4, 2.5, 6.3)		
6. Dons PPE (1.2, 1.4, 1.8, 3.9, 6.4, 9.4)		
7. Assesses the patient and positions them (1.2, 3.2, 4.1, 4.2, 6.4, 7.3, 8.4, 9.4)		
8. Assists with suctioning the tracheostomy tube (1.2, 1.4, 1.8, 3.2, 3.9, 4.4, 6.4, 6.6, 8.4, 9.4)		
9. Remove gloves and performs hand hygiene (1.2, 1.4, 1.8, 3.9, 6.4, 9.4)		
10. Establishes the general aseptic field using a non-touch technique (1.2, 1.4, 3.2, 3.9, 9.4)		
11. Dons gloves, removes the dressing (1.2, 1.4, 1.8, 2.7, 3.2, 3.9, 6.4, 8.4, 9.4)		
12. Removes gloves, performs hand hygiene and dons new gloves (1.2, 1.4, 1.8, 3.9, 6.4, 9.4)		
13. Cleans and dries the stoma (1.2, 1.4, 2.7, 3.2, 3.9, 4.1, 7.1, 8.4, 9.4)		
14. Redresses the stoma site (1.2, 1.4, 2.7, 3.2, 3.9, 8.4, 9.4)		
15. Changes the tracheostomy ties if necessary (1.2, 1.4, 1.8, 3.2, 3.9, 8.4, 9.4)		
16. Removes gloves, performs hand hygiene and dons new gloves (1.2, 1.4, 1.8, 3.9, 6.4, 9.4)		
17. Provides oral hygiene (1.2, 1.4, 2.7, 3.2, 3.9, 4.1, 8.4, 9.4)		
18. Doffs PPE following correct procedure (1.2, 1.4, 1.8, 3.9, 6.4, 9.4)		
19. Performs hand hygiene (1.2, 1.4, 1.8, 3.9, 6.4, 9.4)		
20. Cleans, replaces and disposes of equipment appropriately (1.2, 1.4, 3.9, 6.5, 9.4)		
21. Documents and reports relevant information (1.2, 1.3, 1.8, 3.2, 5.3, 6.6, 7.1, 7.2, 7.3, 7.4, 7.5)		
22. Demonstrates ability to link theory to practice (8.3, 8.4, 8.5, 9.4)		

Student:

Clinical facilitator: Date:

CHAPTER 8.10

ASSIST A PATIENT TO USE CPAP IN THE GENERAL WARD OR COMMUNITY

IDENTIFY INDICATIONS

Patients who have obstructive sleep apnoea or other respiratory problems use continuous positive airway pressure (CPAP) therapy when they sleep to help keep their airways open and breathe more easily. During sleep, the throat muscles of patients with sleep apnoea relax, causing the tissue and the tongue to obstruct the airway. The obstruction becomes an apnoea event, with diminished levels of oxygen in the brain. Oxygen saturation levels also fall. In response, the brain partially awakens the patient to stimulate the person to take a breath. This response then creates a snoring or gasping sound as the patient breathes deeply.

CPAP is a common and accepted standard first-line treatment to help manage sleep apnoea (Miech et al., 2019; Ward et al., 2019). The continuous airway pressure provided by the CPAP machine opens the airway, allowing the patient to breathe normally while asleep. While improving the quality of the patient's sleep, it consequently increases daytime energy and alertness, and also reduces some of the risks created by sleep apnoea, such as cardiac disorders and stroke.

CPAP use is common within the community due to increasing numbers of people being diagnosed with sleep apnoea. When these patients are admitted to hospital, they will need to continue using their CPAP machine. This CPAP therapy differs from the CPAP used in the emergency department or intensive care unit (ICU).

GATHER EQUIPMENT

- *Patient's personal CPAP machine with mask and tubing*
- *Distilled water for the humidifier*

- *Warm soapy water and towel and non-sterile gloves for cleaning the mask and tubing.*

DEMONSTRATE PROBLEM-SOLVING ABILITIES

Ensure the patient has privacy when adjusting and attaching their CPAP machine. The patient will have personal settings and preferences that need to be continued in the hospital environment or community setting where they are using their CPAP. The nurse should also be aware of the expense of this equipment, and ensure no damage occurs to the machine, tubing, straps or mask.

ASSIST THE PATIENT TO USE CPAP

Perform hand hygiene

Perform hand hygiene before touching the patient or the patient's surrounds and prior to any procedure involving patient contact to reduce the possibility of cross-contamination. Hand hygiene is the most effective method of infection control as it removes transient organisms from the hands of the nurse (see Skill 1.1).

Give a clear explanation of the procedure and establish therapeutic communication

Introduce yourself, and check you have the correct patient. Discuss the procedure and gain the patient's consent. Giving a clear explanation is required to gain legal consent and to address policy requirements. It will also assist the patient to cooperate with the procedure, allay anxiety and assist in establishing a therapeutic relationship. Ensure the patient is happy for you to assist them with using their device.

Assist the patient to use their CPAP machine

Complete all required care (e.g. oral hygiene, medication administration) prior to settling the patient and assisting with attaching the CPAP. Assist the patient to a comfortable position. Ensure the CPAP machine is plugged in to the power and close enough to the patient's bed to allow them to move when they are asleep. It needs to be placed on a stable surface where it will not fall. Check that there is water in the humidifier tray or chamber (see next section).

Attach the CPAP tubing to the machine, and the mask to the tubing. Then assist the patient to place the mask over their mouth and nose (under the nose if a nasal mask is being used). Ensure the mask fits comfortably onto the patient's face, with the straps adjusted to their usual position. When turned on, air should blow into the mask and out of the exit ports in the mask. Any leaks around the base of the mask can be noisy and reduce the effectiveness of the therapy.

Depending on the machine, it may turn on automatically now the mask is fitted, or will require switching on. The required pressure is pre-programmed into the machine by a respiratory technician and will not require adjustment. The patient should now be able to settle and sleep.

Humidifier

Humidifiers are part of most devices, and are used to moisten the air and improve comfort when using CPAP. It helps to reduce drying of the mouth, nasal passages and throat. The water should be changed daily (many patients may or may not do this as part of their normal use) to reduce the risk of bacterial growth in the water. Don non-sterile gloves and carefully remove the humidifier tray or chamber and empty it each morning and leave it to dry. Refill the humidifier each night with distilled water when setting up the machine. A weekly wash of the humidifier chamber with warm soapy water will help to reduce the build-up of mineral deposits that can cause long-term damage to the machine.

Maintaining the machine

Wipe over the machine with a damp cloth to remove any surface dust. Disconnect the machine from the power during the day (unless required) and place safely where it will not be dropped or damaged.

Cleaning of masks, straps and tubing

The mask, tubing and straps should be cleaned weekly. Don non-sterile gloves. Separate the parts and disconnect the tubing from the humidifier. Wash gently in mild soapy water, then rinse and leave sitting on a clean towel to air dry. Hang the tubing over a rail to help it dry on the inside. Some patients may prefer to rinse and clean their tubing each day.

Filters

Filters require changing as per the manufacturer's instructions.

Perform hand hygiene

Maintain the 5 Moments for Hand Hygiene and perform hand hygiene after touching the patient and the patient's surrounds.

CLEAN, REPLACE OR DISPOSE OF EQUIPMENT

None of the CPAP equipment is disposable; therefore, it should be cleaned weekly at a minimum as described above.

DOCUMENT AND REPORT RELEVANT INFORMATION

Record the use of CPAP in the patient's care plan. Specific instruction for the patient's preferences can also be added.

CASE STUDY

Fred Travers is a 56-year-old male patient in your ward. As part of your admission, he has stated that he usually uses a CPAP machine at night. He states that he has sleep apnoea.

1. What advice will you give Fred about the use of his machine and his sleep apnoea while he is in hospital?
2. How does the CPAP machine help the patient to breathe, and have a better quality of sleep?

3. Why is it important to ensure the mask and straps are adjusted correctly when assisting Fred to use his CPAP machine?
4. Why should the water in the humidifier be changed each day?

Note: These notes are summaries of the most important points in the assessments/procedures, and are not exhaustive on the subject. The naming of documents or charts may differ from state to state, and facility to facility. In all possible situations the guidelines of the ACSQHC are used when describing national charts or documents (e.g. the ACSQHC Observation and Response Chart is named the Adult Observation and Response Chart in WA, and the Rapid Detection and Response Observation Chart in SA). References of the materials used to compile the information have been supplied. The student is expected to have learned the material surrounding each skill as presented in the references. No single reference is complete on the subject.

CRITICAL THINKING

Thinking of the clinical skills discussed in this skill, what are some of the key components you would need to consider in the following scenario?

During the admission of your patient, he informs you that at home he uses a CPAP machine at night. He has forgotten to bring the machine to the hospital. What actions will you take?

REFERENCES

Miech, E.J., Bravata, D.M., Klar, Y.H., Austin, C., Tobias, L.A., Ferguson, J. & Matthias, M.S. (2019). Adapting continuous positive airway pressure therapy to where patients live: A comparative case study. *Cureus*, 11(2), p. e4078.

Ward, K., Gott, M., & Hoare, K. (2019). Mastering treatment for sleep apnoea: The grounded theory of bargaining and balancing life with continuous positive airway pressure (CPAP), in the context of decisional conflict and change theories. *Forum: Qualitative Social Research*, 20(3), p. 3137.

RECOMMENDED READINGS

Nadal, N., de Batlle, J., Barbé, F., Marsal, J.R., Sánchez-de-la-Torre, A., Tarraubella, N., Lavega, M., Sánchez-de-la-Torre, M. (2018). Predictors of CPAP compliance in different clinical settings: Primary care versus sleep unit. *Sleep and Breathing,* 22(1), pp. 157–63.

Sleep Disorders Australia. (2018). *Sleep Apnea.* https://www.sleepoz.org.au/sleep-apnea

Sleep Health Foundation. (2013). *Fact Sheet: Caring for your CPAP Equipment.* https://www.sleephealthfoundation.org.au/caring-for-your-cpap-equipment.html

ESSENTIAL SKILLS COMPETENCY

Assist a Patient to Use CPAP in the General Ward or Community

Demonstrates the ability to assist the patient to use the personal CPAP device

Criteria for skill performance	Y	D
(Numbers indicate *Enrolled Nurse Standards for Practice*, 2016)	(Satisfactory)	(Requires development)
1. Identifies indication (8.3, 8.4)		

2. Gathers equipment (1.2, 1.6, 4.4, 6.4, 8.4, 9.4):
  ■ personal CPAP machine
  ■ patient's CPAP mask, straps and tubing
  ■ distilled water for humidifier
  ■ warm soapy water, towel and non-sterile gloves for cleaning the CPAP mask and tubing		

3. Demonstrates problem-solving abilities (4.1, 4.2, 8.3, 8.4, 9.4)		
4. Performs hand hygiene (1.2, 1.4, 1.8, 3.9, 6.4, 9.4)		
5. Evidence of effective therapeutic communication with the patient; e.g. gives patient a clear explanation of procedure and confirms patient understanding, gains patient consent (2.1, 2.3, 2.4, 2.5, 6.3)		
6. Assists the patient to set up the CPAP machine and wear the mask; turns on the machine (1.2, 1.4, 3.2, 8.4, 9.4)		
7. Dons non-sterile gloves and adds water to the humidifier; empties the water in the morning (1.2, 1.4, 3.2, 8.4, 9.4)		
8. Dons non-sterile gloves and cleans the mask and tubing (1.2, 1.4, 3.2, 8.4, 9.4)		
9. Performs hand hygiene (1.2, 1.4, 1.8, 3.2, 3.9, 6.4, 9.4)		
10. Cleans, replaces and disposes of equipment appropriately (1.2, 1.4, 3.9, 6.5, 9.4)		
11. Documents and reports relevant information (1.2, 1.3, 3.2, 5.3, 6.6, 7.1, 7.2, 7.3, 7.4, 7.5)		
12. Demonstrates ability to link theory to practice (8.3, 8.4, 8.5, 9.4)		

Student:

Clinical facilitator: Date:

CHAPTER 8.11

NASOGASTRIC TUBE INSERTION

IDENTIFY INDICATIONS

A nasogastric tube (NGT) is a flexible plastic tube that is inserted through the nostrils, down the nasopharynx and into the patient's stomach or the upper portion of the small intestine. It is used for feeding a patient or removing the gastric contents. An NGT is inserted after a doctor's order, and is used for hydration and nutrition for a patient with an impaired gag reflex (see **Skill 8.12**), for those requiring supplemental nutrition (e.g. patients with anorexia nervosa),

to aspirate gastric contents, as a gravity drain (see **Skill 8.5**) or for gastric lavage (i.e. after a drug overdose or poisoning). Facility policy will indicate the frequency of when an NGT is changed, but most short-term tubes should be changed weekly.

This procedure is uncomfortable, but not always painful, for conscious patients. It can sometimes induce vomiting, gagging or coughing.

DEMONSTRATE CRITICAL THINKING AND REVIEW SAFETY CONSIDERATIONS

NGT use is associated with a number of complications, including aspiration and localised tissue trauma. Inserted NGTs create a risk of complications such as aspiration and potential pneumonia (Health Care Safety Investigation Branch, 2021). Fine-bore feeding tubes are used whenever possible as these offer more comfort for the patient than the wide-bore tubes used for gastric drainage. They are also less likely to cause local tissue trauma and irritation (Crisp et al., 2017). Refer to the written orders and reasons for NGT insertion to determine the size of the tube.

The tube will be annoying for some patients, and confused patients may require extra supervision to prevent them from pulling on or removing the tube. Insertion of an NGT will create exposure to body fluids, so standard precautions (and any additional requirements) should be followed when inserting the tube.

VERIFY THE WRITTEN ORDER

Verifying the written order is a legal requirement, and will also identify the reason for the NGT insertion. It may also indicate the size that is needed.

GATHER AND PREPARE EQUIPMENT

Gathering equipment before initiating the procedure is part of effective time management for implementing the procedure and provides an opportunity for the nurse to rehearse the procedure mentally.

- *The nasogastric tube* is a thin, flexible tube with a radio-opaque tip. The smaller gauge tubes are less traumatic to insert and are better tolerated. To increase patient safety, NGTs used for feeding have a coloured (purple or yellow) flange.
- *Lubricant* reduces friction so the tube is more easily inserted.
- *A glass of water with a straw* (if indicated). Water can only be given to patients who are able to swallow, can follow instructions and have no contraindications. The

patient is asked to sip slowly through the straw and swallow the water during insertion as it assists in the process.
- *Personal protective equipment (PPE).* Non-sterile gloves, a plastic apron and goggles are worn to reduce the risk of exposure to body fluids.
- *A 10 or 20 mL syringe (with purple plunger)* is used to remove a small amount of gastric content to test for pH.
- *pH indicator strips.*
- *Kidney dish.*
- *Wooden tongue depressor and penlight torch* are used to visually determine the position of the tube in the oropharynx.
- *Tape* is used to secure the NGT in position.

- *A 'bluey'* keeps the patient and bedclothes clean and dry.
- *Second kidney dish and tissues* (for patient use).
- *Oral hygiene equipment.*

Note: For safety reasons, equipment and disposable items used for giving nasogastric feeds are identified with coloured (e.g. purple or orange) flanges, plungers, tips, etc. **If the tube is inserted as a drain, the tube and other equipment should not have purple colouring**.

INSERT THE NGT

Perform hand hygiene
Perform hand hygiene before touching the patient or the patient's surrounds and prior to any procedure involving patient contact to reduce the possibility of cross-contamination. Hand hygiene is the most effective method of infection control as it removes transient organisms from the hands of the nurse (see **Skill 1.1**).

Give a clear explanation of the procedure and establish therapeutic communication
Introduce yourself, and check you have the correct patient. Discuss the procedure and gain the patient's consent. Giving a clear explanation is required to gain legal consent and to address policy requirements. It will also assist the patient to cooperate with the procedure, allay anxiety and assist in establishing a therapeutic relationship.

Insertion of the NGT is an uncomfortable procedure. If the patient understands the purpose of the procedure and is told what to expect and how to help, they will be more willing to assist in completing the procedure, and this will be accomplished with a minimum of discomfort. Assess the patient's mental status and ability to cooperate, as an extra nurse may be required to assist. An explanation should also be given to an unconscious patient.

Ensure the provision of privacy
Provision of privacy preserves the patient's dignity. This procedure can often distress patients. Family members should be advised to leave the patient's area to minimise their own distress.

Position the patient
The patient is positioned in a semi-upright to upright position if their condition permits. This position facilitates insertion because of the anatomical structure of the nasopharynx and oesophagus. Place a pillow behind the patient to maintain the position.

Ascertain the length to which the NGT is inserted
The length to which the NGT is inserted is determined before initiating insertion to ensure the tube is inserted so that the distal tip rests in the stomach. Open the packaging, uncoil the tube and place the tip of the NGT at the xiphoid process, then stretch the tube to the earlobes and then the patient's nostrils. Note the length, according to the markings on the tube. This length approximates the distance from the nose to the stomach.

Check both nostrils for obstruction
Ask the patient if they have any difficulty in breathing through one nostril or the other, if they have a deviated septum or if they have had nasal surgery. If there are no obstructions, give the patient the choice of which nostril will be used.

Perform hand hygiene
Perform hand hygiene before touching the patient or the patient's surrounds and prior to any procedure involving patient contact to reduce the possibility of cross-contamination. Hand hygiene is the most effective method of infection control as it removes transient organisms from the hands of the nurse (see **Skill 1.1**).

Don PPE
PPE requirements will vary according to the care being delivered. Don plastic apron, goggles and non-sterile gloves to reduce the risk of exposure to body fluids when inserting the tube. Some patients may also vomit when an NGT is being inserted.

Prepare and insert the NGT
Place the 'bluey' on the patient's chest. Prepare tape to secure the NGT when it is positioned, and place it within easy reach. Prepare the syringe and pH test strip for checking placement of the tube. Wrap the initial 10 cm of the tube around your gloved fingers and release to increase the flexibility of tube. Place the tube in the kidney dish and lubricate the NGT for the first 6 to 10 cm from the tip, using the water-soluble lubricant. The use of lubricant will ease insertion by decreasing friction. Leave the end of the tube uncapped during insertion.

Give conscious patients a kidney dish (and tissues) for use during insertion in case they gag or vomit. Gently and steadily insert the tube along the floor of the chosen nostril with the natural curve of the tube towards the patient. Slight resistance may be felt and is normal. If strong resistance occurs, withdraw the tube, relubricate it and reinsert it through the other nostril. The patient is then asked to tilt their head slightly forward so the NGT follows the posterior wall of the nasopharynx more easily and enters the oesophagus rather than the trachea. When the NGT reaches the back of the oropharynx, the patient may begin to gag. Stop advancing the tube momentarily and ask the patient to swallow (or slowly sip water through a straw if not contraindicated) as it will assist in the tube insertion. Finish advancing the tube a little more quickly to the required length (identified with pre-measurement).

The NGT is introduced slowly but steadily, and the patient watched closely during insertion. If the patient begins to choke, cough or become cyanotic, gently pull the tube back a short distance and then resume advancing the tube with each swallow. Observation of coughing, choking or cyanosis indicates that the tube has tracked into the trachea and bronchi. If this occurs, the tube is completely removed and the procedure attempted again, when the patient has regained their breath. Remember that if the patient's level of consciousness is impaired, the cough and gag reflexes will be absent.

Use the tissues to clean any lubricant or mucus from the patient's nose and then secure the tube to the patient's nose by using the prepared tape.

Check the position of the tube

An NGT can coil inside the patient's mouth or throat during insertion. Check the tube by using the tongue depressor and penlight torch to check the patient's mouth and the back of their throat for any coiled tubing.

Attach the 20 mL syringe to the open end of the NGT. Draw back on the plunger to aspirate a small amount of the gastric contents, then (utilising the kidney dish) drip a small amount of the aspirate on the pH indicator strip. A reading of less than 5.0 indicates that the tip of the NGT is in the stomach (Crisp et al., 2017; Royal Children's Hospital Melbourne, 2017). If no aspirate returns, advance the NGT a further 3 to 7 cm and attempt to recover aspirate again. Further assistance from the senior registered nurse (SRN) will be required if suitable aspirate is still not obtained. Read the length of the tube at the nostrils and record the inserted length (i.e. in centimetres) of the tube on the NGT chart. When a positive pH reading is obtained, finish securing the tube to the patient's nose. Ensure the tape is out of the patient's line of vision, and that there is no traction placed on the nares.

Confirmation of NGT placement with an X-ray is required. The tube must be correctly positioned before any further treatment is carried out.

Ensure ongoing patient comfort

Assist the patient to a position of comfort after the tube has been inserted. If the patient is nil orally, offer regular oral care (2- to 4-hourly) with a soft toothbrush and prepackaged foam swabs while the NGT is inserted. Assessment of nasal area should be done frequently for potential pressure injuries and irritation. Replace any tape that comes loose to ensure the NGT does not become dislodged. The nares may need cleansing with a washcloth or normal saline to remove any dried secretions.

Doff PPE

Remove PPE in the following sequence: non-sterile gloves, hand hygiene, eyewear/face shield, plastic apron/gown and mask and then perform hand hygiene (ACSQHC, 2020). Dispose of in the rubbish bag.

Perform hand hygiene

Maintain the 5 Moments for Hand Hygiene and perform hand hygiene after touching the patient and the patient's surrounds.

CLEAN, REPLACE OR DISPOSE OF EQUIPMENT

Dispose of used items (kidney dish, syringe, used pH strip) in the general waste, according to facility policy. Tidy the patient's bed area, and create a tray for oral care (mouth swabs, toothbrush, toothpaste) and another tray for testing the NGT tube placement (20 mL syringe, pH strips, small medication cups).

DOCUMENT AND REPORT RELEVANT INFORMATION

Inform the registered nurse (RN) shift coordinator of the NGT insertion so the confirmation X-ray can be completed. Documentation of this procedure should include the type and size of NGT used and confirmation of placement. A nasogastric chart should be commenced to record the tube length and pH test when the tube is inserted.

CASE STUDY

You are working on a busy medical ward. An 81-year-old woman, Rachel Ullman, had been admitted the day prior, post a stroke that happened at home. She has a past medical history of hypertension and diabetes and has a peripheral intravenous catheter (PIVC) in situ.

Due to Rachel's severely reduced gag reflex, and her inability to swallow fluids, today the doctor has ordered the insertion of an NGT for nutrition and medication administration.

1. Her daughter Ruth is in attendance and asks you why her mother is to have an NGT inserted. What is your response?
2. Why is it important to provide regular oral hygiene for patients with an NGT in situ?
3. List the equipment you will need to perform this NGT insertion, and also the equipment for the subsequent care (e.g. mouth care).

Note: These notes are summaries of the most important points in the assessments/procedures, and are not exhaustive on the subject. The naming of documents or charts may differ from state to state, and facility to facility. In all possible situations the guidelines of the ACSQHC are used when describing national charts or documents (e.g. the ACSQHC Observation and Response Chart is named the Adult Observation and Response Chart in WA, and the Rapid Detection and Response Observation Chart in SA). References of the materials used to compile the information have been supplied. The student is expected to have learned the material surrounding each skill as presented in the references. No single reference is complete on the subject.

CRITICAL THINKING

Thinking of the clinical skills discussed in this skill, what are some of the key components you would need to consider in the following scenario?

While inserting the NGT, you notice that your patient is becoming very distressed. A check of her oral cavity with a torch shows that the tube is curled at the back of the throat. What actions will you take?

REFERENCES

Australian Commission on Safety and Quality in Health Care (ACSQHC). (2020). *Sequence for Putting on and Removing PPE.* https://www.safetyandquality.gov.au/sites/default/files/2020-03/putting_on_and_removing_ppe_diagram_-_march_2020.pdf

Crisp, J., Douglas, C., Rebeiro, G. & Waters, D. (2017). *Potter and Perry's Fundamentals of Nursing – Australian version* (5th ed.). Sydney: Elsevier.

Healthcare Safety Investigation Branch. (2021). *Placement of Nasogastric Tubes.* https://www.hsib.org.uk/investigations-cases/placement-nasogastric-tubes/

Royal Children's Hospital Melbourne. (2017). *Enteral Feeding and Medication Administration.* https://www.rch.org.au/rchcpg/hospital_clinical_guideline_index/Enteral_feeding_and_medication_administration/

RECOMMENDED READINGS

Gray, S., Ferris, L., White, L.E., Duncan, G. & Baumle, W. (2018). *Foundations of Nursing: Enrolled Nurses* (2nd ANZ ed.). Melbourne: Cengage.

Canberra Hospital and Health Services. (2017). *Clinical Procedure Nasogastric Tube (NGT) Management – Adults Only.* https://www.cahs.health.wa.gov.au/-/media/HSPs/CAHS/Documents/Community-Health/CHM/Nasogastric-tube-management.pdf?thn=0

National Health and Medical Research Council (NHMRC). (2019). 3.5.2.4 Enteral feeding tubes. *Australian Guidelines for the Prevention and Control of Infection in Healthcare.* https://www.nhmrc.gov.au/sites/default/files/documents/infection-control-guidelines-feb2020.pdf

WA Country Health Service. (2019). *Enteral Tubes and Feeding – Adults Clinical Practice Standard.* Government of Western Australia. http://www.wacountry.health.wa.gov.au:443/fileadmin/sections/policies/Managed/Enteral_Tubes_and_Feeding_Adults_Clinical_Practice_Standard_TS4KSNFPVEZQ_210_6774.pdf

ESSENTIAL SKILLS COMPETENCY

Nasogastric Tube Insertion
Demonstrates the ability to safely and efficiently insert a nasogastric tube (NGT)

Criteria for skill performance	Y	D
(Numbers indicate *Enrolled Nurse Standards for Practice*, 2016)	(Satisfactory)	(Requires development)
1. Identifies indication (8.3, 8.4)		
2. Demonstrates problem-solving abilities and safety considerations (4.1, 4.2, 8.3, 8.4, 9.4)		
3. Verifies written order (1.2, 1.4, 3.2, 3.9, 5.5, 9.4)		
4. Gathers equipment (1.2, 1.6, 4.4, 6.4, 8.4, 9.4): ■ NGT (appropriate type and size) and lubricant ■ glass of water with straw (if required) ■ PPE – non-sterile gloves, plastic apron, goggles ■ kidney dish × 2, tissues ■ pH indicator strips ■ tongue depressor, penlight torch ■ 10–20 mL syringe with purple plunger ■ hypoallergenic tape cut to appropriate length ■ absorbent pad ('bluey') ■ oral hygiene equipment		
5. Performs hand hygiene (1.2, 1.4, 1.8, 3.2, 3.9, 6.4, 9.4)		
6. Evidence of effective therapeutic communication with the patient; e.g. gives patient a clear explanation of procedure and confirms patient understanding, and gains patient consent (2.1, 2.3, 2.4, 2.5, 6.3)		
7. Positions patient (1.2, 1.4, 3.2, 8.4, 9.4)		
8. Ascertains length of NGT to be inserted (1.2, 1.4)		
9. Checks nostrils for obstruction (1.2, 1.4)		
10. Performs hand hygiene and dons PPE correctly (1.2, 1.4, 1.8, 3.2, 3.9, 6.4, 9.4)		
11. Inserts NGT to appropriate length (1.2, 1.4, 1.8, 2.7, 3.2, 3.9, 4.1, 4.4, 6.4, 7.3, 8.4, 9.4)		
12. Ascertains placement of NGT (1.2, 1.4, 3.2, 3.9, 4.4, 6.4, 8.4, 9.4)		
13. Tapes NGT to patient's nose (1.2, 1.4)		
14. Performs hand hygiene (1.2, 1.4, 1.8, 3.2, 3.9, 6.4, 9.4)		
15. Implements oral hygiene 2–4 hourly (1.2, 1.4, 1.8, 2.1, 2.3, 2.4, 2.7, 3.2, 3.9, 6.1, 6.3, 6.6, 8.4, 9.4)		
16. Removes PPE correctly and performs hand hygiene (1.2, 1.4, 1.8, 3.9, 6.4, 9.4)		
17. Cleans, replaces and disposes of equipment appropriately (1.2, 1.4, 3.9, 6.5, 9.4)		
18. Documents, reports relevant information (1.2, 1.3, 1.8, 3.2, 5.3, 6.6, 7.1, 7.2, 7.3, 7.4, 7.5) and ensures X-ray confirmation of NGT		
19. Demonstrates ability to link theory to practice (8.3, 8.4, 8.5, 9.4)		

Student:

Clinical facilitator:　　　　　　　　　　　　　　　　　　　Date:

CHAPTER 8.12

ENTERAL FEEDING (NASOGASTRIC AND GASTROSTOMY TUBE)

IDENTIFY INDICATIONS

A nasogastric tube (NGT) is a flexible plastic tube that is inserted through the nostrils, down the nasopharynx and into the patient's stomach or the upper portion of the small intestine. An NGT is inserted after a doctor's order and is used for feeding a patient or removing the gastric contents. An NGT is generally used short term and replaced with a gastrostomy tube if a patient requires long-term enteral feeding.

A gastrostomy tube is a soft, flexible tube inserted via a surgical procedure, directly through the abdominal wall and into the stomach, creating a stoma on the outer abdomen. The tube is secured in place by an internal balloon or soft disc (bumper), and a flange on the outside of the abdomen. Different types of tubes are inserted according to the patient's needs.

A percutaneous endoscopic gastrostomy (PEG) tube specifically describes a long gastrostomy tube, with other lower profile gastrostomy tubes having only a flange visible on the abdominal surface.

A jejunostomy tube is a soft plastic tube placed into the jejunum (Medline Plus, 2020). Jejunal feeding is only used in specific circumstances, has an increased infection control risk and is not included in the Diploma of Nursing Training Package, so it is not discussed in this skill. Enteral feeds are implemented when the patient is unable to take adequate nutrition orally. This includes patients who: have an impaired gag reflex; are unconscious; have had oral, facial or neck surgery or trauma; are anorexic; or are seriously ill.

A doctor's written order is necessary to commence a patient on enteral feeds. The order will also indicate the type and amount of enteral feedings required (a dietitian is then usually consulted about the patient's specific nutritional requirements and feed). A patient admitted with a long-term gastrostomy tube will continue their enteral feeding regimen unless it is contraindicated by their medical treatment.

DEMONSTRATE CRITICAL THINKING AND REVIEW SAFETY CONSIDERATIONS

Inserted NGTs and NGT feeding create a risk of patient complications such as aspiration and potential pneumonia (Health Care Safety Investigation Branch, 2021) and localised tissue trauma For a patient receiving an NGT feed there is a risk of the tube dislodging and feed being administered directly into the patient's lungs. Checking placement of the tube is essential prior to a feed or any fluids being administered. For patients receiving NG feeds, a fine-bore feeding tube is used whenever possible as it offers more comfort for the patient than the wide-bore tubes used for gastric drainage. It is also less likely to cause local tissue trauma and irritation (Crisp et al., 2017).

Risks associated with gastrostomy feeds include accidental removal of the tube. Aspiration is also possible if the patient is not placed in the correct position during feeding.

Enteral feeds used over a longer period of time have the potential for further complications such as diarrhoea or constipation, dehydration and electrolyte disturbances.

For safety reasons, equipment and disposable items used for giving NGT feeds are identified with coloured (e.g. purple or orange) flanges, plungers, tips, etc.

If the NGT is inserted as a drain, the tube and other equipment should not have purple or orange colouring.

VERIFY THE WRITTEN ORDER

The written order for the required feed is initially given by the doctor, with the dietitian then prescribing the required type of feed, volume and flush. For a patient already on a long-term feeding routine, record their regular feed, volume and flush in their admission notes and nursing care plan.

GATHER EQUIPMENT

Gathering equipment before initiating the procedure is part of effective time management for implementing the procedure and provides an opportunity for the nurse to rehearse the procedure mentally.

For NGT feeds
- A *20 mL syringe (with safety coloured plunger)* is used to remove a small amount of gastric content to test for pH.
- *pH indicator strips*.
- *Kidney dish and small medication cup*.
- Additional items if full tube aspiration is required including *disposable cups and measuring jug*.

For gastrostomy feeds
- An *extension set* (if required) that is attached for feeding or medication administration and then disconnected when not in use.

For all enteral feeds
- *50 mL syringe* for flushing the tube.
- *The feeding apparatus* (i.e. enteral feeding pump, gravity feed set, 50 mL syringe with purple plunger).
- *Required enteral nutritional fluid and tap water* for flushing and hydration requirements.
- *An adaptor* may be required to connect the tubing to other equipment.
- *An absorbent pad* to keep the patient and bedclothes clean and dry.
- *Non-sterile gloves* (according to facility policy) to reduce the risk of exposure to body fluids.

ADMINISTER THE ENTERAL FEED

Perform hand hygiene
Perform hand hygiene before touching the patient or the patient's surrounds and prior to any procedure involving patient contact to reduce the possibility of cross-contamination. Hand hygiene is the most effective method of infection control as it removes transient organisms from the hands of the nurse (see **Skill 1.1**).

Give a clear explanation of the procedure and establish therapeutic communication
Introduce yourself, and check you have the correct patient. Discuss the procedure and gain the patient's consent. Giving a clear explanation is required to gain legal consent and to address policy requirements. It will also assist the patient to cooperate with the procedure, allay anxiety and assist in establishing a therapeutic relationship.

Prepare the required feed and water flush
Prepare the required feed prior to positioning the patient and checking the placement of the tube. This allows any feed that is cold to be warmed, and to also administer the feed as soon as the position of the tube is confirmed. The patient's nursing care plan and/or the dietitian's chart will state the required amounts of water for flushing and the feeding solution. These are determined on an individual basis to ensure the patient receives the correct amounts of kilojoules, fluids, fibre and nutrients. Times and frequency of feeds will also be stated. The feed should be warmed to room temperature. If it has been stored in the fridge, measure the required volume of feed into disposable cups and then leave to stand for 15 to 30 minutes on the patient's locker to allow the chill to be removed. Measure the required volume for each water flush into a disposable cup (or clean jug from the kitchen) and leave ready by the patient's bed area for adding to the enteral tube.

If the feed is being administered via an enteral feeding pump (e.g. Kanga pump) or NGT feeding set, ensure the giving set is changed every 24 hours. Place a date and time label on the line of each new giving set. Prime the giving set and remove all air from the line. Connect the container and tubing, and turn off the roller clamp. Add extra tap water (50 mL) to the container and hang it from the IV pole. Open the roller clamp and slowly allow the fluid to enter the line and remove the air. Ensure no water is remaining in the container (but fluid is remaining in the line) and turn off the roller clamp. Add the correct volume of feed to the container and hang it from the IV pole ready to connect to the enteral tube.

Ensure the provision of privacy
Provision of privacy preserves the patient's dignity when administering an enteral feed. Patients with an enteral feed may be comfortable with the curtains not being drawn while the feed is administered via an enteral feeding pump or giving set, but privacy should be provided when checking tube placement and initiating the feed.

Position the patient for feeding
The patient's upper body should be raised to at least 45 degrees, or to a sitting position, when a feed is being administered, unless medical treatment excludes this option (patients should then have their head elevated as much as possible). The patient should remain in this position for 30 to 60 minutes after the feed is completely administered. This reduces the risk of reflux and aspiration during a feed and post feeding.

Perform hand hygiene
Perform hand hygiene before touching the patient or the patient's surrounds and prior to any procedure

involving patient contact to reduce the possibility of cross-contamination.

Don personal protective equipment (PPE)

PPE requirements will vary according to the care being delivered. Don plastic apron, goggles and non-sterile gloves to reduce the risk of exposure to body fluids.

Aspirate and check the position of the tube

Coughing and movement in bed can dislodge an NGT, so checking the position of the NGT must be carried out before instillation of every feed or any fluid. Syringe aspiration can also be done to ascertain absorption rates of the previous feed. Refer to the nursing care plan, dietitian's instructions and organisational policies for this action. The type and amount of aspirate must be noted and recorded on the fluid balance chart. Prepare the equipment you will require for aspirating the tube, flushing the tube and connecting the prepared feed immediately after aspirating, and ensure it is within easy reach. Check the expiry date on the pH strips (and the enteral fluids) to ensure they are in date.

Assess the length of the tube at the patient's nares, and compare to the recorded length noted when the tube was inserted and from previous feeds. Record this length on the NGT chart. If this is the same, aspirate the tube to test placement. Kink the end section of the NGT to prevent air entering the tube, then open the flange. Attach the 20 mL syringe (with purple plunger), then unkink the tube and draw back on the plunger to aspirate 5 to 10 mL of the gastric contents. Ensure that you are aspirating more than just fluid from the previous feed that is inside the NGT. Recap the tube. Test the pH by squirting a small amount of the aspirate into the small medication cup and then dipping in the pH indicator strip, or drip a small amount of this aspirate on the pH indicator strip placed in the kidney dish. A reading of less than 5.0 indicates that the tip of the NGT is in the stomach (Crisp et al., 2017; Royal Children's Hospital Melbourne 2017). Note the pH reading on the NGT record chart.

Gastrostomy tubes do not require aspiration for correct placement, but must be checked for position and stability prior to administration of any fluids or medications

If aspiration is to ascertain absorption of feeds, use a 20 to 50 mL syringe (do not use a smaller syringe as this will create too much pressure on the stomach wall) with a safety coloured plunger to aspirate the tube as per the technique for checking the placement of a nasogastric tube. Aspirate the stomach contents until resistance is felt in the syringe and no more fluid can be withdrawn – if necessary, fluid can be placed into a disposable cup and the syringe reconnected. The volume is then measured and recorded on the fluid balance chart. According to the volume withdrawn from the stomach, and facility policy, this aspirate can then be either returned or discarded. When a large volume of aspirate is obtained, it may

be necessary to double-check if the previous feed was administered on time. It will then be necessary to consult with the registered nurse (RN) to determine if the current feed should be adjusted or withheld.

Flush the tube

The enteral tube should be flushed with 10 to 30 mL of room temperature (warm) water prior to administering the feed to clear the tube and ensure tube patency. Flushing the tube between feeds and medication administration also reduces the risk of microbial colonisation within the enteral tube (NHMRC, 2019). Once the correct amount of feed has been administered, the tube is again flushed with a stipulated amount of water to clear it.

Connect a clean 50 mL nasogastric syringe barrel to the end of the tube. So that no air enters the inserted tube, use your fingers to kink the tube when opening the end-cap/spigot and until fluid is placed in the syringe. While keeping the tube kinked, stabilise the syringe with the same hand to prevent spillage when adding fluid into the barrel.

Add the pre-prepared water flush to clear the tube. Move fingers to unkink the tube and allow the fluid to flow down the tube. To enable a slow gravitational flow, keep the syringe at or just above the height of the patient's nose. A syringe plunger must never be used to force fluid down the tube (if the fluid does not flow or the tube is blocked, refer to an RN for further assistance).

Re-kink the tube as the syringe is emptying to prevent air entering the stomach. The feed can now be connected.

Administer feed using correct apparatus

Disconnect the 50 mL flushing syringe (while keeping the tube kinked) and then attach the relevant feeding apparatus as described below. The method and apparatus used will vary according to the dietitian's instructions or facility policy.

Bolus method

Using a nasogastric feeding set or enteral feeding pump with an administration set. While keeping the tube kinked, and avoiding any tension or pulling on the tube, remove the 50 mL syringe used for flushing the tube and attach the end of the prepared feeding set. The clamp on the administration set is then adjusted to allow the feed to be given over the stipulated time. Set the correct flow rate if an enteral feeding pump is being used.

As this can take up to 30 minutes, monitor the patient during administration and while remaining close by. When all of the feed has been administered, the required volume of water is then used to both flush the tubing and to administer enough fluid to maintain the patient's hydration. Turn off the roller clamp and add the required volume of water to the feed container. After this water (i.e. flush) has been administered, the clamp is turned off, the enteral tube is kinked with the fingers and the administration set is disconnected. The cap is then replaced on the tube and then unkinked. Clean the administration set using clean water in a pantry or clean area.

Using syringe method. Maintain the same technique used for flushing the tube. When the water (i.e. flush) has come to the bottom of the syringe, kink the tube and then pour 50 mL of feed into it. Steady the syringe barrel with your fingers to ensure it doesn't spill. Unkink the tube and administer the feed as described in flushing. The barrel must not be allowed to empty, but is continually topped up with the pre-measured amount of feed. When all the feed has been administered, flush the tube with the correct volume of water. After the water flush, the enteral tube is kinked, the syringe is disconnected and the cap closed.

Record fluid intake

After the feed has been administered, the amount of water used to flush is recorded on the fluid balance, as well as the amount of feed. Aspirate should also be recorded on the fluid balance chart, in the output section.

Carry out oral hygiene

Oral hygiene should be carried out every 2 to 4 hours for a patient with an enteral tube. The patient will not be receiving any oral fluids and their mouth will be dry. Oral hygiene using a soft toothbrush and toothpaste should be completed at least twice daily (see **Skill 3.5**). Prepackaged foam mouth swabs with water can be used at other times, and are often kept on a tray next to the patient's bed area. Use lip balm to prevent the lips becoming dry and cracked. Regular mouth care will increase patient comfort, remove plaque and reduce the risk of developing halitosis and gingivitis.

Check insertion-site skin integrity

The NGT insertion-site skin integrity around nostrils must be checked regularly for potential pressure injuries and irritation. Replace any loose tape to ensure the NGT does not become dislodged. The nares may need cleansing with a washcloth or normal saline to remove any dried secretions.

The insertion site of a gastrostomy tube should also be checked for any redness or irritation and to ensure the tube has not been dislodged. The site should also be washed, rinsed and dried daily as part of normal hygiene. Flushing will help remove any encrusted feed or medications, or colonised bacteria

Doffing PPE

Remove PPE in the following sequence: gloves, hand hygiene, eyewear/face shield, plastic apron/gown and mask and then perform hand hygiene (ACSQHC, 2020). Dispose of in the rubbish bag.

Perform hand hygiene

Perform hand hygiene before touching the patient or the patient's surrounds and prior to any procedure involving patient contact to reduce the possibility of cross-contamination.

CLEAN, REPLACE OR DISPOSE OF EQUIPMENT

Dispose of any gastric secretions from tube aspiration in the sluice. Used items should be disposed of in the general waste. The measuring jug, administration set and feed container are washed and rinsed thoroughly between feeds. The giving set should be replaced every 24 hours. It is important that pH indicator strips are kept in their sealed container. Tidy and replace any items on the mouth care tray or any other equipment kept by the patient's bed area for managing the enteral tube.

DOCUMENT AND REPORT RELEVANT INFORMATION

Chart the length of the NGT tube at the nares and the pH of the aspirate on the NGT chart. Record the volume of the feed and water administered via the enteral tube on the fluid balance chart. Any aspirate removed (and discarded) should be recorded on the output section of the fluid balance chart.

CASE STUDY

You are working on a busy medical ward. An 81-year-old woman (Rachel Ullman) had been admitted the day prior, post a stroke that happened at home. She has a past medical history of hypertension and diabetes and has a peripheral intravenous catheter (PIVC) in situ.

Due to Rachel's severe reduced gag reflex, and her inability to swallow fluids, yesterday the doctor ordered the insertion of an NGT for nutrition and medication administration. The NGT is in situ, and confirmed as correctly positioned in the stomach by X-ray.

Rachel has been commenced on NGT feeds every 4 hours, by the dietitian

1. As her nurse, why is it essential to test for the correct location of an NGT prior to administration of any fluids or medication?
2. Describe how you will position Rachel prior to commencing the NGT feeds (she remains in bed).

The dietitian (and doctor) have ordered 4-hourly intermittent feeds (via a syringe), with a 30 mL water flush pre and post NGT feed.

→

3. Why is it necessary to flush an NGT with water prior to and post administering a feed?

4. What will you do during this procedure to ensure air does not enter the NGT tube?

5. After the NGT feed has been completed, where will this information be documented?

6. What other general nursing care should be attended to for Rachel as she is on nil orally?

Note: These notes are summaries of the most important points in the assessments/procedures, and are not exhaustive on the subject. The naming of documents or charts may differ from state to state, and facility to facility. In all possible situations the guidelines of the ACSQHC are used when describing national charts or documents (e.g. the ACSQHC Observation and Response Chart is named the Adult Observation and Response Chart in WA, and the Rapid Detection and Response Observation Chart in SA). References of the materials used to compile the information have been supplied. The student is expected to have learned the material surrounding each skill as presented in the references. No single reference is complete on the subject.

CRITICAL THINKING/LIFESPAN

Thinking of the clinical skills discussed in this skill, and the stages of growth and development, what are some of the key components you would need to consider in the following scenarios?

1. Prior to and after feeding a patient with a recent gastrostomy tube, what additional assessments will you perform?

2. When caring for a 12-year-old patient with a disability who has a long-term gastrostomy tube in situ, identify the importance of parent/carer input when administering regular PEG feeds.

REFERENCES

Australian Commission on Safety and Quality in Health Care (ACSQHC). (2020). *Sequence for Putting on and Removing PPE.* https://www.safetyandquality.gov.au/sites/default/files/2020-03/putting_on_and_removing_ppe_diagram_-_march_2020.pdf

Crisp, J., Douglas, C., Rebeiro, G. & Waters, D. (2017). *Potter and Perry's Fundamentals of Nursing – Australian version* (5th ed.). Sydney: Elsevier.

Healthcare Safety Investigation Branch. (2021). *Placement of Naso-gastric Tubes.* https://www.hsib.org.uk/investigations-cases/placement-nasogastric-tubes/

Medline Plus. (2018). *Jejunostomy feeding tube.* https://medlineplus.gov/ency/patientinstructions/000181.htm#:~:text=A%20

jejunostomy%20tube%20(J%2Dtube,the%20tube%20enters%20the%20body

National Health and Medical Research Council (NHMRC). (2019). 3.5.2.4 Enteral feeding tubes. *Australian Guidelines for the Prevention and Control of Infection in Healthcare.* https://www.nhmrc.gov.au/sites/default/files/documents/infection-control-guidelines-feb2020.pdf

Royal Children's Hospital Melbourne. (2017). *Enteral Feeding and Medication Administration.* https://www.rch.org.au/rchcpg/hospital_clinical_guideline_index/Enteral_feeding_and_medication_administration/

RECOMMENDED READINGS

Agency for Clinical Innovation (ACI) and the Gastroenterological Nurses College of Australia. (2015). *A Clinician's Guide: Caring for People with Gastrostomy Tubes and Devices. From Pre-insertion to Ongoing Care and Removal.* https://www.aci.health.nsw.gov.au/__data/assets/pdf_file/0017/251063/gastrostomy_guide-web.pdf

Canberra Hospital and Health Services. (2017). *Clinical Procedure Nasogastric Tube (NGT) Management – Adults Only.* ACT Government. https://www.health.act.gov.au/sites/default/files/2018-09/Nasogastric%20Tube%20(NGT)%20Management%20Adults%20%E2%80%93%20Only.doc

Feeding Tube Awareness Foundation. (2020). *Gastrostomy Tubes.* https://www.feedingtubeawareness.org/g-tube/

Queensland Health. (2016). *A Guide to Gastrostomy Tubes.* Queensland Government. https://www.health.qld.gov.au/__data/assets/pdf_file/0026/154682/hphe_gastrostomytube.pdf

WA Country Health Service. (2019). *Enteral Tubes and Feeding – Adults Clinical Practice Standard.* Government of Western Australia. http://www.wacountry.health.wa.gov.au:443/index.php?id=1463

ESSENTIAL SKILLS COMPETENCY

Enteral Feeding (Nasogastric and Gastrostomy Tubes)
Demonstrates the ability to safely and efficiently administer an enteral feed

Criteria for skill performance	Y	D
(Numbers indicate *Enrolled Nurse Standards for Practice*, 2016)	(Satisfactory)	(Requires development)
1. Identifies indication (8.3, 8.4)		
2. Demonstrates problem-solving abilities and safety consideration (4.1, 4.2, 8.3, 8.4, 9.4)		
3. Verifies written order (1.2, 1.4, 3.2, 3.9, 5.5, 9.4)		
4. Gathers equipment (1.2, 1.6, 8.4): ■ pH indicator strips ■ kidney dish ■ small medication cups, measuring cups/jug ■ enteric syringes for checking placement and administration; 20 mL and 50 mL (and any connectors if required) ■ disposable cups ■ water for flushing ■ feeding apparatus, appropriate solutions and IV stand, adaptor if required ■ prescribed feed ■ oral hygiene equipment ■ PPE – non-sterile gloves, plastic apron and goggles ■ absorbent pad		
5. Performs hand hygiene (1.2, 1.4, 1.8, 3.2, 3.9, 6.4, 9.4)		
6. Evidence of therapeutic communication with the patient; gives explanation of procedure, gains patient consent (2.1, 2.3, 2.4, 2.5, 3.2, 6.3, 7.3, 7.5)		
7. Feed and water is measured and then warmed to room temperature (1.2, 1.4, 3.2, 3.9, 4.4, 6.4, 8.4, 9.4)		
8. Positions patient sitting up, or at 45 degrees (1.2, 1.4, 3.2, 8.4, 9.4)		
9. Performs hand hygiene (1.2, 1.4, 1.8, 3.2, 3.9, 6.4, 9.4)		
10. Dons PPE in correct order (1.2, 1.4, 1.8, 3.2, 3.9, 6.4, 9.4)		
11. Checks placement and position of enteral tube NGT; measures tube length and aspirates, checking pH with pH test strips to 5.0 or less: ■ and if previous feed was absorbed (1.2, 1.4, 3.2, 3.9, 4.4, 6.4, 8.4, 9.4)		
Gastrostomy tube check insertion site for position and stability		
12. Tube flushed with water pre-feed (1.2, 1.4, 3.2, 3.9, 4.4, 6.4, 8.4, 9.4)		
13. Feed is administered using either bolus syringe or connection to feedline apparatus (7.1)		
14. Tube flushed with water post feed (1.2, 1.4, 3.2, 3.9, 4.4, 6.4, 8.4, 9.4)		
15. Patient remains sitting up, or at 45 degrees, for 30–60 minutes after feed (1.2, 1.4, 3.2, 3.9, 4.4, 6.4, 8.4, 9.4)		
16. Performs oral care (1.2, 1.4, 1.8, 2.1, 2.3, 2.4, 2.7, 3.2, 3.9, 6.1, 6.3, 6.6, 8.4, 9.4)		
17. Doffs PPE in correct order and performs hand hygiene (1.2, 1.4, 3.2, 3.9, 4.4, 6.4, 8.4, 9.4)		
18. Cleans, replaces and disposes of equipment appropriately (1.2, 1.4, 3.9, 6.5, 9.4)		
19. Documents and reports relevant information (1.2, 1.3, 1.8, 3.2, 5.3, 6.6, 7.1, 7.2, 7.3, 7.4, 7.5)		
20. Demonstrates ability to link theory to practice (8.3, 8.4, 8.5, 9.4)		

Student:

Clinical facilitator: Date:

CHAPTER **8.13**

INFECTION CONTROL – STANDARD AND TRANSMISSION-BASED PRECAUTIONS

IDENTIFYING INDICATIONS

Infection prevention and control uses a risk management approach to minimise or prevent the transmission of infection. The two-tiered approach of standard and transmission-based precautions (TBPs) provides a high level of protection to patients, healthcare workers and other people in healthcare settings (Victorian Department of Health, 2018). The world has been dramatically impacted by the COVID 19 pandemic. Infection control, in particular hand hygiene, is paramount to prevent the spread of infection (Australian Government Department of Health, 2020).

EXPLANATION OF TERMS USED IN INFECTION CONTROL

Standard precautions are the primary strategy for minimising the transmission of healthcare-associated infections as part of the treatment and care of all patients. They are used in all patient-care situations and are a first-line approach to infection prevention and control. In situations where standard precautions alone are insufficient, TBPs are added.

The National Health and Medical Research Council states that:

Transmission-based precautions are recommended as additional work practices in situations where standard precautions alone may be insufficient to prevent transmission.

(NHMRC, 2019a)

Infection prevention and control is integral to clinical care and the way it is provided.

Standard precautions

All people potentially harbour infectious microorganisms, and thus all blood and body secretions are potentially infectious. The use of standard precautions aims to minimise and, if possible, eliminate the risk of infection transmission, particularly those caused by blood-borne viruses.

(Victorian Department of Health, 2018)

Standard precautions consist of:

- hand hygiene, before and after every episode of patient contact (the use of gloves should not be considered an alternative to performing hand hygiene)
- the use of personal protective equipment (PPE); for example, gloves, gowns, aprons, masks, eye protection
- the safe use and disposal of sharps
- routine environmental cleaning (environmental control)
- reprocessing of re-usable medical equipment and instruments
- respiratory hygiene and cough etiquette
- aseptic technique
- waste management
- and appropriate handling of linen (NHMRC, 2019a).

Standard precautions should be used in the handling of blood (including dried blood); all other body substances, secretions and excretions (excluding sweat), regardless of whether they contain visible blood; non-intact skin; and mucous membranes (NHMRC, 2019b).

Thus, standard precautions are the work practices required to achieve a basic level of infection prevention and control, and are the minimum infection prevention and control practices that must be used at all times for all patients in all situations.

Transmission-based precautions

Transmission-based precautions (TBPs) are used in addition to standard precautions when standard precautions alone may be insufficient to prevent transmission of infection.

TBPs are applied to patients suspected or confirmed to be infected with agents transmitted by contact (direct or indirect), droplet or airborne routes.

- *Contact transmission.* Indirect or direct contact transmission not able to be contained by standard precautions. This can occur when a healthcare worker's hands or clothing become contaminated, patient-care devices are shared between patients, infectious patients have contact with other patients or environmental surfaces are not regularly decontaminated (e.g. viral gastroenteritis, *Clostridium difficile*, Methicillin Resistant Staphylococcus Aureus [MRSA], scabies).
- *Droplet transmission.* When a healthcare worker's hands become contaminated with respiratory droplets and are transferred to susceptible mucosal surfaces such as the eyes; or when large infectious respiratory droplets are expelled over short distances by coughing, sneezing or talking, and come into contact with another's mucosa (eyes, nose or mouth), either directly or via contaminated hands (e.g. COVID-19, influenza, pertussis [whooping cough], rubella).
- *Airborne transmission.* When attending healthcare workers or others inhale small airborne particles that contain infectious agents (e.g. pulmonary tuberculosis, chickenpox, measles) (NHMRC, 2019a; Victorian Department of Health, 2018).

The combination of measures used in TBPs depends on the route/s of transmission of the infectious agent involved. In the acute-care setting, this will involve a combination of the following measures:

- continued implementation of standard precautions
- appropriate use of PPE (including gloves, aprons or gowns, surgical masks or P2/N95 respirators, and protective eyewear)
- patient-dedicated equipment
- allocation of single rooms or cohorting of patients
- appropriate air management requirements
- enhanced cleaning and disinfecting of the patient environment
- restricted transfer of patients within and between facilities (NHMRC, 2019b).

For diseases that have multiple routes of transmission, more than one TBP category is applied.

Whether used singly or in combination, TBPs are always applied in addition to standard precautions. TBPs remain in effect for limited periods of time until signs and symptoms of the infection have resolved or according to recommendations from infection control professionals specific to the infectious agent (NHMRC, 2019b).

Signage

Signage should be positioned prominently outside the room of a patient with TBPs. This is to ensure staff and visitors do not enter without appropriate PPE. Refer to the facility policies and procedures.

Standardised TBPs signage has been developed by the Australian Commission on Safety and Quality in Health Care (ACSQHC). If a health service uses their own signage, ensure that signage clearly notes the type of TBPs and PPE required (Victorian Department of Health, 2018).

Precautions for immunocompromised patients

Patients who are susceptible to infections (such as the immuno-compromised or burns patients) from microorganisms carried into the environment by hospital personnel, other patients or visitors may need to be separated to protect them from the risk of infection. This is protective isolation (Dougherty & Lister, 2015). Infection control professionals (such as the infection control nurse) within a healthcare facility play a major role in developing specific infection control protocols and the required signage.

In summary, effective work practices to minimise the risk of transmission of infection require consideration of the specific situation as well as appropriate use of standard and TBPs.

IDENTIFY SAFETY CONSIDERATIONS

The nurse should assess the potential risk of infection for the patient, or staff, and implement the appropriate infection control procedures as determined by the health facility. All staff and persons entering the patient's area should be made aware of the required procedures.

GATHER AND PREPARE EQUIPMENT

The equipment required may vary in each facility, and will depend on the reason for the precautions. The facility's guidelines should be followed for each individual case. Before entering the room, the nurse should plan to complete multiple nursing interventions at the one time. All the equipment required, including that which is specific to an individual's nursing care, must be collected prior to entering the patient's room. It is counterproductive to be going in and out of the patient's room repeatedly. Some equipment is left

in the room, and decontaminated or disposed of when the patient vacates the room.

- *Relevant 'Contact, Droplet or Airborne Precautions' poster.* Produced by the ACSQHC and state/territory health departments, each poster specifies the required precautions. These are displayed outside the patient's room.
- *PPE.* According to the required precautions and facility guidelines, PPE may include non-sterile gloves, plastic aprons, disposable gowns, masks or P2/N95 respirators and protective eyewear/face shield that is placed on a

trolley outside the room. Facilities for hand washing and hand hygiene are also required. A waste bin for disposal of used PPE is provided at the doffing station. Hand gel is used for hand hygiene at the appropriate donning and doffing station.

GIVE A CLEAR EXPLANATION OF THE PROCEDURE AND ESTABLISH THERAPEUTIC COMMUNICATION

Prior to implementing infection control procedures, the patient and family should be educated about the disease or condition, the purpose of the precautions and any specific precautions required. Demonstrations by staff relevant to the required procedures also need to be considered. This understanding and participation by the patient and family will increase compliance and can provide a sense of empowerment. It also supports patient understanding with discharge planning and education when continuing these precautions at home (NHMRC, 2019b).

DEMONSTRATE PROBLEM-SOLVING ABILITIES

When a patient is placed in a single room, nurses should be aware that the patient may suffer anxiety, depression or loneliness, as their usual social relationships are disrupted. Activities allowed within the room should be provided to help maintain interaction with others and for intellectual stimulation. They may include a telephone, electronic devices, television, books and magazines. When a patient is discharged after implementing TBPs, some items will still be considered contaminated and are disposed of. Patients and staff need to be aware of this and make relevant informed choices of personal items used in the patient's room.

PERFORM HAND HYGIENE

Perform hand hygiene before touching the patient or the patient's surrounds and prior to any procedure involving patient contact to reduce the possibility of cross-contamination. Hand hygiene is the most effective method of infection control as it removes transient organisms from the hands of the nurse (see **Skill 1.1**).

DONS PPE ACCORDING TO THE REQUIRED TRANSMISSION-BASED PRECAUTIONS

Donning PPE is completed in the following sequence:
- hand hygiene
- gown
- mask (ensure it is fitted correctly over the nose and chin)
- protective eyewear
- non-sterile gloves (ensure they extend to cover the wrist of the gown) (see **FIGURE 8.13.1**).

CARRY OUT APPROPRIATE CARE OF THE PATIENT

The patient is nursed in a single room, and a 'transmission-based precautions' poster is fixed on or near the door stating the types of precautions required and requesting that visitors liaise with nursing or medical staff prior to entering. Protective clothing such as gowns, aprons, masks or masks with face shields, gloves, eyewear and overshoes are utilised (as appropriate) by those providing care or entering the room. Equipment such as a thermometer, stethoscope, sphygmomanometer and pens should be kept in the room. Other equipment (e.g. soiled linen receivers, lined rubbish containers and cleaning materials) is also kept within the room. Double-bagging techniques may be followed when removing contaminated items from the patient's environment. (Double bagging is when the bag with soiled linen or rubbish is tied off within the room, then dropped into another bag held by an assistant who is positioned at the door. Ensure the contaminated bag only touches the inside of the second bag.) Strict attention to hand hygiene is essential.

Within some healthcare facilities, private rooms may have either negative or positive pressure, or laminar airflow to prevent infectious particles from flowing out of the room, as well as high-efficiency particulate air (HEPA) filters when managing some specific infections or immuno-suppressed patients (NHMRC, 2019b). When carrying out the required care, it is important that the nurse utilises the time spent with the patient effectively by listening to the patient's concerns or interests, in order to minimise possible feelings of rejection and isolation.

Doff PPE

Doffing of PPE should occur outside of the patient's room, in the designated zone. PPE is removed in the following sequence.
- Non-sterile gloves – peel off into the waste bin without contaminating hands
- Hand hygiene
- Protective eyewear or face shield – remove by head band or earpieces and place into waste bin
- Gown – unfasten ties, pull away from neck and shoulders touching the inside of the gown only, turn inside out, roll into a bundle and discard into waste bin
- Mask – do not touch the front, grasp the bottom then top ties or elastics to loosen, then bend over waste to let it drop into waste bin
- Hand hygiene – see **FIGURE 8.13.2**.

(ACSQHC, 2020)

SEQUENCE FOR PUTTING ON PPE
Put on PPE before patient contact and generally before entering the patient room

Hand Hygiene

* Wash hands or use an alcohol based hand rub.

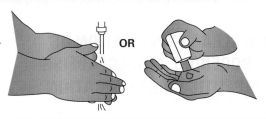

Gown

* Fully cover torso from neck to knees, arms to end of wrists, and wrap around the back.
* Fasten at the back of neck and waist.

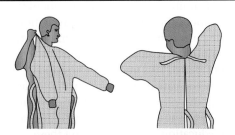

Mask

* Secure ties or elastic bands at middle of head and neck.

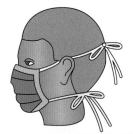

Protective Eyewear Or Face Shield

* Place over face and eyes and adjust to fit.

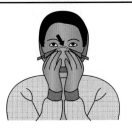

Gloves

* Extend to cover wrist of isolation gown.

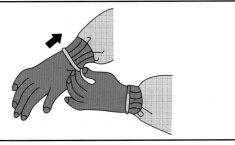

FIGURE 8.13.1 Donning procedure

SOURCE: BASED ON MATERIAL PROVIDED BY THE NATIONAL HEALTH AND MEDICAL RESEARCH COUNCIL (REPRESENTING THE COMMONWEALTH OF AUSTRALIA)

Perform hand hygiene

Maintain the 5 Moments for Hand Hygiene and perform hand hygiene after touching the patient and the patient's surrounds.

CLEAN, REPLACE OR DISPOSE OF EQUIPMENT

Contaminated material is disposed of as per facility policies. Other material is cleaned according to infection control guidelines or replaced as appropriate.

Some dedicated patient-use equipment will remain in the patient's room until discharge. It is then cleaned or disposed of.

DOCUMENT AND REPORT RELEVANT INFORMATION

Any changes in patient condition or relevant information gained during nursing care delivery should be reported so that the healthcare team remains informed.

SEQUENCE FOR REMOVING PPE
Remove PPE at doorway or in anteroon

Gloves

- Outside of gloves is contaminated!
- Grasp outside of glove with opposite gloved hand: peel off.
- Hold removed glove in gloved hand.
- Slide fingers of ungloved hand under remaining glove at wrist
- Peel glove off over first glove.
- Discard gloves in waste container.

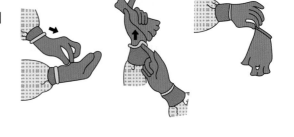

Hand Hygiene

- Wash hands or use an alcohol based hand rub.

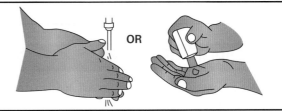

Protective Eyewear Or Face Shield

- Outside of eye protection or face shield is contaminated!
- To remove, handle by head band or ear pieces.
- Place in designated receptacle for reprocessing or in waste container.

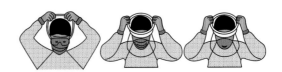

Gown

- Gown front and sleeves are contaminated!
- Unfasten ties.
- Pull away from neck and shoulders, touching inside of gown only.
- Turn gown inside out.
- Fold or roll into a bundle and discard.

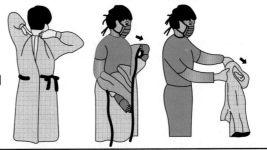

MASK

- Front of mask is contaminated—DO NOT TOUCH!
- Grasp bottom, then top ties or elastics and remove
- Discard in waste container.

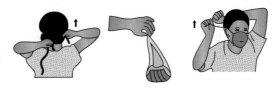

HAND HYGIENE

- Wash hands or use an alcohol based hand rub immediately after removing all PPE.

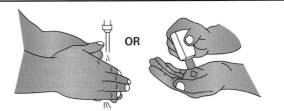

FIGURE 8.13.2 Doffing procedure

CHAPTER 8.13

CASE STUDY

You have received a message from the patient admissions clerk that a new patient is to be admitted to your ward area. The patient is a 57-year-old female with active tuberculosis (TB).

1. Identify the correct type of TBPs this patient will require.

2. Access the guidelines for TBPs on the NHMRC website and identify what precautions should be implemented (e.g. PPE, type of room).

3. You are going to give the patient a saline nebuliser to assist with collecting a sputum specimen. Identify your actions for the use of gloves, gowns and eyewear in this situation.

Note: These notes are summaries of the most important points in the assessments/procedures, and are not exhaustive on the subject. The naming of documents or charts may differ from state to state, and facility to facility. In all possible situations the guidelines of the ACSQHC are used when describing national charts or documents (e.g. the ACSQHC Observation and Response Chart is named the Adult Observation and Response Chart in WA, and the Rapid Detection and Response Observation Chart in SA). References of the materials used to compile the information have been supplied. The student is expected to have learned the material surrounding each skill as presented in the references. No single reference is complete on the subject.

CRITICAL THINKING

Thinking of the clinical skills discussed in this skill, and based on the information available at the following website (https://www.safetyandquality.gov.au/our-work/infection-prevention-and-control), identify how you will maintain standard-based and TBPs in the following scenarios:

- the client's home in the community
- aged care facility – two-bed/twin room with residents sharing the room
- aged care facility – with limited handbasins in the corridor.

REFERENCES

Australian Commission on Safety and Quality in Health Care (ACSQHC). (2020). *Sequence for Putting on and Removing PPE.* https://www.safetyandquality.gov.au/sites/default/files/2020-03/putting_on_and_removing_ppe_diagram_-_march_2020.pdf

Australian Government. (2020). Guidance on the Minimum Recommendations for the use of Personal Protective Equipment (PPE) in Hospitals during the COVID-19 Outbreak. https://www.health.gov.au/sites/default/files/documents/2020/09/guidance-on-the-use-of-personal-protective-equipment-ppe-in-hospitals-during-the-covid-19-outbreak_1.docx

Dougherty, L. & Lister, S. (eds). (2015). *The Royal Marsden Hospital Manual of Clinical Nursing Procedures* (9th ed.). Oxford: Wiley-Blackwell.

National Health and Medical Research Council (NHMRC). (2019a). *Clinical Educators Guide: Australian Guidelines for the Prevention and Control of Infection in Healthcare.* https://www.nhmrc.gov.au/sites/default/files/documents/attachments/Clinical-Educators-Guide-WEB.pdf

National Health and Medical Research Council (NHMRC). (2019b). *Australian Guidelines for the Prevention and Control of Infection in Healthcare (2019).* https://www.nhmrc.gov.au/health-advice/public-health/preventing-infection

Victorian Department of Health. (2018). *Infection Control – Standard and Transmission-Based Precautions.* Victorian State Government. © Copyright State of Victoria 2018. https://www2.health.vic.gov.au/public-health/infectious-diseases/infection-control-guidelines/standard-additional-precautions

ESSENTIAL SKILLS COMPETENCY

Transmission-Based Precautions

Demonstrates the ability to effectively and safely carry out transmission-based precaution procedures

Criteria for skill performance	Y	D
(Numbers indicate *Enrolled Nurse Standards for Practice*, 2016)	(Satisfactory)	(Requires development)
1. Identifies indication (8.3, 8.4)		
2. Identifies safety considerations (1.2, 3.2)		
3. Gathers relevant equipment (4.1, 4.2, 8.3, 8.4, 9.4)		
4. Evidence of effective communication with the patient; e.g. gives patient a clear explanation of procedure, gains patient's consent (2.1, 2.3, 2.4, 2.5, 6.3)		
5. Performs hand hygiene and dons PPE in correct sequence (1.2, 1.4, 1.8, 3.9, 6.4, 9.4)		
6. Carries out appropriate care of the patient; transmission-based precautions followed, including further hand hygiene measures (1.2, 1.4, 1.8, 2.7, 3.2, 3.9, 4.4, 6.1, 6.3, 6.4, 6.5, 6.6, 8.4, 9.4)		
7. Doffs PPE in correct sequence and performs hand hygiene (1.2, 1.4, 1.8, 3.9, 6.4, 9.4)		
8. Cleans, replaces and disposes of equipment appropriately (1.2, 1.4, 3.9, 6.5, 9.4)		
9. Documents and reports relevant information (1.2, 1.3, 1.8, 3.2, 5.3, 6.6, 7.1, 7.2, 7.3, 7.4, 7.5)		
10. Demonstrates ability to link theory to practice (8.3, 8.4, 8.5, 9.4)		

Student:

Clinical facilitator: Date:

CARE OF THE UNCONSCIOUS PATIENT

This section is too brief to discuss the care of the unconscious patient in the detail required. The student is directed to a current medical–surgical textbook for a complete discussion of this vital nursing skill. The care of the unconscious patient is complex. Prioritisation of patient needs is essential. The discussion that follows is, out of necessity, general. It is presented in order of priority; however, care should be individualised and integrated.

IDENTIFY INDICATIONS

Unconsciousness is the:

> interruption of awareness of oneself and one's surroundings, lack of the ability to notice or respond to stimuli in the environment. A person may become unconscious due to oxygen deprivation, shock, central nervous system depressants such as alcohol and drugs, or injury.
>
> (MedicineNet, Inc., 2018)

The depth and duration of unconsciousness span a broad spectrum, from fainting, with a momentary loss of consciousness, to a prolonged coma, lasting weeks, months or even years. When a patient is unconscious for any reason (e.g. following anaesthesia, a cerebrovascular accident, neurological damage, metabolic coma or a drug-induced coma), it is the nurse's duty to provide care that will protect the patient. The nurse must do everything the patient would normally do for themselves. Patients who have suffered traumatic injuries will also receive consequent rehabilitation to maintain and restore maximum function once they are medically stable. The level and type of rehabilitation will depend on the patient's level or stage of recovery (Berman et al., 2020; Dougherty & Lister, 2015). The patient who is unconscious from anaesthetic will require a modification of the following care. The cause of the coma will also impose variations on the care of the unconscious patient. For example, the patient experiencing a hepatic coma, or neuroleptic or neurological coma, would have various different assessments and treatments done on a regular basis. Patients who are mechanically ventilated have additional requirements not addressed in this section.

DISCUSS SAFETY CONSIDERATIONS

Ongoing and regular assessment is necessary to gain a baseline and to determine any small changes. At shift change, the oncoming nurse should complete the first assessment with the nurse who has cared for the patient throughout the shift. This is to ensure consistency. Neurological assessment (including the Glasgow Coma Scale; see **Skill 2.7**) of all unconscious patients (except for those post-anaesthetic) should be done frequently. In the unstable critical patient, vital signs and neurological assessment may be done every 15 minutes. When the patient is more stable, assessment will be done less frequently, but on a regular basis.

Unconscious patients must be protected against injury. Side-rails must be kept up at all times. If the patient has seizures, the side-rails must be padded and kept up at all times. Unconscious patients are unable to protect themselves and therefore the nurse must be aware of, and prevent, injuries that can result from the loss of corneal or blinking reflex, the loss of the swallowing or gag reflex, and the inability to move. Tubes, drains and lines are a potential source of injury (including healthcare-associated infection [HAI]); pressure injuries and care must be taken that they remain intact, unkinked and in situ.

GIVE A CLEAR EXPLANATION OF THE PROCEDURE AND ESTABLISH THERAPEUTIC COMMUNICATION

Although the patient is not responding to you, conversation with the unconscious patient is very important. Evidence suggests unconscious patients are aware of what is happening to them and can hear conversations around them (Dougherty &

Lister, 2015). Hearing is the first sense to return. The patient may not be able to react but may be hearing everything that goes on. This point cannot be emphasised enough. The family must also be made aware, so that conversations in the room do not distress the patient. Since the patient may be able to hear everything that occurs, explanations, respectful treatment and inclusion in conversations are extremely important. Remember to address the unconscious patient with information regarding the proposed nursing care/procedure before you touch them, and while you administer care, to help reduce anxiety and psychological stress.

PERFORM HAND HYGIENE

Perform hand hygiene before touching the patient or the patient's surrounds and prior to any procedure involving patient contact to reduce the possibility of cross-contamination. Hand hygiene is the most effective method of infection control as it removes transient organisms from the hands of the nurse (see **Skill 1.1**).

DON PERSONAL PROTECTIVE EQUIPMENT (PPE)

PPE requirements will vary according to the care being delivered. Don plastic apron, non-sterile gloves and goggles to reduce the risk of exposure to body fluids.

CARRY OUT CARE OF THE UNCONSCIOUS PATIENT

- *Respiratory system.* Respiratory assessment includes monitoring patency of airway; assessing rate, pattern and work of breathing (see **Skill 2.3**); pulse oximetry checks (see **Skill 2.5**); and arterial blood gases to assess gaseous exchange. Positioning is extremely important for the unconscious patient. They are unable to maintain their own airway and so the position in which they are placed must maintain it for them. The recovery or side-lying position with an extended head is most often used unless contraindicated (e.g. acute spinal or head injury). The head of the bed should be slightly elevated to facilitate breathing, as tolerated by the patient. Pillows and other support measures will be required to maintain the position. Frequent turning from side to side facilitates lung expansion and dislodgement of settled secretions in the lungs. Suctioning may be required to remove accumulated secretions (see **Skill 8.8**). Maintaining adequate oxygenation is important, as hypoxia and hypercapnia can contribute to secondary neurological damage. Some patients will require oxygen therapy as per medical documentation. Meet the oxygen requirements of the patient using nasal cannula, masks or ventilators, as indicated (see **Skill 8.1**). Monitor the oxygen levels in the patient's blood with a pulse oximeter (see **Skill 2.5**). Chest physiotherapy may be performed to improve ventilation and reduce pulmonary complications.
- *Cardiac system.* Perfusion should be monitored through the assessment of vital signs (see **Skills 2.3 and 2.4**), peripheral pulses, warmth of peripheries and capillary refill. Cardiac monitoring may be ordered. The risk of deep vein thrombosis and pulmonary embolism is increased due to venous stasis in the legs, hypercoagulability and prolonged pressure from immobility in bed (Dougherty & Lister, 2015). Active and passive exercises should be completed to reduce this risk (see **Skill 3.14**) and anti-embolic stockings applied.
- *Gastrointestinal tract.* Nutrition is vital in the unconscious patient. Fluid balance is equally important. The unconscious patient is usually fed by either nasogastric or gastrostomy tubes (see **Skill 8.12**). The type of feed and delivery times are ordered on an individual basis so that the patient receives the required amounts of kilojoules, fluids and nutrients to support their weight and nutritional requirements. Intravenous fluids or total parenteral nutrition may also be ordered and require constant monitoring. The patient who is unconscious often has problems with bowel functions. Assess the abdomen daily for distension and bowel sounds. Constipation occurs because of immobility and altered dietary intake. Increasing fluids, adding dietary fibre and giving mild aperients or regular suppositories on a schedule will keep the bowels regular. Loose stools can also occur. Assess the patient for the cause of the diarrhoea – it may be the feeding schedule, type of feed or gastroenteritis. The cause must be identified and appropriate treatment commenced.
- *Genitourinary tract.* Unconscious patients are incontinent. Indwelling urinary catheters are common for many unconscious patients and are a source of hospital-associated infection. Closely monitor the urinary output of the patient and perform regular urinalysis. The patient should receive sufficient fluids to keep the urine dilute. Continence promotion aids can be used as an alternative, according to policy, to keep the patient dry. Male patients usually use a urinal (if they are not restless) or an external urine collector/urinary sheath. Perineal care as part of daily hygiene (see **Skill 3.5**), plus following excretion, will help to prevent hospital-associated infections.
- *Musculoskeletal system.* To maintain mobility of joints, range-of-motion and active and passive exercises are carried out regularly (see **Skill 3.14**). Joints should be left in a functional position. Refer to the positioning of a dependent patient in **Skill 3.12**. Padded wrist/hand, ankle and foot splints may be moulded individually for the patient and are applied for 2 hours on and 2 hours off, or as ordered. These help prevent contractures.
- *Integumentary system.* A turning and repositioning schedule is established to avoid extended periods

of pressure on bony prominences and to promote circulation. Pressure-relieving devices such as reactive (constant low pressure) support surfaces or active (alternating pressure) support surfaces are used to reduce pressure. Risk assessments of the skin and for pressure injury should be completed as per hospital policy, and at least every 24 hours (see **Skill 3.13**). Bed linen is kept clean, dry and wrinkle-free. Obtain sufficient assistance when repositioning or moving the patient in bed to avoid shearing forces and friction, and to prevent muscle strain of the nursing staff.

Skin should be kept soft and supple. Take special care with skin folds. Dry them well. If the skin becomes excoriated, complete a skin assessment and implement relevant wound management strategies.

Thermoregulation is often difficult in the unconscious patient. Ambient temperature should be considered to assist the patient to maintain a normal body temperature. Hyperthermia is counteracted using antipyretics, cool sponges, fans and light bedding. Hypothermia can be managed by using a mylar thermal 'space' blanket to help elevate the temperature.

- *Personal hygiene.* The eyes, mouth, nares, ears, hair, nails and skin require assessment and care regularly. Consult the family or significant others as to the patient's routine and preferences. If the patient has an endotracheal tube in place, assess the skin under it (see **Skill 8.9**).
- *Mouth/oral care.* This is required at least every 2 to 4 hours with either a toothbrush and toothpaste, chlorhexidine mouthwash or diluted sodium bicarbonate. The teeth and gums may be brushed using a soft toothbrush and the Yankauer sucker catheter should be used to remove the fluid. Ensure the mouth is rinsed well to remove the toothpaste, which can cause drying. Saliva substitutes can help reduce a dry mouth and the potential for gingivitis (Celik & Eser, 2017). A water-soluble jelly should be applied to lips to prevent drying (see **Skill 3.5**).
- *Eye care.* The loss of the blink reflex means that tears are not blinked across the surface of the eye, so they are at an increased risk of corneal dryness and ulceration. The patient's eyes should be assessed for dryness and polyurethane eye drops applied regularly to reduce the risk of corneal abrasion (Grey et al., 2019). Encrustations of dried tears along the lid margin often occur and should be gently removed with a warm, damp washcloth on a regular basis. The loss of the corneal reflex means that there is no protection for the delicate cornea. Corneal damage can occur very quickly. If the patient's eyes are open, they may be gently taped closed or eye lubricant applied, according to hospital policy (see **Skill 3.5**).
- *Ear care.* The outer ear canal should be checked for earwax and cleansed with a washcloth as necessary. When the patient is turned, check that the pinna is not folded under. The area folded under can quickly become necrotic. The skin behind the pinna is checked regularly to ensure the straps from oxygen masks or nasal prong tubing are not causing pressure injury (see **Skill 3.5**).
- *Nares.* These require cleansing with the washcloth during daily hygiene. Creams/ointments may be used to help prevent drying. Assessment of the skin should be frequently done if the patient has a nasogastric tube in situ.
- *Sensory stimulation.* Find out the patient's preferences for music and radio programs from their family. If appropriate to the patient, play these favourites for part of the day to provide stimulation. Talk to the patient during care. Orient them to the day, the season, the weather and discuss interests that the patient has had in the past. Encourage the family to talk to and touch the patient, telling them about current family events and friends or reading to them. Maintain a normal circadian rhythm with regular sleep patterns and daytime routines (Berman et al., 2020). The lighting and ambient temperature should be lowered during the night period. Minimise sleep interruptions during the night period.

Noisy equipment and the stimuli in an intensive care situation can cause sensory overload. Attempts should be made to reduce these stimuli. Avoid making negative comments about the patient's progress or prognosis within their hearing.

Maintain the patient's dignity when providing care by maintaining privacy.

Family support is vital. Reinforcement of and clarification of information about the patient's condition assists the family to adapt. Support their decision-making process. Tolerate and support them as they vent negative emotions. This permits them to come to terms with the situation. Involvement in the patient's care permits the family to cope with their feelings of helplessness.

DOFF PPE AND PERFORM HAND HYGIENE

Remove PPE in the following sequence: gloves, hand hygiene, eyewear/face shield, plastic apron/gown and mask and then perform hand hygiene (ACSQHC, 2020). Dispose of PPE in the rubbish bag.

DOCUMENT AND REPORT RELEVANT INFORMATION

Documentation for the patient who is unconscious depends on the diagnosis, patient's stability and the length of time that they have been unconscious. All observations should be recorded on a patient observation and response chart and neurological observations chart. Nursing care should be recorded in the nursing care plan and patient progress notes. Risk assessment tools for pressure injury, falls risk and skin assessment should all be completed as per facility policy and kept in the patient's file.

CASE STUDY

You are an enrolled nurse working in a neurological ward, and have been allocated the care of 22-year-old Troy Machin, who was admitted 5 days ago following an unprovoked assault outside a city nightclub. He has remained unconscious since his admission, and requires all assistance with his nursing care needs. His girlfriend and parents visit regularly each day and stay for extended time periods by his bedside, keeping vigil. They have asked their religious minister to visit Troy regularly.

They are keen to participate in his care while they are visiting.

1. Access a nursing care plan and complete this care plan for Troy, recognising the requested family input into his care.
2. Review all the care you have listed in the care plan and identify the rationale/reasons for each of your care actions.

Note: These notes are summaries of the most important points in the assessments/procedures, and are not exhaustive on the subject. The naming of documents or charts may differ from state to state, and facility to facility. In all possible situations the guidelines of the ACSQHC are used when describing national charts or documents (e.g. the ACSQHC Observation and Response Chart is named the Adult Observation and Response Chart in WA, and the Rapid Detection and Response Observation Chart in SA). References of the materials used to compile the information have been supplied. The student is expected to have learned the material surrounding each skill as presented in the references. No single reference is complete on the subject.

CRITICAL THINKING

Refer to the clinical skills discussed, and identify the key components you would need to consider in the following scenarios.
   When caring for people who are unconscious reflect on the importance of:
- communicating directly with the client (e.g. informing them of planned care actions)
- not having a casual personal conversation with a colleague in the unconscious patient's room while ignoring the patient.

REFERENCES

Australian Commission on Safety and Quality in Health Care (ACSQHC). (2018). *Selected Best Practices and Suggestions for Improvement for Clinicians and Health System Managers: Hospital-acquired Complication 3 Healthcare-associated Infections.* https://www.safetyandquality.gov.au/sites/default/files/migrated/SAQ7730_HAC_Factsheet_HealthcareAssociatedInfections_LongV2.pdf

Berman, A., Frandsen, G., Snyder, S., Levett-Jones, T., Burston, A., Dwyer, T., Hales, M., Harvey, N., Moxham, L., Langtree, T., Reid-Searl, K., Rolf, F. & Stanley, D. (2020). *Kozier & Erb's Fundamentals of Nursing, Volumes 1–3.* (5th ed.) Melbourne: Pearson.

Celik, G. & Eser, I. (2017). Examination of intensive care unit patients' oral health. *International Journal of Nursing Practice,* 23(6), e12592. doi:10.1111/ijn.12592

Dougherty, L. & Lister, S. (eds). (2015). *The Royal Marsden Hospital Manual of Clinical Nursing Procedures* (9th ed.). Oxford: Wiley-Blackwell.

Gray, S., Ferris, L., White, L.E., Duncan, G. & Baumle, W. (2018). *Foundations of Nursing: Enrolled Nurses* (2nd ANZ ed.). Melbourne: Cengage.

MedicineNet, Inc. (2018). Medical definition of unconscious. https://www.medicinenet.com/script/main/art.asp?articlekey=11852

RECOMMENDED READINGS

Australian Commission on Safety and Quality in Health Care (ACSQHC). (2019). *Comprehensive Care Standard.* https://www.safetyandquality.gov.au/standards/nsqhs-standards/comprehensive-care-standard

Berman, A., Snyder, S., Levett-Jones, T., Burton, T. & Harvey, N. (2021). *Skills in Clinical Nursing* (2nd ed.). Melbourne: Pearson.

Koutoukidis, G. & Stainton, K. (2020). *Tabbner's Nursing Care: Theory and Practice* (8th ed.). Sydney: Elsevier.

Vivek. P. (2019). *Unconscious Patients: Sense of Hearing (Evidence Summary).* AN: JBI15085. Joanna Briggs Institute.

PART 8

ESSENTIAL SKILLS COMPETENCY

Care of the Unconscious Patient

Demonstrates the ability to effectively and safely care for the patient who is unconscious

Criteria for skill performance	Y	D
(Numbers indicate *Enrolled Nurse Standards for Practice*, 2016)	(Satisfactory)	(Requires development)
1. Identifies indication (8.3, 8.4)		
2. Discusses safety considerations (1.2, 1.4, 1.8, 3.2, 3.9, 7.3, 8.4, 9.4)		
3. Evidence of effective communication with the patient; e.g. talks to the patient during care (2.1, 2.3, 2.4, 2.5, 6.3)		
4. Performs hand hygiene and dons PPE as appropriate (1.2, 1.4, 1.8, 3.9, 6.4, 9.4)		
5. Respiratory care (1.2, 1.4, 1.8, 2.3, 2.4, 2.7, 3.2, 3.3, 3.7, 3.9, 4.1, 4.2, 4.3, 4.4, 5.2, 6.1, 6.2, 6.4, 6.6, 7.1, 7.2, 7.3, 7.4, 7.5, 8.4, 9.4)		
6. Cardiac care (1.2, 1.4, 1.8, 2.3, 2.4, 2.7, 3.2, 3.3, 3.7, 3.9, 4.1, 4.2, 4.3, 4.4, 5.2, 6.1, 6.2, 6.4, 6.6, 7.1, 7.2, 7.3, 7.4, 7.5, 8.4, 9.4)		
7. Gastrointestinal tract care (1.2, 1.4, 1.8, 2.3, 2.4, 2.7, 3.2, 3.3, 3.7, 3.9, 4.1, 4.2, 4.3, 4.4, 5.2, 6.1, 6.2, 6.4, 6.6, 7.1, 7.2, 7.3, 7.4, 7.5, 8.4, 9.4)		
8. Genitourinary tract care (1.2, 1.4, 1.8, 2.3, 2.4, 2.7, 3.2, 3.3, 3.7, 3.9, 4.1, 4.2, 4.3, 4.4, 5.2, 6.1, 6.2, 6.4, 6.6, 7.1, 7.2, 7.3, 7.4, 7.5, 8.4, 9.4)		
9. Musculoskeletal system care (1.2, 1.4, 1.8, 2.3, 2.4, 2.7, 3.2, 3.3, 3.7, 3.9, 4.1, 4.2, 4.3, 4.4, 5.2, 6.1, 6.2, 6.4, 6.6, 7.1, 7.2, 7.3, 7.4, 7.5, 8.4, 9.4)		
10. Integumentary system care (1.2, 1.4, 1.8, 2.3, 2.4, 2.7, 3.2, 3.3, 3.7, 3.9, 4.1, 4.2, 4.3, 4.4, 5.2, 6.1, 6.2, 6.4, 6.6, 7.1, 7.2, 7.3, 7.4, 7.5, 8.4, 9.4)		
11. Personal hygiene (1.2, 1.4, 1.8, 2.3, 2.4, 2.7, 3.2, 3.9, 6.1, 6.6, 8.4, 9.4)		
12. Sensory stimulation (1.2, 1.4, 1.8, 2.3, 2.4, 2.7, 3.2, 3.3, 3.7, 3.9, 4.1, 4.2, 4.3, 4.4, 5.2, 6.1, 6.2, 6.4, 6.6, 7.1, 7.2, 7.3, 7.4, 7.5, 8.4, 9.4)		
13. Doffs PPE and performs hand hygiene (1.2, 1.4, 1.8, 3.9, 6.4, 9.4)		
14. Documents and reports relevant information (1.2, 1.3, 1.8, 3.2, 5.3, 6.6, 7.1, 7.2, 7.3, 7.4, 7.5)		
15. Demonstrates ability to link theory to practice (8.3, 8.4, 8.5, 9.4)		

Student:

Clinical facilitator: Date:

PALLIATIVE CARE AND END-OF-LIFE CARE

DEFINING PALLIATIVE CARE

The World Health Organization defines palliative care as:

> an approach that improves the quality of life of patients and their families facing the problems associated with life-threatening illness, through the prevention and relief of suffering by means of early identification and impeccable assessment and treatment of pain and other problems, physical, psychosocial and spiritual.

> (WHO, 2021)

As the population ages and advancements are made in all areas of medicine, nurses are increasingly exposed to patients with a plethora of chronic diseases requiring palliative management. Nurses have a key role in caring for patients with a life limiting illness throughout the palliative care trajectory, including end-of-life care, as they spend more time with patients than any other members of the health profession (Gallagher et al., 2014).

Palliative patients are admitted to all wards and care is provided by a variety of health professionals, depending on the illness and the needs of the patient, their family and caregivers (Palliative Care Australia [PCA], 2017). This multidisciplinary team may include:

- specialist palliative care doctors and nurses
- general practitioners
- specialist doctors (e.g. cardiologists and oncologists)
- allied health professionals (e.g. pharmacist, occupational therapist, physiotherapist, speech pathologist)
- pastoral care workers
- social workers
- counsellors.

The focus of palliative care is to maintain an individual's quality of life while meeting the needs of the individual and their family/carer. Palliative care clinicians and others who care for seriously ill patients nearing the end of life seek to balance enough care to ensure comfort while avoiding care that could diminish quality of life (Ferrell, 2020). As the illness advances and the patient enters the terminal phase, the focus shifts from curative to comfort care. There is no single specific point in an illness when end-of-life care/terminal care begins. It very much depends on the individual and their illness. An Advanced Care/Health Directive will guide any decision making at this time. They are legally written documents that specify the patient's wishes, either consenting or refusing future care relating to health decisions (Department of Health, 2019).

While a *Voluntary Assisted Dying Act* is now in place in Victoria and has commenced in Western Australia in July 2021, these will not be discussed in this skill. VAD does not replace the need for exemplary palliative care that should be delivered to all patients.

DEFINING END-OF-LIFE (TERMINAL) CARE

End-of-life (terminal) care is a broad term for care that is planned for, negotiated with or provided to people at the end of their lives, lasting usually only a few days (CareSearch, 2017).

IDENTIFY INDICATIONS FOR END-OF-LIFE CARE

Nursing care and support for the dying patient and their family includes the need for an accurate assessment of the physiological signs of approaching death (Berman et al., 2020). The main characteristic changes include loss of muscle tone, slowing of the circulation, sensory impairment, altered level of consciousness and changes in respirations and pattern.

COMMON SYMPTOMS OBSERVED IN END-OF-LIFE CARE

- *Dyspnoea*. A common symptom in the terminal phase. It is distressing for both the patient and family members.
- *Respiratory tract secretions*. These can be manifested as gurgling, bubbling noises (often referred to as the 'death rattle'). It occurs when patients are

unable to clear their oral secretions due to the loss of swallowing or coughing reflex.

- *Nausea and vomiting.* These can be caused by many factors (e.g. medications, intestinal obstruction, anxiety).
- *Pain.* There is a need to consider physical as well as emotional factors.
- *Terminal restlessness and/or agitation.* This is an agitated delirium that may occur in some patients in the last days of life (CareSearch, 2020).

IMPLEMENT END-OF-LIFE CARE

Perform hand hygiene
Perform hand hygiene before touching the patient or the patient's surrounds and prior to any procedure involving patient contact to reduce the possibility of cross-contamination. Hand hygiene is the most effective method of infection control as it removes transient organisms from the hands of the nurse (see **Skill 1.1**).

Don personal protective equipment (PPE)
Don PPE as appropriate. PPE requirements will vary according to the care being delivered and the patient's health status: plastic apron/gown, eyewear/faceshield, mask and non-sterile gloves – to reduce the risk of exposure to bodily fluids.

Give a clear explanation of the procedure and establish therapeutic communication
An understanding of the cultural values, beliefs and practices of the patient/family relevant to death and dying are especially important during this time. Open and honest communication skills are vital. Both the patient and family members need to be kept informed regularly and may need to have this new information repeated on more than one occasion. Many patients and their families fear the unknown. The nurse's role is to prepare the patient and their family for what may lie ahead, allowing both the patient and family time to absorb and reflect on the information delivered.

Implement nursing care of the patient
In order to deliver the most appropriate nursing care, the nurse first needs to carry out an impeccable assessment of the patient's symptoms.

- *Pain.* Pain is not something that should be accepted as part of the dying process; therefore, a thorough pain assessment needs to be conducted on a regular basis (see **Skill 2.9**). The patient may be experiencing different pains (e.g. visceral pain and/or neuropathic pain) and the nurse needs to administer appropriate interventions. This may be pharmacological or non-pharmacological. When administering any intervention, a pre- and post-intervention pain assessment should be conducted.

- *Respiratory.* As the patient enters the terminal phase, respiratory changes may be noticed. Respirations may become irregular, shallow and very slow. The patient may no longer be able to clear respiratory secretions due to the loss of the swallow and cough reflex. Medications may be prescribed to assist. The unconscious/ semiconscious patient is positioned on their side with the head slightly elevated to promote drainage of excess secretions. Good mouth care at this time is essential. Oral suctioning at this stage is usually contraindicated and can be distressing to the patient.

- *Cardiac.* As the patient enters the terminal phase, the peripheries of the limbs may become cold and mottled, as in peripheral shutdown. The radial pulse gradually fails. Increasing the frequency or completing regular vital signs may not be required because often no intervention will be implemented for alterations in cardiac function.

- *Gastrointestinal.* As the patient's condition deteriorates, the need for food and fluid declines. Giving the patient fluids at this time can be harmful as the gag reflex disappears. Family members often find the withholding of diet and fluids very distressing. Encouraging the family to perform regular mouth care can be a way of involving the family in the patient's care. Even though the patient may not be eating and drinking, the body will still produce waste. It is important that effective bowel care is given. Oral aperients are inappropriate if the patient cannot swallow, and rectal interventions are used to prevent constipation.

- *Genitourinary.* Maintaining the patient's dignity and comfort is important. As the sphincters relax, the patient will become incontinent. This can be managed with regular washes and incontinence pad changes. Alternatively, the patient may suffer from retention of urine and the insertion of an indwelling catheter (for comfort) (see **Skill 8.6**) may be required if a bladder scan shows significant urinary retention.

- *Musculoskeletal.* As the musculoskeletal system fades, there are changes in the patient's muscle strength. The patient may experience inability to move or swallow, and the jaw may sag. The nurse needs to assess the patient on a regular basis, so that the appropriate intervention, such as repositioning (see **Skill 3.12**) or mouth care (see **Skill 3.5**), may be implemented.

- *Integumentary.* It is important to keep the patient's body in alignment to promote comfort. The use of special mattresses or pillows to support limbs is beneficial. Regular pressure area care and inspection of the skin for redness is essential as the patient deteriorates. Many patients will be nursed on air/alternating pressure air mattress so that moving of the patient is minimal, but the risk of a pressure injury is reduced (see **Skill 3.13**).

- *Personal hygiene.* The eyes, mouth, nares, ears, hair, nails and skin require assessment and care. Skin care is particularly important in response to incontinence of urine and faeces, or if the patient is diaphoretic. Bed linen and patient clothing are changed as often as needed, and the room is kept as odour free as possible. At all times the dignity and privacy of the patient is maintained (see **Skill 3.5**).
- *Spiritual, cultural and emotional needs.* The patient and their family will require support and respect for their personal beliefs. Assist with contacting a spiritual leader (e.g. priest, imam, rabbi, monk, minister, healer) at the patient's request, or create privacy for other rituals and prayers. Patients may request specific icons or items to be kept close. Ensure that any culturally specific needs for personal care, diet, clothing or death and dying are also respected and maintained within the care delivered. Support the family by creating an environment that allows frequent visiting of the family, including an area for them to take a short break. Family members may also implement rosters for someone to always stay with the patient, including overnight.

DOCUMENT AND REPORT RELEVANT INFORMATION

Document relevant patient information on care plans and the patient's notes, particularly any observed deterioration in the patient status and any family concerns. Facility policy should also be considered. Ensure there are also contact numbers for family and preferred religious or spiritual leaders. Details for the preferred funeral director may be noted in some facilities. A patient observation and response chart to record observations may be maintained in some acute care areas, but notation should be made by the doctor to accommodate the anticipated variances in the dying patient's observations. Many facilities use Goals of Care documentation that promotes shared decision making.

LAST OFFICES

Once the patient has been certified deceased (usually by a medical doctor), the nurse is required to follow the facility's practices/policies regarding documentation and the implementation of the 'last offices'. As this is an expected death, there generally should be no need to follow the limitations or requirements for a coroner's case. The Salisbury NHS Foundation Trust (2017) state that the last offices is the care given to a deceased patient and their family/ carer from the time of death in hospital until release of the body to the funeral director.

The process described for last offices is applicable to all patients. Each facility will have specific policies that need to be followed, including specific documentation requiring completion by different members of the healthcare team. For non-terminal patients, also refer to specific guidelines for any patient that may be classified as a coroner's case, as the washing of the patient's body plus the removal of any drains, peripheral intravenous catheter (PIVC), clothing and other items is not permitted. The actions of making the environment clean and as presentable as possible for the family to view the body should still be followed.

GATHER AND PREPARE EQUIPMENT

- *Equipment for patient hygiene needs –* sponge bowl, towels, disposable flannel, toothbrush, hairbrush or comb, clean pyjamas, electric shaver.
- *Clean bed linen.*
- *Last offices tray/box –* depending on the facility, this box may contain documents, body bag and other items to assist with implementing last offices.

- *PPE –* non-sterile gloves, plastic apron, eyewear/ faceshield and mask.
- *Tape and non-sterile gauze.*
- *Extra sheet and tape, or body bag –* used for wrapping the patient after the family has left.

IMPLEMENT LAST OFFICES

Last offices are implemented after a patient has been certified as deceased by the doctor. This care will generally include attention to hygiene needs (washing/ cleansing of the body and oral care/denture care); combing of the hair; dressing the body in a clean gown, pyjamas, or nightie; and placing the body in alignment with the head on a pillow. Follow a process similar to sponging the patient and implementing patient hygiene needs (see **Skill 3.5**). If the patient has been recently sponged or showered (i.e. within the last 3 to 4 hours) and they do not have excess secretions or other body fluids on their skin, a briefer process of grooming and cleaning the patient can be implemented. After washing and changing, the patient's jaw may require propping with a rolled towel under the chin. This should be removed when the family comes into the room. Wearing non-sterile gloves, remove any drains, catheters, PIVC, oxygen masks and other tubing from the patient. Seal the removal site with tape and gauze, if required. If soiled, change the patient's sheets and make the patient's bed (see **Skill 3.2** for making an occupied bed). It is not necessary to cover the patient's face until the family has left as it can increase their grief.

The nurse should maintain respect for the patient and their belongings when completing these actions, with some nurses preferring to maintain communication similar to that for an unconscious patient. It is often less distressing to complete last offices soon after the patient has died, when the body is still warm and relaxed. The original patient identification bands must be maintained on the body. The overall appearance of the patient and environment should be as clean and pleasant as possible, as it is usual for family to view the body.

Remove excess clutter and equipment from the patient's area, and bring in chairs for the family to sit on. The patient's personal belongings should also be packed neatly, and any valuables recorded. According to facility policy, valuables may be signed for and collected by family/next of kin or sent to the facility safe.

After the family has completed the viewing of the patient, the body is placed in a body bag or wrapped in a sheet and externally tagged as per facility policy (name, date of birth etc.), then either transported to the hospital morgue or kept in the room until the arrival of the funeral director (Grey et al., 2019). Some families and carers may wish to assist with the last offices and, unless this is contraindicated, they should be supported in doing this as it may help to facilitate their grieving process.

DOFF PPE

Remove PPE in the following sequence: gloves, hand hygiene, eyewear/face shield, plastic apron/gown and mask and then perform hand hygiene (ACSQHC, 2020). Dispose of in the rubbish bag.

PERFORM HAND HYGIENE

Maintain the 5 Moments for Hand Hygiene and perform hand hygiene after touching the patient and the patient's surrounds.

CLEAN, REPLACE OR DISPOSE OF EQUIPMENT

Clean any used equipment by wiping with disinfecting wipes recommended by your facility, and return to the storage area. Disposable items should be discarded in either the general waste or in the relevant sharps and biohazard containers, according to facility policy. The patient's bed area will be cleaned by the support staff after the patient has been sent to the morgue or collected by the funeral director.

DOCUMENT AND REPORT RELEVANT INFORMATION

Specific documentation for the death of the patient will be completed by the doctor and the registered nurse. Some of the patient's valuables and other items may need to be recorded according to facility policy. This is to prevent potential legal issues. Collect any notes and documentation to be sent with the patient, if working in an acute care facility. Record that last offices have been implemented in the nursing notes.

CASE STUDY

Gino Bertoloni is a 68-year-old Italian man who was recently been diagnosed with late-stage inoperable gastric cancer. Up until his diagnosis, he worked in his own successful business. Initially he was treated with immunotherapy and then chemotherapy, as a hospital outpatient, but had been admitted overnight or for a few days when his condition required extra care and monitoring.

Gino has four adult children, and although divorced, has a partner who lives with him and is very supportive. His children visit him regularly, are very upset regarding his rapid health deterioration and have found this difficult to accept.

He is now in the final stages of his illness, and wishes to remain at home with his partner and have community palliative care to assist. He is weak and frail, and prefers to rest during the day on his bed. He often feels nauseous, eats and drinks very little, requires frequent pain management medication, and at times is confused. Due to his frailty and lack of mobility, he had difficulty with regular toileting, and now requires the use of continence aids for his urinary

incontinence and constipation. He is an agnostic, and as such does not want spiritual support.

1. Use the above information and access other relevant information to create a plan of care appropriate to Gino and his family's needs. Use the following headings.
   a. Pain
   b. Respiratory needs
   c. Cardiac needs
   d. Gastrointestinal needs
   e. Genitourinary needs
   f. Musculoskeletal needs
   g. Integumentary needs
   h. Personal hygiene
   i. Cultural and spiritual needs.
2. What bereavement support is available for Gino's partner and children?
3. As this is your first experience with a dying/deceased patient and bereaved family, what support services are available for you to access at this time?

Note: These notes are summaries of the most important points in the assessments/procedures, and are not exhaustive on the subject. The naming of documents or charts may differ from state to state, and facility to facility. In all possible situations the guidelines of the ACSQHC are used when describing national charts or documents (e.g. the ACSQHC Observation and Response Chart is named the Adult Observation and Response Chart in WA, and the Rapid Detection and Response Observation Chart in SA). References of the materials used to compile the information have been supplied. The student is expected to have learned the material surrounding each skill as presented in the references. No single reference is complete on the subject.

CRITICAL THINKING

We talk of patients being palliative and how to support the patient through their journey.
1. What is the difference between palliative care and end-of-life care?
2. Research voluntary assisted dying/euthanasia in your state/territory and familiarise yourself with the rules and regulations.

REFERENCES

Australian Commission on Safety and Quality in Health Care (ACSQHC). (2020). *Sequence for Putting on and Removing PPE.* https://www.safetyandquality.gov.au/sites/default/files/2020-03/putting_on_and_removing_ppe_diagram_-_march_2020.pdf

CareSearch. (2020). *Care of the Dying Person.* https://www.caresearch.com.au/caresearch/ClinicalPractice/Physical/EndofLifeCare/tabid/738/Default.aspx

Department of Health. (2019). *Advance Care Directive.* Australian Government. https://www.health.gov.au/health-topics/palliative-care/planning-your-palliative-care/advance-care-directive

Ferrell, B.R. (2020). Treating infections near the end of life. *Medscape.* 3 February. https://www.medscape.com/viewarticle/924395

Gallagher, O., Saunders, R., Tambree, K., Alliex, S., Monterosso, L. & Naglazas, Y. (2014). Nursing student experiences of death and dying during a palliative care clinical placement: teaching and learning implications. *Transformative, Innovative and Engaging: 23rd Annual Learning Forum.* Perth, Western Australia, 23, pp. e1–10.

Gray, S., Ferris, L., White, L.E., Duncan, G. & Baumle, W. (2018). *Foundations of Nursing: Enrolled Nurses* (2nd ANZ ed.). Melbourne: Cengage.

Palliative Care Australia (PCA). (2017). *What is Palliative Care?* http://www.palliativecare.org.au

Salisbury NHS Foundation Trust. (2017). *End of Life Care – Last Offices.* http://www.icid.salisbury.nhs.uk/ClinicalManagement/EndOfLifeCare/Pages/EndofLife.aspx

World Health Organization (WHO). (2021). *Palliative care.* http://www.who.int/cancer/palliative/definition/en/

RECOMMENDED READING

Australian Commission on Safety and Quality in Health Care (ACSQHC). (2019). *Comprehensive Care Standard.* https://www.safetyandquality.gov.au/standards/nsqhs-standards/comprehensive-care-standard

Australian Commission on Safety and Quality in Health Care (ACSQHC). (2019). *End-of-life Care.* https://www.safetyandquality.gov.au/our-work/end-life-care

Berman, A., Frandsen, G., Snyder, S., Levett-Jones, T., Burston, A., Dwyer, T., Hales, M., Harvey, N., Moxham, L., Langtree, T., Reid-

Searl, K., Rolf, F. & Stanley, D. (2020). *Kozier & Erb's Fundamentals of Nursing, Volumes 1–3.* (5th ed.) Melbourne: Pearson.

World Health Organization (WHO). (2018). *Integrating Palliative Care and Symptom Relief into Primary Health Care: A WHO Guide for Planners, Implementers and Managers.* Geneva: World Health Organization. https://apps.who.int/iris/handle/10665/274559

PART 8

ESSENTIAL SKILLS COMPETENCY

Palliative Care and End-of-Life Care

Demonstrates the ability to effectively and safely care for the end-of-life/terminal patient

Criteria for skill performance	Y	D
(Numbers indicate *Enrolled Nurse Standards for Practice*, 2016)	(Satisfactory)	(Requires development)
1. Identifies indication (8.3, 8.4)		
2. Discusses safety considerations (1.2, 1.4, 1.8, 3.2, 3.9, 7.3, 8.4, 9.4)		
3. Evidence of effective communication with the patient and family and gains consent (2.1, 2.3, 2.4, 2.5, 6.3)		
4. Performs hand hygiene and dons appropriate PPE as required (1.2, 1.4, 1.8, 3.9, 6.4, 9.4)		
5. Assesses and manages pain (1.2, 1.4, 3.2, 4.1, 4.2, 4.4, 6.3, 6.4, 6.6, 7.1, 8.4, 9.4)		
6. Respiratory care (1.2, 1.4, 1.8, 2.3, 2.4, 2.7, 3.2, 3.9, 4.1, 4.2, 6.1, 6.6, 7.1, 8.4, 9.4)		
7. Cardiac care (1.2, 1.4, 1.8, 2.3, 2.4, 2.7, 3.2, 3.9, 4.1, 4.2, 6.1, 6.6, 7.1, 8.4, 9.4)		
8. Gastrointestinal tract care (1.2, 1.4, 1.8, 2.3, 2.4, 2.7, 3.2, 3.9, 4.1, 4.2, 6.1, 6.6, 7.1, 8.4, 9.4)		
9. Genitourinary tract care (1.2, 1.4, 1.8, 2.3, 2.4, 2.7, 3.2, 3.9, 4.1, 4.2, 6.1, 6.6, 7.1, 8.4, 9.4)		
10. Musculoskeletal system care (1.2, 1.4, 1.8, 2.3, 2.4, 2.7, 3.2, 3.9, 4.1, 4.2, 6.1, 6.6, 7.1, 8.4, 9.4)		
11. Integumentary system care (1.2, 1.4, 1.8, 2.3, 2.4, 2.7, 3.2, 3.9, 4.1, 4.2, 6.1, 6.6, 7.1, 8.4, 9.4)		
12. Personal hygiene care (1.2, 1.4, 1.8, 2.3, 2.4, 2.7, 3.2, 3.9, 6.1, 6.6, 8.4, 9.4)		
13. Recognises and responds to spiritual, cultural and emotional needs of patient and family (1.2, 1.4, 1.8, 2.3, 2.4, 2.7, 3.2, 3.9, 4.1, 4.2, 6.1, 6.6, 7.1, 7.3, 8.4, 9.4)		
14. Doffs PPE and performs hand hygiene (1.2, 1.4, 1.8, 3.9, 6.4, 9.4)		
If performing last offices		
15. Gathers equipment for last offices (1.2, 1.6, 4.4, 6.4, 8.4, 9.4)		
16. Performs hand hygiene and dons PPE as required (1.2, 1.4, 1.8, 3.9, 6.4, 9.4)		
17. Implements last offices (1.2, 1.4, 1.8, 2.3, 2.4, 2.7, 3.2, 3.9, 6.1, 6.6, 8.4, 9.4)		
18. Doffs PPE and performs hand hygiene (1.2, 1.4, 1.8, 3.9, 6.4, 9.4)		
19. Cleans, replaces and disposes of equipment appropriately (1.2, 1.4, 3.9, 6.5, 9.4)		
20. Documents and reports relevant information (1.2, 1.3, 1.8, 3.2, 5.3, 6.6, 7.1, 7.2, 7.3, 7.4, 7.5)		
21. Demonstrates ability to link theory to practice (8.3, 8.4, 8.5, 9.4)		

Student:

Clinical facilitator: Date:

MENTAL HEALTH CARE

Note: These notes are summaries of the most important points in the assessments/procedures and are not exhaustive on the subject. References of the materials used to compile the information have been supplied. The student is expected to have learnt the material surrounding each skill as presented in the references. No single reference is complete on each subject.

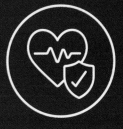

CHAPTER 9.1

MENTAL STATE EXAMINATION

Mental state examination (MSE) is part of an overall mental health assessment, and a generalised MSE should be completed as part of general history taking for all consumers/clients (Hercelinskyj & Alexander, 2020). Within the mental health setting, a mental status is the counterpoint of a physical assessment in the general care setting (Moxham et al., 2017). The purpose is to gather information to make an informed judgement about an individual's mental state and if there is a need for follow-up psychiatric care. Use of an MSE at different points during the consumer's care also provides a reference for comparison of future assessments (Evans et al., 2016). A more focused MSE and other assessments such as risk assessment and substance screening are completed for consumers admitted to a psychiatric care area and are part of an ongoing comprehensive mental health assessment completed by different members of the mental health team. The MSE will help identify a consumer's care requirements and involves a semi-structured interview to assess their neurological and psychological function. It can also be used within general care delivery to gather and then share information about a consumer's status with other members of the healthcare team or implement further risk assessment processes. Hercelinskyj and Alexander (2020) point out that the (MSE) is a 'snapshot' of the person being assessed on a particular day, and that over time, there may be changes or improvements.

DEMONSTRATE PROBLEM-SOLVING ABILITIES

The person's age, culture (including religion) and language require consideration when assessing the mental status, since each of these impact on their ability to process information and respond to questions posed by the healthcare worker (Warren, 2013). A further example of the impact of culture is transgressions of cultural law and subsequent fear of punishment that may present as anxiety, depression or psychosis. Educational level and attainment could impact on the client's vocabulary as well as on their ability to process mathematical concepts. Having English as a second language would reduce their ability to display their knowledge, to display their ability to reason in the abstract and in some cases their ability to adequately demonstrate reasoning and judgement. Consequently, an official interpreter will be required for admission and other key assessments. The healthcare environment should be culturally safe and inclusive, respecting each individual's cultural and religious background (Barkway & Nizette, 2018).

When completing an MSE it is important to be aware of and work within the workplace role and scope of the enrolled nurse. A more in-depth or comprehensive assessment may be the responsibility of a senior registered nurse (RN) or other mental health team member. It may also be relevant to involve the assistance of an RN or urgently advise them of the person's mental health status if there is any assessment data that is unusual or indicative of a potential risk to the consumer, other clients or staff, and the nurse. This is particularly relevant if there is any disturbed perception or thought processes.

Some facilities may use a mnemonic (e.g. PAMSGOTJIMI – perception, affect, mood, speech, general behaviour, orientation, thought, judgement, insight, memory, intelligence) as a prompt for what to include when assessing a client (Evans et al., 2016; Moxham et al., 2017). Hercelinskyj & Alexander (2020) use 'BATOMIPJR' – behaviour and appearance, affect, thought, orientation, mood, insight, perception, judgement and risk. These are separate to, and should not replace, a standardised workplace tool for MSE.

GIVE A CLEAR EXPLANATION OF THE PROCEDURE AND ESTABLISH THERAPEUTIC COMMUNICATION

Effective and therapeutic communication skills are a vital part of mental health nursing. Provide a quiet and private area, and use open communication skills to help establish a positive therapeutic relationship (refer to **Skill 9.2**). Introduce yourself and give the person a clear explanation of the procedure to help gain their cooperation and trust. Allow personal space, listen carefully and focus on the content of the person's conversation and feelings, as well as their body language. Be aware that the person may be anxious or fearful.

PERFORM ASSESSMENT ACCORDING TO FACILITY PROTOCOLS

Use the following guidelines to gather information about the person being assessed, and their current mental health status. Any formal mental health assessments should be conducted according to the facility's standards and protocols.

- *Appearance.* General appearance provides information about an individual's self-care ability, lifestyle and daily living skills. The way the person dresses, their facial expression, their posture and gait, their general mannerisms and their apparent age, gender and race are all included in general appearance. Observe the person's clothing for style, cleanliness, appropriateness and character. Note any peculiarities of choices in clothing, jewellery, hairstyle and cosmetics. Take note of the level of personal hygiene. Clean skin, hair, nails and minimal body odour are expectations of our culture; however, take the circumstances into consideration. For example, the individual who is admitted to the accident emergency department straight from a work-related injury at a factory or construction site could not be expected to be clean or without body odour created by their manual work. Illness, both mental and general, often affects the person's ability for self-care.
- *Behaviour.* Note what the person is doing during the assessment as well as their manner, attitude and non-verbal communication, as this can reveal information about their emotional attitude. Identify their level of activity, posture, gait and gestures, plus their rapport and level of social engagement. For example, is the person calm, aggressive or agitated? Are they underactive or hyperactive?

  Posture and gait reflect self-concept, body image and self-esteem. Mannerisms will often reflect a person's underlying emotions. Assess the person's facial expression and level of eye contact. Facial expressions provide clues about the person's mood. Is their expression alert, vacant, sad, pleasant, hostile or mask-like? Eye contact is culturally determined, so be aware of the culture of the person when assessing this.
- *Mood and affect.* Mood can be defined as a person's own description of their feelings or emotion, and affect as the feeling or emotional state inferred from the client's statements, appearance and behaviour (Barkway & Nizette, 2018).

To assess mood, ask the person to describe their feelings and reasons for these feelings. Identify emotions such as feeling depressed or happy. Is the client crying, irritable, angry, calm, neutral, apathetic, fearful and/or euphoric? Assess a person's affect by observing their appearance, body language, behaviour and any inconsistencies between this and emotions they express. Description of affect can include:
- appropriate to inappropriate
- range: grandiose, flat, blunted, restricted, full range (normal)
- stability: labile, stable.

- *Speech/conversation.* Speech is important in revealing the person's presentation. Assessment should include a person's speech behaviour as well as its content. Use the following as a guide to assess speech.
  - Is the rate fast, slow, interrupted, uneven or steady?
  - Is the volume loud, inaudible or normal?
  - Is the tone moderate, calm or hostile?
  - Does the conversation flow, have clarity (slurred, monosyllabic, pressured), is interrupted or stays on topic?
  - Does the content include references to disordered, negative or unrealistic thoughts?
  Slurring, extremely rapid or slow speech, or poorly intoned speech may indicate neurological dysfunction or a mental disorder. Be careful to ascertain that the person being assessed does not have a speech disorder (e.g. teeth or palate problems) or a hearing disorder.
- *Cognition.* Cognitive function assesses the person's level of consciousness and their orientation to time, person and place, and helps determine a person's capacity to process information.
- *Level of consciousness.* Determine if the individual is fully alert, confused, lethargic, unresponsive or intoxicated. A fully alert person will have clear and organised thoughts, appropriate flow of speech and no attention drifting.
- *Orientation.* Ask the person being assessed: 'What day/date is it (or recent event/current affairs)?', 'Where are you?' or 'What is your name?' Remember that it is common for people who are hospitalised to lose track of the exact date.
- *Memory.* Short-term memory, long-term memory and memory of other recent events is assessed. If there appear to be large gaps in memory, or the person being assessed is forgetful, formal evaluation is required.
  - *Immediate memory.* The nurse recites a list of items and asks the person to repeat them immediately.
  - *Recent memory.* Ask about something that happened today or a recent news story.
  - *Long-term/remote memory.* Ask the person to give a coherent story about events in their life.
- *Attention and concentration.* Assess this by asking the person to do simple addition or subtraction

exercises, such as counting backwards from 100 by sevens, or asking them to spell 'world' backwards.

■ *General knowledge*. This usually becomes apparent in the history taking. This can be further assessed by asking questions that would be within an individual's frame of reference.

■ *Language*. Ask the person to name objects or follow instructions.

■ *Thought processes and content*. Thinking should be logical, coherent and relevant.
  – *Processes*. These are the individual's thoughts: frequently changing topic or fragmented, irrelevant or loosely associated, excessively vague, hesitant, blocked or nonsense.
  – *Content*. Refers to topics or nature of content. Thought content should be assessed for obsessive or repetitive thinking, delusions (uncompromising false beliefs not consistent with the person's background), distorted perceptions, religious or grandiose ideas, phobias, depressive thoughts, anxiety, self-harm or aggressive ideas.

■ *Perception*. Perception is the person's experience and interpretation of their world through their senses. Identify if they are experiencing:
  – *hallucinations*, which are a false sensory perception that does not have an actual external stimulus and the sufferer cannot distinguish them from reality; they can involve all five senses – auditory, visual, touch, smell and taste
  – *illusions*, which are misinterpretations of an external stimulus
  – *derealisation*; that is, the sense that the external world feels unreal
  – *depersonalisation*; that is, a feeling of self being different, unfamiliar or being detached.

■ *Insight*. This is the person's ability to understand or identify their symptoms and acknowledge their mental health problems. Ask them about their understanding of their mental illness, treatment options and how it is affecting their life.

■ *Judgement and abstract thinking*. Assess judgement by evaluating the person's ability to use appropriate thought processes to problem-solve and make sensible decisions for everyday activities and social situations. Present an everyday problem. The individual should show their ability to consider a range of options and apply sound reasoning. Abstract thinking is the ability to generalise information, and to evaluate it. This can be ascertained by asking the person to explain the meaning of a proverb such as 'the early bird catches the worm' or 'there is no place like home'.

DOCUMENT AND REPORT RELEVANT INFORMATION

The MSE requires formal documentation in the client's progress notes and admission forms (for admissions). Most areas use a specific data collection tool. In some instances (e.g. distressed , unusual thought processes), verbatim reports of what was said should be included and any deviations from previous MSEs should be noted. The documentation of an MSE in a psychiatric setting will be more comprehensive than in the general setting and should be documented at least once per shift.

Gain the assistance of other experienced or senior staff if the consumer becomes distressed or agitated. Report any changes to their behaviours or information that is different to other recently noted mental state/health assessments or examinations, or indicates a potential risk (e.g. self-harm, aggression) for the consumer or others, to the RN. This is particularly relevant if the consumer has any disturbed perception or thought processes.

Note: Please refer to facility policy and/or a specific mental health text such as Hercelinskyj & Alexander (2020) for other screening tools such as substance use or risk assessment.

CASE STUDY

Access a mental state examination tool from your clinical work area, or use the headings in this skill to create your own data collection tool.

1. What specific communication skills (see therapeutic communication skills) will be useful to help obtain an accurate MSE of a client with a psychiatric illness?

2. Using these communication skills, practise the collection of information for an MSE on a family member or one of your fellow students. Your practice partner may choose to role-play a client with a psychiatric illness, and express emotions or thought processes relevant to this illness.

3. Document the information you collect, and then write a brief report that you would include in the client's progress notes.

Note: These notes are summaries of the most important points in the assessments/procedures, and are not exhaustive on the subject. The naming of documents or charts may differ from state to state, and facility to facility. In all possible situations the guidelines of the ACSQHC are used when describing national charts or documents (e.g. the ACSQHC Observation and Response Chart is named the Adult Observation and Response Chart in WA, and the Rapid Detection and Response Observation Chart in SA). References of the materials used to compile the information have been supplied. The student is expected to have learned the material surrounding each skill as presented in the references. No single reference is complete on the subject.

REFERENCES

Barkway, P. & Nizette, D. (2018). *Mosby's Pocketbook of Mental Health* (3rd ed.). Chatswood: Elsevier.

Evans, K., Nizette, D. & O'Brien, A. (2016). *Psychiatric and Mental Health Nursing* (4th ed.). Chatswood: Elsevier.

Hercelinskyj, G. & Alexander, L. (2020). *Mental Health Nursing: Applying Theory to Practice.* Melbourne: Cengage.

Moxham, L., Hazelton, M., Muir-Cochrane, E., Heffernan, T., Kneisl, C.R. & Trigoboff, T. (2017). *Contemporary Psychiatric-Mental Health Nursing: Partnerships in Care.* Melbourne: Pearson.

Warren, B.J. (2013). How culture is assessed in the DSM-5. *Journal of Psychosocial Nursing & Mental Health Services,* 51(4), pp. 40–45.

RECOMMENDED READINGS

Department of Health. (2021). *What We're Doing About Mental Health.* https://www.health.gov.au/health-topics/mental-health-and-suicide-prevention/what-were-doing-about-mental-health?utm_source=health.gov.au&utm_medium=callout-auto-custom&utm_campaign=digital_transformation

Royal Children's Hospital Melbourne. (2018). *Clinical Practice Guidelines.* http://www.rch.org.au/clinicalguide

ESSENTIAL SKILLS COMPETENCY

Mental State Examination

Demonstrates the ability to effectively assess a client's mental status

Criteria for skill performance	Y	D
(Numbers indicate *Enrolled Nurse Standards for Practice*, 2016)	(Satisfactory)	(Requires development)
1. Identifies indication (8.3, 8.4)		
2. Demonstrates problem-solving abilities; e.g. person's age, culture and language require consideration when assessing the mental status; works within own scope of practice; gains assistance of RN or senior staff when required (1.1, 1.2, 1.6, 2.3, 2.4, 3.7, 4.1, 4.2, 8.3, 8.4, 9.4)		
3. Evidence of effective and therapeutic communication with the person; e.g. gives person a clear explanation of procedure, gains relevant consent, establishes trust, listens carefully (1.2, 1.4, 2.1, 2.3, 2.4, 2.5, 6.1, 6.3, 6.6, 7.3, 7.5, 8.4, 9.4)		
4. Performs hand hygiene (1.2, 1.4, 1.8, 3.9, 6.4, 9.4)		
5. Assesses person according to protocols (1.1, 1.2, 1.3, 2.2, 2.5, 4.1, 4.2, 7.1, 7.2, 7.3, 8.4, 9.4)		
6. Performs hand hygiene (1.2, 1.4, 1.8, 3.9, 6.4, 9.4)		
7. Documents relevant information; reports unusual data or potential risks to RN (1.2, 1.3, 1.8, 3.2, 3.9, 5.3, 6.6, 7.1, 7.2, 7.3, 7.4, 7.5)		
8. Demonstrates ability to link theory to practice (8.3, 8.4, 8.5, 9.4)		

Student:

Clinical facilitator: Date:

CHAPTER 9.2

ESTABLISHING A 'THERAPEUTIC RELATIONSHIP' IN THE MENTAL HEALTH SETTING

IDENTIFY INDICATIONS

The focus of mental health care is to facilitate a consumer's mental health, minimise the impact of mental illness, focus on an individual's resilience and manage the symptoms. Care should support consumers to achieve the best outcomes while living with their illness and focus on their future. Nursing care is based on being and interacting with a consumer and establishing a therapeutic relationship, not 'doing' (e.g. implementing actions such as wound care) or being disease oriented. Establishing rapport and a therapeutic relationship between the nurse, the consumer and the family is the cornerstone of mental health care (Barkway & Nizette, 2018; Moxham et al. 2017). It requires the use of well-developed communication skills, plus

empathy and trust. Applying these skills to deliver recovery-oriented practices and person-centred care will help establish emotional safety and a safe environment for the consumer.

Nursing care will also include the delivery of general nursing care actions for other health problems, as many consumers with mental illness may have other medical conditions. This co-morbidity of illness can be related to side effects of psychotropic medications, lifestyle factors such as smoking or other substance use, inactivity and diet, or the age of the consumer. People with chronic illness are also at increased risk of developing problems such as depression or anxiety.

INTERACT WITH THE CONSUMER AND ESTABLISH A THERAPEUTIC RELATIONSHIP

A therapeutic relationship (or nurse–consumer relationship) is the process for providing care to consumers in a mental health setting. It uses theoretical understanding, personal attributes and appropriate clinical techniques to provide and sustain positive emotional experiences for consumers within a mental health area, and is built over a period of time (Moxham et al., 2017). This therapeutic relationship helps a client to feel understood, explore their interpersonal problems or gain insight to their own behaviour and work towards problem solving and developing coping skills. It helps the consumer to identify their personal strengths and draw on them in the recovery journey, and relates specifically to the Australian College of Mental Health Nurses' standards of practice (standard 3), which states the need for a therapeutic relationship to be respectful of the consumer's choices, experiences and circumstances (Australian College of Mental Health Nurses [ACMHN], 2010). Establishing trust and a therapeutic alliance with the consumer will:
- enable the completion of a full assessment and care plan
- encourage the consumer to define their problems and perceptions of their distress

- help the consumer to adapt, rebound, grow, define a sense of self and become resilient
- facilitate the consumer to learn and develop coping skills
- assist the consumer to understand and find their personal interests, strengths and skills.

Good communication skills are the tools for delivering appropriate consumer care. Be aware that different forms of communication will be used for each client and their needs. Follow the communication and interaction strategies stated in the client's care plan.

SELF-AWARENESS

The enrolled nurse (EN) working in a mental health area needs to be conscious of their own values, beliefs and identity. Understanding and being aware of your own emotional reactions, thoughts and communication skills will help you be able to manage them and then focus on those of the person and their family. You can also consciously manage your use of 'self' to interact and establish a therapeutic relationship with the client. Be aware of how you use your non-verbal behaviours, such as tone of voice, body language and ability to respond calmly. Avoid your own personal behaviours and communication actions that are distracting, annoying or provocative (Moxham et al., 2017).

Self-awareness does require time to develop and can be assisted by receiving feedback from mentors and clinical supervisors or keeping a reflective journal when working in the mental health setting.

PROFESSIONAL BOUNDARIES

Professional boundaries refer to verbal and non-verbal actions and interactions between individuals or groups. It is important to recognise that care actions in mental health involve the emotions of the consumer, which can create some confusion if the boundaries between a professional relationship and over-involvement with a client are not understood. The nurse–client therapeutic relationship is not a social relationship and it is essential to establish and maintain professional boundaries to ensure a safe therapeutic connection (Moxham et al., 2017; NMBA, 2018). The importance of professional boundaries is not only for personal safety, but breaching these will impair the nurse–client relationship and the client's care outcomes (Barkway & Nizette, 2018). To help maintain the appropriate boundary between a therapeutic relationship and a personal relationship, the communication and interaction with the client should be based on plans and goals that are therapeutic (NMBA, 2010).

Introduce yourself and your role to the consumer. Use their preferred name or title, and respond respectfully and thoughtfully when interacting with them. Be professional in your responses and avoid including your personal information, views or feelings (excessive self-disclosure). Maintain open and non-judgemental communication, using clarification of what the client said. The nurse's own self-care is important in this care environment. Discuss any unexpected feelings (e.g. guilt, worry, attraction, feelings of friendship, over-involvement) you may experience with your supervisor (Barkway & Nizette, 2018; Evans, Nizette & O'Brien, 2016).

Professional boundaries and codes of conduct/ethics specified by the Nursing and Midwifery Board of Australia (2018) reinforce the importance of not sharing personal contact details with clients or establishing interaction via social media. No contact in any form should take place outside of work time. Disciplinary actions can be implemented by the workplace and/or the NMBA if these guidelines are breached.

COMMUNICATION SKILLS

Good communication and interpersonal skills are what the mental health nurse uses as a nursing intervention. It is important to not only interact with a client, but to know why some specific communication strategies are used, and to be able to skilfully change or implement a new communication action as a client situation requires. Each individual also requires different communication interventions as part of their individualised client care. Refer to the client's nursing and overall care plan to identify the correct communication and interaction that should be implemented. Purposeful interaction and communication is also used to elicit information from a consumer, express empathy and provide feedback to them.

Good therapeutic communication skills are focused on the individual, and include both the nurse's verbal and non-verbal communication. Make yourself available and show interest towards the client (e.g. 'I am happy to walk with you. Can I do this with you?'). Face the person (preferably sitting) when communicating and have an open posture. Maintain an appropriate use of personal space. Encourage the client to lead the conversation.

The following skills are used as part of interacting with a consumer, and varied according to their care needs.

- *Listening.* Use active listening to observe, hear and understand what the consumer has said. Use your verbal remarks, facial expression and verbal encouragers (e.g. 'uh-huh', 'go on') to clarify their comments and encourage further communication. An appropriate use of silence helps the client to think about what is being discussed and to be able to say more. Listening is a core skill in caring for consumers with a mental illness.
- *Clarification.* Clarify what the person has said to determine that the message being sent is what you are hearing or understanding.
- *Paraphrasing.* Use paraphrasing to gain clarification or validation of what the client has said. It can also be used to reflect back on what they have said, to help them feel accepted and recognised.
- *Feedback and summarising.* Feedback as part of the client interaction should remain neutral by restating or summarising what they have said. Verbalise observed behaviour and information from the client (e.g. you sound upset). Summarise the overall points that have been discussed.
- *Questioning.* Questions should be open-ended to encourage spontaneous responses and promote discussion. According to your role, or the types of discussion, use questions to explore information from the client. Ensure the questions are clear, concise and easily understood.
- *Non-verbal communication.* The EN needs to use their personal body language and non-verbal communication to create comfort and ease in the consumer and help them feel accepted. Maintain an open and relaxed posture, with a friendly tone of voice. Eye contact should recognise cultural boundaries, and be used to show interest in the current interaction. You will also need to be skilled at deciphering an individual's body language and non-verbal behaviour. What body posture, rate of speech, tone of voice, gestures, pauses, and so on is the person using? These will help you to assess a client's status, plus become able to predict their responses and interactions.

- *Focus*. Identify the main or recurrent themes in what the client has been saying.

There are types of input and communication that should be avoided in a therapeutic relationship. These include giving advice or your opinions, talking about yourself, telling the consumer they are wrong, giving false reassurance, entering into their hallucinations or changing the subject. Be careful not to be too quiet and unresponsive, or ignore or avoid a client who interacts with you. Work closely with the registered nurse (RN) when making any assessments or decisions about changes of care, and don't jump to conclusions about a client's behaviour or make quick assumptions.

CLIENT ASSESSMENT

A mental state examination (see **Skill 9.1**) is used for assessing the consumer when interacting with them. Be observant of their communication and behaviour. Observe non-verbal behaviour such as posture, facial expressions, eye and hand movements. Personal care, grooming and choice of clothing is also important in understanding the person's wellbeing and mental status. Verbal communication should be assessed for things such as content, rate and tone.

Assess the information gathered from the client when interacting with them. It will influence how the EN continues the current interaction and communication with them.

LEGAL CONSIDERATIONS AND SCOPE OF PRACTICE

National practice standards for the mental health workforce and the World Health Organization Action Plan for 2013–2020 state the need for all areas of care delivery in the mental health setting to maintain a consumer's rights, dignity and respect, including respect for values, belief and culture (Department of Health, 2013; Kanna et al., 2020). Individual human rights for both voluntary and involuntary consumers should be respected in all communication and interaction.

While developing a therapeutic relationship and using communication skills as part of care implementation, the role of the EN is to participate as part of a team. Listening to the guidance of the RN and other team members, as well as working within the scope of practice guidelines, is essential. National practice standards for the mental health workforce recognise that it can take an extended period of time (up to 2 years) to develop effective skills specific to the mental health setting (Department of Health, 2013).

DOCUMENT AND REPORT RELEVANT INFORMATION

Communicating and interacting with the consumer are part of the care provision which will be recorded in nursing care plans and the progress notes. Any other relevant charts or tools should also be completed. Any information about the client's status such as client behaviour, thoughts or emotion should be reported verbally to the RN. The written record of interactions and the client's verbal content provide data used to assess their status and response to treatment. The content should be descriptive and directly quote the client where relevant. Any client verbalisation of risks such as violence, self-harm or suicidal idealisation should be documented and reported to the appropriate staff member immediately.

CASE STUDY

You are working within the mental health ward of an acute care city hospital.

1. What actions could you implement to increase your ability to understand your own communication skills and establish a therapeutic relationship with your clients?

2. Why is listening, not judging, and encouraging the client to do most of the talking the preferred approach to client care?

3. Identify where you would find the communication skills and other planned activities or interactions that are part of each consumer's care.

4. During handover you note that one of the clients in the ward is actually an old work colleague. You are interested to learn more about his background and history of mental illness and read his medical notes, even though your allocation is in a different section. You also stop to chat with him during the shift and have a great catch-up about time you shared while working together in the past. You also exchange personal stories and contact information. Identify how and why this situation is in breach of professional boundaries for the EN.

5. Another client in your ward tells you about his Instagram account and asks if you want to become a 'follower' or 'like' his page on Facebook. How will you manage this request?

Note: These notes are summaries of the most important points in the assessments/procedures, and are not exhaustive on the subject. The naming of documents or charts may differ from state to state, and facility to facility. In all possible situations the guidelines of the ACSQHC are used when describing national charts or documents (e.g. the ACSQHC Observation and Response Chart is named the Adult Observation and Response Chart in WA, and the Rapid Detection and Response Observation Chart in SA). References of the materials used to compile the information have been supplied. The student is expected to have learned the material surrounding each skill as presented in the references. No single reference is complete on the subject.

CRITICAL THINKING/LIFESPAN

Thinking of the clinical skills discussed in this skill, and the stages of growth and development, what are some of the key components you would need to consider in the following scenarios?

Establishing therapeutic boundaries and a therapeutic relationship will have some variations between different care settings, although some therapeutic boundaries do not change. They must also always adhere to guidelines from the NMBA. Describe how you could establish professional boundaries and a therapeutic relationship in each of the following settings:

- a 16-year-old boy who is self-harming in a paediatric mental health setting
- a 19-year-old woman with a long history of anorexia nervosa, recently discharged from an acute facility and now being managed in a community care environment
- a 35-year-old woman with schizophrenia being managed in her community clinic, and has a long-term therapeutic relationship with her community nurses and doctors
- a 76-year-old female client with a long-term history of mental illness who is now a resident of a mental health aged care facility.

REFERENCES

Australian College of Mental Health Nurses (ACMHN). (2010). *Standards of Practice in Mental Health Nursing.* http://members.acmhn.org/publications/standards-of-practice

Barkway, P. & Nizette, D. (2018). *Mosby's Pocketbook of Mental Health* (3rd ed.). Sydney: Elsevier.

Department of Health. (2013). *National Practice Standards for the Mental Health Workforce.* Australian Government. https://www1.health.gov.au/internet/publications/publishing.nsf/Content/mental-pubs-n-wkstd13-toc

Evans, K., Nizette, D. & O'Brien, A. (2016). *Psychiatric and Mental Health Nursing* (4th ed.). Sydney: Elsevier.

Kanna, S., Faraaz, M., Shekhar, S. & Vikram, P. (2020). An end to coercion: rights and decision-making in mental health care. *Bulletin of the World Health Organization*, 98(1), pp. 52–8. Geneva: World Health Organization.

Moxham, L., Hazelton, M., Muir-Cochrane, E., Heffernan, T., Kneisl, C.R. & Trigoboff, T. (2017). *Contemporary Psychiatric-Mental Health Nursing: Partnerships in Care.* Melbourne: Pearson.

Nursing and Midwifery Board of Australia (NMBA). (2010). *A Nurse's Guide to Professional Boundaries.* http://www.nursingmidwiferyboard.gov.au

Nursing and Midwifery Board of Australia (NMBA). (2018). *Code of Conduct for Nurses.* http://www.nursingmidwiferyboard.gov.au

RECOMMENDED READINGS

Eliassen, B.K., Sørlie, T., Sexton, J. & Høifødt, T.S. (2016). The effect of training in mindfulness and affect consciousness on the therapeutic environment for patients with psychoses: an explorative intervention study. *Scandinavian Journal of Caring Sciences*, 30(2), pp. 391–402.

Hercelinskyj, G. & Alexander, L. (2020). *Mental Health Nursing: Applying Theory to Practice.* Melbourne: Cengage.

Queensland Health. (2010). *Queensland Mind Essentials – Mental Illness Nursing Documents.* https://www.health.qld.gov.au/__data/assets/pdf_file/0029/444773/mindessentialsfinal.pdf

Thompson, R., Valenti, E., Siette, J. & Priebe, S. (2016). To befriend or to be a friend: a systematic review of the meaning and practice of 'befriending' in mental health care. *Journal of Mental Health*, 25(1), pp. 71–7.

ESSENTIAL SKILLS COMPETENCY

Establishing a 'Therapeutic Relationship' in the Mental Health Setting

Demonstrates the ability to effectively assess a client's mental status

Criteria for skill performance	Y	D
(Numbers indicate *Enrolled Nurse Standards for Practice*, 2016)	(Satisfactory)	(Requires development)
1. Identifies indication (8.3, 8.4)		
2. Able to establish and work within professional boundaries when interacting with consumers, including legal/ethical implications (1.2, 1.4, 1.8, 2.3, 2.4, 2.5, 3.2, 3.9, 6.1, 6.3, 7.3, 8.4, 9.4)		
3. Recognises importance of self-awareness, self-care and own communication skills (1.2, 3.2, 3.9, 7.3)		
4. Establishes therapeutic relationship, showing empathy, recognition of cultural values or beliefs; creates comfortable and trusting environment for consumer to communicate (1.2, 1.4, 2.1, 2.3, 2.4, 2.5, 6.1, 6.3, 6.6, 7.3, 7.5, 8.4, 9.4)		
5. Uses appropriate communication and interpersonal skills, according to client's plan of care and situation; includes listening, appropriate non-verbal communication, clarification, reflection, focus on client's content etc.; communication is client centred (1.2, 1.4, 2.1, 2.3, 2.4, 2.5, 6.1, 6.3, 6.6, 7.3, 7.5, 8.4, 9.4)		
6. Recognises consumer's rights, behaviour and needs when interacting (1.2, 1.4, 2.1, 2.5, 3.2, 3.9, 4.1, 4.2, 6.1, 6.6, 8.4, 9.4)		
7. Implements planned communication and interaction strategies (1.2, 1.4, 2.1, 2.3, 2.5, 6.1, 6.3, 7.3, 7.5, 8.4, 9.4)		
8. Maintains safety of self, client and others (1.2, 1.4, 1.8, 2.5, 3.2, 3.9, 6.1, 8.4, 9.4)		
9. Liaises and works with RN and other team members when interacting with clients; recognises own scope and role within the team (1.2, 1.4, 1.5, 1.6, 1.7, 1.10, 2.5, 3.2, 3.7, 3.9, 6.1, 6.2, 6.3, 6.6, 8.4, 9.4)		
10. Reports and documents relevant information (1.2, 1.3, 1.8, 3.2, 5.3, 6.6, 7.1, 7.2, 7.3, 7.4, 7.5)		
11. Demonstrates ability to link theory to practice (8.3, 8.4, 8.5, 9.4)		

Student:

Clinical facilitator: Date:

CHAPTER 9.3

MANAGEMENT OF A CLIENT WITH CHALLENGING BEHAVIOUR (AGGRESSIVE OR VIOLENT)

Challenging behaviour can occur in any clinical setting, and:

> is any behaviour with the potential to physically or psychologically harm another person, or self, or property. It can be deliberate or unintentional and ranges from verbal abuse through to threats or acts of physical violence.

(SA Health, 2021)

The behaviour may result from medical illness (e.g. brain injury, dementia, confusion, trauma, sepsis, constipation, urinary tract infection and medication side effects), some psychiatric illnesses or drug intoxication/withdrawal. Pain, discomfort, fatigue, hunger, memory difficulties or the need to go to the toilet can trigger irritability and stress. The environment can also trigger changes in a client's behaviour. This includes overstimulation that can easily be caused in the clinical area by factors such as noise, hospital machinery, staff interactions and client chatter. It is essential for nurses to be aware that client behaviours will be influenced by staff attitudes, waiting times and consumer's perceived expectations. Cross-cultural factors and a consumer's needs must be understood by the enrolled nurse (EN).

Challenging behaviour can include:

- *non-verbal*; for example, wandering, pacing, being socially disruptive, making intimidating facial expressions, withdrawal from specific activities
- *verbal*; for example, shouting, swearing, offensive speech, repeated questioning, hallucinations
- *physical*; for example, disinhibition, overactivity, excessive rocking, scratching, self-harm, spitting, punching, property damage.

Challenging behaviour can occur within any clinical setting and the strategies for managing the behaviour are relevant to all areas. The focus of the skill in this section is for more acute or immediate risks related to aggression and violence that may occur in any clinical setting, although there is a focus on the skill being applied in the mental health setting. Management of other events such as a psychotic episode, suicide/self-harm risk and panic attack may have some similar principles but are not necessarily covered by the skills described herein. In addition to the general guidelines discussed, facilities and health services will have specific policies based on the state/territory mental health Act, and the facility's own client base (or location). It is essential in managing challenging behaviour to know and adhere to the facility policy.

IDENTIFY INDICATIONS

Aggression and violence are two common forms of challenging behaviour that can occur in a consumer. Barkway and Nizette (2018) link clients behaving in an aggressive or violent manner to unmet needs caused by fear, intimidation or frustration. In the aged care setting, residents with dementia have a higher incidence of aggressive behaviour.

Client behaviours that can indicate the potential for violence include a client who is exhibiting one or more of the following:

- pacing and restless, abnormal levels of activity
- swearing, being verbally threatening or sarcastic
- shouting or talking rapidly
- staring or exhibiting prolonged eye contact
- dilated pupils
- poor concentration
- delusions or hallucinations with violent content.

When interacting with the client or completing a risk assessment, it is important to distinguish between the person's usual language and verbal aggression, as well as recognise culturally influenced behaviours or responses (Evans et al., 2016; Queensland Health, 2010). Also be aware that mental illness can lead to diminished control and lack of ability to self-regulate behaviour, making some of the listed behaviours routine actions for some clients. Zero-tolerance policies (i.e. facility policies that state any aggressive behaviour is not acceptable) require special consideration in mental health areas. Aggressive situations do not have to escalate to an emergency situation. The consumer may be releasing their anxiety and frustrations, and the role of the healthcare team is to manage the situation and restore calm. The primary goal is to act as soon as possible to stop the consumer's behaviour from escalating and keep their agitation under control with maximum safety.

LEGAL CONSIDERATIONS AND SCOPE OF PRACTICE

Principles of maintaining a consumer's rights, dignity and respect when delivering care in a mental health setting should be maintained when managing a client experiencing a violent or aggressive episode (Department of Health, 2013; Kanna et al., 2020). Principles and standards stated in the Standards of Practice for Mental Health Nurses (Australian College of Mental Health Nurses, 2010) should be adhered to, as well as the relevant state/territory mental health act.

The role of the EN is to assess risks for challenging behaviours, plus respond to and manage client's situations according to their workplace role and scope of practice. In some more acute situations, the EN may identity the client's behaviour, call for assistance (implement a code black if relevant), initiate risk assessment and establish initial communication strategies with the client or assist as a member of the team. More senior and experienced staff members will manage the overall situation. However, in some workplaces (e.g. community, aged care) the EN may be the most senior member of staff and will be required to manage the scenario and make decisions based on the risk assessment.

PREVENTION STRATEGIES

When a consumer is recognised as potentially becoming distressed or aggressive, a range of therapeutic interventions should be implemented to help minimise and manage the behaviour. Most consumers will exhibit early warning signs of distress, and it is important to recognise and respond to these before a situation escalates. Verbal expressions of emotional distress can produce changes in behaviour in a similar way that extreme pain will change a client's behaviour, especially for those with dysfunctional coping skills. Maintaining a calm demeanour and a relaxed posture may help the client to regain control of their actions. Some specific prevention strategies include the following.

- Spend one-to-one time with the client and actively engage with them.
- Speak clearly, using short sentences. Use active listening skills to hear what the client is saying. Be non-judgemental and use a friendly tone of voice.
- Modify environmental conditions (e.g. noise, lighting, overstimulation) that may be potentiating the behaviour.
- Reduce any demands being made on the person. Distract the person's attention to another task (go for a walk, eat, read a magazine).
- Review the client's care plan for specific risk management interventions.

If the client does not respond to these actions, a call for assistance and a further risk assessment will be necessary.

Strategies to manage the situation may also include de-escalation actions such as 'leave and return', especially if a client is resisting care. This skill requires good judgement, but is effective in situations when required care is not urgent.

MANAGING RISK

A risk assessment to determine the possible risk to the health and safety of the client should be completed by the EN on admission to any mental health service and also when a client is showing signs of challenging behaviour. A second risk assessment may be completed when more experienced staff respond to a call for assistance. This assessment will help to determine the level of risk (low, medium or high) and an appropriate plan of action, and reduce the likelihood of an adverse event. Assess the situation using the following questions.

- What is the risk?
- Who is at risk?
- What is the chance of the risk occurring?
- How immediate is the risk (stressors, people, situation)?
- What factors can increase or decrease the risk?
- What needs to be done to reduce or manage the risk? (Barkway & Nizette, 2018)

Many facilities use a formal aggression scale or risk assessment tool, so these should be completed where appropriate. Accessing and using these tools may not be possible in urgent situations.

SAFETY CONSIDERATIONS

Managing a client displaying aggression requires skill and confidence. As an EN, allow experienced staff to take over the leadership and management of the challenging behaviour. To maintain the safety of other staff and clients, the following actions should be implemented.

1. Carefully minimise the danger, as well as the risk of injury to the client and others around them (staff and other clients). Other clients should be calmly removed from the area.
2. Call for assistance (and security) using the facility duress alarms or other protocols. Request this assistance early, before a situation escalates, and wait for assistance to arrive before approaching the client.
3. Always maintain a safe distance from the client and have an open door or exit behind you. Be aware of your possible escape routes. Specific mental health assessments may need to be conducted in a room with two exit doors.
4. Attend facility in-service and induction training sessions to keep up to date, and enhance your skills for managing consumers with challenging behaviour. Learn appropriate communication and 'de-escalation' skills.

DE-ESCALATION

De-escalation focuses on reducing the tension in a situation and preventing it from deteriorating. The goal is to avoid violence and stop people from being traumatised or hurt. When implementing these processes, ensure principles of safety are followed. Never approach an angry client before assistance arrives, and do not attempt to restrain someone on your own. All staff should maintain a calm demeanour. A member of staff will be required to take the lead of managing the environment by creating space, reducing noise, removing excess staff or bystanders and managing security. Another experienced member of staff will communicate and interact with the client to help manage their behaviour. All other clients should be asked quietly but firmly to leave the area. Staff members are responsible to help move them to a safer space. The EN can assist with this process.

Client communication and interaction: while using the communication skills described in the following list, the goal is to redirect the client's attention to deflect their anger and identify the possible cause of their distress, then problem solve this with them.

- Use an empathetic, non-confrontational approach. Speak calmly, clearly and slowly.
- Introduce yourself to the client and explain your actions. Give brief, clear instructions.
- Allow more personal space than usual. Do not touch the client.
- Avoid aggressive postures – be relaxed, with your arms by your side.
- Ensure you can also retreat if necessary.
- Eye contact should be intermittent and not prolonged.
- Listen carefully. Acknowledge their feelings, and respect their feelings, thoughts and views.
- Use open questions to encourage the client to talk and try to determine what the problem is. This may help them to calm down.
- Treat medical issues such as pain or discomfort.
- Be patient and breathe slowly. Allow the person to 'let off steam'.
- Offer realistic options, and do what you say you will do.
- Don't disagree, make threats or tell the client to calm down.

Queensland Health (2017) use the mnemonic DEESCALATION to summarise these actions.

INFORM THE MEDICAL OFFICER

Some situations may require further intervention to help settle the client, or a medical review to assess and manage an underlying cause of their behaviour. Restraint and sedation (and seclusion) should only be considered as a last resort, and implemented only in an emergency situation when there is threat of harm to the client and others, and all other interventions and management strategies have been used (SA Health, 2020; WA Country Health Service, 2020). The EN may be the most senior member of staff in some work areas (e.g. aged care setting or hostel), but otherwise the RN, most experienced mental

health practitioner or attending medical officer will implement these decisions. Clients within the non-mental health areas who experience an episode of challenging behaviour with an unknown cause may be referred by the medical officer for further assessment by a psychiatrist.

POST-INCIDENT CARE AND DEBRIEF

Following an incident, managers may ensure staff involved have time-out or undertake alternative duties. The incident will also be documented and an incident review conducted. The incident review should be conducted by a senior member of staff, when and where appropriate. As part of the team, the EN may contribute information about the event, the risk assessment and client responses. Some areas may include the client and/or family in this process to help understand the behaviour or provide them with further support.

A debrief will be implemented for situations that have escalated. Participation is essential to create the opportunity to reflect, and to share reactions and feelings about what has occurred. A debrief will help the EN deal emotionally with what has happened, and reduce their own stress or concerns from the experience.

Following an incident, the consumer should be monitored to ensure they remain calm. Check for and implement any personal care requirements (e.g. diet, fluid, rest, pain management). Further medical review (if required) should be implemented. As part of their ongoing care, a long-term risk assessment will be completed. Risk assessment tools (according to facility policy or underlying disorder) should be used alongside the care plan and cross-referenced (SA Health, 2020) with individually tailored management plans to prevent, identify and manage challenging behaviour. Simplifying and adapting the environment, music (relevant to the client and their age), exercise and activity programs help reduce challenging behaviours in clients with dementia.

DOCUMENTATION

The event should be recorded on an incident form and in the progress notes, although senior staff involved in the incident may complete most of this paperwork. If present from the beginning of the event, the EN will need to assist with completing the documentation, but otherwise would contribute any other relevant information. Care plans may require editing to include strategies to prevent future episodes of challenging behaviour.

Some situations may require reporting of severe incidents to the police. Refer to facility policies.

Many facilities will use an aggression scale or other challenging behaviour assessment tool that relates specifically to the type of clinical setting or underlying disorder, as part of risk assessment. Refer to facility's policies for completing these correctly.

CASE STUDY

You are working in an acute adult mental health facility. Your client Ron Johnson, is an 'involuntary patient' who has become aggressive and disruptive.

1. Describe the actions you will implement to maintain the safety of yourself, other clients and staff.
2. Follow the link to the Queensland Health website and define each of the words in the mnemonic,

DEESCALATION: https://www.health.qld.gov.au/__data/assets/pdf_file/0025/665314/qh-gdl-452.pdf

3. What is the purpose of de-escalation?
4. List six communication skills you should be using to help de-escalate the situation.
5. What prevention strategies could be used to prevent similar situations of challenging behaviour for Ron?

Note: These notes are summaries of the most important points in the assessments/procedures, and are not exhaustive on the subject. The naming of documents or charts may differ from state to state, and facility to facility. In all possible situations the guidelines of the ACSQHC are used when describing national charts or documents (e.g. the ACSQHC Observation and Response Chart is named the Adult Observation and Response Chart in WA, and the Rapid Detection and Response Observation Chart in SA). References of the materials used to compile the information have been supplied. The student is expected to have learned the material surrounding each skill as presented in the references. No single reference is complete on the subject.

CRITICAL THINKING/LIFESPAN

Thinking of the clinical skills discussed in this skill, and the stages of growth and development, what are some of the key components you would need to consider in the following scenario?

Many people with dementia or mental illness may respond negatively to a nurse's requests or communication skills when the nurse is busy and not carefully consider their own actions or communication skills. Think about the nurse's possible non-therapeutic verbal communication and interactions in the following scenarios, and how they might negatively influence each client's behaviour or response. Add an alternative response by the nurse to de-escalate or prevent the situation.

- Aged care resident with dementia who believes you are in his house when you enter his room without knocking. He becomes verbally agitated and defensive in protecting his home when the nurse continues to enter his space and administer his medications.
- A client with anxiety and an unstable mental health situation is requesting food and a cigarette in a busy emergency department. Staff respond by telling them to sit down and wait for the doctor. This situation starts to escalate as the client says they are hungry and have been waiting for a long time.

REFERENCES

Australian College of Mental Health Nurses. (2010). *Standards of Practice in Mental Health Nursing.* http://members.acmhn.org/publications/standards-of-practice

Barkway, P. & Nizette, D. (2018). *Mosby's Pocketbook of Mental Health* (3rd ed.). Sydney: Elsevier.

Department of Health. (2013). *National Practice Standards for the Mental Health Workforce 2013.* Australian Government. https://www1.health.gov.au/internet/publications/publishing.nsf/Content/mental-pubs-n-wkstd13-toc

Evans, K., Nizette, D. & O'Brien, A. (2016). *Psychiatric and Mental Health Nursing.* Chatswood: Elsevier.

Kanna, S., Faraaz, M., Shekhar, S. & Vikram, P. (2020). An end to coercion: rights and decision-making in mental health care. *Bulletin of the World Health Organization.* 98(1), pp. 52–8. Geneva: World Health Organization.

Queensland Health. (2010). *Queensland Mind Essentials – Mental Illness Nursing Documents.* http://www.health.qld.gov.au/mentalhealth/mindessentials.asp

Queensland Health. (2017). Acute behavioural disturbance management (including acute sedation) in Queensland health authorised mental health services (adults). Mental Health Alcohol and Other Drugs Branch. Queensland Government. https://www.health.qld.gov.au/__data/assets/pdf_file/0025/665314/qh-gdl-452.pdf

SA Health. (2020). *Challenging Behaviour Strategic Framework.* Government of South Australia. https://www.sahealth.sa.gov.au/wps/wcm/connect/eaabdfa9-3eaf-4f96-ab3a-01b6c31391f5/20082.2+Challenging+Behaviour+Strategic+Framework_FINAL_v2.pdf?MOD=AJPERES&CACHEID=ROOTWORKSPACE-eaabdfa9-3eaf-4f96-ab3a-01b6c31391f5-nwKxjXC

SA Health. (2021). *Challenging Behaviour for Health Professionals.* Government of South Australia. https://www.sahealth.sa.gov.au/wps/wcm/connect/public+content/sa+health+internet/clinical+resources/clinical+programs+and+practice+guidelines/safety+and+wellbeing/challenging+behaviour/challenging+wbehaviour+for+health+professionals

WA Country Health Service. (2020). *Prevention of Workplace Aggression Procedure.* Government of Western Australia. http://www.wacountry.health.wa.gov.au:443/fileadmin/sections/policies/Managed/Disturbed_Behaviour_Management_Clinical_Practice_Standard_TS4KSNFPVEZQ_210_6722.pdf

RECOMMENDED READINGS

Abraha, I., Rimland, J.M., Trotta, F.M., Dell'Aquila, G., Cruz-Jentoft, A., Petrovic, M., Gudmundsson, A., Soiza, R., O'Mahony, D., Guaita, A. & Cherubini, A. (2017). Systematic review of systematic reviews of non-pharmacological interventions to treat behavioural disturbances in older patients with dementia. (the SENATOR-OnTop series). *BMJ Open, 7*(3).

Anderson, P. (2014). Reducing need to restrain vulnerable patients. *NursingTimes.Net,* 110(29), pp. 24–5.

Curyto, K.J., McCurry, S.M., Luci, K., Karlin, B.E., Teri, L. & Karel, M.J. (2017). Managing challenging behaviors of dementia in veterans: Identifying and changing activators and consequences using STAR-VA. *Journal of Gerontological Nursing,* 43(2), pp. 33–43.

Department of Health and Wellbeing. (2021). *Challenging Behaviour for Health Professionals* . Government of SA. https://www.sahealth.sa.gov.au/wps/wcm/connect/public+content/sa+health+internet/clinical+resources/clinical+programs+and+practice+guidelines/safety+and+wellbeing/challenging+behaviour/challenging+behaviour+for+health+professionals

Department of Mines, Industry Regulation and Safety. (2014). *Guide to Working Safely with Challenging Behaviours in Health Care.* Government of Western Australia. https://www.commerce.wa.gov.au/publications/guide-working-safely-challenging-behaviours-health-care

Hercelinskyj, G. & Alexander, L. (2020). *Mental Health Nursing: Applying Theory to Practice.* Melbourne, Cengage.

Jones, S. & Mitchell, G. (2015). Assessment of pain and alleviation of distress for people living with a dementia. *Mental Health Practice,* 18(10), p. 32.

Schaefer, R., Broadbent, M. & Bruce, M. (2016). Violent typologies among women inpatients with severe mental illness. *Social Psychiatry and Psychiatric Epidemiology,* 51(12), pp. 1615–22.

ESSENTIAL SKILLS COMPETENCY

Assist with the Management of a Client with Challenging Behaviour (Aggressive or Violent)
Demonstrates the ability to effectively assess a client's mental status

Criteria for skill performance	Y	D
(Numbers indicate *Enrolled Nurse Standards for Practice*, 2016)	(Satisfactory)	(Requires development)
1. Identifies indication (8.3, 8.4)		
2. Able to discuss legal and safety implications (1.2, 1.8, 3.2, 3.9, 7.3, 8.4, 9.4)		
3. Recognises potential signs of a client having challenging behaviour, and advises other staff/calls for assistance (1.2, 1.4, 1.8, 1.10, 2.5, 3.2, 3.9, 5.2, 6.1, 6.6, 7.3, 8.4, 9.4)		
4. Implements planned strategies to prevent or reduce risk of challenging behaviour escalating (1.2, 1.4, 1.8, 2.1, 2.3, 2.4, 2.5, 3.2, 3.9, 4.1, 4.2, 4.3, 8.4, 9.4)		
5. Maintains safety of self and others; assists with removing other clients from environment and reducing other possible environmental factors (1.2, 1.4, 1.8, 2.2, 2.5, 3.2, 3.9, 6.1, 6.3, 6.6, 8.4, 9.4)		
6. Supports and assists senior staff in managing situation; maintains calm demeanour; also displays evidence of effective and therapeutic communication when interacting with the clients; e.g. gives a clear explanation of what is happening, establishes trust, listens carefully, speaking calmly and uses short sentences (1.2, 1.4, 1.8, 2.3, 2.4, 2.5, 3.2, 3.6, 3.9, 6.1, 6.2, 6.3, 6.6, 8.4, 9.4)		
7. Participates in post-incident debrief (when implemented) and incident review (1.2, 1.4, 3.2, 3.9, 7.3, 8.4, 8.6, 9.4)		
8. Documents relevant information (1.2, 1.3, 1.8, 3.2, 5.3, 6.6, 7.1, 7.2, 7.3, 7.4, 7.5)		
9. Demonstrates ability to link theory to practice (8.3, 8.4, 8.5, 9.4)		

Student:

Clinical facilitator:

Date:

CHAPTER 9.4

ASSIST WITH THE MANAGEMENT OF A CLIENT IN SECLUSION

IDENTIFY INDICATIONS

Seclusion is an action that may be implemented within an authorised mental health setting. It is used only if necessary and as a last resort for the protection or wellbeing of a consumer or others with whom the consumer may come into contact, and can become the final response to emergency situations. It is not a treatment intervention. Seclusion is described as confining a person in a room and it is not within their control to leave (Hercelinskyj & Alexander, 2020).

It should be differentiated from time-out, where a consumer is asked to seek voluntary social isolation for a minimum period of time. Seclusion is deemed acceptable only to prevent injury to the consumer or others (including staff), and after other implemented actions are not effective. The seclusion room is an environment with low sensory stimuli and has respite from the excess stimuli that occur in a general area. In seclusion the person does not have to relate to other people when such relationships are pathologically intense because of their illness.

Seclusion is used:
- when all other actions to de-escalate have not been successful
- when the person has lost control and is destructive, or not responding to verbal command or physical contact
- when the person is overstimulated by the environment and needs time to regain control.

Seclusion should not be used if the consumer is:
- medically unstable and requires frequent physical assessment
- suicidal and is on a one-to-one observation schedule.

Consumers in seclusion are alone, and must be carefully monitored by members of the nursing staff, including the use of closed-circuit TV.

LEGAL CONSIDERATIONS

The United Nations Principles for the Protection of Persons with a Mental Illness identifies seclusion as being used only when it is the only means available to prevent immediate or imminent harm to the client or others (McSherry, 2014). Commonwealth and state/territory legislation and related Acts have requirements that must be fulfilled in order to use seclusion or restraint. The relevant Act and guidelines for the use of seclusion must be followed when assisting with the skill described in this section. Authorisation for using seclusion is according to individual state legislation that identifies the relevant health practitioner (i.e. psychiatrist or authorised medical practitioner). Some states permit authorisation from a senior mental health practitioner or registered nurse (RN) in an emergency. Any medication administered must be for a therapeutic purpose and not as a punishment.

National practice standards for the mental health workforce and the *World Health Organization 2013–2020 Action Plan* (Kanna et al., 2020) recognise the need to respect the human rights of consumers when delivering care in a mental health setting and minimising the use of involuntary treatment (Department of Health, 2021). They reinforce the need to follow relevant Commonwealth and state or territory mental health legislation when implementing all types of restraint and seclusion.

SAFETY CONSIDERATIONS

There are several aspects of safety to consider when seclusion is required for a client who is out of control or overstimulated.

1. Identify that an emergency situation is occurring and call for assistance, according to facility guidelines.
2. Other clients should be asked quietly but firmly to leave the area. Staff members are responsible for removing clients from the immediate area to a safer space.
3. Maintain a calm demeanour; requesting assistance and then waiting for this to arrive promotes safety for the nurse/s. Providing the client with space and awaiting adequate assistance before attempting restraint (if it is required) enhances client safety.

4. One team member will be designated as the team leader and their directions should be followed to reduce the chance of miscommunication. The team leader will be the person who talks to the client. Staff who assist in restraining a client for seclusion should have training in dealing with aggressive or overstimulated clients so that neither the client nor staff member are injured.

5. If restraint is required, it should be accomplished without hesitation. This show of unity and determination helps prevent the client from exhibiting out-of-control behaviour.

6. The use of restraint should be minimal, but when required, the client should be adequately restrained to enable staff intervention while placing them in seclusion and until any neuroleptic medication has begun to take effect.

7. When the client is left in a seclusion room, all items are to be removed and all staff are to leave the room before the door is securely locked. Ensure the CCTV is activated and the room meets safety requirements.

8. Clients in seclusion require constant monitoring via CCTV, frequent visual observation through the observation window, plus close observation in the seclusion room to ensure the client is conscious. This will vary according to each state/territory's mental health Act, but is generally at least every 10 to 15 minutes. WA Country Health describes best practice as continual monitoring of the client in seclusion (2020).

GATHER EQUIPMENT

Each area should have a psychiatric emergency box that contains materials, medications and equipment required for neuroleptisation (as per the process outlined in this skill). This emergency box is kept in a prominent but locked position on the ward, and should be taken to the seclusion room as required.

GIVE A CLEAR EXPLANATION OF THE PROCEDURE AND ESTABLISH THERAPEUTIC COMMUNICATION

Effective and therapeutic communication skills are a vital part of mental health nursing. Explaining what is happening during the entire seclusion procedure helps to calm the client. When implementing seclusion, the nurse should maintain an attitude that recognises consumer's rights and is as respectful and compassionate as possible. Giving reassurance about the necessity of seclusion, client safety and the availability of the nurse for assistance and observation will help to reduce the client's potential hostility and fear.

Use short sentences, a normal volume and relay only relevant information to the client. The behaviours that have necessitated the use of seclusion should be explained to the client and their family. The standard of behaviour to terminate seclusion should also be explained. A contract for maintaining control of their behaviour may be implemented with the client. Instruction and guidance on self-control methods may also be appropriate.

ASSIST WITH/IMPLEMENT RESTRAINT OF THE CLIENT

Only experienced and specifically trained staff should implement restraint and seclusion of a client (Evans et al., 2016). When adequate assistance is available, follow facility policies and state/territory legislation to restrain the client. Avoid causing harm to other clients, staff or the client. Restraint should be as minimal as required. When the client is restrained, remove them to the seclusion room. They may need to be transported to the seclusion room if unable to walk.

Remove all personal items from the client's pockets and other objects or personal possessions which may potentially cause harm to themselves or the attending staff. This includes any belts, shoes, necklaces, tie and spectacles.

INFORM THE MEDICAL OFFICER

A medical order is required to place and keep the client in seclusion. According to state/territory legislation, a medical officer is required to authorise the seclusion. Within some states, a senior mental health care professional or RN can authorise seclusion in an emergency situation if a medical practitioner is not available. In this situation, the medical officer should be contacted as soon as possible to authorise, vary or revoke the seclusion (Queensland Health, 2017; Victorian Department of Health, 2017). The chief psychiatrist will also have to approve periods of restraint longer than 2 to 3 hours, or repeated episodes longer than 1 week (Chief Psychiatrist of Western Australia, 2016; Queensland Health, 2017). The medical officer must assess the client within a specified time limit, and may also order neuroleptic medication if required.

ASSIST WITH NEUROLEPTISATION

Medication may be ordered to reduce the person's agitation, or to assist with other needs impacting on their health status. Medication should be administered following the rights of medication administration. Frequently this may be an intramuscular injection, and quick safe administration will be required to reduce the risk of harm to the nursing staff during the administration process. Staff experienced in managing difficult clients should be involved in giving the medication.

MONITOR THE CLIENT

Clients in seclusion require frequent monitoring by both nursing staff and a psychiatrist or medical officer. The specific types of monitoring, timeframes for the frequency and specific observations should be determined by the local state/territory mental health Act. Nursing observation of the client is generally every 10 to 15 minutes, and for medical practitioners every 1 to 2 hours.

The client must be assessed visually to check for changes in their condition, conscious state and any potential self-harm that may have occurred. It may be necessary to enter the seclusion room (follow local policies for safety when doing this) for close observation, such as checking conscious state. Each check must be documented. Ensure the client's rights, dignity and privacy are respected by not being unnecessarily exposed to those not directly involved in their care.

ASSIST THE CLIENT WITH BASIC CARE NEEDS

All the client's basic needs including bedding food, drink, appropriate clothing, toileting and bathing should be met while in seclusion. Adequate (at least two) staff must attend the client when assisting with these needs to ensure the safety of both the person and staff. Food and fluids must be in non-breakable containers. The environment must be monitored and adjusted to ensure client comfort (e.g. room temperature) and the room should be routinely cleaned.

ENGAGE IN THERAPEUTIC INTERACTION AND ASSESS THE CLIENT

Use appropriate communication skills of listening, speaking calmly and using short sentences when interacting with the client. Listening and talking with the client helps to re-establish a therapeutic relationship and assist them in gaining control of their behaviour. Also observe their behaviour, non-verbal communication and verbal responses to evaluate their mental health status. Contribute collected data from client interaction to the team so that as the client becomes calm and able to reason, verbal contracts for behaviour can be made with the relevant mental health practitioner. Seclusion can slowly be lifted as they are able to fulfil these.

MOVE THE CLIENT TO A HIGH DEPENDENCY UNIT

As soon as the client is stable and able to interact with others, they can be involved in making decisions to move to a less restrictive environment. When assessment by the mental health team identifies that the client is stable and able to interact with others, they can be moved to a high dependency unit where there are fewer restrictions and they can continue to be closely observed for any recurrence of their behaviour. A behaviour contract may also be negotiated if one is not already in place.

REPLACE USED EQUIPMENT

The emergency psychiatric box should be restocked and replaced in its locked location. The enrolled nurse (EN) may assist in checking the contents of the box.

FOLLOW-UP ACTIVITIES

Debriefing should occur with both the team and the client. The EN can contribute relevant information to the team during the review of the events that occurred, and help the staff become more aware of the situation, stimuli, events and clients who require attention and strategies to prevent recurrence. Participation in debriefing also enables the EN and other staff to discuss their feelings about what has occurred to reduce their own stress or concerns from the experience.

Debriefing with the client (and co-clients) will also be implemented by a senior team member. This aims to allay fears and develop trust between the client and others in the ward area. The EN may also participate or assist in discussion with the person about issues that led to the seclusion and alternative methods of coping that can prevent seclusion in the future.

DOCUMENT AND REPORT RELEVANT INFORMATION

Forms authorising the seclusion will need to be completed, submitted to the relevant authority (according to state/territory mental health Act requirements) and filed in the notes. These forms will require completion by specific medical and nursing staff. A seclusion form will be used to document the client's response to seclusion, as well as times and observations, physical and psychological status of the client, medications and nursing care. The EN should complete the relevant sections when administering any basic care needs or completing client observations. The event should also be clearly documented in the progress notes, although senior staff involved in the incident may complete most of this paperwork. The EN would contribute relevant information.

CASE STUDY

You are working in an acute adult mental health facility. Your client Jane Morris, is an 'involuntary patient' who has become agitated, aggressive and abusive . Attempts by senior nursing staff to de-escalate the situation have not been successful.

The medical team have attended to the event, leading to Jane being placed in seclusion.

Refer to your state/territory mental health Act and the requirements for a client in seclusion.

1. What forms are required to report the placement of Jane in seclusion?
2. How frequently do you need to observe the client?
3. What types of observations need to be made?
4. How long can Jane be left in seclusion before further authorisation is required?
5. What assistance should be given to ensure Jane's basic care needs are being met?
6. How many staff members should be assisting Jane with these basic care needs?

Note: These notes are summaries of the most important points in the assessments/procedures, and are not exhaustive on the subject. The naming of documents or charts may differ from state to state, and facility to facility. In all possible situations the guidelines of the ACSQHC are used when describing national charts or documents (e.g. the ACSQHC Observation and Response Chart is named the Adult Observation and Response Chart in WA, and the Rapid Detection and Response Observation Chart in SA). References of the materials used to compile the information have been supplied. The student is expected to have learned the material surrounding each skill as presented in the references. No single reference is complete on the subject.

REFERENCES

Chief Psychiatrist of Western Australia. (2016). *Reporting Episodes of Seclusion & Restraint*. Government of Western Australia. http://www.chiefpsychiatrist. wa.gov.au/monitoring-reporting/reporting-episodes-of-seclusion-restraint/

Department of Health. (2021). *Mental Health Statement of Rights and Responsibilities*. Australian Government. https://www1.health.gov.au/internet/publications/publishing.nsf/Content/pub-sqps-rights-toc~pub-sqps-rights-4

Evans, K., Nizette, D. & O'Brien, A. (2016). *Psychiatric and Mental Health Nursing*. Sydney: Elsevier.

Hercelinskyj, G. & Alexander, L. (2020). *Mental Health Nursing: Applying Theory to Practice*. Melbourne: Cengage.

Kanna, S., Faraaz, M., Shekhar, S. & Vikram, P. (2020). An end to coercion: rights and decision-making in mental health care. *Bulletin of the World Health Organization*. 98(1), pp. 52–8. Geneva: World Health Organization.

McSherry, B. (2014). *Australia's International Human Rights Obligations*. Mental Health Commission of New South Wales.

https://nswmentalhealthcommission.com.au/sites/default/files/assets/File/NSWMHC-InternationalHumanRights%20report%20cover.pdf

Queensland Health. (2017). *Seclusion, Mechanical Restraint and Other Restrictive Practices*. Queensland Government. https://www.health.qld.gov.au/clinical-practice/guidelines-procedures/clinical-staff/mental-health/act/resources/videos/restrictive-practices

Victorian Department of Health. (2017). *Restrictive Interventions – Bodily Restraint and Seclusion*. Victorian State Government. https://www2.health.vic.gov.au/mental-health/practice-and-service-quality/mental-health-act-2014-handbook/safeguards/restrictive-interventions-bodily-restraint-and-seclusion

WA Country Health Service. (2020). *Mental Health Restraint Policy*. Government of Western Australia. http://www.wacountry.health.wa.gov.au/fileadmin/sections/policies/Managed/Mental_Health_Restraint_Policy_TS4KSNFPVEZQ_210_19489.pdf

RECOMMENDED READINGS

Moxham, L., Hazelton, M., Muir-Cochrane, E., Heffernan, T., Kneisl, C.R. & Trigoboff, T. (2017). *Contemporary Psychiatric-Mental Health Nursing: Partnerships in Care*. Melbourne: Pearson.

Queensland Health (Mental Health Alcohol and Other Drugs Branch). (2017). *Acute Behavioural Disturbance Management (Including Acute Sedation) in Queensland Health Authorised Mental Health Services (Adults)*. Queensland Government. https://www.health.qld.gov.au/__data/assets/pdf_file/0025/665314/qh-gdl-452.pdf

SA Health. (2021). *Challenging Behaviour for Health Professionals*. Government of South Australia. https://www.sahealth.sa.gov.au/wps/wcm/connect/public+content/sa+health+internet/clinical+resources/clinical+programs+and+practice+guidelines/safety+and+wellbeing/challenging+behaviour/challenging+behaviour+for+health+professionals

Victorian Department of Health. (2017). *Definitions – Mental Health Act 2014 Handbook*. Victorian State Government. https://www2.health.vic.gov.au/mental-health/practice-and-service-quality/mental-health-act-2014-handbook/definitions

ESSENTIAL SKILLS COMPETENCY

Assist with the Management of a Client in Seclusion

Demonstrates the ability to effectively assess a client's mental status

Criteria for skill performance	Y	D
(Numbers indicate *Enrolled Nurse Standards for Practice*, 2016)	(Satisfactory)	(Requires development)
1. Identifies indication (8.3, 8.4)		
2. Able to discuss legal and safety implications in the use of seclusion (1.2, 1.8, 3.2, 3.9, 7.3, 8.4, 9.4)		
3. Evidence of effective and therapeutic communication when interacting with the client; e.g. recognises client's rights, gives a clear explanation of procedure, establishes trust, listens carefully, speaking calmly and using short sentences (1.2, 1.4, 2.1, 2.3, 2.4, 2.5, 6.1, 6.3, 6.6, 7.3, 7.5, 8.4, 9.4)		
4. Gathers equipment (1.2, 1.6, 4.4, 6.4, 8.4, 9.4)		
5. Assists with restraint (1.2, 1.4, 1.8, 2.2, 2.5, 3.2, 3.9, 6.1, 6.3, 6.6, 8.4, 9.4)		
6. Assesses client according to legal protocols (1.1, 1.2, 1.3, 2.2, 2.3, 2.4, 2.5, 4.1, 4.2, 7.1, 7.2, 7.3, 8.4, 9.4)		
7. Assists client with basic care needs (hygiene, diet, fluids, etc.); maintains protocols for safety when administering this care (1.2, 1.4, 1.8, 2.3, 2.4, 2.5, 2.6, 2.7, 3.2, 3.9, 4.1, 4.2, 6.1, 6.6, 8.4, 9.4)		
8. Assists with cleaning, replacing and disposing of equipment appropriately (1.2, 1.4, 3.9, 6.5, 9.4)		
9. Documents relevant information. (1.2, 1.3, 1.8, 3.2, 3.9, 5.3, 6.6, 7.1, 7.2, 7.3, 7.4, 7.5)		
10. Demonstrates ability to link theory to practice (8.3, 8.4, 8.5, 9.4)		

Student:

Clinical facilitator: Date:

CHAPTER 9.5

ELECTROCONVULSIVE THERAPY (ECT) – CLIENT CARE PRE- AND POST-TREATMENT

IDENTIFY INDICATIONS

Electroconvulsive therapy (ECT) is an effective treatment for mood disorders including severe depression, and has a strong evidence base (Hercelinskyj & Alexander, 2020; Queensland Health, 2018; RANZCP, 2019). Older adults, who often suffer side effects from antidepressant medication, can respond well to this treatment. ECT is a procedure where modified seizures are induced by the selective passage of an electrical current through the brain (RANZCP, 2019). To prevent the client from experiencing pain or convulsing, it is performed under general anaesthetic.

For most consumers, ECT is given in a series of 6 to 12 treatments. It can include two or three treatments per week, over a series of weeks (Hercelinskyj & Alexander,

2020; Stergiopoulou, 2016). This schedule varies with the consumer's response, the effect on memory impairment, the severity of the condition and the client's medical condition (Stergiopoulou, 2016). It can be given to inpatients and outpatients. It is usually given in the morning, as the person is required to fast. The key part of the nurse's role is to provide clinical care and emotional support prior to, during and after the ECT procedure. Reducing stress and providing information about the procedure are also important (Stergiopoulou, 2016). Staff working regularly within an ECT suite will require specialist training to maintain competency and consumer safety (Queensland Health, 2018).

LEGAL AND ETHICAL CONSIDERATIONS

ECT is designated a 'regulated treatment' and its use is governed by the mental health Act for each state or territory. Each mental health Act will stipulate requirements that must be met in the administration of ECT. This will include guidelines for administration of ECT, who can administer ECT, ensuring informed consent for all consumers receiving ECT, recognising cultural parameters and requiring the approval or authorisation processes for involuntary clients receiving ECT. It is essential for the enrolled nurse to refer to and understand the mental health Act for their state/territory and the requirements for ECT.

The rights, privacy, dignity and confidentiality of the clients receiving ECT should be maintained at all times. The nature of the treatment must not be disclosed to others.

CLIENT ASSESSMENT PRIOR TO ECT

The complete history, physical examination and neurological examination must be completed prior to ECT. Blood tests, urinalysis, X-rays and an electrocardiogram are done to rule out pre-existing physical illnesses, as this may compromise the procedure and the client's wellbeing. Systemic effects such as headaches, nausea, muscle aches, soreness,

weakness, drowsiness, anorexia and amenorrhoea can occur following ECT. These can be managed symptomatically with simple analgesia, if required (Queensland Health, 2018). Cognitive effects of confusion and memory disturbance (of both past and recent events) are commonly discussed side effects of ECT. They do usually subside after the treatment course, although some consumers have reported longer memory losses, including recall of the days prior to and during the course of the ECT treatment.

SUPPORT, PREPARE AND ASSIST THE CLIENT RECEIVING ECT

Perform hand hygiene
Perform hand hygiene before touching the client or the client's surrounds and prior to any procedure involving client contact to reduce the possibility of cross-contamination. Hand hygiene is the most effective method of infection control as it removes transient organisms from the hands of the nurse.

Give a clear explanation of the procedure and establish therapeutic communication
ECT is often perceived by the consumer initially with dread and trepidation. Educating the client and their family about the benefits of this procedure and

discussing their fears are dependent on the therapeutic relationship that has been established. Giving sound concrete explanations of the procedure and offering realistic reassurance will help to reduce anxiety and allay fears. Supply them with a brochure about ECT (available from each state/territory health department) or help them access state/territory health websites that explain the procedure.

Complete pre-procedure safety checklist

Preoperative care is the same as for any pre-anaesthetic client, and a pre-ECT/procedure checklist is completed. Anaesthetic and muscle relaxing drugs are given (to prevent convulsions), so fasting is important. The client must void prior to the ECT to prevent incontinence and possible damage to the bladder from distension. Baseline vital signs are documented. Clear informed consent should be given by voluntary clients and state/territory guidelines followed for involuntary clients.

Accompany the client to the treatment area

Clients may be apprehensive and the company of a trusted nurse will help to reduce that fear. They can come to the treatment area either in a wheelchair or they may walk. Introduce them to the registered nurse (RN), anaesthetist and doctor who will be involved with the treatment, to reduce stress. Assist the client onto the bed and remain with them throughout the treatment (depending on facility policies). As with any procedure, the client's ID band is again checked with the consent form, along with verbal clarification from the client (ACSQHC, 2019; Queensland Health, 2018).

Assist the client to remain comfortable and safe

The support of the nurse throughout the procedure is important to the client, who will be anxious and frightened. The nurse should offer reassurance by explaining every step of the procedure as it is happening, emphasising the benefits of the treatment and listening and responding appropriately to their fears. The side rails should be raised to prevent injury.

Observe the process of ECT

Once an intravenous (IV) line is established, the anaesthetic is administered and then the muscle relaxant. Once the client is asleep, a mouth guard is used to protect the teeth and tongue during the procedure. Use of a Guedel airway can be dangerous (Queensland Health, 2018). Skin is prepared with an alcohol wipe and electrodes are applied to the relevant areas. A weak electrical current is passed across the brain, and causes a brief generalised seizure. A seizure lasting 30 to 60 seconds is considered adequate to produce a therapeutic effect. The nurse must record the time from onset to cessation of fasciculations (muscle twitching).

Observe or assist with positioning the client in the left lateral position

Position the client in the left lateral position following all seizure activity to maintain an open airway until the client regains consciousness. Oxygenation has been maintained throughout the period of anaesthesia by the anaesthetist. This continues until the effects of the anaesthetic and muscle relaxant are fully worn off and the client is breathing spontaneously. Following recovery, the client will expel the Guedel airway (if used post-procedure to help maintain airway) when sufficiently awake to do so. Oxygen, as ordered, may be continued via a mask during the entire recovery period and until the client's oxygen saturation is returned to normal parameters (Queensland Health, 2018; WA Country Health Service, 2019).

Transfer the client to recovery area

Transfer the client to the recovery area as soon as the vital signs are stable. An experienced theatre recovery RN should be involved in the post-procedure care (Queensland Health, 2018). Monitor the client's vital signs, peripheral oxygen concentration and general condition until they are fully awake. There is a need to be aware of the potential for falls from the trolley/bed, and safety measures such as side rails must be utilised. As soon as the client is awake, orient them and provide frequent reassurance. Repetition of this information at frequent, regular intervals is necessary until the client retains it. The IV access device is removed.

Return the client to the ward

Return the client to the ward, usually in a wheelchair, although some may prefer to walk. Oxygen saturation, vital signs and mental status will have returned to an acceptable level. If treatment is in the morning, the client's breakfast and morning medications should be given after establishing that the gag reflex has returned. Clinical handover (see **Skill 7.3**) given to the ward staff includes medications administered, any adverse vital signs, changes in the procedure and the client's response to treatment that may affect their recovery and behaviour. Observation may need to continue for several hours following the procedure, similar to any post-procedure observations. If the client is drowsy, allowing them to sleep often hastens the recovery. When they first get out of bed, they may require assistance because of the remaining effects of the muscle relaxant. Orientation should be assessed every 30 minutes after the client wakes and until their mental status returns to baseline. Potential side effects that may require treatment include headache, muscle soreness and nausea. Confusion and disorientation respond well to restricted environmental stimulation. Frequent nursing contacts reminding the client about ECT treatment, frequent reorientation and reassurance help address memory loss.

If the client is being treated as an outpatient, they will require a carer and a transport plan for returning home, once their condition is stable post-treatment.

Perform hand hygiene

Maintain the 5 Moments for Hand Hygiene and perform hand hygiene after touching the client and the client's surrounds.

CLEAN, REPLACE OR DISPOSE OF EQUIPMENT

The treatment room and recovery area must be cleaned and all equipment and drugs used must be replaced so they are available for the next time the treatment is carried out. This is a time-management strategy as well as a courtesy to other healthcare professionals involved.

DOCUMENT AND REPORT RELEVANT INFORMATION

Documentation is recorded in four areas. The preoperative period is documented on a preoperative checklist or specific ECT procedure checklist and chart. Assessment, both physical and psychological, is recorded in the progress notes. The peri-operative period – that is, the time in the treatment room – is usually recorded on an ECT treatment chart. The recovery period is recorded on a recovery room chart where notations and observations are made frequently, using designated observations. Post-treatment nursing care is usually recorded on the progress notes and summarises the client's response to treatment, side effects, nursing care for those side effects and other observations made. The nursing care plan should also be completed, and observations recorded on the client's observation and response chart.

CASE STUDY

You are an enrolled nurse (EN) working in an acute adult mental health unit. Clients treated in this area include both voluntary and involuntary client. Greg Anders (a voluntary client) is a 47-year-old man who has been admitted for the treatment of severe depression. His psychiatrist has recommended he have a series of ECT treatments.

1. What information can you supply to Greg to help him understand what ECT is and how it works? Locate information and resources from your state/territory health department.
2. How many treatments with ECT are usually recommended?
3. Greg is currently a voluntary client. Why is it important to gain his informed consent prior to administering this treatment? Use an internet search to locate the specific ECT consent form for your state/territory health department. (Alternatively, use the consent form for WA Health or Queensland Health.)
4. Greg asks you why the doctor completed a thorough physical assessment and other tests on him prior to commencing his ECT. What will you explain to him?
5. List the pre-procedure nursing care actions you would implement for Greg.
6. Why is it important to:
   a. administer oxygen post ECT treatment
   b. perform vital signs and assessment of the client's conscious state post procedure?

Note: These notes are summaries of the most important points in the assessments/procedures, and are not exhaustive on the subject. The naming of documents or charts may differ from state to state, and facility to facility. In all possible situations the guidelines of the ACSQHC are used when describing national charts or documents (e.g. the ACSQHC Observation and Response Chart is named the Adult Observation and Response Chart in WA, and the Rapid Detection and Response Observation Chart in SA). References of the materials used to compile the information have been supplied. The student is expected to have learned the material surrounding each skill as presented in the references. No single reference is complete on the subject.

CRITICAL THINKING

Thinking of the clinical skills discussed in this skill, and the stages of growth and development, what are some of the key components you would need to consider in the following scenarios?

1. ECT is found to have higher rates of response and remission in the treatment of major depressive disorders in older adults (over 60). Consider how this treatment might help an otherwise fit and well elderly consumer with depression regain their independence and live in the community.
2. ECT is a controversial therapy that can create fear in the consumer being prescribed the therapy or their family. Review the following online resources for information you could potentially use as part of a consumer education plan about ECT.
   - https://www.beyondblue.org.au/the-facts/depression/treatments-for-depression/medical-treatments-for-depression/electroconvulsive-therapy-ect#:~:text=Electroconvulsive%20therapy%20(ECT)%20is%20a,ECT%20is%20safe%20and%20effective
   - https://www.ranzcp.org/news-policy/policy-and-advocacy/position-statements/electroconvulsive-therapy-(ect)
   - https://www.psychiatry.org/patients-families/ect
   - https://www.mayoclinic.org/tests-procedures/electroconvulsive-therapy/about/pac-20393894

REFERENCES

Australian Commission on Safety and Quality in Health Care (ACSQHC). (2019). *Patient Identification.* https://www.safetyandquality.gov.au/our-work/communicating-safety/patient-identification

Hercelinskyj, G. & Alexander, L. (2020). *Mental Health Nursing: Applying theory to Practice.* Melbourne: Cengage.

Queensland Health. (2018). The administration of electroconvulsive therapy. Queensland Government. https://www.health.qld.gov.au/__data/assets/pdf_file/0028/444763/2018_Guideline-for-the-administration-of-Electroconvulsive-Therapy-v0.7.pdf

Royal Australian and New Zealand College of Psychiatrists (RANZCP). (2019). *Electroconvulsive Therapy (ECT). Position Statement 74.* October. https://www.ranzcp.org/news-policy/policy-and-advocacy/position-statements/electroconvulsive-therapy-(ect)

Stergiopoulou, A. (2016). Electroconvulsive therapy effects on cognition and memory and nurse's role. *Perioperative Nursing,* 5(2), pp. 103–12.

WA Country Health Service. (2019). *Electroconvulsive Therapy Procedure.* WACHS Great Southern. Albany Hospital Acute Psychiatric Unit. http://www.wacountry.health.wa.gov.au/index.php?id=1414

RECOMMENDED READINGS

Barkway, P. & Nizette, D. (2018). *Mosby's Pocketbook of Mental Health* (3rd ed.). Chatswood: Elsevier.

Brown University. (2016). Continuation ECT with medication improves outcomes in geriatric depression. *The Brown University Psychopharmacology Update,* 27(11), pp. 1–5, doi:10.1002/pu.30181.

Chief Psychiatrist of Western Australia. (2021). *Electroconvulsive Therapy (ECT).* Government of Western Australia. http://www.chiefpsychiatrist.wa.gov.au/monitoring-reporting/electroconvulsive-therapy-ect/

Department of Health. (2021). *What We're Doing About Mental Health.* Australian Government. https://www.health.gov.au/health-topics/mental-health-and-suicide-prevention/what-were-doing-about-mental-health?utm_source=health.gov.au&utm_medium=callout-auto-custom&utm_campaign=digital_transformation

Eid, M. (2016). Electroconvulsive therapy use among depressive inpatients: Position Statement. *Middle East Journal of Nursing,* 10(2), pp. 16–21.

Evans, K., Nizette, D. & O'Brien, A. (2016). *Psychiatric and Mental Health Nursing.* Chatswood: Elsevier.

Hamzelou, J. (2016). Can tainted treatment make a shock return? *New Scientist,* 231(3087), pp. 16–17.

Maric, N.P., Stojanovic, Z., Andric, S., Soldatovic, I., Dolic, M. & Spiric, Z. (2016). The acute and medium-term effects of treatment with electroconvulsive therapy on memory in patients with major depressive disorder. *Psychological Medicine,* 46(4), pp. 797–806.

Stergiopoulou, A. (2015). Electro convulsive therapy: a therapeutic choice in psychiatry. *Perioperative Nursing,* 4(1), pp. 3–9.

ESSENTIAL SKILLS COMPETENCY

Electroconvulsive Therapy (ECT) – Client Care Pre- and Post-Treatment
Demonstrates the ability to effectively and safely manage a client who is pre- and post-ECT

Criteria for skill performance (Numbers indicate *Enrolled Nurse Standards for Practice*, 2016)	Y (Satisfactory)	D (Requires development)
1. Identifies indication (8.3, 8.4)		
2. Recognises pre-procedure client assessment (1.2, 1.4, 1.8, 2.6, 2.7, 3.2, 4.1, 4.2, 4.3, 4.4, 6.4, 7.1, 7.3, 8.4, 9.4)		
3. Performs hand hygiene (1.2, 1.4, 1.8, 3.9, 6.4, 9.4)		
4. Evidence of effective communication; e.g. respects rights, educates client about procedure, gives reassurance and explanation (1.2, 1.4, 2.1, 2.3, 2.4, 2.5, 6.1, 6.3, 6.6, 7.3, 7.5, 8.4, 9.4)		
5. Completes pre-ECT procedure checklist (1.2, 1.4, 3.2, 4.1, 4.2, 4.4, 7.1, 7.3, 7.5, 8.4, 9.4)		
6. Accompanies client to treatment room; ensures identification of client and safety check completed (1.2, 1.4, 2.7, 3.2, 3.9, 4.4, 6.4, 8.4, 9.4)		
7. Assists client to remain safe and comfortable (1.2, 1.4, 2.5, 2.7, 3.2, 3.9, 4.4, 6.4, 8.4, 9.4)		
8. Assists with positioning the client; applies oxygen (1.2, 1.4, 1.8, 2.7, 3.2, 3.9, 4.4, 6.4, 8.4, 9.4)		
9. Assists with transferring client to the recovery area and monitors them (1.2, 1.4, 2.7, 3.2, 3.9, 4.4, 6.4, 8.4, 9.4)		
10. Accompanies client to ward, provides breakfast and morning medication, when gag reflex returns (1.2, 1.4, 1.8, 2.2, 3.2, 3.9, 6.1, 8.4, 9.4)		
11. Performs hand hygiene (1.2, 1.4, 1.8, 3.9, 6.4, 9.4)		
12. Cleans, replaces and disposes of equipment appropriately (1.2, 1.4, 3.9, 6.5, 9.4)		
13. Documents and reports relevant information (1.2, 1.3, 1.8, 3.2, 5.3, 6.6, 7.1, 7.2, 7.3, 7.4, 7.5)		
14. Demonstrates ability to link theory to practice (8.3, 8.4, 8.5, 9.4)		

Student:

Clinical facilitator: Date:

APPENDIX

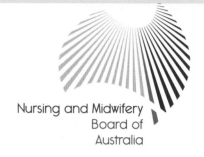

Nursing and Midwifery Board of Australia
Board of
Australia

Nursing and Midwifery Board of Australia
standard for Enrolled nurses

STANDARDS FOR PRACTICE:
ENROLLED NURSES

1 January 2016

NMP00006

STANDARDS FOR PRACTICE: ENROLLED NURSES

Introduction

The *Enrolled nurse standards for practice* are the core practice standards that provide the framework for assessing enrolled nurse (EN) practice. They communicate to the general public the standards that can be expected from ENs and can be used in a number of ways including:

- development of nursing curricula by education providers,

- assessment of students and new graduates,

- to assess nurses educated overseas seeking to work in Australia, and

- to assess ENs returning to work after breaks in service.

In addition, they may also be used by the Nursing and Midwifery Board of Australia (NMBA) and relevant tribunals or courts to assess professional conduct or matters relating to notifications.

The *Enrolled nurse standards for practice* replace the *National competency standards for the enrolled nurse* (2002).

These contemporary standards reflect the role of the EN within the health environment. The standards for practice remain broad and principle-based so that they are sufficiently dynamic for practising nurses to use as a benchmark to assess competence to practise in a range of settings.

The EN works with the registered nurse (RN) as part of the health care team and demonstrates competence in the provision of person-centred care. Core practice generally requires the EN to work under the direct or indirect supervision of the RN. At all times, the EN retains responsibility for his/her actions and remains accountable in providing delegated nursing care. The need for the EN to have a named and accessible RN at all times and in all contexts of care for support and guidance is critical to patient safety.

Although the scope of practice for each EN will vary according to context and education, the EN has a responsibility for ongoing self and professional development to maintain their knowledge base through life-long learning, and continue to demonstrate the types of core nursing activities that an EN would be expected to undertake on entry to practice. Therefore the core standards in this document are the *minimum*

standards that are applicable across diverse practice settings and health care populations for both beginning and experienced ENs. They are based on the Diploma of Nursing being the education standard.

ENs engage in analytical thinking; use information and/or evidence; and skilfully and empathetically communicate with all involved in the provision of care, including the person receiving care and their family and community, and health professional colleagues.

The EN standards are clinically focused and they reflect the EN's capability to:

- provide direct and indirect care;

- engage in reflective and analytical practice; and

- demonstrate professional and collaborative practice. ENs, where appropriate, educate and support other (unregulated) health care workers (however titled) related to the provision of care.

ENs collaborate and consult with health care recipients, their families and community as well as RNs and other health professionals, to plan, implement and evaluate integrated care that optimises outcomes for recipients and the systems of care. They are responsible for the delegated care they provide and self-monitor their work.

How to use these standards

The EN standards for practice are intended to be easily accessible to a variety of groups, including ENs, governments, regulatory agencies, educators, health care professionals and the community. It should be noted that the 'indicators' (refer to glossary) written below the statements are indicative of EN behaviours, they are not intended to be exhaustive. Rather, they are examples of activities that demonstrate the specific standard.

The standards should be read in conjunction with the following relevant documentation, including, but not limited to:

- Decision-Making Framework (NMBA 2013),

- Nursing practice decisions summary guide (NMBA 2010),

STANDARDS FOR PRACTICE:
ENROLLED NURSES

- Nursing practice decision flowchart (NMBA 2013),

- Code of professional conduct for nurses in Australia (NMBA 2008),

- Code of ethics for nurses in Australia (NMBA 2008), and

- Professional boundaries for nurses in Australia (NMBA 2010).

They should also be read in conjunction with the attached glossary, which describes the way in which key terms are used in the standards.

There are three domains, namely:

- professional and collaborative practice,

- provision of care, and

- reflective and analytical practice.

The indicators are expressed through knowledge (capabilities)[1], skills[2], and attitudes[3] inherent within these clinically focused domains. All are variable according to the context of practice.

Domains

Professional and collaborative practice

The professional and collaborative practice domain relates to the legal, ethical and professional foundations from which all competent ENs respond to their environment. The domain reflects the responsibilities of the EN to maintain currency and to demonstrate best practice. The standards are:

- functions in accordance with the law, policies and procedures affecting EN practice,

- practises nursing in a way that ensures the rights, confidentiality, dignity and respect of people are upheld, and

- accepts accountability and responsibility for own actions.

Provision of care

The provision of care domain relates to the intrinsic care of individuals or groups entrusted to the EN. It encompasses all aspects of care from assessment to engaging in care, and includes health education and evaluation of outcomes. The standards are:

- interprets information from a range of sources in order to contribute to planning appropriate care,

- collaborates with the RN, the person receiving care and the healthcare team when developing plans of care,

- provides skilled and timely care to people receiving care and others whilst promoting their independence and involvement in care decision–making, and

- communicates and uses documentation to inform and report care.

Reflective and analytical practice

The reflective and analytical practice domain relates to the ability of the EN to reflect on evidence-based practice and ensure currency of essential knowledge and skills, to care for the personal, physical and psychological needs of themselves and others. The standards are:

- provides nursing care that is informed by research evidence,

- practises within safety and quality improvement guidelines and standards, and

- engages in ongoing development of self as a professional.

---

1 *Knowledge (capabilities)* refers to information and the understanding of that information to guide practice.
2 *Skills* refers to technical procedures and competencies
3 *Attitudes* refers to ways for thinking and behaving

STANDARDS FOR PRACTICE: ENROLLED NURSES

Professional and collaborative practice

Standard 1: Functions in accordance with the law, policies and procedures affecting EN practice

Indicators:

1.1 Demonstrates knowledge and understanding of commonwealth, state and /or territory legislation and common law pertinent to nursing practice.

1.2 Fulfils the duty of care in the undertaking of EN practice.

1.3 Demonstrates knowledge of and implications for the NMBA standards, codes and guidelines, workplace policies and procedural guidelines applicable to enrolled nursing practice.

1.4 Provides nursing care according to the agreed plan of care, professional standards, workplace policies and procedural guidelines.

1.5 Identifies and clarifies EN responsibilities for aspects of delegated care working in collaboration with the RN and multidisciplinary health care team.

1.6 Recognises own limitations in practice and competence and seeks guidance from the RN and help as necessary.

1.7 Refrains from undertaking activities where competence has not been demonstrated and appropriate education, training and experience has not been undertaken.

1.8 Acts to ensure safe outcomes for others by recognising the need to protect people and reporting the risk of potential for harm.

1.9 When incidents of unsafe practice occur, reports immediately to the RN and other persons in authority and, where appropriate, explores ways to prevent recurrence.

1.10 Liaises and negotiates with the RN and other appropriate personnel to ensure that needs and rights of people in receipt of care are addressed and upheld.

Standard 2: Practises nursing in a way that ensures the rights, confidentiality, dignity and respect of people are upheld.

Indicators:

2.1 Places the people receiving care at the centre of care and supports them to make informed choices.

2.2 Practises in accordance with the NMBA standards codes and guidelines.

2.3 Demonstrates respect for others to whom care is provided regardless of ethnicity, culture, religion, age, gender, sexual preference, physical or mental state, differing values and beliefs.

2.4 Practises culturally safe care for (i) Aboriginal and Torres Strait Islander peoples; and (ii) people from all other cultures.

2.5 Forms therapeutic relationships with people receiving care and others recognising professional boundaries.

2.6 Maintains equitable care when addressing people's differing values and beliefs.

2.7 Ensures privacy, dignity and confidentiality when providing care.

2.8 Clarifies with the RN and relevant members of the multi-disciplinary healthcare team when interventions or treatments appear unclear or inappropriate.

2.9 Reports incidents of unethical behaviour immediately to the person in authority and, where appropriate, explores ways to prevent recurrence.

2.10 Acknowledges and accommodates, wherever possible, preferences of people receiving nursing care.

STANDARDS FOR PRACTICE:
ENROLLED NURSES

Standard 3: Accepts accountability and responsibility for own actions.

Indicators:

3.1 Practises within the EN scope of practice relevant to the context of practice, legislation, own educational preparation and experience.

3.2 Demonstrates responsibility and accountability for nursing care provided,

3.3 Recognises the RN[4] as the person responsible to assist EN decision-making and provision of nursing care.

3.4 Collaborates with the RN to ensure delegated responsibilities are commensurate with own scope of practice.

3.5 Clarifies own role and responsibilities with supervising RN in the context of the healthcare setting within which they practice.

3.6 Consults with the RN and other members of the multidisciplinary healthcare team to facilitate the provision of accurate information, and enable informed decisions by others.

3.7 Provides care within scope of practice as part of multidisciplinary healthcare team, and with supervision of a RN.

3.8 Provides support and supervision to assistants in nursing (however titled) and to others providing care, such as EN students, to ensure care is provided as outlined within the plan of care and according to institutional policies, protocols and guidelines.

3.9 Promotes the safety of self and others in all aspects of nursing practice.

Provision of care

Standard 4: Interprets information from a range of sources in order to contribute to planning appropriate care

Indicators:

4.1 Uses a range of skills and data gathering techniques including observation, interview, physical examination and measurement.

4.2 Accurately collects, interprets, utilises, monitors and reports information regarding the health and functional status of people receiving care to achieve identified health and care outcomes.

4.3 Develops, monitors and maintains a plan of care in collaboration with the RN, multidisciplinary team and others.

4.4 Uses health care technology appropriately according to workplace guidelines.

Standard 5: Collaborates with the RN, the person receiving care and the healthcare team when developing plans of care

Indicators:

5.1 Develops and promotes positive professional working relationships with members of the multi-disciplinary team.

5.2 Collaborates with members of the multi-disciplinary healthcare team in the provision of nursing care.

5.3 Contributes to the development of care plans in conjunction with the multidisciplinary healthcare team, the person receiving care and appropriate others[5].

5.4 Manages and prioritises workload in accordance with people's care plans.

5.5 Clarifies orders for nursing care with the RN when unclear.

5.6 Contributes to and collaborates in decision-making through participation in multidisciplinary healthcare team meetings and case conferences.

---

4 Where an enrolled nurse is working in maternity services setting it is expected that they will be supervised by a midwife.

5 Appropriate others include those in direct association with the person receiving care (with his/her consent) such as family, unpaid and paid carers, volunteers and clergy.

STANDARDS FOR PRACTICE:
ENROLLED NURSES

Standard 6: Provides skilled and timely care to people whilst promoting their independence and involvement in care decision–making

Indicators:

6.1 Provides care to people who are unable to meet their own physical and/or mental health needs.

6.2 Participates with the RN in evaluation of the person's progress toward expected outcomes and the reformulation of plans of care.

6.3 Promotes active engagement and the independence of people receiving care within the health care setting by involving them as active participants in care, where appropriate.

6.4 Demonstrates currency and competency in the safe use of healthcare technology.

6.5 Exercises time management and workload prioritisation.

6.6 Recognises when the physical or mental health of a person receiving care is deteriorating, reports, documents and seeks appropriate assistance.

Standard 7: Communicates and uses documentation to inform and report care

Indicators:

7.1 Collects data, reviews and documents the health and functional status of the person receiving care accurately and clearly.

7.2 Interprets and reports the health and functional status of people receiving care to the RN and appropriate members of the multidisciplinary healthcare team as soon as practicable.

7.3 Uses a variety of communication methods to engage appropriately with others and documents accordingly.

7.4 Prepares and delivers written and verbal care reports such as clinical handover, as a part of the multidisciplinary healthcare team.

7.5 Provides accurate and appropriate information to enable informed decision making by others.

Reflective and analytical practice

Standard 8: Provides nursing care that is informed by research evidence

Indicators:

8.1 Refers to the RN to guide decision-making.

8.2 Seeks additional knowledge/information when presented with unfamiliar situations.

8.3 Incorporates evidence for best practice as guided by the RN or other appropriate health professionals.

8.4 Uses problem-solving incorporating logic, analysis and a sound argument when planning and providing care.

8.5 Demonstrates analytical skills through accessing and evaluating healthcare information and quality improvement activities.

8.6 Consults with the RN and other relevant health professionals and resources to improve current practice.

Standard 9: Practises within safety and quality improvement guidelines and standards

Indicators:

9.1 Participates in quality improvement programs and accreditation standards activities as relevant to the context of practice.

9.2 Within the multi-disciplinary team, contributes and consults in analysing risk and implementing strategies to minimise risk.

9.3 Reports and documents safety breaches and hazards according to legislative requirements and institutional policies and procedures.

9.4 Practises safely within legislative requirements, safety policies, protocols and guidelines.

STANDARDS FOR PRACTICE: ENROLLED NURSES

Standard 10: Engages in ongoing development of self as a professional

Indicators:

10.1 Uses EN standards for practice to assess own performance,

10.2 Recognises the need for, and participates in, continuing professional and skills development in accordance with the NMBA's Continuing professional development registration standard.

10.3 Identifies learning needs through critical reflection and consideration of evidence-based practice in consultation with the RNs and the multidisciplinary healthcare team.

10.4 Contributes to and supports the professional development of others.

10.5 Uses professional supports and resources such as clinical supervision that facilitate professional development and personal wellbeing.

10.6 Promotes a positive professional image.

Glossary

Accountability/accountable: Nurses and midwives must be prepared to answer to others, such as people in receipt of healthcare, their nursing and midwifery regulatory authority, employers and the public for their decisions, actions, behaviours and the responsibilities that are inherent in their roles. Accountability cannot be delegated. The RN or midwife who delegates an activity to another person is accountable, not only for their delegation decision, but also for monitoring the standard of performance of the activity by the other person, and for evaluating the outcomes of the delegation. However, they are not accountable for the performance of the delegated activity.

Best practice: A technique, method, process, activity or incentive which has been proven by evidence to be most effective in providing a certain outcome.

Core practice: The day-to-day or regular activities or policies of a health service provider that fundamentally guide the service as a whole.

Decision-making framework: The NMBA expects all nurses and midwives to practise within the relevant standards for practice and decision-making frameworks.

Delegation/delegate: A delegation relationship exists when one member of the health care team delegates aspects of care, which they are competent to perform and which they would normally perform themselves, to another member of the health care team from a different discipline, or to a less experienced member of the same discipline. Delegations are made to meet people's needs and to ensure access to health care services — that is, the right person is available at the right time to provide the right service to a person. The delegator retains accountability for the decision to delegate and for monitoring outcomes.

Duty of care/standard of care: A responsibility or relationship recognised in law. For example, it may exist between health professionals and their clients. Associated with this duty is an expectation that the health professional will behave or act in a particular way. This is called the standard of care, which requires that a person act toward others and the public with watchfulness, attention, caution and the prudence that would be made by a reasonable person in those circumstances. If a person's actions do not meet this standard of care, whereby they fall below the acceptable standards, any damages resulting may be pursued in a lawsuit for negligence.

Enrolled nurse (EN; Division 2): A person with appropriate educational preparation and competence for practice, who is registered under the Health Practitioner Regulation National Law.

Evidence-based practice: Assessing and making judgements to translate the best available evidence, which includes the most current, valid, and available research findings and the individuality of situations and personal preferences as the basis for practice decisions.

Indicators: Key generic examples of competent performance. They are neither comprehensive nor exhaustive. They assist the assessor when using their professional judgement in assessing nursing practice. They further assist curriculum development.

Midwife/midwifery practice: A midwife is a person with appropriate educational preparation and competence for practice who is registered by the NMBA. This term includes endorsed midwives for the purposes of this document.

STANDARDS FOR PRACTICE:
ENROLLED NURSES

The NMBA has endorsed the ICM definition of a midwife (that includes the statement below on scope of practice) and applied it to the Australian context.

The <u>International Confederation of Midwives (ICM)</u> defines a midwife as follows:

A midwife is a person who has successfully completed a midwifery education programme that is duly recognised in the country where it is located and that is based on the ICM essential competencies for basic midwifery practice and the framework of the ICM global standards for midwifery education; who has acquired the requisite qualifications to be registered and/or legally licensed to practise midwifery and use the title 'midwife'; and who demonstrates competency in the practice of midwifery.

Scope of practice[6]

The midwife is recognised as a responsible and accountable professional who works in partnership with women to give the necessary support, care and advice during pregnancy, labour and the postpartum period, to conduct births on the midwife's own responsibility and to provide care for the newborn and the infant. This care includes preventative measures, the promotion of normal birth, the detection of complications in mother and child, the accessing of medical care or other appropriate assistance and the carrying out of emergency measures. The midwife has an important task in health counselling and education, not only for the woman, but also within the family and the community. This work should involve antenatal education and preparation for parenthood and may extend to women's health, sexual or reproductive health and child care.

A midwife may practise in any setting including the home, community, hospitals, clinics or health units (ICM international definition of the midwife 2012). www.internationalmidwives.org

Nursing and Midwifery Board of Australia (NMBA): The national body responsible for the regulation of nurses and midwives in Australia.

Person/people: Refers to those individuals who have entered into a relationship with an enrolled nurse.

Person/people encompass patients, clients, consumers and families that fall within the EN scope and context of practice.

Person-centred practice: A collaborative and respectful partnership built on mutual trust and understanding. Each person is treated as an individual with the aim of respecting people's ownership of their health information, rights and preferences while protecting their dignity and empowering choice. Person-centred practice recognises the role of family and community with respect to cultural and religious diversity.

Plan of care: Outlines the care to be provided to an individual/ family/ community and includes the nursing component. It is a set of actions the nurse will implement to resolve/ support nursing diagnoses identified by nursing assessment. The creation of the plan is an intermediate stage of the nursing process. It guides in the ongoing provision of nursing care and assists in the evaluation of that care.

Professional boundaries: Professional boundaries in nursing are defined as "limits which protect the space between the professional's power and the client's vulnerability; that is they are the borders that mark the edges between a professional, therapeutic relationship and a non-professional or personal relationship between a nurse and a person in their care" (NMBA, 2010, page 1).

Quality: Refers to characteristics and grades with respect to excellence.

Refer/referral: Referral is the transfer of primary health care responsibility to another qualified health service provider/health professional. However, the nurse or midwife referring the person for care by another professional or service may need to continue to provide their professional services collaboratively in this period.

Registered nurse (RN; Division 1): A person who has completed the prescribed educational preparation, demonstrated competence to practise, and is registered under the Health Practitioner Regulation National Law as a registered nurse in Australia. For the purposes of this document the term also includes nurse practitioners.

---

6   Scope of practice forms a part of the ICM definition of a midwife.

STANDARDS FOR PRACTICE:
ENROLLED NURSES

Risk assessment/risk management: An effective risk management system is one incorporating strategies to:

- identify risks/hazards,

- assess the likelihood of the risks occurring and the severity of the consequences if the risks do occur, and

- prevent the occurrence of the risks, or minimise their impact.

Scope of practice: Is that in which nurses are educated, competent to perform and permitted by law. The actual scope of practice of individual practitioners is influenced by the settings in which they practise, the health needs of people, the level of competence and confidence of the nurse and the policy requirements of the service provider.

Standards for practice: Set the expectations of enrolled nurse practice. They inform the education standards for enrolled nurses; the regulation of nurses and determination of nurses' fitness for practice; and guide consumers, employers and other stakeholders on what to reasonably expect from an enrolled nurse regardless of the area of nursing practice or years of nursing experience. They replace the previous *National competency standards for the enrolled nurse.*

Supervision/supervise: Supervision can be either direct or indirect:

- **Direct supervision** is when the supervisor is actually present and personally observes, works with, guides and directs the person who is being supervised.

- **Indirect supervision** is when the supervisor works in the same facility or organisation as the supervised person, but does not constantly observe their activities. The supervisor must be available for reasonable access. What is reasonable will depend on the context, the needs of the person receiving care and the needs of the person who is being supervised.

For the purpose of this document, supervision is defined as access, in all contexts of care, at all times, either directly or indirectly to professional supervision to a named and accessible RN for support and guidance of the practice of an EN.

INDEX